A History of
Chiropractic Education
in North America

Report to the Council on Chiropractic Education

Joseph C. Keating, Jr., Ph.D., Professor
Los Angeles College of Chiropractic

Alana K. Callender, M.S., Director
Palmer Foundation for Chiropractic History

Carl S. Cleveland, III., D.C., President
Cleveland Chiropractic Colleges

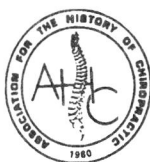

The Association for the History of Chiropractic

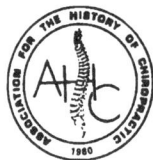

The Association for the History of Chiropractic

Project Manager: Alana Callender
Printer: Clinch Valley Printing, North Tazewell, Virginia

Copyright: Council on Chiropractic Education, 1998
Published through a grant from the NCMIC Group, Inc.

ISBN: 0-9659131-1-2
Library of Congress Catalog Card Number: 98-72099

FOREWORD

The history of chiropractic education is rich indeed, as varied and colorful as the story of the wider profession. The evolution of our training institutions is the natural outgrowth of those wider historical developments in our profession, and events within chiropractic education have reciprocally shaped and influenced most other areas of our maturation. To understand the one is to better appreciate the other.

The story of the Council on Chiropractic Education (CCE) is an important piece of the saga of chiropractic education. The earliest efforts to standardize and upgrade the training of doctors date back to World War I. By the mid-1930s this movement took the form of a national commitment, to accreditation, and in the years following World War II, to the formation of the first "Council on Education," a division of the old National Chiropractic Association. By the decade of the sixties, a time when most state and national chiropractic organizations and agencies were well established, the need to bring chiropractic colleges into the realm of federally recognized higher education in North America became paramount. The Council was the vehicle for this important step in the maturation of the chiropractic profession.

All professions, if they hope to move into the mainstream of our society, have several tasks that are key to their development. They must: 1) create an educational infrastructure; 2) form state and national associations; 3) pursue research in order to expand knowledge related to the purposes for which the profession exists; and 4) attend to legislative matters that authorize and regulate the profession's activities in the interest of the welfare of society.

The story of the CCE and its Commission on Accreditation pertains to the first of these goals, the formation of methods for guaranteeing the quality of training for doctors of chiropractic. The tale encompasses the early years of the Council's formation, the struggles involved in its refinements, the leaders who sought excellence in all of its undertakings, and the thrilling achievement of its approval, in August of 1974, by the United States Office of Education (USOE). Federal recognition of the CCE was accomplished despite extensive efforts to obstruct the Council from assuming its rightful place among professional accrediting agencies. The CCE had to overcome obstacles to its approval that few if any agencies ever had to face, either before or since.

Our own internal professional struggles have presented additional challenges. The pursuit of recognized accreditation was sometimes hampered by internecine disputes over priorities, methods and goals. At various times during the chiropractic century two or more agencies competed for recognition as the preeminent standard-setter for chiropractic education. Not surprisingly, therefore, this history of chiropractic reveals the duality (and more) of efforts in each endeavor attempted by this young and optimistic profession. The struggles culminated with the final battle before the United States Office of Education (USOE) from which the selection of the CCE's Commission on Accreditation emerged. Since then the Council has placed its imprimatur on the profession. Those who worked so long and hard to achieve USOE approval and to bring the CCE to its current status deserve not so much appreciation or special respect, but rather a recognition of their Herculean and successful efforts. Their tale, as histories of any walk of life are wont to do, suggests a direction for the chiropractic profession's future.

Of course, the challenges continue. The profession and its educational enterprise still lack consensus in terms of common goals and objectives. To this day, the single most significant obstacle to progress remains the lack of agreement on a "shared vision" of the chiropractor. How ironic, inasmuch as the early pioneers in chiropractic, who themselves often possessed little formal training, many of whom lacked advanced academic degrees, shared a passion for the profession. That passion may never again be realized; whether this will aid or deter us from finding a common vision of "the chiropractor" remains to be seen.

Let us hope that we may learn from history, or else, as the saying goes, we may be doomed to repeat it. And what can be learned from this carefully documented text is the story of a profession in struggle, a profession challenged but undaunted by obstacles, a profession determined to achieve its rightful place in society and to secure its benefits for the patients it serves. We may take some measure of hope in realizing that ours is a tale of very self-directed people, colorful and idiosyncratic individuals who nonetheless pulled together in times of crisis and conflict, and worked to achieve common objectives.

Once characterized as "Lost, Strayed or Stolen,"[1] the history of our profession has recently become the focus of increasing scholarly attention, much of it centered within the leadership and members of the Association for the History of Chiropractic (AHC). They have worked hard to detail and analyze our early struggles and achievements, and this text is one example of this initiative. I wish to take this opportunity to thank Joe Keating, Ph.D., Carl Cleveland, D.C., Alana Callender, M.S. and the entire AHC for their tireless efforts on behalf of this project.

The CCE is a tribute to the vision of those who saw the significance of the accreditation goal long before it was achieved; to those who unselfishly provided the pathway for the profession to begin the journey toward the year 2000 and beyond. Perhaps from personal reflection on this valuable history will come the necessary vision to bring chiropractic together as we move toward a new millennium.

As a field practitioner, past president of CCE and past chairman of CCE's Commission on Accreditation, I am pleased to have been a small part of the CCE's history and am honored to be able to introduce the reader to this contribution to the profession's literature. Read, enjoy, learn!

Marino Passero, D.C.
Past President, Council on Chiropractic Education
Director, NCMIC Group, Inc.
Norwalk, Connecticut
31 March 1998

1 Gibbons, Russell W. Chiropractic history: lost, strayed or stolen. ACA Journal of Chiropractic 1976 (Jan); 13(1): 18-24

A Note of Appreciation

Perhaps because National Chiropractic Mutual Insurance Company (NCMIC) is directed by members of the chiropractic profession, there is a special commitment to protecting the profession. As the leading chiropractic insurance company they protect the doctor against malpractice claims. As a partner with the profession they have made a special effort to insure the profession against the loss of its heritage, with annual grants to the Association for the History of Chiropractic, to enable them to maintain their diligence in documenting chiropractic history. Through their generosity to the Council on Chiropractic Education, the NCMIC Group has underwritten the cost this publication, in order to preserve this record of chiropractic education's journey through its first century. We are indebted to NCMIC for this act of preservation.

Alana Callender, M.S.
Past President, Association for the History of Chiropractic
Director, Palmer Foundation for Chiropractic History
Davenport, Iowa

PREFACE

> History is not some past from which we are cut off. We are merely at its forward edge as it unrolls. And only if one is without historical feeling at all can one think of the intellectual fads and fashions of one's own time as a "habitation everlasting." We may feel that at last, unlike all previous generations, we have found certitude. They thought so, too. (Conquest, 1993)

The training of doctors of chiropractic occupies a unique niche in the annals of higher education in the United States. Constituting a few months of apprenticeship at its outset, the evolution of the educational enterprise to a fedrally recognized health care discipline would parallel developments in other professions in terms of expansion of curricula, growth in number and diversity of faculty, overcoming the intrinsic impediments of proprietary schools, and meeting the financial challenges created by ever growing demands from state and federal regulators. Unlike rival institutions in medicine and dentistry in the post-Flexner (1910) period, chiropractic schools adapted to these changing requirements without the external support from government and private philanthropy (Starr, 1982) that was lavished upon the "regular school." Moreover, this climb from an apprenticeship model to the federal recognition exemplified by the Council on Chiropractic Education (CCE) occurred within a combative environment fueled by severe dissension among chiropractors themselves and by sustained efforts by organized medicine to contain and eliminate chiropractic. As Gibbons (1980a) has suggested, the evolution of chiropractic education is a tale of extraordinary "bootstrapping" and self-improvement, and one that is still generally unrecognized and unappreciated by historians and scholars outside the profession.

The evolution of chiropractic education in North America constitutes a significant portion of the story of the profession. Throughout chiropractic's first century, school leaders have exercised great influence over the definition of the profession and over the political organizations created to sustain the rank and file. This has been a source both of strength and of weakness. Disputes among school leaders over the nature of chiropractic would reverberate throughout the profession for most of its first century. The earliest feuds set the stage for the intra-professional disputes which have impeded many of the profession's efforts to establish legitimacy in the wider social and political arena. The rhetoric of prominent college administrators would help to shape not only the content of chiropractic education, but also such issues as scope of practice, legislation and licensure, and chiropractors' relations with other disciplines, most notably allopathic medicine. In a very real sense the study of the history of chiropractic education provies a window on the entire chiropractic saga.

Chiropractic schools historicaly remained isolated from most of mainstream higher education and continue to depend almost exclusively upon tuition to meet their operating expenses. Among the consequences are a relatively modest level of scholarly activity among the faculties and the inability to be selective in student admissions; these deficiencies are seemingly not widely recognized. Ironically, chiropractors' bootstrapping self-improvements of the educational enterprise in chiropractic, with which the profession takes justifiable pride, have become a liability. Among the challenges now confronting the colleges and the profession are greater integration with other disciplines and greater productivity in scholarship and scientific research. To approach these goals the schools must grow out of the fierce independence and professional xenophobia which has in the past served them so well.

New demands for accountability in education and practice also challenge the limited resources of the tuition-driven colleges. Chiropractic education will have to respond to the emerging dicta of a new health care marketplace wherein economy and efficiency have become watchwords. Students will have to be better prepared to function in association and in collaboration with other health care providers. The next generation of chiropractors must be ready to find the appropriate balance between integration with the wider health care system and the need to maintain professional identity and autonomy. Perhaps a review of the history of chiropractic education will assist in planning for these sea changes.

In this, as in any scholarly treatise, the "facts" are necessarily embedded in the world views and biases that we as authors bring to the subject. Moreover, as the stories we relate here draw closer to the present, this work necessarily becomes less a history and more a reporting of current events. We do not apologize for our biases, but acknowledge that we cannot escape them, and remind the reader that they are present. We have done our best to report the realities of the history of chiropractic education as we understand them, but realize that others may look at the same information sources and arrive at a different interpretation of the "truth." There is room for reasonable people to disagree.

Joseph C. Keating, Jr., Ph.D.
Professor, Los Angeles College of Chiropractic
Past President, Association for the History of Chiropractic
Vice President, National Institute of Chiropractic Research
Whittier, California
October 1997

In Memory Of...

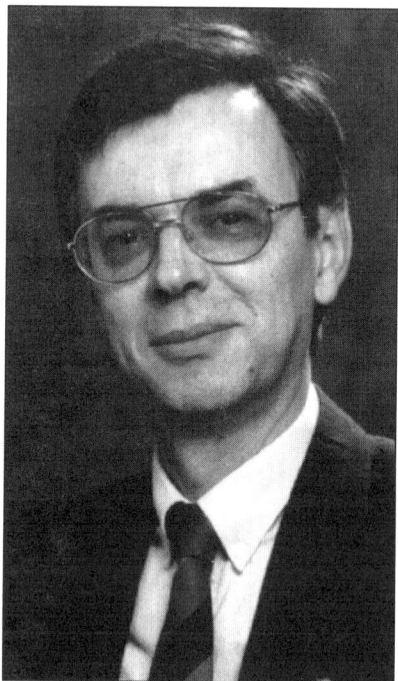

This work is dedicated to the memory of Pierre-Louis Gaucher-Peslherbe, D.C., Ph.D. Chiropractor, historian and scholar, he left this world on May 22, 1996. Born March 23, 1943, in Le Mans, France, Dr. Gaucher-Peslherbe earned his chiropractic degree from the Anglo-European Chiropractic College in 1972 and his doctorate in the history of medicine from the *Ecole des Hautes Etudes en Sciences Sociales* in Paris in 1983. His doctoral dissertation, a consideration of D.D. Palmer's theories within the context of nineteenth century neurophysiology, was a landmark in chiropractic literature. The dissertation was translated into English and published by the National College of Chiropractic as *Chiropractic: Early Concepts in Their Historical Setting.*

The Association for the History of Chiropractic conferred *in absentia* its Lee-Homewood Award for lifetime contributions to chiropractic on Dr. Gaucher-Peslherbe at the Association's 1996 Conference on Chiropractic History at Sherman College of Straight Chiropractic. At the time of his death, Dr. Gaucher-Peslherbe was under indictment for unlicensed practice in his native land, which still restricts the practice of chiropractic to medical physicians.

ACKNOWLEDGMENTS

We wish to thank Robert T. Anderson, Ph.D., D.C., M.D.; Fred Barge, D.C.; Edwin D. Follick, Ph.D., J.D., D.C.; Thomas A. Gelardi, D.C.; Friedhelm Kirchfeld, M.L.S.; Jerome McAndrews, D.C.; Gary Miller, Ph.D.; Ralph G. Miller, Ed.D.; Jean Moss, D.C., M.B.A.; Paul Smallie, D.C.; and Randy L. Swenson, M.H.P.E., D.C. for their thoughtful contributions. We thank the William Alfred Budden Library, the Council on Chiropractic Education, the Los Angeles College of Chiropractic, the National College of Chiropractic, the David D. Palmer Health Sciences Library and the Stockton Foundation for Chiropractic Research for access to their valuable archives. We thank the American Chiropractic Association, the Foundation for Chiropractic Education and Research, the publisher of the *American Journal of Chiropractic Medicine* and the editors of *Chiropractic History, Chiropractic Technique*, the *Journal of the Canadian Chiropractic Association*, and the *Journal of Manipulative and Physiological Therapeutics* for permission to reprint selected items.

Thanks are also due to Bernard A. Coyle, Ph.D.; Meredith A. Gonyea, Ph.D.; Bart Green, D.C.; David B. Koch, D.C.; Jerome McAndrews, D.C.; Reed B. Phillips, D.C., Ph.D.; W. Heath Quigley, D.C., M.S.; Frederik E. Schultz; David Sikorski, D.C. and Herbert J. Vear, D.C. for their critical reviews of preliminary drafts of this manuscript. We are grateful to the National Institute of Chiropractic Research, the Los Angeles College of Chiropractic, Palmer College of Chiropractic, and the Cleveland Chiropractic Colleges of Kansas City and Los Angeles for their support of this project.

TABLE OF CONTENTS

Chapter 1

THE FIRST DECADE
1896-1906

D.D. Palmer's chiropractic evolved from a variety of metaphysical concepts which were popular in the nineteenth century (Donahue, 1987). Chiropractic education began in 1896 as an outgrowth of Palmer's practice and teaching of magnetic healing. Magnetic healing, derived from the work of Austrian-trained physician Anton Mesmer (Mesmer, 1776), proposed that the diseases of living organisms could be influenced by an electromagnetic force generated by or transmitted through healers. Mesmer's theories and practices were carried to North America, where they became quite popular. The form of magnetic healing practiced by Palmer probably derived from the teachings of the Caster family, who operated a large infirmary for magnetic treatment in Burlington, Iowa (Beck, 1991), and from Palmer's extensive readings on the subject. Palmer came to believe that he could cool and relieve inflamed tissues in his patients by laying on hands and imparting his personal, excess vital magnetic energy to the sufferer (Keating, 1991b, 1992a).

Although some historians (and Palmer himself) have dated the birth of the educational process to D.D.'s near fatal railroad accident in Fulton, Missouri, in 1897, Palmer had been teaching his magnetic methods (Palmer, 1896) prior to the "discovery" of chiropractic. Moreover, despite Palmer's dating of the first chiropractic adjustment to September 1895, the earliest known account, published by Palmer, gave a slightly later time for the event. According to Harvey Lillard (1897), somewhere between January and April of 1896, the father of chiropractic administered that first thrust:

> THE CHIROPRACTIC.
> PUBLISHED MONTHLY BY
> PALMER'S
> School of Magnetic Cure
> *(Incorporated under the Laws of the State of Iowa)*
> FOR THE PURPOSE OF
> Teaching How to Get Well and Keep Well
> Without Taking Poisonous Drugs
>
> ———
>
> Office, School and Place of Publication:
> Fourth Floor, Ryan Block, Corner Second
> and Brady Streets
> DAVENPORT, IOWA

Figure 1-1: From the first issue of Palmer's flier, *The Chiropractic*, 1897

> I was deaf 17 years and I expected to always remain so, for I had doctored a great deal without any benefit. I had long ago made up my mind to not take any more ear treatments, for it did me no good.
>
> Last January Dr. Palmer told me that my deafness came from an injury in my spine. This was news to me; but it is a fact that my back was injured at the time I went deaf. Dr. Palmer treated me on the spine; in two treatments I could hear quite well. That was eight months ago. My hearing remains good. (Lilliard, 1897)

On June 17, 1896, perhaps less than six months after his treatment of Harvey Lillard, Palmer applied to incorporate his Palmer's School of Magnetic Cure and on July 10, 1896, the charter was granted (Wiese, 1986). By the time of the January 1897 issue of his school paper, *The Chiropractic* (see Figure 1-1), previously called *The Magnetic Cure*, Palmer could include testimonials from several of his students. His $100 per month magnetic instruction (Palmer, 1896) had evolved into a $500, three-month program of training in the new method:

> $500 will get you an education in three months which will better fit you for a healer of disease than any medical education in the world. Above does not include medicine, surgery, chemistry or obstetrics.

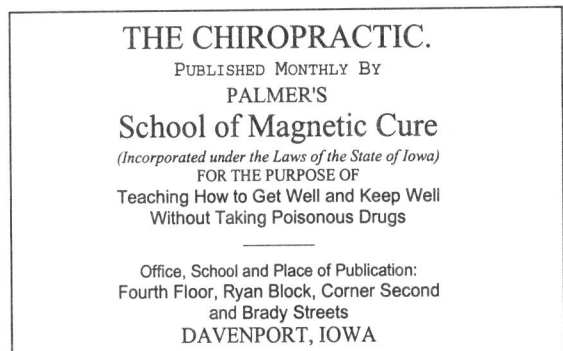

CAN THE NEW IDEA BE LEARNED?

> There are many who can learn and do just what we are doing - how to fix the human machine and make it run smooth.
>
> How long will it take to learn what we know? That depends upon the ability of the student, how much they know of anatomy and how much attention he or she will give to the business. Some will learn it in a month; it will take others 3 months, and some would never make it a success. Those that can't learn to do what Dr. Palmer is doing in 3 months better not try (Palmer, 1897a, p.1).
>
> We have always dones our business under the head of Magnetic Cure. Our ideas and business have so improved and expanded that we raise another flag. Chiropractic from two Greek words, means hand-fixing; a hand practitioner -- which is quite appropriate, as our work is all done by the hands. Not that we have ceased to believe in magnetic treatment, but that we have so much improved our method that magnetic does not fully cover our work. Under the chiropractic we can cure many cases which the magnetic would not reach. Every intelligent person can learn to be a chiropractic (Palmer, 1897a, p.3).

Palmer's formal preparation as an educator was extremely limited, but his knowledge base was exceptionally strong. His biographer credits him with "the equivalent of an eighth grade education" (Gielow, 1981a, p. 4), and notes that the future chiropractor had earned a living teaching grade school in various counties in Iowa and Illinois during the 1860s and 1870s (Gielow, 1981a, pp. 7, 8, 11, 15). An American Medical Association (AMA) publication noted that a "Dr. D. Palmer, Magnetic Healing" was listed as a faculty member during 1897-98 at the Independent Medical College in Chicago, one of a number of poor quality institutions that flourished in the Windy City prior to the Flexner report (Cramp, 1921, pp. 777-8). Many authors have noted that "Old Dad Chiro" (D.D.'s preferred self-designation) was extremely well read in the biology of his times (e.g., Gaucher-Peslherbe, 1994; Terrett, 1986), and the founder's writings reveal a grasp of the contemporary biological literature that would have been very unusual for the typical M.D. at the turn of the century.

The prominent position given in his earliest chiropractic advertising to his offer to train others suggests that education was no less a part of Old Dad's business plan than was patient care (e.g., Palmer 1897a&b, 1899, 1900, 1902). Lerner (1954, pp. 321-2) has noted the financial incentives available to Palmer for teaching chiropractic at that time:

> As a doctor who cared for patients, he earned a moderate fee. He charged so much a visit and that was all he could earn from his practice.
>
> But, as a teacher, he found that he could "command" a different kind of fee. He could get a "tuition fee" from a student who was willing to pay him many times more than any patient would ever consider paying him.
>
> Whereas a patient would give him from $2.00 to $5.00 a visit, and over a period of treatment lasting about a month, for example, the doctor could earn about $50.00 from his patient -- a student would be willing to give him $500.00 -- ten times as much -- for learning about his discovery during the same period of time approximately.
>
> In addition to this alluring situation, he found that teaching a student did not carry with it the responsibilities that he had when caring for a patient. As a doctor, he had to make certain promises to his patient....and making a promise, meant fulfilling it. If he did not succeed in getting his patient well, it was as though he had failed to fulfill his promise. If the patient did not get well, the patient left the doctor and he would go somewhere else. The loss of any patient is naturally a factor in any doctor's earning capacity.
>
> But as a teacher he was not obliged to make any promises or guaranties to a student. As a teacher he merely represented that he had found new knowledge about the body -- knowledge that was not known to anyone before. He offered to give this knowledge to anyone who wanted to learn it for a price. The temptation to the student, naturally, was that he could use this knowledge to prepare himself for a new way to earn money.

The earliest training provided at the first chiropractic school was similar to the apprenticeship training in medicine that had been common in the nineteenth century. Gibbons (1980b) suggests that training under Old Dad Chiro may at first have been limited to as few as three weeks of instruction in "anatomy, physiology, symptomatology, pathology, diagnosis, chiropractic philosophy and adjusting technique." However, some thirty years after his own chiropractic training, Oakley G.

Smith (see Figure 1-2), an 1899 graduate of Palmer's school and founder of the rival profession of naprapathy (Beideman, 1994; Zarbuck, 1986), described an even more meager educational experience at Palmer's school:

> ...I was taken to Davenport, Iowa, where I took chiropractic treatment for five months. I was convinced of the fact that cures could be made by manipulation. A few days before I was 19 my tuition of $500.00 was paid for a course of instruction in Chiropractic. The first thing I learned was that there was no instruction to be given. There were no blackboards, no text books, no notes, not a single lecture. For six days I witnessed the giving of a number of treatments. That was the sum total of information that was transferred in exchange for the tuition paid. The diagnosis as I witnessed it consisted of a quick gliding pressure from upper dorsal to middle lumbar to detect the position of apical prominences. That was the sum total of examination that was given to any patient. The treatment consisted of giving a single forceful lunge on that prominent apex, using the flat of the hand as a contact. That was the sum total of the treatment. Nothing else was done. The patient's treatment for that day was finished. These treatments were given daily. There were no charts made, no histories taken, and no records made. After being permitted to watch this identical form of treatment on a number of patients for six days, I was told that I knew all that was necessary for me to know, and that I should do the treating myself thereafter.

> As patients who could not pay applied for treatment they were turned over to me. In a room set apart for me I began to dispense the form of treatment that I have just described. There were no more instructions given to me. I was left wholly to my own devices. Thus left to myself, I soon began to make notes, to keep records. I adopted an ambition - an ambition to make a science out of manipulation. To this end I applied every energy I had. I kept on treating and improving my technique, in that same room set aside for me, for the next eight months (Smith, 1932, pp. 5-6).

Palmer granted a diploma which indicated that the graduate had "taken a course in Chiropractic as taught in this school and has passed the examination required. I consider (him/her) competent to *Teach* and *Practice* the same" (Gibbons, 1981a). Although the founder obviously expected that his graduates were going to spread his teachings and methods to others, he had apparently not considered the possibility that this would mean further development in theory and technique, and competition in the school business. Before the end of the first decade of chiropractic, Old Dad Chiro was embroiled in a number of disputes with his professional progeny, disputes which influenced the practice and theories of chiropractic, the training of chiropractors and the profession's legal standing. Palmer himself may have inadvertently encouraged some of the early proliferation of chiropractic schools by his general unwillingness to cooperate with his graduates.

Palmer's earliest known rival in chiropractic instruction was the National School of Neuropathy and Psycho-Magnetic Healing, Inc., which advertised a course in neuropathy which included "chiropractice, osteopathy, massage, Swedish movement, hypnotism, hydropathy, magnetism, hygiene, psychic sciences, mental sciences, Etc." The advertisement appeared in a Minneapolis directory for 1899; officers of the school included Irving J. Eales, N.D., D.O., President; Uriah H. Thomas, M.D., N.D., C.D., Vice-President; C. Wilbur Taber, N.D., Secretary and Manager; and Andrew G. Williams, N.D., Treasurer. The school proposed to cure "All forms of acute and chronic diseases, Habits of all kinds, Mental Characteristics changed or strengthened, Nervous diseases, and Sexual Weakness in both sexes a specialty. Absent Treatment if desired. No Drugs or Knife Used." Nothing more is known of this school, and it seems probable that the offer to teach "chiropractice" involved little if any knowledge of Palmer's work.

Another of the earliest rival educators was Solon Massey Langworthy who had earned his chiropractic diploma from Palmer in September 1901 (Zarbuck, 1988c). Langworthy immediately established his Chiropractic Cure and School in Cedar Rapids, Iowa. Three months later he wrote to the founder's son, B.J. Palmer, to propose a collaborative venture wherein the Palmers would:

> ...sell me an interest in the Davenport plan at rock bottom, you to take the active management and I to give you some of my time each week? My idea would be to run the infirmary for all it is worth and then incorporate the Western School of Chiropractic securing as stock holders D.D. Palmer, Thomas Storey, Oakley Smith, B.J. Palmer, Dr. Sutton, Dr. Jones, Dr. Strouder, Miss Olcutt, and Solon Langworthy, each to own an equal amount of stock and each (except D.D. Palmer) to send all students to the school, all sharing alike in the profits of the school (Langworthy, quoted in Zarbuck, 1988c).

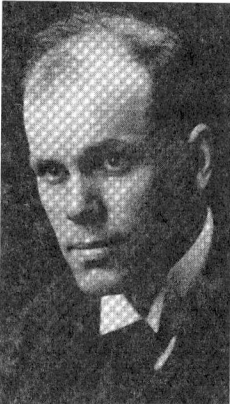

Figure 1-2: Oakley G. Smith, D.C., c1930

Langworthy's concept of a unified chiropractic educational enterprise was shared by Oakley Smith (see Figure 1-2):

> Clarinda, Iowa, June 16, 1902
>
> Old Chiro --
>
> Say, Doc, if we take things just cool and saw wood faithfully, we will see Chiropractic the leading system of treatment or fixment. What we need is one school with Dr. Palmer at the head. Chiropractic will never be taught right in any other way. As it is going now, it will degenerate. OAKLEY (Lerner, 1954, pp. 379-80)

Langworthy's idea of chiropractic training and practice included elements of osteopathy, hydropathy and naturopathy. He shared several books on "Nature Cure" with the younger Palmer during the latter's visit to Cedar Rapids, Iowa, in April 1902. However, the father of chiropractic indicated that he had "no use for those books on 'natural cure,' as I have been over the whole field and have outgrown them" (Zarbuck, 1988c). Palmer went on to specifically reject:

> ...all "Natural Methods," whether they be "Hypnotism, Homeopathy, X-rays, Ozone, Electricity, Oil, Variations of Diet, Gymnastics, Massage, Magnetism, Bacteria Remedies, Baths, Medical Herbs, or Kneipp's Water Cure...Every physician, no matter of what schools, says and believes that his means are the "natural Methods." Chiro. is not benefited by mixing it with any other method, if there is a positive excuse for mixing, it is to fool the patient, belittling Chiro., deceiving the patient and losing confidence in ourselves (D.D. Palmer, quoted in Zarbuck, 1988c).

However, by June 1902, D.D. had departed from Davenport for the West Coast, presumably to avoid the legal consequences of his feud with former student H.H. Reiring (Lerner, 1954, pp. 254-66; Zarbuck & Hayes, 1990). Old Dad Chiro took most of the infirmary equipment, down to the bedsheets, with him. In his absence B.J. strove to re-establish the Palmer School with financial assistance from Howard Nutting. Langworthy's competing institution, renamed the American School of Chiropractic and Nature Cure (ASC&NC), enjoyed a period of ascendancy. Gibbons (1981a) credits Langworthy (see Figure 1-3) as the "Keeper of the Flame During the 'Lost Years' of Chiropractic."

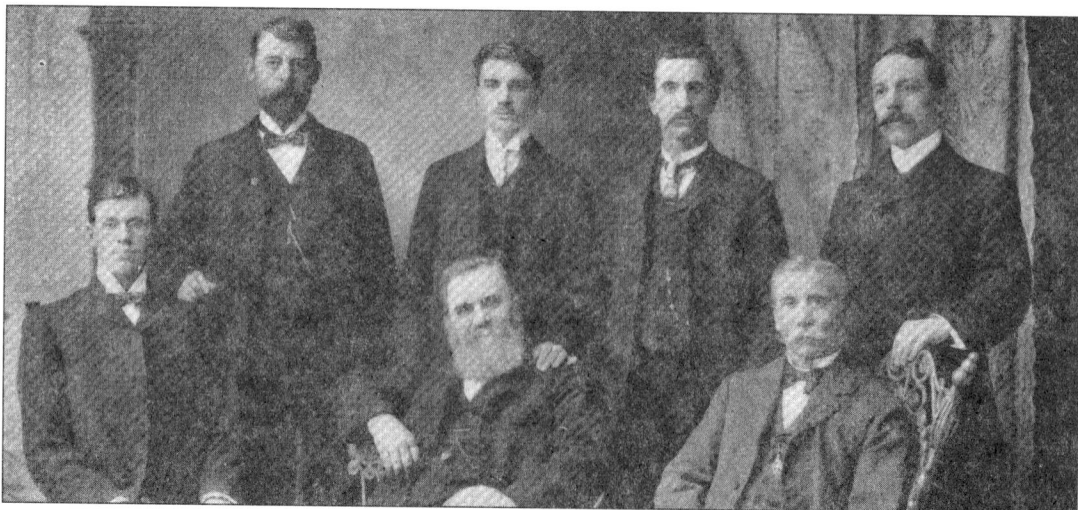

Figure 1-3: From D.D. Palmer's 1910 *The Chiropractor's Adjuster* (p.886): early Palmer graduates gathered for this December 1902 photo with Old Dad Chiro. Left to right, standing: E.E. Sutton (Class of 1901), B.J. Palmer (1902), O.B. Jones (1900), Solon M. Langworthy (1901). Left to right, seated: Oakley G. Smith (1899), D.D. Palmer, Thomas H. Storey (1901). Langworthy and Smith would serve as president and dean, respectively, of the American School of Chiropractic and Nature Cure in Cedar Rapids, Iowa; Storey taught chiropractic to Charles A. Cale in Los Angeles, where Cale founded the Los Angeles College of Chiropractic in 1911.

Palmer's feud with Reiring is worthy of mention, because it illustrates the early antagonistic influence of the medical community upon the chiropractic educational enterprise. Unlike many of the other students with whom the founder would do battle, Reiring appears to have been planted in the school by Davenport's Henry Matthey, M.D., an orthodox physician with whom Palmer had publicly feuded (Lerner, 1954). Reiring enrolled at Palmer's School in March 1900, and soon thereafter began to complain to other students that he had been defrauded. Palmer summoned the local police to remove the irate student from the campus, but did not subsequently press charges against the young man. Reiring brought suit for false arrest; his complaint against Palmer included:

> ...a charge that Palmer had defrauded his student; that he had been induced by misrepresentations
> on the part of Palmer to pay $500 for taking a course in Chiropractic which was not a real science;
> which was based upon quackery, etc.; that Palmer himself was ignorant and knew nothing about
> anatomy and physiology, etc. (Lerner, 1954, p. 262).

With D.D. Palmer temporarily out of the picture and young B.J. Palmer struggling to keep his father's institution going, Solon Langworthy's Cedar Rapids institution came to the fore. Zarbuck (1986) credits Langworthy's American School as the first "mixer" institution, a designation which, at least in the early years of the profession, referred to the use of other treatment methods in addition to manual adjusting. Founded in 1903 in conjunction with Langworthy's Health Home, the school is remembered for a number of innovations. The ASC&NC began publication of the profession's first journal, *Backbone*, in 1903, and graduated seven students in 1904 (Gibbons, 1981a). Langworthy is also credited with the first use of the term "subluxation" in the chiropractic literature, and with the first mention of the role of gravity in the creation of spinal dysfunc-

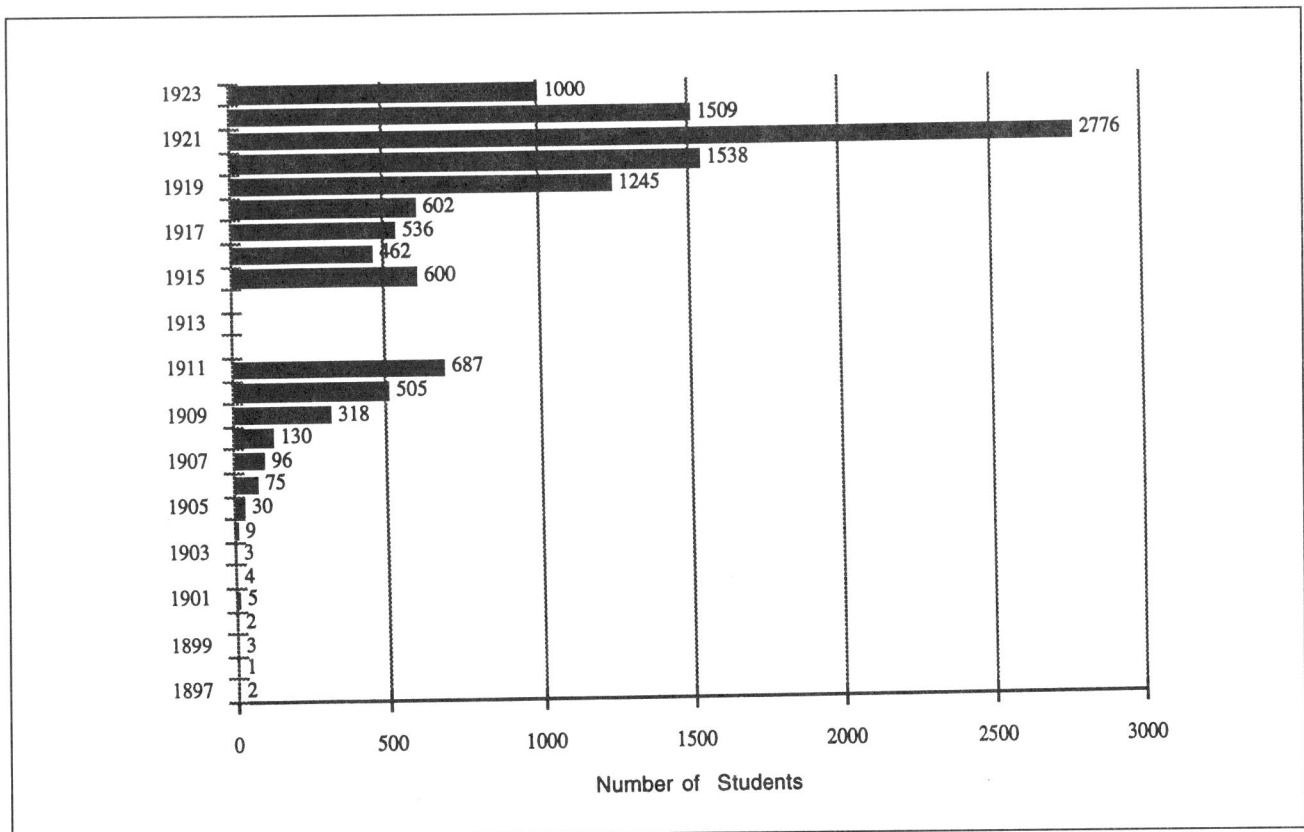

Figure 1-4: Annual student enrollment at the Palmer School of Chiropractic during its first quarter century of operations; two students were mentioned by D.D. Palmer in his 1897 publications of *The Chiropractic*; data for 1898-1910 are from *The Chiropractor* (Palmer, 1911; Will, 1910) and Lerner (Wardwell 1992, p.69); the 1911 figure of 687 students is from Brennan (1983); enrollment in 1915 is based on information provided by Turner (1931, p.34); data for 1916-1922 are based on information provided by B.J. Palmer in the *Fountain Head News* 1923 (Oct 20); 13(4):8-9; 1,000 student figure for 1923 is an estimate. Most of these data probably err in the liberal direction, and authors and historians disagree on exact numbers.

tions. Smith, Langworthy and Minora Paxson, (another early Palmer graduate) are also credited with the first textbook of chiropractic in 1906, *Modernized Chiropractic*. The ASC&NC is also noteworthy for implementing the first structured curriculum, which involved four five-month terms (Gibbons, 1981a). When Langworthy and his apprenticeship-trained associate, Daniel W. Reisland, D.C., were successful in moving a bill to license chiropractors through both houses of the Minnesota legislature in 1905, the proposed law specified a twenty-month program of instruction rather than the short course offered in Davenport. Had the legislation been passed, only Langworthy's graduates would have been eligible to sit for the licensing examination. Opposition from the medical community and a personal visit by D.D. Palmer to Governor Johnson led to a veto of what would probably have been the first chiropractic statute (Gibbons, 1993).

Old Dad Chiro had returned from California in 1904 to a revitalized institution, and now became a partner to the son who had earned his D.C. just before the father's departure in 1902. B.J. had done well. With the assistance of Howard Nutting (Gielow, 1981a, p. 130), an uncle of D.D. Palmer's attorney (Willard Carver, LL.B.), the younger Palmer had secured a bank loan for the school, had expanded the student body (see Figure 1-4 and Table 1-1), and had relocated the Palmer School from its origins in D.D. Palmer's fourth floor infirmary in the Ryan Block Building to a modest house in the 800 block of Brady Street. Although B.J. had been threatened with prosecution for unlicensed practice in Davenport, he had discovered that the Iowa laws did not prevent his teaching of the new health care method. Just across the Mississippi River the young D.C. apparently found that Illinois authorities were less hostile toward his practice of chiropractic.

The Palmers met the competition from Langworthy's school by establishing *The Chiropractor,* a "Monthly Journal Devoted to the Interests of Chiropractic," which continued in publication into the 1960s. The curriculum was expanded to nine months, although, as *The Chiropractor* noted in its first issue (p. 5), shorter courses were still offered: "six months, $400; three months, $300; one month, $200, ten days, $100." In this first issue (December 1904) Old Chiro also wrote about several aspects of his West Coast sojourn, most importantly about his experience in Santa Barbara (see Figure 1-5). There, on July 1, 1903, Palmer had revealed to his students his discovery that the body is "heated by nerves and not by blood" (Palmer, 1904b).

This evolution of Palmer's theories (see Table 1-2) may have been prompted in part by the continuing criticism that the founder of chiropractic had been receiving in the osteopathic literature. It is indeed ironic that this evolution of Old Dad Chiro's theories helped to give rise to the diversity of theories and techniques in the profession. Those who graduated during various periods of Palmer's conceptual metamorphosis took what they had learned as the "true" theory of chiropractic. B.J. Palmer, for example, who had trained under his father prior to D.D.'s departure from the Palmer School in 1906, always after taught that nerves were pinched or compressed in the intervertebral foramina. The founder of chiropractic, on the other hand, abandoned the compression theory in favor of "nerve stretching" in his final version of chiropractic. Similarly, D.D.

1.	H.D. Reynard	15.	Dr. Oas	29.	S.M. Hunter	43.	F.B.C. Eilersficken
2.	Ira H. Lucas	16.	Dr. Hananska	30.	Andrew Coleman	44.	W.L. Bowers
3.	O.G. Smith	17.	Dr. Evans	31.	Dr. Bennett	45.	Chas. G. Munro
4.	Minora C. Paxsion	18.	G.B. Danelz	32.	C.D. Sprague	46.	R.P. Rold
5.	A.B. Wightman	19.	Selma Doelz	33.	C.E. Ashwill	47.	W.F. Booth
6.	M.A. Collier	20.	E.E. Sutton	34.	A.P. Davis	48.	D.W. Resiland
7.	A.S. Dresher	21.	O.B. Jones	35.	P.W. Hammerle	49.	Dr. Raymond
8.	S.D. Parrish	22.	J.L. Hirely	36.	Thomas Francis	50.	Ernie Simon
9.	A. Henry	23.	S.M. Langworthy	37.	Ella Bon	51.	D.B. Baker
10.	T.H. Story	24.	W.J. Robb	38.	C. Wright Dodd	52.	Miss Eliza Murchison
11.	Henry Gross	25.	E.E. Jones	39.	C.W. Konkler	53.	Ray Stouder
12.	J.E. Marsh	26.	E.D.B. Newton	40.	Mrs. M. Gould French	54.	Dr. Schooley
13.	Martha Brake	27.	E. Ellsworth Schwartz	41.	Edward D. Schoffman	55.	Ralph Graham
14.	J.J. Darnell	28.	A.G. Boggs	42.	C.H. Fancher	56.	Chas. Ray Parker

Table 1-1: B.J. Palmer's list of Palmer graduates druing 1895-1905. From Palmer BJ (1919b). There is no apparent order to this numbering of graduates, and some of them earned their D.C. degrees from D.D. Palmer during his 1902-1903 visit to the West Coast, rather than from the Palmers' Davenport institution.

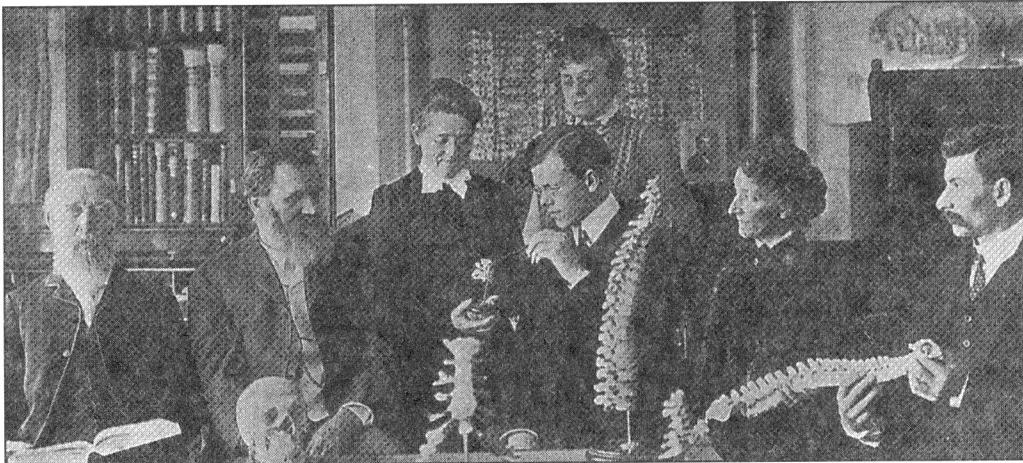

Figure 1-5: From *The Chiropractor* 1904; 1(1):13. Original caption reads, "Note - the cut on Page 13 was the class present when nerve heat was first announced. From left to right they were: Lucas, Old Chiro, Collier, Smith, Wright, Paxson, Reynard."

Palmer's abandonment of the terms "diagnosis" and "therapeusis" in favor "analysis" and "adjustment" was accepted by some as genuine conceptual developments, although other early students, such as 1906 Palmer graduate John Howard, (founder of the National School of Chiropractic), understood these changes in terminology as "garments to protect the child until legal clothing could be secured" (Beideman, 1983).

Palmer's new ideas in the post-1903 era were consistent with his notions of the vibratory transmission of neural impulses (Donahue, 1987) and with his idea of inflammation as the essence of disease (Keating, 1991b). The newly limited focus on the nervous system was reinforced, ironically, by Langworthy's exclusive interest in the spine, and with Langworthy's proposition that the brain was the source of an unseen life force. Palmer (1910a) later proposed that Innate Intelligence could direct human physiology through any nerve ganglion. When Langworthy's textbook, *Modernized Chiropractic*, helped to win the first acquittal of a chiropractor arrested for unlicensed practice of osteopathy (Rehm, 1986), the theoretical reduction to a concern for neural-interference-only was carved in stone. Chiropractors ever since have suggested that osteopathic theory is exclusively concerned with the "rule of the artery," while chiropractors are solely interested in the nervous system. This historical revisionism (cf. Schiller, 1971) was incorporated in the curricula of most schools.

Concept:	The Chiropractic (1897-1902)	The Chiropractor (1904-06)	The Chiropractor Adjuster; The Chiropractor's Adjuster (1908-10)
circulatory obstruction?	Yes	No	No
nerve pinching?	Yes	Yes	No
foraminal occlusion?	?	Yes	No
nerve vibration?	?	?	Yes
therapeusis?	Yes	No	No
method of intervention?	manipulation	adjustment	adjustment
innate/educated?	absent	nerves; Intelligence	Intelligence
religious plank?	absent	absent	optional?
machine metaphor?	Yes	Yes	Yes & No

Table 1-2: D.D. Palmer's concepts during three periods of publications. *The Chiropractic* was the title of D.D. Palmer's journal during the early years of his practice in Davenport, Iowa. *The Chiropractor* was the title of the journal published by D.D. Palmer and B.J. Palmer beginning in December 1904 from the Palmer School. *The Chiropractor Adjuster* was the title of D.D. Palmer's journal published in Portland by the D.D. Palmer College of Chiropractic, while the *Chiropractor's Adjuster* was the title of his book. Reprinted by permission from Keating JC. Old Dad Chiro comes to Portland, 1908-10. *Chiropractic History* 1993; 13(2):36-44.

Pacific School of Chiro-Practic

Old Dad's several years on the West Coast during 1902-1904 helped to spread the new healing art. One of the students present (see Figure 1-5) at the Santa Barbara discovery was Harry Reynard (Zarbuck, 1988b&c), who opened the Pacific School of Chiro-Practic in Oakland, California, in 1904 (Gillespie, 1925). The program of instruction was only about half as long as that offered by Langworthy's ASC&NC, but still exceeded what was offered in Davenport at that time (see Table 1-3). Clinical instruction included access to both in-patients and out-patients. Tuition was $500 in total. By 1907, with the assistance of Carl V. Schultz, M.D., N.D., LL.B., the school had expanded its curriculum to include naturopathic instruction, and its faculty and trustees sought to establish the first board of naturopathic examiners in California (Gillespie, 1925). Schultz, a German immigrant who had arrived in Los Angeles in 1885, had established the Naturopathic Institute of California in Los Angeles in 1905 (Stanford, 1960, p. 215), and earned his law degree to better cope with the persecution he experienced from the orthodox medical community. California had passed its first medical practice act in 1876; Schultz and associates were successful in having a naturopathic act passed in 1909. Harry Reynard later served as vice-president of the state's naturopathic society. Schultz is recalled as "the father of naturopathy in California."

Chiropractic schools continued to proliferate in these first years of the twentieth century (Gibbons,1993). Palmer's earliest graduates offered apprenticeship training to others, who in turn opened schools; 1901 Palmer graduate Thomas Storey is exemplary, and trained new chiropractors in several states by preceptorship. Minnesota became very fertile ground for this growth, and prompted derisive comments from the Palmers (Gibbons, 1993). In California, the Sinclair College of Chiropractic began operations in Santa Rosa in 1900 (Stanford, 1960).

Table 1-3: Curriculum of the Pacific School of Chiro-Practic, Inc.
COURSE OF STUDY
The course of study covers a period of one year, divided into two terms of five months each. Students may matriculate at the beginning of each term.
First Term
Anatomy. Urinalysis. Toxicology. Physiology. Pathology. Symptomatology. Lectutres on the Principles and Practices of Chiro-Practic.
Second Term
Anatomy. Physiology. Symptomatology. Pathology. Minor Surgery. Medical and Chiropractic diagnosis compared. Chiropractic Technique, Clinical Demonstrations, Diagnosis and Practic. Hygiene and dietetics.

Board of Trustees.
 Harry D. Reynard, D.C., President
 Rev. J.J. Marrall, Vice-President
 William F. Booth, D.C., Secretary
 Elza L. Lichty, D.C., Treasurer
 I.W. Bridenbecker

Faculty
 Harry D. Reynard, D.C., Maude L. Reynard, D.C., William F. Booth, D.C., Elze L. Lichty, D.C., Ruby A. Lichty, D.C., W.E. Ledyard, M.D., D.C.

From the *College's Announcement, Session of 1905* and from Gillespie (1925)

Western States Chiropractic College

Ritter (1991) attributes the first chiropractic education in Oregon to John and Eva Marsh, graduates of "The Brainiard School in Minnesota." In 1904 the couple established an apprenticeship program in their offices in Portland; the school was known variously as the Chiropractic School and Cure, as the Pacific Chiropractic College, and as "a branch of Dr. Lynch's school of the Brainiard College" in Minnesota (Ritter, 1991). Through a series of mergers and amalgamations the Marsh School eventually combined with the remnant of the D.D. Palmer College of Chiropractic to become today's Western States Chiropractic College (see Figure 1-6).

Old Dad Chiro's December 1904 return to the leadership of his Davenport school was brief. Although he apparently was not bothered any further by his former student Reiring, he soon began to be hounded by the local allopathic community. Late in 1905 he was charged with unlicensed medical practice based upon his advertised offer to heal the sick. After a brief trial in April 1906, during which he offered no defense except to insist that in practicing chiropractic he was not practicing medicine, he was convicted and incarcerated in Scott County Jail. His relationship with son B.J., which had always been stormy, reached a new low following D.D.'s release from jail. The father was forced to sell his interest in the school, and soon relocated with his wife to Medford, Oklahoma, where his brother Thomas helped him to establish a grocery business. The father of chiropractic was once more without a facility wherein he could teach his theories and methods.

With his wife, Mabel H. Palmer, D.C., in control of the school's assets, B.J. assumed the presidency of his father's former institution and changed its corporate title to the Palmer School and Infirmary of Chiropractic (PSIC) (Wiese, 1986). Without his father's consent he published D.D.'s collected papers as *The Science of Chiropractic*, thereby further alienating the elder Palmer (Donahue, 1986; Palmer, 1910a). This 1906 volume was probably released in response to the challenge posed by Smith, Langworthy and Paxson's (1906) *Modernized Chiropractic*.

National School of Chiropractic

Dissatisfaction with the policies of the new president of the PSIC began to grow, perhaps in reaction to D.D. Palmer's departure from the school, but apparently owing also to B.J.'s vision for chiropractic education. A number of students approached John F.A. Howard, D.C., with the idea of establishing a competing chiropractic school (Beideman, 1983). Howard, a 1906 graduate who had begun his studies prior to Old Dad Chiro's departure from the school, had dabbled in naturopathic remedies prior to enrolling at the Palmer School. Howard was interested in seeing a more academically rigorous training for D.C.s than B.J. was prepared to offer. With a letter of encouragement from D.D. that also recounted the founder's delight in an impromptu lecture and clinical demonstration delivered to a local medical society (see Table 1-4), Howard established the National School of Chiropractic (NSC) in Davenport in 1906.

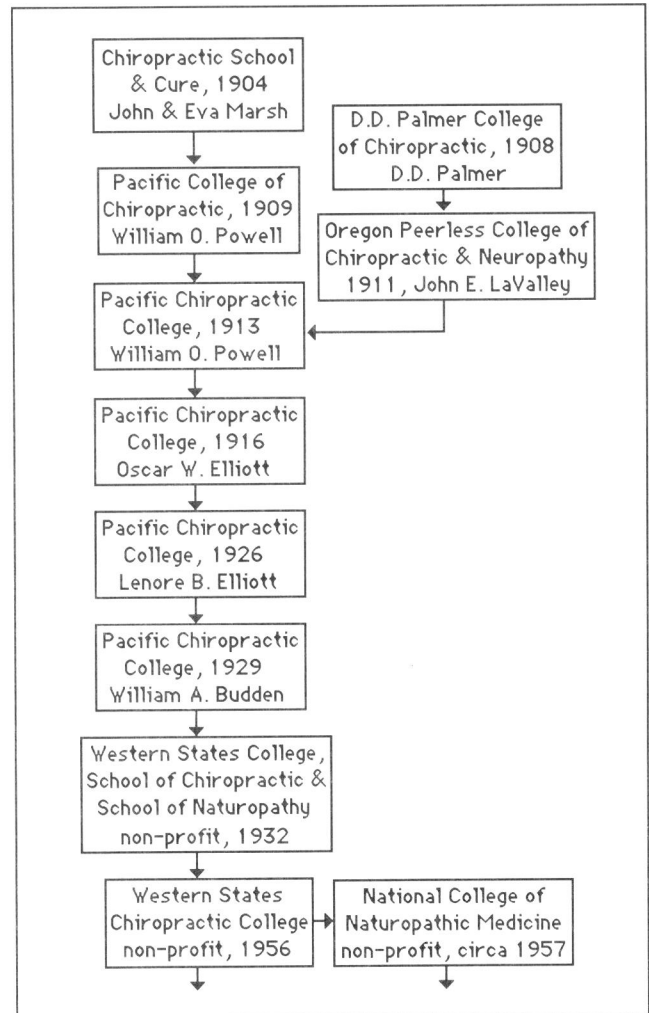

Figure 1-6: Geneaology of today's Western States Chiropractic College, including title and date of founding, re-sale, owner or establishment of non-profit status; based on Ritter (1991) and Naturopathic (1957).

The first "campus" of the NSC consisted of several rooms in the same building where D.D. Palmer had practiced magnetic and chiropractic during the 1880s and 1890s. However, owing to restrictions on access to cadavers imposed by Iowa statutes at that time, the NSC relocated to Chicago in 1908. Here the broad-scope school could more easily expand its curriculum to include anatomical instruction by dissection. Within a few years Howard had attracted several medical physicians to his faculty, most notably Rush Medical College graduate William C. Schulze, M.D. (Eleventh, 1918; Keating & Rehm, 1995a&b) and Arthur L. Forster, M.D., a graduate of the Medical Department of the University of Illinois (Eleventh, 1918). Forster's role in the early history of the National is sadly under-recalled. Although provocative in his war of words with B.J. Palmer (each as editor of his respective school's journal), Forster also infused a scholarly attitude within the early literature of the profession. He found room both for praise and criticism in the work of D.D. Palmer, and in his criticism echoed the sentiments of Palmer's short-time school partner, Alva Gregory, M.D., D.C., that the founder's lack of education had seriously hindered his theory development:

...Palmer, however, fell into one serious error. He did as so many before him have done. He became overzealous. He claimed that all disease is due to subluxations of the vertebrae and that all diseases could be eradicated by adjustment of the vertebrae. Naturally, such views could not be subscribed to by anyone with a liberal training in the sciences underlying the art of healing, and

John F. Howard
Davenport, Iowa
Dear Sir and Friend:

Kansas City, Mo.
May 28, 1906

You have been on my mind for several days, therefore I will write you a few lines.

Why should I not approve of your teaching the science of chiropractic; when I consider you a capable and qualified teacher....In practice and as a teacher I consider you qualified.....

I cannot let your letter go until I tell you of the M.D.'s meeting yesterday. They have a county society which meets once each month. I attended. Did not do so at home (Davenport). A paper was read; each member discussed its merits. I asked to have a say. They reluctantly voted me 5 minutes. When the 5 minutes were up several said, "Go on." So they voted me another 5 minutes. By that time all the rules were forgotten and I occupied most of the afternoon....Dr. Martin said that he had a headache. I offered to cure it by one touch. He accepted. I seated him in front of the audience. He showed his surprise and admitted that the headache was gone. Several questions were asked for me to answer. Chiropractic captured the meeting....
With best wishes,

D.D. Palmer

Table 1-4: National College of Chiropractic advertisement. *The Chiropractic Journal* (NCA), March 1936. Caption reads: "The following are brief excerpts from letters written in 1906 by D.D. Palmer to John F. Howard, Founder, National College of Chiropractic. One letter was written from Kansas City, Missouri; several others from Medford, Oklahoma."

especially, one with a knowledge of pathology. This preliminary training Palmer lacked; and it goes without saying that had he possessed such knowledge, he would not have made the claims which he did. He derided all other forms of therapy, and persisted in his original views to the end. Nevertheless, while the advancement made in chiropractic technique has been very great, and broader views now obtain among the profession as a whole, still to Palmer must be given the credit for furnishing the impetus which carried chiropractic to a recognition of its wonderful possibilities (Forster, 1915, p. 7).

Together these men, Howard, Schulze and Forster, created the major rival to the Palmer institution for most of the twentieth century, and firmly established physiotherapeutic and naturopathic theories and methods within the profession (Beideman, 1983; Keating & Rehm, 1995; Ransom, 1984). The National College of Chiropractic (renamed in 1920) absorbed a great number of other institutions during the coming decades (see Figure 1-7).

Figure 1-7: Name, date of founding or reorganization, and owner of some of the ancestor institutions of today's National College of Chiropractic.

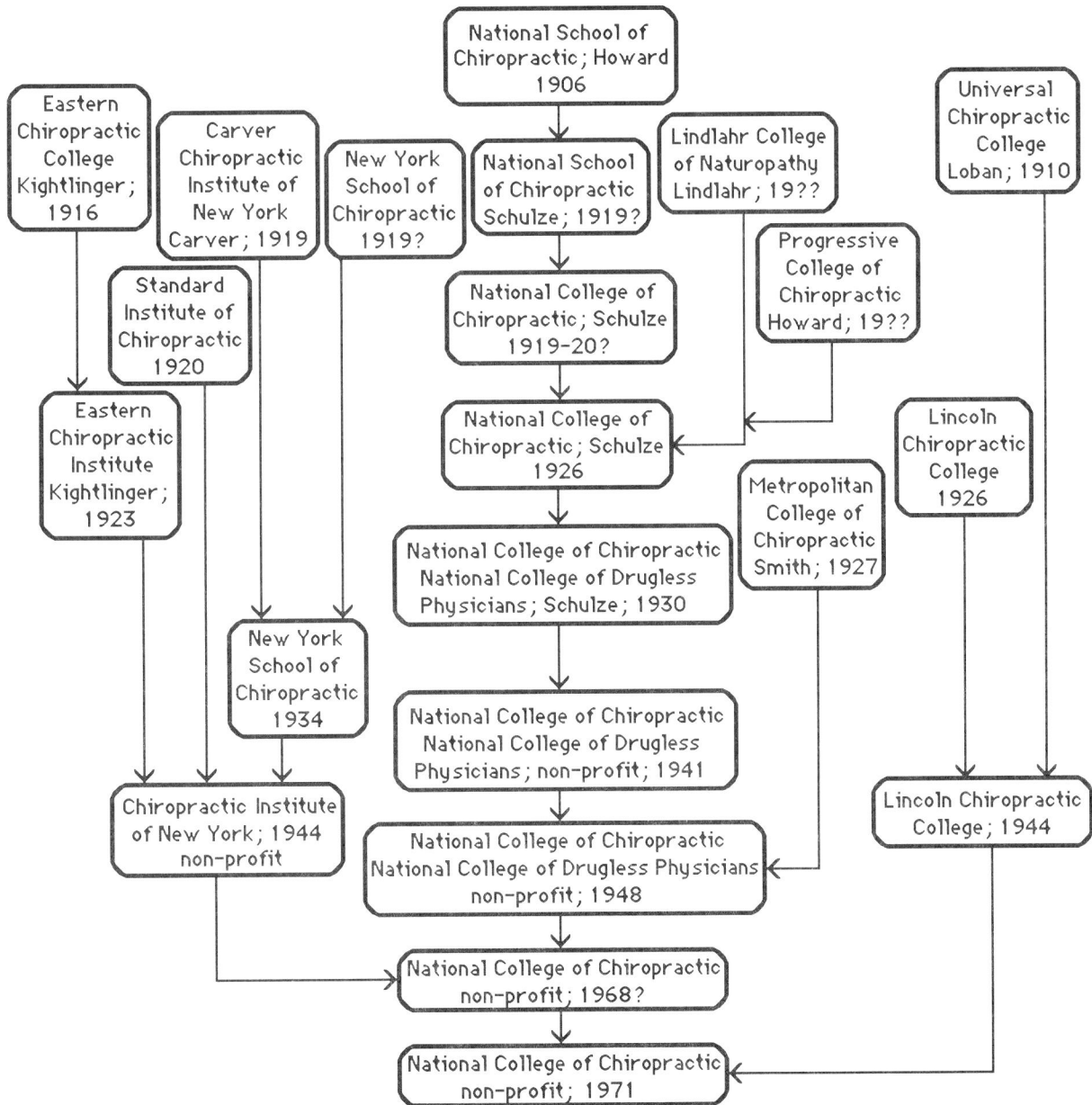

Chapter 2

EARLY MEDICAL PRESENCE IN CHIROPRACTIC EDUCATION

The role of medical physicians within the ranks of early faculties and student bodies was by no means unique to the National School of Chiropractic (e.g., Gromala, 1986; Gibbons, 1981a&b, 1991). The guiding influence of Carl V. Schultz at the Pacific School of Chiro-Practic has already been mentioned, but an earlier medical presence was apparent at the Palmer School. Among D.D. Palmer's first graduates (1898) were A.P. Davis, M.D., D.O., D.C., N.D., Oph.D., and William A. Seeley, M.D. (Palmer, 1909d, p. 25; Rehm, 1980, p. 271). M.P. Brown, M.D., D.C. served on the faculty and as clinic director of the PSIC in the 1900s, and A.B. Hender, M.D., D.C. served for decades as dean of the institution while maintaining his obstetrical practice in Davenport (Gibbons, 1981b).

A.P. Davis played unique roles in both chiropractic and osteopathy. He was born in New York State in 1835, raised in Indiana, and trained at both homeopathic and allopathic (Rush Medical College) schools. Davis studied under Andrew T. Still at the latter's American School of Osteopathy (ASO) in Kirksville, Missouri, where he earned his D.O., graduating from Still's first class in March 1893 (Booth, 1924, p. 81; Davis, 1915). After teaching at the ASO he apparently relocated to Davenport to study under Old Dad Chiro in 1898, and meanwhile completed the first osteopathic text, *Osteopathy Illustrated*. He graduated from the Palmer institution on October 18, 1898, and set up practice in Rock Island and Moline, Illinois. An "itinerant healer and schoolman" (Gibbons, 1991), Davis spent the next several decades teaching and practicing a mixture of the theories and methods of chiropractic, osteopathy and medicine which he called "Neuropathy" (Davis, 1905, 1915). Although he established his own schools in several cities, most notably the Davray Neuropathic Institute of Battle Creek, Michigan in 1901 (Gibbons, 1991) and the Bullis and Davis School of Neuropathy, Ophthalmology and Chiropractic in Los Angeles during 1911 (Zarbuck, 1988b), he was unsuccessful in establishing neuropathy as a viable health profession. He also served as dean of the Union College of Osteopathy in Pittsburgh circa 1910 (Gibbons, 1991; Zarbuck, 1988b). Despite Davis' lack of success as a "founder" in his own right, his broad-scope, "mixer" concepts were widely disseminated among chiropractors and other drugless healers through his several books, his lecture tours, and through D.D. Palmer's publication of their correspondence in the latter's 1910 volume.

American School of Chiropractic, New York

The American School of Chiropractic (ASC) in New York City began operations as the American School of Naturopathy on March 1, 1901 (Kirchfeld & Boyle, 1994, p. 200). Founded by Benedict Lust, (see Figure 2-1), the "father of naturopathy in America," the institution continued to produce drugless healers, including chiropractors and naturopaths, until 1942. The school was chartered in New York as the American School of Naturopathy in 1905, was chartered in the District of Columbia as the American School of Chiropractic in 1919, and was re-chartered as the ASC in Maryland in 1940 (Application, 1941). Lust, who held degrees in homeopathic and eclectic medicine as well as chiropractic and was licensed as a medical physician in Florida, was an arch-mixer. Although he found some favor from super-straight B.J. Palmer (Kirchfeld & Boyle, 1994, p. 213), a 1922 inspection of the ASC by Palmer's Universal Chiropractic Association was not favorable:

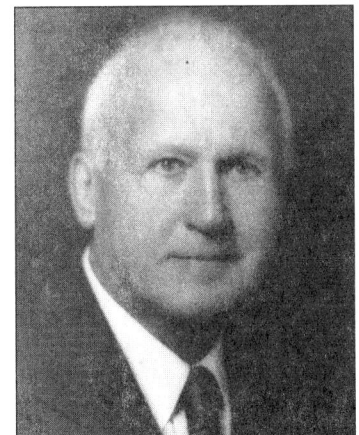

Figure 2-1: Benedict Lust, M.D., N.D., courtesy of Friedhelm Kirchfeld, M.L.S.

...My opinion, with relation to Chiropractic is that they have taken on this subject for its commercial possibilities and are not devoting any of their time to specializing on it... Nevertheless their graduates are being turned out and practicing their mode under the name of Chiropractic (Ferguson & Wiese, 1988).

Lust's school, his many books, and his journal (at various times known as either the *Naturopath*, the *Herald of Health* or both), exerted a widespread influence not only upon chiropractors and chiropractic school leaders (e.g., J.S. Riley, F.W. Collins, A.A. Gregory), but also upon the general public, who learned about chiropractors and chiropractic education as well as the schools and methods of various other drugless practitioners. Predictably, the AMA's 1928 report on chiropractic and naturopathic education were not kind to Lust's American School:

This school...is the famous (?) institution founded by Benedict Lust, N.D., D.O., D.C., M.D., and is now a night school only. It is located in an old apartment house at 236 East Thirty-Fifth Street, New York, where it makes use of two floors and a portion of the third. It has two small lecture rooms each containing about a dozen chairs, a very small demonstration room containing a McMannis osteopathic table, a small clinic room into which five chiropractic adjusting tables have been crowded, and a little chemical laboratory with one table (offering room for two or three students)...Quite a number of chiropractic adjusting tables were said to be stored - evidence of the balmier days that once were known.

There were said to be twenty students at present. Fifteen were graduated last year. The school does not publish a catalogue: it is too expensive. A four-year course is offered, covering nine months of the year, the classes being in session from 7 to 10:30 p.m....

The tuition is $250 annually. Textbooks and other supplies are offered to students at discounts; Lust has a book store at his business and publishing office...

Benedict Lust is the great national organizer of naturopathy. He is now in Florida and the inspector did not meet him personally, but his school is a very sorry looking affair. Aside from the giving of chiropractic adjustments the instruction must be almost altogether didactic. The dean, whose name is Sinai Gershanek, is dear, nervous and thick headed (Schools, 1928).

Lust's contributions to chiropractic have been overlooked, perhaps partly because of the 1940s and 1950s efforts of broad-scope D.C.s to distance themselves from naturopathy. Yet he set an example for other broad-scope chiropractic institutions before the 1935 onset of educational reform in the profession, and his institution participated in early efforts at educational standardization, such as those of the International Chiropractic Congress in the 1920s and early 1930s.

Mecca College of Chiropractic

Frederick W. Collins, M.D., D.O., D.C. earned the enmity not only of organized medicine, but also of B.J. Palmer, who labeled the New Jersey drugless physician a "mountebank" and a "chiropractic fraud" (Gibbons, 1989). Collins claimed chiropractic degrees from D.D. Palmer, from Benedict Lust's ASC in New York City (Kirchfeld & Boyle, 1994, p. 213) and from J.N. Stone's Texas Chiropractic College. He operated his school in Newark under a number of names (see Table 2-1). Collins' curriculum provided the broadest of offerings in chiropractic, osteopathy and naturopathy, and seems to have specialized in iridology, for which Collins authored *Disease Diagnosed by Observation of the Eye* in 1919 (Jensen, 1976, p. iii). However, an AMA report in 1928 noted:

The school has no electrical apparatus because it is too expensive, yet it gives (nominally) both naturopathic and physiotherapeutic courses and grants degrees of "Doctor" in both lines (Schools, 1928).

Collins' reputation was widened by his legal battles with the local medical community in New Jersey, which was led by William A. Tansey, M.D. of Newark (Collins, 1923; Newspaper, 1923), and involved repeated arrests and jailings of the school leader. He wrote a number of other books and pamphlets, including *System of Painless Adjusting* (1924),

New Jersey College of Chiropractic and Naturopathy (1910-1916)	Modern School of Electrotherapeutics
	Newark School of Arts and Applied Psychology - Registred
The Famous Mecca College of Chiropractic, the Shrine of Chiropractic (1916-1943)	American Academy of Medicine Inc.
American School of Naturopathy	White Cross School of First Aid
United States School of Naturopathy	American College of Spectro-Chrome Therapy Inc.
American School of Iridiology	American College of Electronic Reactions and Radio Activity Inc.
New Jersey School of Osteopathy	
National School of Neuropathy	Naturopathic Health School of Chicago
Union School of Physical Culture and Gymnastics	First National University of Naturopathy

Table 2-1: Chartered institutions comprising F.W. Collins' First National University of Naturopathy and Allied Sciences. From Collins (1924a&b), Jensen (1976 p.iv) and Ferguson & Wiese (1988).

Naturopathic Tonic Treatment (1924) and *Original Osteopathic Techniqu*e. Collins also served as vice-president of the American Naturopathic Association and as secretary of the National Association of Drugless Practitioners (Collins, 1924a). Despite the enmity he received from broad-scope chiropractors, he participated at least peripherally in the American Chiropractic Association in the 1920s (National, 1926). The AMA included a review of Collins' enterprises in its 1928 critique of "Schools of chiropractic and naturopathy in the United States":

> The First National University of Naturopathy is supposedly the result of a merging of the Mecca College of Chiropractic, the New Jersey College of Osteopathy, and the United States Schools of Naturopathy, a year or more ago. The fact seems to be that these three are creations of F.W. Collins, who also chartered the United States School of Physiotherapy, the American Academy of Medicine and Surgery, and about fifteen other similar paper colleges....The twenty or more institutions are all crowded into the one building, and there are now said to be twenty-six students.

> Two or three diplomas are given each graduate, from as many different "schools." The tuition is $600. In short, for this price a student may get all the diplomas the walls of one small office will offer space for, and have them with no great effort on his part, with no preliminary education insisted on, and with the school frankly cooperating in the faking of everything that can be conveniently faked in this preparation to fool the public (Schools, 1928).

Palmer-Gregory College of Chiropractic

Another early medical influence within chiropractic education was that of Alva Gregory, M.D., D.C., a graduate of the University of Texas Medical School (Gibbons, 1991) and of the Carver-Denny School of Chiropractic in Oklahoma City. Willard Carver, LL.B., D.C., Old Dad Chiro's former attorney, had earned his doctorate in 1906 from 1905 Palmer graduate Charles Ray Parker of Ottumwa, Iowa. Carver established the first of his five schools (Gibbons, 1991; Jackson, 1994) in the capital of the future state of Oklahoma (then known as the Indian Territory). When Carver learned that D.D. Palmer had relocated to nearby Medford, he invited his friend and former client to join him as a partner or faculty member. Palmer proceeded to Oklahoma City, but instead of joining Carver's institution, he went into partnership with Gregory. The Palmer-Gregory College of Chiropractic continued in operation for several years, but Palmer and the Texas physician had a falling out (ostensibly over theory and technique) after only a few months, and dissolved their partnership (Gielow, 1981a, p. 118). Palmer relocated to Portland, where he established the D.D. Palmer College of Chiropractic in November 1908 (Keating, 1993b). Gregory retained the Palmer-Gregory name for his school, which was an undoubtedly useful marketing strategy. Palmer was irritated, not only by Gregory's teaching of what the father of chiropractic considered medical content, but also by Gregory's continued use of the Palmer name to compete with the Portland school:

If Dr. D.D. Palmer's connection with the Gregory School as a teacher for nine weeks is of such importance to justify the continuance of advertising "Palmer-Gregory Chiropractic College," how much more is it worth to you as a student to be under the personal instruction of D.D. Palmer for nine months? During that nine weeks much of my Chiropractic teaching was sidetracked, owing to the teaching of medical ideas which were not Chiropractic (Palmer, 1909a, p. 62).

Old Dad Chiro proposed that subluxation correction was the sole concern of the chiropractor. Gregory, on the other hand, taught that percussion of various spinal segments, known as spondylotherapy, could have therapeutic value whether or not a subluxation was present. He also differed with Palmer over the nature of the lesion that chiropractors treated, and disparaged Palmer's educational limitations:

> ...It might be well to state that the practice of spinal adjustment was introduced into his country by a man almost wholly unacquainted with Pathology, Symptomatology, or Etiology, and one who knew practically nothing of Anatomy and but little of Physiology. Consequently so many of the teachings in connection with the philosophy and science of spinal adjustment have been freely mixed with error and superstition and this fact has greatly hindered its investigation and reception by the medical world. Some of the medical profession and others of the better educated class of people have felt that because spinal adjustments were first introduced by a man who was wholly uneducated in therapeutic lines, he could not have made any discovery of much consequence or importance as a therapeutic auxiliary; but this does not, by any means, follow (Gregory, quoted in Gibbons, 1981b).

Gregory offered various electronic and pneumatic percussive instruments ("concussors") for sale, and characterized Palmer as an uneducated practitioner who had no grasp of modern biology. Gregory also became an activist on behalf of mixer chiropractic. He served as editor of the widely read *American Drugless Healer,* a monthly periodical published by the Oklahoma City-based American Chiropractic Association (ACA) during 1911-1913. Among Gregory's most prominent graduates were Joe Shelby Riley, D.O., D.C., who founded schools in Boston, Detroit and Washington, D.C. (Gibbons, 1991), Albert W. Richardson, D.C., founder of several of the broad-scope California Chiropractic Colleges and a central player in the medical-chiropractic and straight-mixer feuds in California during the second decade of this century (Keating et al., 1994), and C. Sterling Cooley, D.C. of Enid, Oklahoma (Godzway, 1934), who served as president and board member of the broad-scope National Chiropractic Association (NCA) during the 1930s and 1940s (Keating & Rehm 1993).

Table 2-2: Advertisement from the *American Drugless Healer* 1913; 3(4): 96 for the instructional program of the combined St. Louis Chiropractic College and the Palmer-Gregory College of Chiropractic.

St. Louis Chiropractic College
Incorporated and Chartered Under the Laws of the State of Missouri

Our full two years course of graded instruction covers Anatomy, Embryology, Histology, Physiology, Pathology, Symptomatology, Diagnosis, Neurology, Nerve Palpation and Nerve Tracing. We teach the latest methods of spinal adjustment and concussion. Our course leads to the degree of DOCTOR OF CHIROPRACTIC AND RATIONAL THERAPY.

Our course is so thorough that our graduates can pass the most critical examinations that may be given by any State Board for drugless physicians.

OUR FACULTY is composed of such leaders in the science of Chiropractic spondylotherapy as the world famous authors, Dr. Alva Emery Gregory our vice-president, and Dr. Irvin J. Eales and other regularly graduated physicians and experienced Chiropractors.

STUDENTS may begin course at any time. Patients may arrange to be treated at the College.

NIGHT CLASSES are held so that students may earn while they learn.

PARTIAL CORRESPONDENCE COURSES may be had in special cases where gentlemen or ladies cannot attend full term.

SPECIAL POST GRADUATE COURSES FOR PHYSICIANS who desire to build up a large and paying office practice and MAKE MORE MONEY than ever before and make it easier than by old worn-out methods, for if you "Know How" you will succeed by the aid of Rational Therapy Methods.

Act Today and Write to

L. WILLIAM RAY, A.M., M.D., D.C., Pres. • ALVA EMERY GREGORY, M.D., D.C., Vice-President
New Grand Central Theatre Building, Cor. Grand and Lucas Avenues, St. Louis, Missouri

---

Gregory effected a temporary merger of his Palmer-Gregory College with the St. Louis Chiropractic College in 1913 (see Table 2-2). The St. Louis College, founded by L. William Ray, A.M., M.D., D.C., offered an 18-month program in "progressive chiropractic" and "Rational Therapy Methods" (including "anatomy, chemistry (urinalysis, blood tests, stomach fluid tests) and bacteriology," and proposed to qualify its graduates for licensure as drugless practitioners (D.P.s) in several states, such as California, Illinois, Michigan and Washington (Consolidation, 1913). The school advertisement also noted that the combined St. Louis/Palmer-Gregory course of instruction

> ...will enable their graduates to qualify by examination and to receive regular medical license in
> several different states, where the state law does not require graduation from an AMA medical col-
> lege before admittance to examination.

Gregory's continuing influence derived from several sources, including his role as administrator at several schools, his extensive lecture tours throughout the United States, and from his numerous publications. His books included *Spinal Adjustment* (1910), *Spinal Treatment* (1912), *Rational Therapy* (1913) and *Spondylotherapy Simplified* (1914). His eclectic orientation to chiropractic and drugless healing struck a responsive chord among many who found favor with Gregory's motto: "...the true principle of progress in the healing art, namely, try all things with an open mind, and hold fast to that which is found to be good" (Gregory, 1912).

Columbia Institute of Chiropractic

Born in 1891 in Easton, Pennsylvania, Frank E. Dean earned his medical degree (Bachelor of Medicine) from the University of Warsaw, and later studied in "Heidelberg, The Sorbonne, and the Imperial Institute of Russia," where he specialized in neurology (Rehm, 1980, p. 298). The enigmatic future founder of the Columbia Institute of Chiropractic (CIC) took his chiropractic degree from the Standard School of Chiropractic in New York City circa 1917. He incorporated the CIC in Delaware on November 19, 1919, but the main branch of the school was always in New York. The CIC (renamed the New York Chiropractic College in 1977) was one of the earliest, if not the first, non-profit chiropractic educational institution, and Dean served as its president until his death in 1958 (Wardwell, 1992, pp. 94-5). Apparently something of a maverick, Dean affiliated his college with the egalitarian International Chiropractic Congress in the 1930s, but resisted the broad-scope educational reform efforts of the National Chiropractic Association. In the 1940s Dean served on the B.J. Palmer's board of control for the International Chiropractors' Association. A Maryland branch of the school, the Columbia College of Chiropractic in Baltimore, operated from 1946 though 1954 (Rehm, 1980, p. 298). Dean was assisted in operating the CIC and the Baltimore satellite by his wife and former student and patient, Lorraine Welch, D.C., who earned a Ph.D. in education from New York University in 1955 (Wardwell, 1992, pp. 94-5). Under the guidance of its second president, 1942 Palmer graduate Ernest G. Napolitano, D.C., LL.B., the CIC absorbed the Atlantic States Chiropractic Institute in 1964 (Columbia, 1964, 1969), when chiropractors were first licensed in the state.

Texas Chiropractic College

The Texas Chiropractic College (TCC) claims yet another MD-DC school founder in the early years of chiropractic education. Dr. J.N. Stone is described as a medical doctor (Rhodes, 1978, p. 112) and graduate of either the PSC in Davenport or the Carver Chiropractic College in Oklahoma City (Rhodes, 1978, p. 112; Smithers, 1996). However, a report in the *American Drugless Healer* mentioned that Stone had "excited the jealousy of some of the allopath physicians, hence has had to defend himself in the courts of the state" (Special, 1911). This suggests, at least, that Stone was not licensed as a medical physician in Texas. The TCC was opened in San Antonio in September 1908.

Offering a 12-month program from its outset (Rhodes, 1978, p. 112), the TCC's first graduate was A.R. Littrell, M.D. (Hariman, 1970; Rhodes, 1978). Stone and Littrell practiced together in San Antonio during 1911-12 (Directory, 1911b-d,

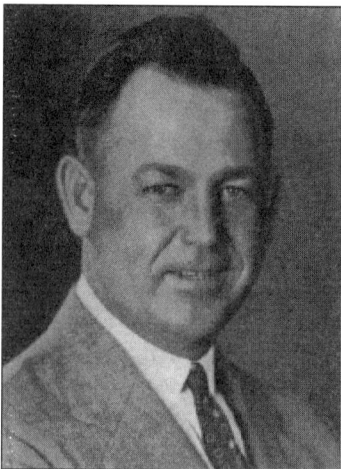

Figure 2-2: James R. Drain, D.C.

1912a&b). On April 16, 1913, the TCC was chartered as "THE CHIROPRACTIC COLLEGE of San Antonio" by Littrell as president, Stone as secretary, and F.S. Hayes, treasurer (Articles, 1913). The probably broad-scope influence of TCC's early administration is also suggested by another early alumnus, Frederick W. Collins, D.O., D.C., founder and president of the Mecca College of Chiropractic in New Jersey, who, as noted earlier, may have been a November 1912 graduate of the TCC (Gibbons, 1989).

The college was purchased in 1918 by J.M. McLeese, D.C. and associates, several of whom held both chiropractic and medical degrees. McLeese was a graduate of the National School of Chiropractic in Chicago, and a friend of its administrator, Arthur L. Forster, M.D., D.C. The TCC's new owner and dean advocated a 12-month curriculum and a broad-scope of instruction, even to include surgery (McLeese, 1919). McLeese's short term (about 18 months) as leader of the institution was described as "mercenary" in orientation (Drain, 1920). During this period also the college operated a "branch" facility in Louisville, Kentucky (Dunn, 1920; Palmer, 1920b). The TCC was sold to B.F. Gurden, D.C., Flora Gurden, D.C. and James Riddle Drain, D.C. on March 13, 1920 (Smithers, 1996). The purchase precipitated an expansion of facilities and faculty; anatomy was taught by dissection as an elective course during 1921-24 by a medical physician, P.D. Brown (Smithers, 1996).

The Gurdens departed Texas for California in 1924, and their shares in the corporation were purchased by Charles B. Loftin, D.C., H.E. Weiser, D.C., and Clarence Weiant, D.C. Weiant, who served in later years as the dean of the Eastern Chiropractic Institute and as research director of the National Chiropractic Association (NCA) and the Chiropractic Research Foundation (now renamed the Foundation for Chiropractic Education and Research), departed for New York State in 1925.

Drain, a straight chiropractor and 1912 Palmer graduate (Rehm, 1980, pp. 286-7), led the school for nearly three decades (see Table 2-3), and became well known throughout the profession. Among his published works were *Chiropractic Thoughts* (1927) and *Man Tomorrow* (1949). After succeeding Gurden as president of TCC in 1924 (Smithers, 1996), Drain (see Figure 2-2) was active in the struggle among straight and mixer schools over length of training, scopes of practice and instruction, and non-profit status (Keating et al., 1991, 1992; Keating & Rehm, 1993). He sided with straight college leaders B.J. Palmer, Carl Cleveland and T.F. Ratledge, but in the late 1940s became an enthusiastic promoter of Concept-Therapy, a broad-scope form of chiropractic health care devised by 1935 TCC graduate Thurman Fleet. H.E. (Buddy) Weiser, D.C. and Charles B. Loftin, D.C. joined the faculty in 1921 and 1924, respectively, and became prominent within the profession. The trio (Drain, Weiser and Loftin) became co-owners of the institution, and struggled throughout the Depression years to keep the school afloat. Following the college's 1948 purchase by its alumni association and its re-chartering as a non-profit institution, TCC wandered in and out of the orbit of the broad-scope national professional association, NCA.

Term	President	Term	President
1908-1918	J.N. Stone, M.D., D.C.	1966-1976	William D. Harper, D.C.
1918-1920	J.M. McCleese, D.C.	1977-1985	John B. Barfoot, D.C.
1920-1924	B.F. Gurden, D.C.	1985-1986	Hugh McDonald, D.C.
1924-1954	James R. Drain, D.C.	1986-1990	Lewis W. Ogle, Ed.D.
1955-1959	E.B. Hearn, D.C.	1990-	Shelby M. Elliott, D.C.
1962-1966	Julius C. Troilo, D.C.		

Table 2-3: Presidents of the Texas Chiropractic College. (Hocking, 1996; Smithers, 1996).

Nebraska Chiropractic College

Another important but dimly recalled medical influence in chiropractic education was that of the Crabtrees. H.C. Crabtree, M.D., D.C. founded his first school in Coffeyville, Kansas, which was relocated to Lincoln, Nebraska and renamed the Nebraska Chiropractic College (NeCC) in 1911 (Mawhiney, 1984, p. 247; Metz, 1965, p. 12). The school was conducted by Crabtree, his wife Rosalie Crabtree, D.C. and her brother John Calamore, D.C., all of whom were graduates of Willard Carver's school in Oklahoma City (Hariman, 1970, p. 13). Although Metz (1965) and Rehm (1995) describe the Crabtree's Kansas operation as somewhat scandalous, the NeCC was a pioneer in pushing for higher standards for chiropractic education. The NeCC offered a 27-month program (three years of nine months each), and may have had an articulation with the nearby University of Nebraska to provide basic science coursework to its students (Beaumont, unpublished).

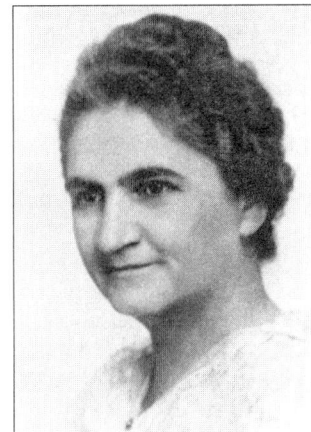

Figure 2-3: Sylva L. Ashworth, D.C., 1918

The Crabtrees were influential in obtaining Nebraska's first licensing law for chiropractors circa 1919. The law required the 27 months of training then available perhaps only at the NeCC, which meant that the PSC's 18-month graduates were ineligible to take the licensing examination. H.C. Crabtree served on the first board of examiners, and earned public condemnation within and outside the profession for his strict and self-serving enforcement of the licensing statutes (Keating & Cleveland, 1992). A tremendous feud among chiropractors peaked in June 1921, when Palmer graduates Sylva Ashworth (see Figure 2-3), Lee W. Edwards, M.D., D.C., B.J. Palmer and other of his disciples walked out of the annual convention of the Nebraska Chiropractic Association in Omaha (Keating & Cleveland, 1992; Not, 1921) and formed an opposition society. The pages of B.J.'s *Fountain Head News* filled with animosity toward the Crabtree clan and their ally, O.G. Clark, D.C. of Columbus, Nebraska, who actively sought prosecutions of unlicensed Palmer graduates who practiced in the state. Hostilities continued until 1922, when the Crabtrees apparently sold their interest in the school to a "Dr. Dorothy Stonesifer and associates" (Hariman, 1970, p. 13). In 1923, when Nebraska lowered its educational requirements for licensure to 18 months, largely in response to the successful political campaign of the Palmer graduates, led by Sylva L. Ashworth. To our knowledge, Nebraska was the only state ever to lessen educational standards for D.C.s. The reaction from Crabtree and the Nebraska Chiropractic Association was by now predictable:

> WHEREAS, the Department of Public Welfare of the State of Nebraska has seen fit to reduce the educational qualifications from twenty-seven months to eighteen months and in some instances twelve months college training, and

> WHEREAS, said Department has offered to license chiropractors who have violated the law for twelve months in Nebraska by practicing without a license, thereby favoring law-breakers, and consenting that they may be licensed after having taken twelve months' course, and

> WHEREAS, we believe that the educational standard of twenty-seven months which has been maintained for about ten years is necessary for the protection of the public and should be kept without change, and

> WHEREAS, the reputable chiropractors of the State of Nebraska and this Association have firmly and steadfastly refused to countenance or approve such a backward step and such favoritism.

> NOW, THEREFORE, BE IT RESOLVED by the Nebraska Chiropractic Association that it continue to keep up the fight to prevent thus lowering the qualifications for admission to practice and that we continue the fight to prevent the licensing of incompetent, inexperienced, convicted person until the State Department shall see the error of its ways.

> BE IT FURTHER RESOLVED that we lend every assistance possible in the case now pending in the Supreme Court to the end that the Chiropractic profession may be kept upon a high plane (Resolution, 1924b).

The Palmer group's victory was short-lived. In 1927 Nebraska enacted basic science legislation which effectively barred any further licensing of chiropractors during 1929 through 1950 (Metz, 1965, p. 100). Perhaps in response to this legal barrier, the NeCC closed its doors in 1929. Its most famous graduate, Major B. DeJarnette, D.O., D.C. (Class of 1924), became renowned as the developer of Sacro-Occipital Technique and as editor and publisher of the *Journal of Bloodless Surgery*.

Missouri Chiropractic College

Although he did not earn his medical degree until after his co-founding of the Missouri Chiropractic College (MCC), Henry C. Harring must be counted among those early physician-chiropractors who exerted a significant, if forgotten, influence upon chiropractic education. After earning his chiropractic credential in 1918, and dissatisfied with the training he had received at L. William Ray's St. Louis College of Chiropractic (Harring, 1924), Harring pursued the M.D. at the St. Louis College of Physicians and Surgeons (Rehm, 1980, p. 300; Reinert, 1992). Meanwhile, with chiropractors Robert Colyer and Oscar W. Schulte, the MCC was chartered as a for-profit institution in 1920, with Harring as its secretary-treasurer. Colyer was the school's first president, and was later succeeded by Harring.

The school opened in St. Louis with a five-room campus and 12 students (Progress, 1922), each of whom paid $375 in tuition. Although Reinert (1992) suggested that the school commenced with a 27-month curriculum, as late as 1924 Harring was opposed to requiring that length of training in any law passed by the state of Missouri (Harring, 1924). As noted in discussing the curriculum of the Nebraska College of Chiropractic, the 27-month curriculum was unusually long in that era, and half again longer than what B.J. Palmer insisted was the only acceptable length of training for chiropractors. However, when the state of Missouri finally passed a chiropractic law in 1927, MCC graduates were among the few who became license-eligible without "grandfathering."

Harring was a "straight" chiropractor in the sense that he emphasized adjusting as the primary focus of the chiropractor's work, and initially, at least, he supported the straight chiropractic policies of B.J. Palmer. Early chiropractic historian Chittenden Turner noted that the MCC president did not approve of "modalities" in the chiropractor's practice, but felt that "if used only where indicated and with the clear understanding that such methods are not chiropractic they will do no harm" (Turner, 1931, p. 269). Harring was also at first opposed to the requirement of four years of high school education as a condition for entering chiropractic college (Harring, 1924). On the other hand, the MCC president was among the earliest of college leaders to encourage a research orientation, to bemoan the lack of selectivity in the recruitment of students to chiropractic colleges (Harring, 1925a), to encourage greater standards for basic science training (Harring, 1950) and to call for the abolition of proprietary schools:

> ...The fundamentals of chiropractic are based on scientific truths and there is no healing science today that can surpass it. But, we have not developed these fundamentals sufficiently to be accurate in our application or positive in our assertions. For advancement we must rely on the few who possess the genius and initiative to prove our contentions. The facilities for this, however, are inadequate and the support of the profession is not manifested. Many schools exist, yet if you would ask each of them to submit their curriculum and the reasons why certain subjects are taught, there would be a great difference of opinion and no chance to arrive at a logical conclusion.
>
> Dogmatism is a detriment to the scientific development of anything, and as long as this can creep into the control of the individually owned schools we will not see any great advancement...Support will not be forthcoming so long as we have individual and privately owned schools...There are two things we need; the first is a more scientific study of chiropractic principles, and second, we need a united support of Chiropractic by chiropractors. These can be accomplished by a merging of all standard schools under the control of a selective body representing the entire profession (Harring, 1925b).

In the late 1930s the MCC became an accredited school within the orbit of the broad-scope National Chiropractic Association. Harring continued as president of the MCC until the early 1960s, when he was succeeded by MCC alumnus, Otto C. Reinert. However, by this time the MCC's status with the NCA Council on Education was lost. Reinert led the MCC into merger with the former Logan Basic College of Chiropractic in September 1965 (Reinert, 1992).

Chapter 3

The Second Wave: School Proliferation During 1908-1920

D.D. Palmer College of Chiropractic

D.D. Palmer's unsuccessful attempts to establish new schools in Oklahoma (i.e., the Palmer-Gregory College and the equally short-lived Fountain Head School) appear only to have whetted his appetite. Late in 1908, perhaps at the request and with the financial support of practitioners in the Northwest (Keating, 1993b), he relocated to Portland to try again. The D.D. Palmer College of Chiropractic held its first classes on November 9, 1908, in downtown Portland. The proposed curriculum included instruction in dissection, obstetrics and minor surgery. Although Willard Carver later claimed that his Oklahoma school had been first (in 1906) to offer coursework in obstetrics and gynecology (Carver, 1931), Palmer's 1908 curriculum was undoubtedly among the first to offer such subjects, and probably helped to influence the broad-scope chiropractic tradition in Oregon. Old Chiro (see Figure 3-1) proposed to prepare his students as primary care providers:

> ...A Chiropractor should be able to care for any condition which may arise in the families under his care, the same as a physician; this we intend to make possible in a two year's course (Palmer, 1910a, p. 789).

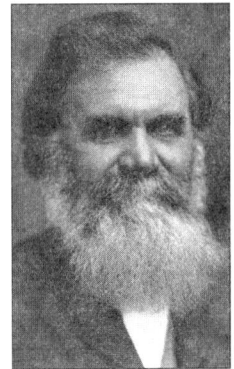

Figure 3-1: D.D. Palmer, c1910

Palmer's curriculum was noteworthy also in that it proposed two years of nine months each (see Table 3-1), although Palmer probably awarded certificates to his first Portland class after only one year (LaValley, 1955; Palmer, 1909d, p. 3). His first partner in the school, PSC graduate Leroy M. Gordon, was replaced by John E. LaValley, D.C. Palmer and LaValley had a falling out sometime in 1910 or 1911, which resulted in the founder's abandonment of yet another school, and his departure for Los Angeles. LaValley renamed the institution the Oregon Peerless College of Chiropractic and

---

Table 3-1: Description of the curriculum at the D.D. Palmer College of Chiropractic in Portland, Oregon, as noted in the College's journal, *The Chiropractor Adjuster* 1909 (Jan); 1(2): 58

...Students at this school receive instructions under the direct supervision of Dr. D.D. Palmer, the man who found the cause of disease and developed a unique method of adjustment for correcting the same.

The course at this school covers a period of two years; nine months to the year.

The first year is devoted to Chiropractic and all that pertains to it, including a short course in dissection on the cadaver.

The second year, minor surgery, obstetrics, forensic jurisprudence and a full course of dissection.

Tuition, per year $250.00

Adjustments at the D.D. Palmer College of Chiropractic in ordinary cases $10.00 each week for the first six weeks, payable in advance, or the first six weeks paid in advance $50.00, following weeks $5.00.

Special cases, as Cancers, Tumors and Epilepsy, $20.00 first week, $10.00 each week thereafter in advance.

Address all communications to L.M. Gordon, D.C., Secretary, 205 Oregonian Building, Portland

---

Neuropathy (perhaps part of the A.P. Davis influence), and claimed to have offered the first course in dissection at any chiropractic school in the state. However, Oregon Peerless was merged in 1913 with the Pacific Chiropractic College (see Figure 1-6) (Ritter, 1991).

Palmer's second brief stay in the Northwest (1908-1911) is noteworthy also for the journal that his college published. The *Chiropractor Adjuster* magazine has been forgotten by many, but formed the basis for Old Dad Chiro's classic volume, *The Chiropractor's Adjustor: The Science, Art and Philosophy of Chiropractic* (Palmer, 1910a). As their names imply, the journal and the book were intended to "adjust" what Palmer considered to be the mistaken ideas of many of his followers and professional descendants, most especially those of son B.J., against whom the founder issued many stinging criticisms. Although also intended as a textbook for students in his Portland school (see Table 3-2), its rambling style could hardly be expected to introduce the novice to chiropractic. Palmer's book was essentially a compilation of many of the articles that had appeared in the Portland periodical.

D.D. Palmer joined the faculty of the Ratledge System of Chiropractic Schools in Los Angeles in 1911-1912. T.F. Ratledge, president and owner of the Ratledge school and a 1907 Carver College graduate, recalled in later years that Old Dad Chiro "...grieved over the termination with the PSC, at Davenport, and I believed that he was planning (or perhaps dreaming would better express it) to open another school of his own" (Smallie, 1963).

Palmer lectured at several other schools before his death in 1913, most notably the Davenport Chiropractic College and the Universal Chiropractic College, both of which competed with the PSIC for students in the birthplace of chiropractic.

Table 3-2: Promotion for D.D. Palmer's 1910 book which appeared in the D.D. Palmer College of Chiropractic journal, *The Chiropractor Adjuster* 1909 (Dec); 1(7): 56

CHIROPRACTIC TEXTBOOK

For the first time in the history of Chiropractic, the Founder of the science has consented to issue a textbook. Heretofore, he felt that the science had not been sufficiently developed to warrant such an undertaking.

This book will be designed as a textbook for the school room. The author is now using advanced sheets for his classes with much satisfaction. It will also be adapted for the practitioner of Chiropractic.

It will teach Physiology, Pathology, Nerve Tracing, the Principles of the Science and the Art of Adjusting Vertebrae.

The author defines each disease, gives its etiology, symptoms, degeneration and the locality of vertebral impingement.

To more fully elucidate the principles of the science, they are contrasted with those of the old school.

This textbook of Chiropractic, a medical dictionary and an anatomy comprises the books used in the Portland school.

It will contain information needed by the student and practitioner. The usual gush will be omitted.

In undertaking the preparation of this work, the author realizes to the fullest extent the great importance attached to its production, inasmuch as it will be referred to and quoted as authority on Chiropractic, being written by the Founder.

Ratledge System of Chiropractic Schools

As noted above, Palmer's employer during 1911-1912 was Tullius de Florence Ratledge, D.C. Born in Hartsville, Tennessee in 1881 (Rehm, 1980), the tall, gangly young man was the son of itinerant school teacher parents who settled in the Indian Territory in the early years of the century. He apparently followed his mother, who had graduated from the first class at the Carver-Denny School in Oklahoma City, into chiropractic in 1907. While enrolled at the Carver school he also took lectures from D.D. Palmer, possibly at the Palmer-Gregory College, and considered Palmer and Carver his mentors (Keating et al., 1991, 1992).

Immediately upon graduation in 1907 he collaborated with Willard Carver in the latter's efforts to obtain a licensing law for D.C.s through the legislature of the newly established State of Oklahoma (Jackson, 1994). Ratledge and Carver created a free clinic or "adjustory" for members of the state legislature and their families in the state's first capital city, Guthrie. Here in 1908 he created the first of four or five branches of his Ratledge System of Chiropractic Schools. In true missionary fashion he started schools in Arkansas City, Kansas and in the Kansas capital of Topeka, and then moved on. His Arkansas City branch graduated several members of the Foy family (Keating et al., 1992); Anna Foy, D.C. was instrumental in 1913 in having the first chiropractic law passed in Kansas, and served for many years as president of the state's board of chiropractic examiners. Foy and her chiropractor husband purchased Ratledge's Topeka college (Keating et al., 1992), which continued for a number of years as the Kansas School of Chiropractic.

Figure 3-2: T.F. Ratledge, D.C., c1930

In 1911, Ratledge visited southern California for the first time, and was inspired to commence his career as the "missionary of straight chiropractic in California" (Keating et al., 1991):

> ...Upon looking over the situation here in California, where at that time chiropractic was only available through the "bootleg" channel and had received some very bad and recent publicity, all of which was medically inspired propaganda, I decided that where chiropractic was not, there I should be, so, I decided to open a school in California and establish chiropractic in California. That was in 1911, March. In September that year I opened the Los Angeles branch of the Ratledge System of Chiropractic Schools which I conducted continuously until Dr. Cleveland of Kansas City, Mo. bought me out in 1951 (Ratledge, 1955).

He soon earned the ire of organized medicine in the unlicensed Golden State:

> ...Believing in American principles and knowing that Chiropractic was NOT the practice of medicine and not based upon medical principles and/or superstitions, I knew that I was not violating any medical statutes when I was applying the principles of Chiropractic, so I, never having been accustomed to being considered an outlaw or engaged in illegal business, I set out to establish chiropractic as a separate and legal science and practice in California. Opening my office and advertising the fact through newspapers and the distribution of hundreds of thousands of pamphlets telling the people about the great truths of this new science, soliciting patients, etc., I was soon visited by representatives of official medicine in California and told to remove my signs and cease the "practice of medicine" or face arrest. I defied them and served several communities, personally, after the similar threats had driven other chiropractors to discontinue their practices. Such brazenry did not raise me in the eyes of the medical authorities, but it did make them hesitate, and for two years they held off any attempt to stop me by legal procedures.... (Ratledge, 1955).

Ratledge and his school were players in the struggle for licensure in California which culminated in the initiative act of 1922. He feuded with broad-scope chiropractors, with the Board of Chiropractic Examiners he had helped to create and with the Board of Medical Examiners throughout his 40 year ownership of the Los Angeles school. At one point prior to the passage of the chiropractic law he chose 90 days in Los Angeles county jail rather than accept a license as a "drugless practitioner" from the Board of Medical Examiners, on the grounds that the medical board was not qualified to judge his competence as a D.C., and that to accept such a license would be fraud against the people of the state. Ratledge (see Figure 3-2) railed against naturopathy and broad-scope chiropractic no less vehemently than against organized medicine, and was more than once threatened with bodily harm when he expressed his opinions at various chiropractic meetings.

The Ratledge Chiropractic College of Los Angeles was always a meager operation. The basic sciences were taught exclusively through lecture and readings, since the school had no laboratory facilities. Unlike his mentors, Carver and Palmer, Ratledge did not permit M.D.s to serve as faculty members nor to enroll as students, because, he believed, they were incapable of understanding chiropractic. Like many school founders and presidents of his period, Ratledge taught his students his own technique system, but it is recalled that he was not dogmatic about this. His clinical goal was the relief of "obstructive nerve pressure" (Keating et al., 1991), and any procedures which accomplished this purpose were acceptable to him.

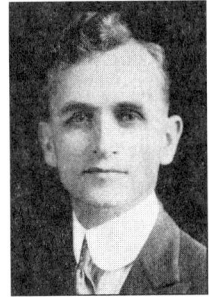

Carver Chiropractic College

Ratledge's first chiropractic instructor was Willard Carver, who had known D.D. Palmer as a boy, prior to Palmer's magnetic healing days in Davenport (Jackson, 1994). Carver earned his law degree from the Iowa College of Law in Des Moines in May 1891, and maintained his friendship with D.D. Palmer. In later years Carver claimed to be the oldest student of chiropractic, this on the grounds that he had been a confidante of the founder during D.D.'s transition from magnetic to chiropractic. However, his formal training in the new healing system came a decade later. He graduated from Charles Ray Parker's school in June 1906 (Jackson, 1994; Zarbuck, 1988d), and immediately opened his own school in Oklahoma City.

The Oklahoma school (see Table 3-3) was surely among the first (in 1906) to include minor surgery in its curriculum, although this subject had been included in the instructional program of the Pacific School of Chiro-Practic in 1905 (see Table 1-3). Carver's original falling out with the Palmers revolved around his recommendation of suggestive therapeutics (Carver, 1909; Zarbuck, 1988d), which Old Dad Chiro considered an unjustified therapeutic intrusion upon his chiropractic. Carver introduced other theoretical and technical innovations to the profession, including his "structural approach" to spinal analysis (Cooperstein, 1990; Montgomery & Nelson, 1985; Rosenthal, 1981), which proposed that many "disrelations" of spinal joints were compensatory, that is, were adaptations produced by other subluxations. This "systems theory" of subluxation stood in contrast to the "segmentalist" position adopted by the Palmers, which proposed that spinal joints subluxate independently of one another. Despite these variations, Carver imparted a firm belief in "obstructive nerve pressure" to his students.

Styling himself the "Constructor of Chiropractic," in contrast to B.J. Palmer's self-designation as the "Developer," Carver engaged in many nasty battles with D.D.'s son. He established the *Scientific Head News* to challenge B.J.'s *Fountain*

Table 3-3: Excerpt from the *Twentieth Annual Catalog* of the Carver Chiropractic College of Oklahoma City, 1928-1929

THE DOCTOR'S COURSE
Entrance Requirements
Persons of good moral character; whose physical condition will reasonably permit their mastering the science and art of Chiropractic; and who have a high school education, or have had experience which may be considered equivalent to a high school education, or can bring their education up to that standard by the time they finish the Doctor's Course, are eligible to matriculate for this course.
Time
The Doctor's Course consists of four semesters of five months each. During these twenty calendar months we spend more than 3,500 class hours in actual school work. We require an attendance of not less than 80 per cent of time in each of the various departments. This easily satisfies the legal requirement of 2,100 sixty-minute hours.
Grades
Carver College requires a grade of not less than 80 per cent on each subject taught in the entire course, and a grade of not less than 75 per cent on the general final examination which is given at the end of the course.
Books
Books for the entire Doctor's Course are the following:

Cunningham's anatomy	$11.00
Stedman's Medical Dictionary	7.50
Carver's Scientific Catechism	6.50
Carver's Psycho-Bio-Physiology	10.00
Carver's Chiropractic Analysis, Volume 1	7.00
Carver's Chiropractic Analysis, Volume 2	8.00
Total cost of Books for entire course	$50.00

These prices are publishers' prices. Carver College handles the books only for the benefit of the student.
Tuition

Tuition for Freshman semester	$150.00
Tuition for Sophomore semester	150.00
Tuition for Junior semester	150.00
Tuition for Senior semester	150.00
Tuition for entire course	$600.00

To those who pay the tuition for the entire course at the time of matriculation, we give the $50.00 set of books free. Otherwise tuition is payable at the beginning of each semester.

Head News. Each accused the other of lies and distortions in the pages of their college magazines (Jackson, 1994; Palmer, 1919b), and generated considerable disgust over college leaders among the rank and file of the profession. Despite this decades-long feud with the younger Palmer, by the later 1930s and early 1940s the pair had found a common foe in the educational reform efforts of the broad-scope National Chiropractic Association, and Carver even served on the Board of Control of B.J. Palmer's International Chiropractors' Association (ICA).

Following World War I students became plentiful owing to the vocational training benefits granted to veterans; the number of chiropractic colleges mushroomed (Keating, 1994a). Carver established schools in Wichita, Kansas (1917), New York City (1919), Montgomery, Alabama (1920), Washington, D.C. (1922) and Denver (1923) (Carver-Colorado, 1994; Jackson, 1994; Rehm, 1980, p. 278). His New York Institute merged with several others, eventually to become one of the ancestors of the Chiropractic Institute of New York (see Figure 1-7), which closed its doors in 1968. Carver's school in the nation's capital was apparently sold, and operated as the Chiropractic Research University in the 1920s under the direction of A.B. Chatfield, another attorney-chiropractor. Carver's Colorado Chiropractic University, which became the non-profit University of Natural Healing Arts (UNHA) in 1934 under the direction of Homer G. Beatty, D.C., N.D. (University, 1939), closed its doors in the 1950s after Beatty's passing, and transferred its records to the National College in 1965 (Rehm, 1980, p. 312). The UNHA offered degree programs in chiropractic, naturopathy and physiotherapy, and operated as a non-profit institution, one of the early chiropractic schools to do so. The Carver Chiropractic College of Oklahoma City continued under its founder's personal supervision until his death in 1943. The institution continued under the supervision of Paul O. Parr, D.C. until the mid-1960s, when the school closed its doors and its registry and alumni were affiliated with the Logan College of Chiropractic.

Universal Chiropractic College

At the PSIC in 1910, a rebellion against B.J. Palmer took place for reasons that are not entirely clear. Joy M. Loban, D.C. (see Figure 3-3), who had traded adulatory comments with B.J. in the 1908 period, when Palmer appointed him chairman of philosophy, led a dissident group of Palmer students to form the Universal Chiropractic College (UCC). Following a dramatic exit from one of B.J.'s lectures, the students strode down Brady Street to organize the new school (Dye, 1939; Gibbons, 1991). The possibility that B.J.'s 1910 introduction of x-ray technology at the PSC was a cause of this revolt has been debated, some suggesting that Loban may have objected to the new assessment method because it exceeded the notion of "done by hand," and was therefore a form of "mixing," others mentioning other "philosophical divisions" (Rehm, 1980, p. 280). Others note that the dispute may have been more personally directed at B.J.'s authoritarian manner; in a somewhat oblique release the new school indicated that:

> ...Previous to the organization of the Universal Chiropractic College, the need was strongly felt by the profession for an institution where certain results could be obtained and certain conditions prevail, which are not, at that time, existing. So, on April 23, 1910, a committee of graduated and student chiropractors met and perfected plans for a liberal and democratic institution, founded upon the broad altruistic principle of the greater good to the greater number, and not upon the ideas of any one man...It is the aim of the institution to teach all that is good and ennobling in the universe of Chiropractic and thereby fit its students to be of the greatest possible service to suffering humanity; it is constructive rather than destructive; its purpose always to elevate and never denigrate (Canterbury & Krakos, 1986).

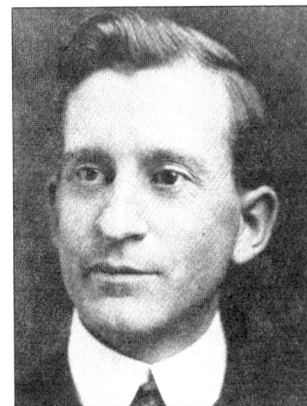

Figure 3-3: Joy M. Loban, D.C., from the *14th Annual Catalog* of the Universal Chiropractic College (WSCC Library Archives)

Within a few years the UCC established a reputation for excellence in chiropractic roentgenology. This development seems to undermine the contention that rejection of the new modality, which became an elective course at the PSC in 1911 and a required

Figure 3-4: Letter published in the NCA's *The Chiropractic Journal*, January 1936, p.41.

UNIVERSAL CHIROPRACTIC COLLEGE
ALUMNI ASSOCIATION

Our Dear Alma Mater:

We congratulate you on your contributions to Chiropractic progress.

1910-You began your educational work, incorporating in your course of training such necessary subjects as Symptomatology, Pathology, and Diagnosis;

1911-You increased your course of training from nine to twelve months;

1915-You inaugurated a course of training of eighteen months duration;

1921-You developed the vertical position for spinal examination;

1923-At your request and with your cooperation the Englen Company built the first vertical X-ray unit. In the college bulletin of November, 1923, you gave to the profession the principle of the ERECT SPINOGRAPH;

1927-You gave to us, the Alumni, the control of the college, making Universal the first professionally-owned Chiropractic College;

1931-You announced the development of the subject of Spinal Hygiene, the result of ten years of intensive research work. In the college bulletin of August, 1931, you urged the profession to establish an institute of Spinal Hygiene;

1934-You increased your teaching staff;

1935-Your Silver Anniversary. Your teaching staff was again increased and your college quarters enlarged;

1936-The twenty-fifth anniversary of the graduation of your first class. We respectfully ask the Faculty to cooperate in observing this occasion fittingly in June by presenting an intensive post graduate course to which chiropractors from the entire world can be invited.

The death in 1913, of Dr. Daniel David Palmer, took from your Faculty a man who could not be replaced. We are happy and proud that his guiding influence has been lasting and that, through the years, you have kept faith with Dr. Palmer, abiding always by the principles and ideals given to you by him, without deviating to the teaching of other therapeutic measures.

We express our undying gratitude to the many brilliant teachers who have aided you. We pledge our continued cooperation toward further true Chiropractic progress. We invite UNITY OF EFFORT from all Chiropractic colleges and associations and from all chiropractors.

Devotedly yours,
Universal Chiropractic College Alumni Association

Dr. H.E. Olsen, Secretary
211 Wilkinson Ave., Jersey City, New Jersey

component of the D.C. program in 1924, was a critical factor in the PSC/UCC schism (Canterbury & Krakos, 1986). What is incompletely remembered, however, is that the respective leaders of the PSC and the UCC traded charges of homicide, charges which would reverberate through an entire generation (Gibbons, 1994; Keating, 1994b; Peters & Chance, 1993). The vicious dispute between B.J. Palmer and Joy M. Loban occupied the bulk of the UCA's 1910 convention (Universal, 1910). It saturated the pages of the two schools' respective magazines, and amplified a growing distrust of educators among the members of the profession.

The UCC nonetheless earned respect for scholarship and research within the profession, and gained the respect of its graduates (see Figure 3-4). Exemplary were Loban's *Technique and Practice of Chiropractic* (1912), *Diet and Exercise* (1928) and *Textbook of Neurology* (1929), the latter co-authored with Charles R. Bunn, D.C. By 1916 Loban had relocated to Pittsburgh, where he headed the Pittsburgh College of Chiropractic; a new leadership (see Table 3-4) was in place at the Davenport institution. However, financial considerations forced the UCC to relocate in 1918 from Davenport to Pennsylvania, where it merged with the Pittsburgh College of Chiropractic, and Loban headed the amalgamated school. In the same year, college faculty member Leo J. Steinbach, D.C. produced "the first postural or upright films of the spinal column in order to demonstrate the effects of unequal leg lengths, pelvic distortion and body stress under the influence of gravity," the results of which were published in the college's journal in August 1924 (Rehm, 1980, pp. 281, 296-7), just as B.J. was formally introducing his neurocalometer at the PSC. A 1916 graduate of the UCC, Steinbach became dean of his alma mater in 1921, and led the UCC into merger with the Lincoln Chiropractic College in 1944 (see Figure 1-7).

Table 3-4: Administration and faculty of the Universal Chiropractic College in 1916 (Carter, 1916)

W.F. Ruehlman, President
C.A. Barnes, Vice-President
W.E. Carter, Secretary-Treasurer
G.M. Otto, Assistant Secretary-
  Treasurer
H.A. Hackett
W.E. Runnells
J.H. Denlinger

Ross Chiropractic College

Yet another school which exerted a significant influence on the profession's early development was the Ross Chiropractic College of Fort Wayne, Indiana. Founded in 1908 in Grand Rapids as the Michigan College of Chiropractic (Rehm, 1980, p. 289), the school was later renamed for its founder, N.C. Ross, D.C. (see Figure 3-5), who relocated the institution to Fort Wayne in 1911. Ross became a central player in the National Federation of Chiropractors (NFC), an organization formed during World War I to seek commissioned officer status for D.C.s in the military and federal reimbursement for chiropractic services to veterans (Keating & Rehm, 1993). The NFC may have been the springboard for the 1922 formation of the broad-scope American Chiropractic Association (ACA), for it demonstrated that a national society of D.C.s could operate successfully without B.J. Palmer at the helm (B.J. served on a three-man executive committee with Ross and Willard Carver). Ross served as founding president of the NFC, and was succeeded by one of his alumni, Albert B. Cochrane, D.C. of Chicago, who also later served as vice-president and president of the ACA. Significantly, when the ACA was established in competition with Palmer's Universal Chiropractors' Association (UCA), it promoted its independence from "school control" (Keating & Rehm, 1993; Sauer, 1925).

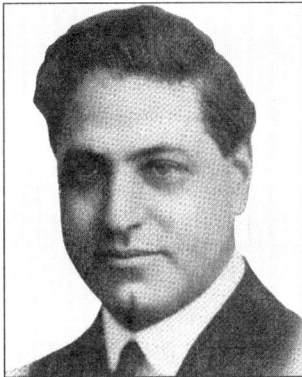

Among the best remembered of the Michigan/Ross College was Archie W. Macfie, D.C., who graduated from the institution in 1914. He practiced for decades in London and Toronto, Ontario, and served for many years as the secretary-treasurer of the Drugless Practitioner's Association of Ontario (Biggs, 1989; Rehm, 1980, p. 291).

In 1929 the Ross College was purchased by another alumnus, George M. O'Neil, D.C. (Class of 1913), and was renamed the O'Neil-Ross College of Chiropractic. Ironically, under O'Neil's supervision the school came within the orbit of B.J. Palmer's International Chiropractors' Association (ICA) during the 1940s, and O'Neil served on the ICA Board of Control. The college closed its doors in the mid-1950s, just a few years after O'Neil's passing in 1951.

Figure 3-5: N.C. Ross, D.C., M.C.

Los Angeles College of Chiropractic

A more enduring influence in chiropractic education has been the Los Angeles College of Chiropractic (LACC). The LACC was launched in October 1911, only a few months after T.F. Ratledge founded his Los Angeles school (Keating et al., 1994). Unlike Ratledge, LACC's founder, Charles A. Cale, had studied in the broad-scope tradition of chiropractic. Cale earned his degree through apprenticeship to Thomas H. Storey, a former "vitapathic physician" from Duluth, Minnesota who had studied under D.D. Palmer in 1901. Cale earned a license as a drugless healer during a short-lived (1909-1910) naturopathic law in California, and gave as purposes for his school:

> ....the teaching of chiropractic, anatomy, histology, gynecology, pathology, obstetrics, bacteriology, chemistry and toxicology, physiology, general diagnosis, hygiene, and naturopathy, and the conferring of the degree of Doctor of Chiropractic upon those completing the course (Articles, 1911).

Charles Cale's wife, Linnie A. Cale, was among the first graduates of the LACC, and immediately joined the faculty upon her graduation in 1912 from the school's nine-month curriculum. The Cales were both professional educators, and had met while attending Terra Haute Normal School in Indiana in the 1890s. In 1914 they suspended operations of the LACC and enrolled at the College of Osteopathic Physicians and Surgeons in Los Angeles. After graduation in 1916, they reactivated the LACC's corporate charter and graduated another class of D.C.s in 1917 (see Figure 3-6). The curriculum expanded at this time to 12 months. B.J. Palmer's *Fountain Head News* offered a derisive description of the LACC's program:

BARGAIN DAY IN CALIFORNIA

LOS ANGELES CHIROPRACTIC COLLEGE. The curriculum includes X-ray, anatomy, physiology, diagnosis, urine analysis, histology, chemistry, bacteriology, geneology, pathology, toxicology, hygiene, minor surgery, obstetrics, medical, Spanish, chiropractic technique. Ten teachers, day and evening classes. Clinic and private treatments. Dr. CHARLES A CALE, President, 931 S. Hill Street. Classes and treatments from 8 a.m. to 10 p.m. Our regular $300, 2,400 hour course, is now given for $125, payable $1 down and $1 a week. Forty-one students now attending. The tuition price will positively be increased to $130 May 1. The present Legislature is practically certain to legalize chiropractic. Enroll now and be ready. — Los Angeles Examiner.'

The ad is sent us with this remark: 'The legislature slipped up on this so I presume the fee will be $1.05 down and $1.05 a week.'

Come when you please, stop when you like. Your credit is good. No wonder only 'Forty-one students now attending' when the possibilities could be for four hundred and forty-one.

Cheap methods, cheap business. You are just what you are. You place the valuation and others follow your lead. No wonder THE PSC away over in Iowa pulls more students per year, from California, than the schools in California have themselves (Bargain, 1917).

The Cales and their LACC, and T.F. Ratledge and his straight school, were antagonists over issues of the appropriate scope of practice for chiropractors, and competitors for the available pool of students for their tuition-driven institutions. However, they were able to set aside their differences during 1921-1922 for just long enough to unite for the campaign that saw California pass a chiropractic law by means of the initiative process. Charles Cale subsequently established two more broad-scope chiropractic colleges in the Golden State,

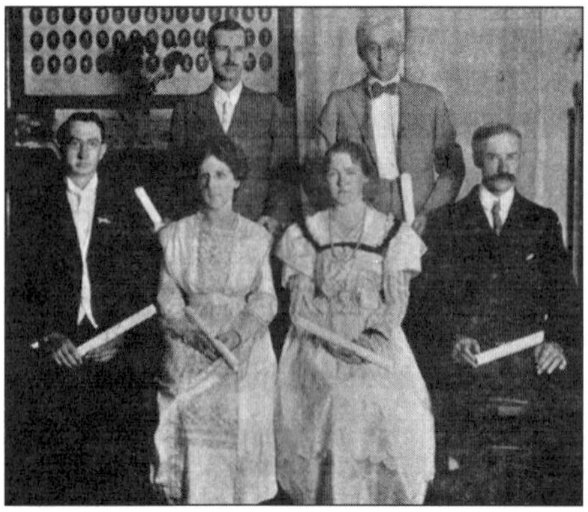

Figure 3-6: LACC Class of 1917

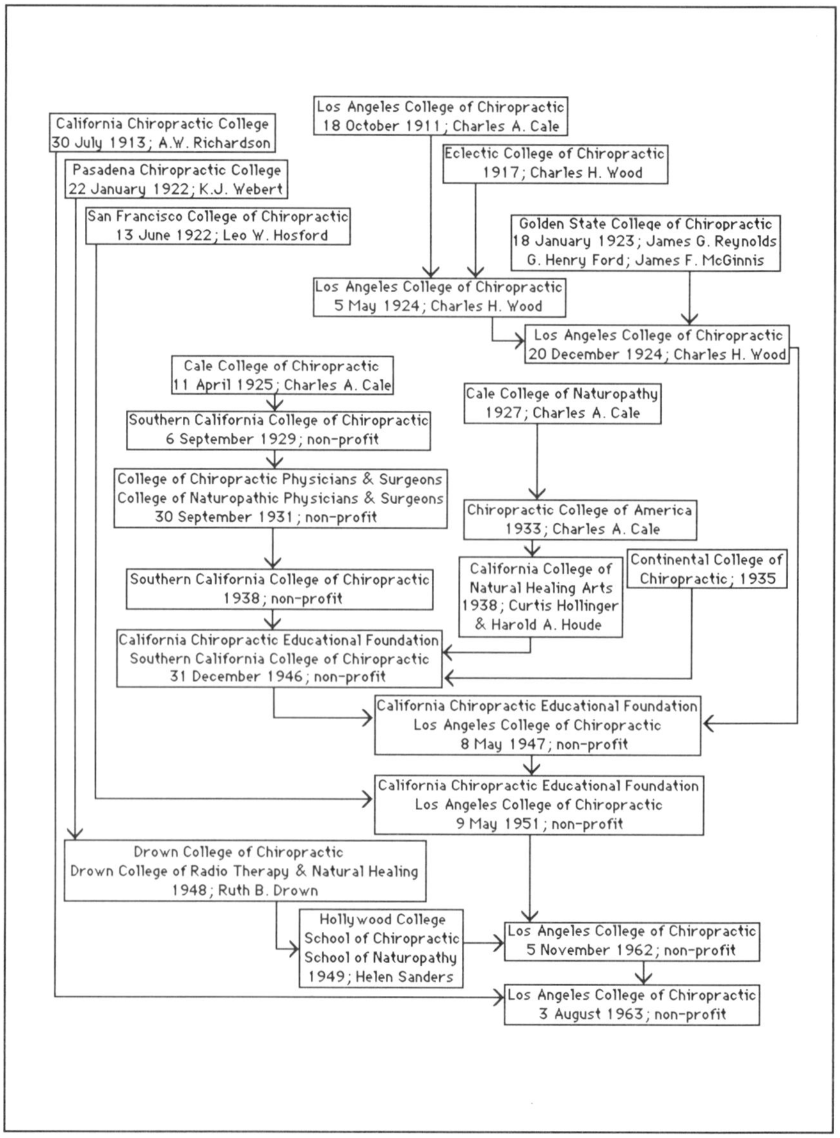

Figure 3-7: Name, date of founding or reorganization, and owner or status of the ancestor institutions of the Los Angeles College of Chiropractic

most notably the non-profit Southern California College of Chiropractic (sometimes known as the College of Chiropractic Physicians and Surgeons), all of which merged in the decade following Charles Cale's death in 1938 (Keating et al., 1993). This amalgamated LACC became a non-profit institution in 1947 (see Figure 3-7) , and became the first regionally accredited chiropractic college in California in 1993.

New England College of Chiropractic & the Washington School of Chiropractic

The chiropractic career of Joe Shelby Riley began at the Palmer-Gregory College of Chiropractic in Oklahoma City, where Riley earned his D.C. and subsequently (1911) served as a senior administrator. Riley established his own school, the New England College of Chiropractic, in Boston in 1912 (Wardwell, 1992, p. 122), and quickly ran afoul of the local medical establishment. He was charged with violation of the state law that required authorization to grant degrees, when he awarded the D.C. to his graduates. Riley relocated to the District of Columbia, where in 1914 he established the Washington School of Chiropractic, an institution that may have lasted as late as 1926 (Ferguson & Wiese, 1988).

Riley was among those early college leaders who were enamored of academic degrees. Riley's 1919 *Science and Practice of Chiropractic with Allied Sciences* listed his credentials as "M.D., Ph.D., M.S., D.M.T., D.O., D.P., D.C., Ph.C." Although the American Chiropractic Association (1991, p. 17) characterizes Riley as a "prominent medical man," most accounts of this itinerant school man imply that Riley's degrees

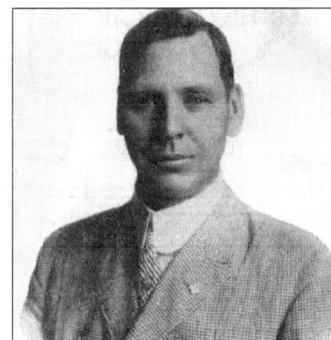

Figure 3-8: A.W. Richardson, D.C.

were as questionable as his colleges' curricula. His educational program involved a part-time faculty of 15, including two medical doctors, and provided the then standard three years of six months each. Instruction was provided in a variety of alternative healing methods, including spondylotherapy, instrument adjusting (concussors) and naturopathic remedies. Riley was the maximum mixer of his era, and he earned the scorn of both the straight community and of elements of broad-scope chiropractic.

Riley's peer group, as suggested by his 1911 listing in the directory of the *American Drugless Healer* magazine, included Charles A. Cale and A.W. Richardson, D.C. (see Figure 3-8) of the Los Angeles and California Chiropractic Colleges, his mentor Alva Gregory and George H. Patchen, M.D., D.C. of New York City. In later years he became a "philosophical" ally of F.W. Collins' Mecca Chiropractic College in Newark, New Jersey, and Benedict Lust's naturopathic-chiropractic institution in New York City (Briggs, 1924). Riley's 1918 text on *Zone Therapy* went through at least 12 editions, which bespeaks an appeal despite the censure of the chiropractic establishment. However, Willard Carver, LL.B., D.C. had little respect for Riley's published work, suggesting that "statements in this book...were not based upon provable scientific facts," and denied the popularity of Riley's contribution (Carver, 1936, p. 60).

Eastern Chiropractic Institute

The Eastern Chiropractic College was founded in Newark, New Jersey in 1918 by Craig M. Kightlinger, M.A., D.C., Ph.C. Kightlinger earned his bachelor's and master's degrees from Valparaiso University in Indiana in 1903 and 1905 respectively, and later added a credential as a pharmacist (Rehm, 1980, pp. 298-9). In 1917 he was awarded the D.C. from F.W. Collins' New Jersey College of Chiropractic in Newark, and he earned the Ph.C. from Palmer in 1919. Kightlinger's Eastern College was relocated from Newark to New York City in 1923, and was renamed the Eastern Chiropractic Institute (ECI) (see Figure 3-9).

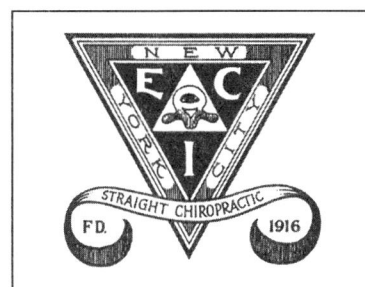

Figure 3-9: Symbol of the Eastern Chiropractic Institute

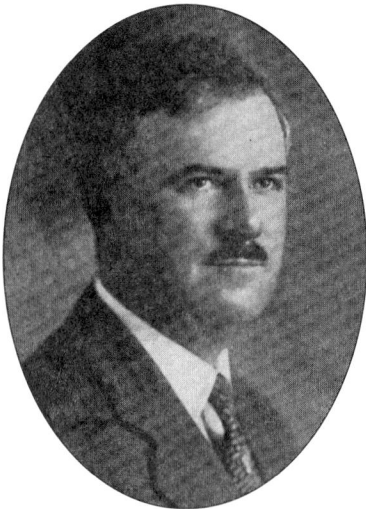

Figure 3-10: Craig M. Kightlinger, D.C., from the *Annual Catalogue* of the ECI, 1929-30

"Kight" was one of that interesting breed of "straight" chiropractors with a scholarly bent and the academic credentials to match. The diagnostic sciences received stronger attention at his school than at most others, and he attracted faculty members with similar convictions about the importance of the fundamental sciences to chiropractors. Among these were Julius Dintenfass, a 1936 alumnus of the ECI, and Clarence Weiant, a 1921 Palmer graduate who joined the ECI faculty in 1928 and would earn a Ph.D. in anthropology from Columbia University in 1943.

Although initially a strong supporter of B.J. Palmer, Kightlinger (see Figure 3-10) was gravely disenchanted by the introduction of the NCM and by Palmer's autocratic rule over the Universal Chiropractors Association (UCA). These sentiments led to his 1925 resignation as vice-president of the UCA in order to join the American Chiropractic Association (Keating & Rehm, 1993; Kightlinger, 1925, 1928). However, he maintained his ties with straight chiropractic education, and joined with college presidents Carl S. Cleveland, T.F. Ratledge and James R. Drain to form the Associated Chiropractic Colleges of America in 1937 (Keating et al., 1991, 1992), a group organized to oppose the educational reform efforts of the broad-scope National Chiropractic Association (NCA). Nonetheless, by 1944 he would, at the urging of the NCA, preside over the merger of his school with several others (see Figure 1-7) to form the Chiropractic Institute of New York (CINY). In the same year he participated in the formation of the Chiropractic Research Foundation (CRF), a forerunner of today's Foundation for Chiropractic Education and Research, and provided laboratory facilities for Weiant's research work (1945-1948) as CRF Director of Research (Keating et al., 1995).

Early Canadian Schools

Chiropractic education came to Canada at least as early as 1909, when the Robbins School of Chiropractic was established in Sault Ste. Marie in central Ontario (Biggs, 1989, S6.1). Medical physicians W.J. Robbins and W.E. Lemon of Plainwell, Michigan, were recruited to start a chiropractic school in the Founder's native land by Archibald B. West, who graduated in the class of 1910 (see Figure 3-11). John A. Henderson, a 1911 alumnus of the Robbins Institute (Lee, 1981c), subsequently served on the faculty of the Hamilton-based Canadian Chiropractic College, and in 1945 became a founder and administrator of today's Canadian Memorial Chiropractic College (CMCC). Another important alumnus of the school (in 1912) was S.F. Sommacal (Lee, 1981d; Rehm, 1980, p. 288), who practiced for 53 years in Toronto and served as chairman of the board of governors and president of the CMCC during 1947-1951. The Robbins Institute, which was probably a "straight" college, closed circa 1914 (Biggs, 1989, S6.1).

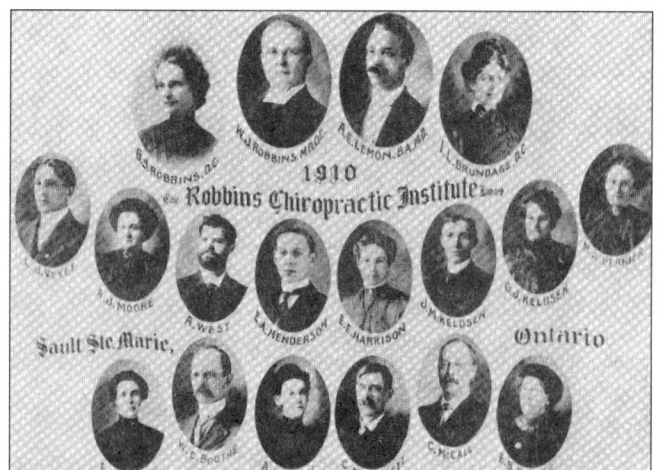

Figure 3-11: Early graduation photo of the Robbins Chiropractic Institute (Chiropractic, 1985)

Henderson is credited with encouraging Ernst DuVal, D.C. (see Figure 3-12) to relocate from Davenport, Iowa, to Hamilton, Ontario, to establish the Canadian Chiropractic College (CCC) in 1914 (Rehm, 1980, p. 285). DuVal was a 1911 or 1912 graduate of the Palmer School, where "on graduation, he was prevailed upon to accept the Chair of Chiropractic Philosophy, which he occupied to the evident satisfaction of all until he accepted the Chair of Philosophy and Anatomy at the U.C.C. for about a year, from which he resigned to establish the Canadian Chiropractic College in his own Country, that he thought needed his services. Chiropractic is too vast to be confined to one Country" (Canadian, 1922, p. 7). Declaring his institution the "MOTHER SCHOOL OF CHIROPRACTIC in Canada" (Canadian, 1922, p. 3), president and dean DuVal effected a B.J. Palmer appearance and a straight chiropractic philosophy which, with B.J.'s help (Sutherland, 1985), convinced the commissioner/author of a devastating report (Biggs, 1985; Hodgins, 1918) on chiropractic for the provincial government of Ontario that the new healing art was:

> ...a system which denies the need of diagnosis, refers 95 per cent of disease to one and the same cause, and turns its back resolutely upon all modern scientific methods as being founded on nothing and unworthy even to be discussed (Sutherland, 1985).

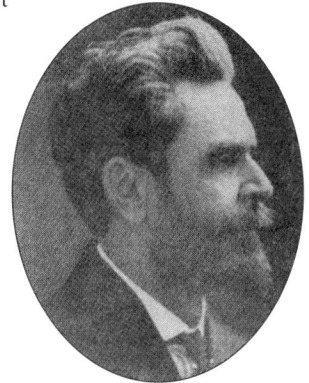

Figure 3-12: Ernst DuVal, D.C.

During most of its life the CCC was a "family run operation" (Biggs, 1989, S6.1), with many of the faculty and staff drawn from DuVal's sons and in-laws. By 1922 the school had relocated from Hamilton to Toronto (see Figure 3-13), and continued to offer a 12-month curriculum which eschewed and denigrated everything but straight chiropractic. The college catalogue proclaimed: "We have no course in Photography, Chemistry, Bacteriology or any other 'Bugology' that take the time, waste the money, and tax the energy of our students" (Canadian, 1922, p. 29). However, DuVal, who fancied himself a skilled orator and debater, offered a course in:

> THE POLEMICS OF CHIROPRACTIC. This is a unique, special study, and exclusively taught at the Canadian Chiropractic College at the present, until other schools adopt it and follow the lead.
>
> This consists of the presentation of numerous logical arguments to defend the science controversal-ly [sic] when attacked by opponents; but especially to convince skeptic, though intelligent, professional and lay prospective patients. It is one of the most useful accomplishments of the practising Chiropractor. Patients, especially the chronics, who know much about their diseases, are loath to believe that Chiropractic is applicable to their special cases and the Chiropractor must demonstrate and convince them... (Canadian, 1922, pp. 35-6).

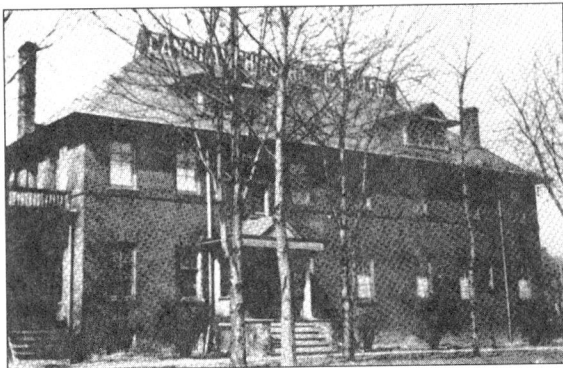

Figure 3-13: Campus of the Canadian Chiropractic College (Biggs, 1985)

The requirement for admission to CCC was the ability to read and write (Canadian, 1922). Tuition for the 12-month program was $300 cash, with discounts made for husband-wife, siblings and parent-child matriculations. Veterans could earn the D.C. for $200, and deferred (installment) payments of tuition were only slightly higher, and payable at the rate of $25 per month. DuVal and his institution participated in the 1917 formation of the International Association of Chiropractic Schools and Colleges during the Palmer lyceum in Davenport. We do not know exactly when the CCC terminated its operations, but it probably was not later than 1928, when the province's Drugless Practitioners Act (DPA) was passed.

Perhaps the best remembered graduate of the CCC was John S. Clubine, D.C., another straight chiropractor who earned his degree in 1919. The following year he and J.A. Cudmore, D.C. organized the Toronto College of Chiropractic (Rehm, 1980, p. 302), one of several Toronto-based competitors to DuVal's CCC in the early 1920s (including the Imperial Chiropractic College and the Ontario Chiropractic College). Clubine served as the first president of the Toronto Chiropractic College (TCC). While president of TCC, he played an active role in provincial efforts to secure licensure for chiropractors in Ontario (Biggs, 1985), but resigned in 1926 (Rehm, 1980, p. 302). He is recalled as one of the founding fathers and the first president of the CMCC in 1945.

Biggs (1989, S6.1) notes that the TCC was a rather successful competitor to DuVal's school, and that it graduated 76 new chiropractors in 1922. However, graduation class sizes had already begun to decline (54 in 1923, 44 in 1925-26) before the passage of the DPA in 1928, which Biggs attributes to "the uncertain legal position of chiropractic, generated by the controversy surrounding the legislative battles of the 1920s" (Biggs, 1989, S6.1). She further indicates:

> The TCC closed in 1928 as a result of the regulations of the DPA. The Board of Regents, the newly formed licensing body, was dominated by "mixer" chiropractors who implemented legislation which required junior matriculation as a pre-entrance requirement. The TCC did not require junior matriculation since this acted as an entrance barrier for prospective students. Since the TCC was the only chiropractic school in existence, these regulations worked effectively to eliminate straight chiropractic...The three chiropractic schools in operation in the years from 1910 to 1927 trained a very small proportion of practising chiropractors.   By far the majority practising in Ontario were trained in the United States (Biggs, 1989, S6.1)

   With the closing of TCC, nearly two decades would pass before a permanent presence for chiropractic education would be established in Canada.

Chapter 4

EARLY EFFORTS AT EDUCATIONAL REFORM

When Abraham Flexner wrote his critique of medical education on behalf of the Carnegie Foundation (Flexner, 1910), he mentioned chiropractic schools only in passing, suggesting they were best dealt with by prosecuting attorneys and grand juries (Brennan, 1983). Flexner reserved the bulk of his critique for the preponderance of proprietary medical schools then in operation, many of them little more than diploma mills (Jochims, 1982). But in this same period, chiropractic training centers were beginning to proliferate, each with its own idea of chiropractic, its scope of practice, methods of training, and with homegrown notions about the appropriate content of a chiropractic curriculum. Instruction in such fundamental subjects as anatomy might include supervised experience in human dissection (such as at Howard's Chicago-based National School of Chiropractic) or involve little more than lectures and study from textbooks (for instance at the Ratledge School in Los Angeles). Supervised clinical training might be non-existent, or could require many hundreds of adjustments (such as at the LACC) and might even involve hospital experience, such as that offered to National students through the Cook County General Hospital in Chicago (Gibbons, 1982), at the Mecca College and Hospital in Newark, New Jersey (War, 1917), and at A.E. Field's Chiropractic University in Kansas City (Eighth, 1915-16; Miscellany, 1988).

As if this diversity of offerings were not enough, the second decade of chiropractic also saw the emerging "menace" (Bethea, 1927) of correspondence schools, which provided chiropractic "education" through the mail. Several authors (Carver, 1936; Rehm, 1992b) report that the Howard System of Chiropractic, taught by the National School of Chiropractic since its first year of operation, continued to be offered as correspondence training toward the "Diplomat of Chiropractic" degree until 1918, or roughly until the school was taken over by William C. Schulze, M.D., D.C. [However, Schulze was the former owner and dean of the American College of Mechano-Therapy (Nostrums, 1912, pp. 480-6), and had operated correspondence courses in manipulation, psychotherapy and other "drugless" methods prior to his involvement with the chiropractic profession.] The "Doctor of Chiropractic" degree at National was reserved for those who took the "resident course." National's founder, John F.A. Howard, later rationalized the home study program by suggesting that in this early, missionary phase of chiropractic, his most important goal had been to disseminate chiropractic as widely as possible.

The National School was not alone in training "mail-order" doctors. Despite the ridicule that D.D. Palmer heaped upon his son for presuming to train chiropractors through the mail, B.J. established the Palmer School of Correspondence circa 1911 (Lessons, 1911; Lerner, 1954, p. 533; Rehm, 1992b), by which students might study "chiropractic philosophy" and earn advanced standing in the Davenport school. The birth of the correspondence program at Palmer could not have been much earlier than 1908, for this was the moment when B.J.'s faculty awarded him the first "Philosopher of Chiropractic" (Ph.C.) degree, presumably a consequence of the success that a "separate and distinct philosophy" enjoyed in winning the day in the Morikubo trial for unlicensed practice in LaCrosse, Wisconsin, in 1907 (Lerner, 1954; Rehm, 1986). Rehm (1992) reproduces an undated advertisement from the "Palmer School of Chiropractic" (not the School of Correspondence) which explicitly indicates that "You can become a competent Doctor of Chiropractic by studying at home."

The most flagrant example of correspondence degree programs of study in chiropractic was that offered by the American University in Chicago during 1913-1935 (Rehm, 1992b). Operated by initially by Dr. D.E. Wood and later by Denton Higbe, M.D., D.C., American University offered a variety of diplomas, including chiropractic and osteopathic doctorates. The headquarters of the "University" consisted primarily of a mail room, from which Higbe ruled over his swindle, disseminated extraordinary claims to prospective students, and continuously enticed "matriculants" to pay their "tuition" at a faster rate. American University advertised widely, and infuriated chiropractic reformers for decades. Medical critics of chiropractic hammered away at this major sore point for decades after American University had closed, indiscriminately painting all chiropractic training with this taint of fraud. Willard Carver recalled the chiropractic correspondence schools less harshly:

> The National School of Chiropractic gradually receded from the idea that Chiropractic could be taught by correspondence, and with the casting off of those unworthy garments, it became recognized as a standard institution of Chiropractic learning.
>
> The National School from the beginning had quite a large business, and that fact resulted in many correspondence schools springing up in Chicago, some in Newark, New Jersey, some in New York City, and one, it must be said with deep regret, was conducted for some time in Oklahoma City.
>
> Generally speaking, however, the correspondence school idea faded very rapidly, and to the eternal praise of the profession, it should be said, Chiropractors have frowned upon attempts to teach Chiropractic by correspondence from the very first (Carver, 1936, pp. 55-6).

To be sure, there was as much to criticize in chiropractic education during the first quarter century of the profession (Lerner, 1954) as Flexner had found in medicine. Standards for admission to chiropractic institutions were minimal or non-existent (Schools, 1928). The Palmer School required only a "common school education" in 1920, which may have meant only the ability to read and write (Miscellany, 1993); the National College of Chiropractic required only a "high school equivalency" for admission as late as 1927 (Advertisement, 1927; Schools, 1928). The absence of any prior study in fundamental subjects, such as physics, biology and chemistry, was no deterrent for the prospective chiropractor. Chiropractic faculty members came in for harsh criticism from organized medicine as "uneducated louts," although such rebuke was not necessarily justified (Miscellany, 1993). As Gibbons has pointed out, several of the Palmer faculty were trained in the liberal arts and/or held baccalaureate degrees, and a number were also graduates of medical schools (e.g., M.P. Brown and A.B. Hender). By 1918 the majority of faculty members at the National School in Chicago held degrees in multiple disciplines (see Table 4-1).

Many early schools offered a continuous curriculum which allowed students to enroll on any day, to commence their studies at whatever point in the curriculum was being taught at that moment, and to walk away with a diploma when sufficient time had been spent at the school or when the curriculum came around to where the student had begun (Keating et al., 1991, 1992; Schools, 1928). Duration of training necessary to receive a chiropractic diploma varied from a few dozen lectures delivered by itinerant seminar instructors such as Alva Gregory (Ratledge, 1915) to the 27 months required at Crabtree's Nebraska school. Moreover, computation of the number of hours in a chiropractic curriculum was obfuscated by schools leaders' willingness to designate a 30-minute instructional period as a class hour. Such shenanigans were not missed by medical critics (Brennan, 1983).

The proliferation of schools took place concurrently with the field's early efforts to free itself from the threat of prosecution for unlicensed practice through the introduction of distinctively chiropractic legislation. Lyndon E. Lee, D.C., of New York, a 50-year crusader for a chiropractic licensing law in his state, railed against the correspondence programs that served to humiliate the profession, and urged his state government to license chiropractors so as to eliminate unqualified practitioners. The rapid growth (1913-1925) in the number of states licensing D.C.s occurred during the "golden age of medical attacks on chiropractic education" (Brennan, 1983), and encouraged educational reform from within the profession.

Table 4-1: Officers and Faculty of the National School of Chiropractic in 1918, as listed in the college's *Eleventh Annual Catalog*

John F. A. Howard, D.C., President, Professor of Principles and Practice of Chiropractic
William C. Schulze, M.D., D.C., Dean, Professor of Gynecology and Obstetrics
Arthur L. Forster, M.D., D.C., Secretary-Manager, Professor of Symptomatology and Diagnosis
Erik Juhl, B.Sc., M.D., D.C., Professor of Anatomy and Dissection
Edward B. Rispin, M.D., D.C., Professor of Chemistry and Pathology
C. Bernhard Herrmann, B.Sc., M.D., D.C., Professor of Physiology
Richard J. Morrison, M.D., D.C., Professor of Histology
Rosemary Rooney, D.C., Dean of Women Students, Professor of Hygiene and Sanitation
Winfield S. Whitman, D.C., Professor of Chiropractic Technique, Post-Graduate Department
Eugene P. Heinze, D.C., Instructor, First Aid
Nels M. Lundberg, Professor of X-Ray and Spinography

Although D.D. and B.J. Palmer had been attempting to impose their visions of what was and was not legitimate chiropractic since the turn of the century, the first suggestion for a formal, organized effort to standardize chiropractic training probably did not appear until 1914 (Palmer, 1917). Palmer was still opposed to licensing laws in this early era (Keating & Rehm, 1993; Palmer, 1924; Wardwell, 1992, p. 110), and so may have been unconcerned about the sort of educational reforms that might assist in obtaining legislation. However, with the passage of the first chiropractic bill (Hariman, 1970, p. 13) in Kansas in 1913, followed quickly by similar legislation in Arkansas, Michigan, North Dakota, Ohio and Oregon, Palmer apparently began to see the wisdom in attempting to direct such legislation, and the problem of the schools came into focus. The educational qualifications of chiropractors were a central issue in all licensing legislation. By 1915 straight college president T.F. Ratledge of Los Angeles, who then offered a 2,400 hour, 20-month curriculum, was attempting to influence who would be licensed by Arkansas' state board of examiners on the basis of the school from which they graduated (Ratledge, 1915); he particularly sought to prevent the licensing of graduates of competitor, broad-scope schools, such as the LACC and the California Chiropractic College.

In 1917, at the Palmer School's annual lyceum, held in conjunction with the yearly meeting of the UCA, one of the earliest attempts to organize and standardize chiropractic education was made (see Table 4-2). In a meeting chaired by UCA attorney Tom Morris, three officers of a society of chiropractic schools were elected: Willard Carver as president, N.C. Ross as secretary, and B.J. Palmer as treasurer (Carver, 1936). Carver later wrote:

> Schools were organized so rapidly that by August 1917, there were 32 chiropractic schools and colleges. By the end of 1917, 19 of these institutions joined the International Association of Chiropractic Schools and Colleges, which was organized at Davenport, Iowa on August of that year, by eight of the leading schools and colleges of Chiropractic (Carver, 1936, p. 56).

The International Association of Chiropractic Schools and Colleges (IACSC) represented a fairly broad spectrum of the colleges then operating, including both "mixer" and "straight" institutions. The political bond which held members together, and presumably excluded certain other schools, is not entirely clear. Turner described the IACSC as:

> ...an attempt to reconcile the educational policies of all schools of recognized standing, presumably in accordance with the regime of the "Fountain Head", the Palmer School of Chiropractic. A close affiliation, however, proved difficult to bring about, although some advance was made towards unifying educational methods in several important schools (Turner, 1931, pp. 168, 288).

College:	Location:	Representative:
[1] Canadian Chiropractic College	Hamilton, Ontario	Ernest G. DuVal, D.C., President
Ross College of Chiropractic, Inc.	Fort Wayne, Indiana	N.C. Ross, D.C., President
Palmer School of Chiropractic	Davenport, Iowa	B.J. Palmer, D.C., President; Frank W. Elliott, D.C., Registrar
Carver Chiropractic College	Oklahoma City	Willard Carver, LL.B., D.C., President
St. Louis Chiropractic College, Inc.	St. Louis, Missouri	L.W. Ray, M.D., D.C., President
Davenport School of Chiropractic	Davenport, Iowa	R. Trumand Smith, D.C., President
[1] National School of Chiropractic	Chicago, Illinois	William C. Schulze, M.D., D.C., President & Dean; Arthur L. Forster, M.D., D.C., Secretary
Universal Chiropractic College	Davenport, Iowa	W.F. Ruehlmann, D.C., M.C., President & Dean; George Otto, D.C., Secretary
[2] University of Chiropractic	[2] unknown	[2] unknown
Kansas Chiropractic College	Topeka, Kansas	Andrew C. Foy, D.C., President

Table 4-2: Membership of the International Association of Chiropractic Schools and Colleges (IACSC), Tom Morris, LL.B., Chairman; as noted in the *Fountain Head News* 1917; 7(1-2): 1, and in Carver (1936, p. 66)

[1] Not mentioned by Carver

[2] Not mentioned in *Fountain Head News*; possibly the "Chiropractic University" operated by A.E. Field, M.D., D.C. in Kansas City since 1907 (Seventh, 1914-15)

College leader Willard Carver's *History of Chiropractic* described the IACSC's intended purpose as

> ...to unify and standardize the conceptions of Chiropractic leaders as to what Chiropractic actually is, and to determine what should be conceived to be a standard Chiropractic education...(Carver, 1936, p. 67).

Carver also suggests that the Association adopted policies that went "a little further than the majority of schools organizing it. Never one to avoid taking a poke at B.J., Carver also noted that Palmer had been among the first to violate IACSC policy, but is unclear about the nature of the Davenport leader's violations (Carver, 1936, p. 66). The Oklahoma chiropractic leader also mentioned resistance to implementing the Association's policies by all schools except his own Carver College:

> The other member schools had not changed their literature, and were going on with their old definitions and procedures, just as they had before organizing the association...So, as executive officer, Dr. Carver felt that the association was a failure (Carver, 1936, p. 67).

Table 4-3: Membership of the Associated Colleges and Schools of Chiropractic (ACSC), as noted in the *Fountain Head News* 1917 (Nov 3); 8(8): 2

New Jersey College of Chiropractic amalgamated with the Mecca College of Chiropractic
New England College of Chiropractic amalgamated with the Washington School of Chiropractic
St. Paul College of Chiropractic
Palmer-Gregory College of Chiropractic
Empire College of Chiropractic
New York School of Chiropractic
Davenport School of Chiropractic

What is known with certainty is that a second confederation of schools, the Associated Colleges and Schools of Chiropractic (ACSC), was organized two months after the IACSC's formation (see Table 4-3), and that one of the ACSC's leaders, Francis W. Allen, D.C. of the Mecca College (who was also an associate of naturopathic leader Benedict Lust), compared B.J. to the German Kaiser (Palmer, 1917). This reinforces Turner's notion that Palmer's involvement (and presumable dominance) may have been an important stumbling block to the formation of one, unified association of schools. The IACSC's developed an explicit concept of chiropractic:

> Chiropractic is hereby defined to be the science that teaches health in anatomic relation, an disease or abnormality in anatomic disrelation; and teaches the art of restoring anatomic relation by a process of adjusting by hand. No other means of securing health shall be construed to be Chiropractic except the application of the inherent qualities at the time in the patient, or appertaining to the Chiropractor (Carver, 1936, p. 56).

The IACSC was either succeeded by or remembered incorrectly as the Federation of Chiropractic Schools and Colleges (Resolution, 1919), and its recommendations, including a call for a "standard education" involving 18 months of training, were endorsed by a meeting of representatives of the state boards of chiropractic examiners of Arkansas, Connecticut, Florida, Kansas, Minnesota, Montana, Nebraska, North Carolina, North Dakota, Vermont and Washington. Among the co-signatories to this resolution were Sylva Ashworth and Lee W. Edwards, M.D., D.C. of the Nebraska board, and Anna Foy of the Kansas board:

> Whereas, It appears that the educational requirements in the various states having laws governing the practice of Chiropractic are so widely at variance;

> Whereas, some state laws require a three years course of six months each, or more or its equivalent, others require a three year course of nine months each, while others have intermediate requirements;

> Whereas, the non-uniformity of laws governing the practice of Chiropractic tends to create confusion between the various Schools and Colleges of Chiropractic to establish a uniform course of education to meet the requirements of different state Chiro Laws.

> Whereas, There is a Federation of Chiropractic Schools and colleges who have adopted a standard course of study of three years of six months each and

> Whereas, This Federation of Chiropractic Schools and Colleges maintain and consider that the course of three years of six months each of sufficient length of time to produce capable and competent Chiropractors, due to the fact that the course of Chiropractic study is devoted primarily to the study of subjects that bear directly on the Science of Chiropractic and does not include the extended study of Materia Medica, surgery and kindred subjects,
>
> Now, Therefore, Be It Resolved by the undersigned representatives of the following state boards of Chiropractic Examiners, assembled in conference at Davenport, Iowa, on the 23rd day in August, 1919, that it is the agreed consensus of opinion that a uniform course of study of three years of six months each is of sufficient length, and should be adopted as the standard of education to be required by all states now having laws governing the practice of Chiropractic, and be it further resolved that a standard educational requirement of a course of study of three years of six months each should hereby be adopted as a standard for future Chiropractic legislation (Resolution, 1919).

Carver reported that the association did not survive for much beyond its first annual meeting; only four schools sent representatives to the IACSC's first annual meeting, held in Cincinnati. He described what he saw as the principal barrier to organizing chiropractors, be they educators, licensing board members or field practitioners:

> ...the trouble with the whole matter of organization has been that there is a pronounced lack of unanimity in the objects to be accomplished by the profession. There had been a fear and distrust, coupled with a failure to understand each other, that has made successful organization impossible (Carver, 1936, p. 69).

Another effort to bring order to the chaos of chiropractic education in the first 25 years of the profession was the creation of a National Board of Chiropractic Examiners (NBCE), which was apparently first proposed by B.J. Palmer (1920). Palmer recommended that the examining boards in those states which then licensed chiropractors subscribe to a UCA-organized agency which would create a rigorous national examination process. The state boards would have the option of accepting passage of this national test in lieu of a state examination, but would maintain control of the licensing process in their own jurisdiction.

Palmer's proposal quickly received heated opposition from Arthur L. Forster, then secretary (later, dean) of the renamed National College of Chiropractic in Chicago. Forster indicated that he was not opposed to the concept of a NBCE, but rather to the control that might come to rest within Palmer's UCA (Forster, quoted in Palmer, 1920). Palmer's newsletter also reprinted a number of letters from various state boards, many of whom approved the plan in principal. However, a number of these letters also revealed substantive misunderstanding of the nature and purpose of the NBCE. A common mistake was the notion that a National Board would issue a national license, thereby undermining the authority of individual state boards.

Occasional criticism was heard that the NBCE, like the IACSC before it, proposed to set a maximum limit on education (i.e., 18 months), rather than to set minimum standards for chiropractic curricula. The Palmer School had only recently announced that it would require future students to register for an 18-month program, and still required only 12 months of training to qualify for a diploma:

Important Announcement

> Beginning January 1, 1920, we will accept no more students for less than a three-year course of study...Students enrolling at The P.S.C. for a three-year term WILL BE PERMITTED TO GRADUATE AT THE END OF A TWO-YEAR (12 MONTHS) PERIOD upon application, with the understanding that they may or can return to school within five years from taking a two-year diploma, to complete the remaining year. After returning to complete their third year (of six months) they shall deposit their two-year diploma, and upon completion of the course will be granted a three-year course diploma (D.C.), and if during their course they have made all "A" grades they will be granted a (Ph.C.) diploma.
>
> This change is made necessary by the standardization of various Chiropractic State Boards, who are agreed that eighteen months shall be the maximum time required to graduate a Chiropractor. Many students not conversant with these requirements enroll for a two-year course and do not take the extra work required in our three-year course, hence they have not completed enough work to meet the requirements of some Chiropractic State Boards, and a Post Graduate course of six months does not meet these requirements in all instances. So, the faculty of this school has decided that it is for the best interests of the school and its graduates to require all students to complete

at least two years of the three years' course before graduation, so that they may return at some future date, IF DESIRED, and complete a full three-year course.

Ninety per cent of students now enrolling at The P.S.C. are taking a three-year course under above conditions. The only change after Jan. 1st in this announcement is, that after that date, ALL matriculations shall be for a three-year course and a slight advance in the tuition fee made necessary by the constantly increasing price of all things used in our work (Important, 1919).

Objections to the NBCE from those few college leaders who were offering longer programs, such as H.C. Crabtree, president of the Nebraska Chiropractic College, emphasized the Developer's disdain for education. Palmer had made his views plain:

Any chiropractor who plays to the higher educational qualifications, either willingly or unwillingly, deliberately or unconsciously plays the medical man's game just as he plays it and does just what the medical man wants done; except that the chiropractor does it against his own and saves the medical man the trouble of doing it for himself...

Why does the chiropractor succeed and why does not the medical man? The medical man puts in too much time in school; he muddles his mind; he complexes his subject; he knows too much that isn't so and won't work. He HAS SPENT TOO MANY YEARS BEHIND FOUR WALLS. If he could but reverse his school time, cut it as short as he has lengthened it, he would come out knowing something and be able to do something...

"Time" behind college walls is the great intermediary which kills right ideas, initiative, ability to think and reason, ability to do it. It has ruined many a good chiropractor by making a fool of a physician out of him; and, just as fast as we force Chiropractic schools into a "time" medical educational system, just that fast will we be ruining many a good chiropractor into a fool of a physician (Palmer, 1919a)

It should be noted that curricular limits were not the basis for resistance to the NBCE in most cases. The National College, for example, had only recently discontinued its correspondence courses and still offered an 18-month program as its "standard" (Carver, 1936, p. 190; Palmer, 1920; Rehm, 1992b). Despite these objections, the "original NBCE," unrelated to today's organization by the same name, was created in 1921 during the Palmer School's homecoming in August. Turner (1931, p. 168) recalled that "J. Ralph John, D.C. was elected president of the new board, and for two years examinations were held, then the undertaking was abandoned." In a February 1922 note to Nebraska's secretary for the Department of Public Welfare, B.J. Palmer noted that the NBCE was also involved in school inspections, and that Crabtree was resisting these efforts:

The National Board of Chiropractic Examiners have had an examiner trotting about getting facts on schools. Crabtree refused to co-operate in ANY way. He simply refused to give any information, any dates, refused to let this inspector visit his classes or anything else. He was discourteous, etc. I thought perhaps you would like to know this in advance of his report which will be made at the next coming conference which will be held immediately AFTER Lyceum this year (Palmer, 1922).

This first NBCE also adopted the "House Cleaning" policies of the UCA (Report, 1922), which were intended to eliminate "mixer" members from state societies. To enforce this policy, the UCA threatened that:

...if the State Associations refuse to clean then the UCA will voluntarily come into the respective state and organize a branch in opposition to the State Association, requiring affidavits from members they are straight chiropractors, also the complete endorsement of UCA Principles.

The National Board of Examiners countenance no mixers...Nebraska, Minnesota and New York as well as other States are due for UCA Cleaning...

The UCA is willing to allow the different organizations as well as Chiropractors a reasonable amount of time to Clean House... (Report, 1922)

The UCA's punitive contingency, the creation of rival state societies, was implemented in several instances, such as in New York and Nebraska. As we noted earlier, Palmer's forces were successful in 1923 in having the state board of chiropractic examiners roll back the educational requirements for licensure from 27 to 18 months of training, thereby making Palmer graduates eligible for license. So far as is known, Nebraska was the only state to lower its educational requirements for licensure.

Chapter 5

AFTER THE GREAT WAR

The second quarter of chiropractic's first century commenced in the wake of the First World War. While Europe had been dealt a severe blow, the United States had been largely unharmed by this "war to end all wars." Newly elected in 1920, Warren G. Harding called for a return to "normalcy" in his presidential inauguration address in 1921. It would hardly be that, neither for the nation nor for the chiropractic profession.

The war had several direct and indirect effects upon the profession. For chiropractors' orthodox medical rivals, the war marked the beginning of increased government funding of medical research and education. Modest government investment in the medical profession augmented the massive infusion of private philanthropy that allopathic institutions had begun to enjoy in the aftermath of the 1910 Flexner report and the subsequent campaign to improve medical education (Starr, 1982). Although larger financial contributions from the federal government were not seen until the end of World War II, the medical community had no difficulty in gaining compensation for care to veterans, as did the chiropractors. The war also gave rise to the physical therapy profession, which had begun as the Army Reconstruction Corps, and was focused on rehabilitation of the many maimed, crippled and otherwise disabled veterans (Keating, 1994a; Kranz, 1986).

In the Roaring '20s chiropractors enjoyed none of this private and public investment in health care educational reforms, and were outraged at the government's refusal to reimburse for chiropractic services to veterans (Keating, 1994a). Many D.C.s had served their country valiantly along the front lines and in the trenches in Europe, and now were to be humiliated on the home front. A fighting spirit was aroused among D.C.s.

However, chiropractic institutions, most notably the Palmer School of Chiropractic (PSC) in Davenport, the First National University of Naturopathy in Newark, New Jersey (which included the Mecca College of Chiropractic) and Carver College in Oklahoma City, were approved for "vocational training" by the Veterans' Bureau (a forerunner of the Veterans' Administration), and trained thousands of new chiropractors in the immediate years following the war. In a 1921 survey of chiropractic schools in the New York City and Newark, New Jersey area some 1800 students were noted (Stowe, 1921). Ferguson and Wiese (1988) note an all-time record number of schools operating in the post-war period, and perhaps as many as 82 schools were open in 1925. Although Turner (1931, pp. 34-6) reported a temporary decrease in student enrollments during America's participation in the war (1917-1918), this fall-off was not apparent at the Palmer School. Indeed, the Davenport mecca's enrollment catapulted to over 1,000 students in the immediate post-war period, and reached an all-time high of 2,776 in 1921, a

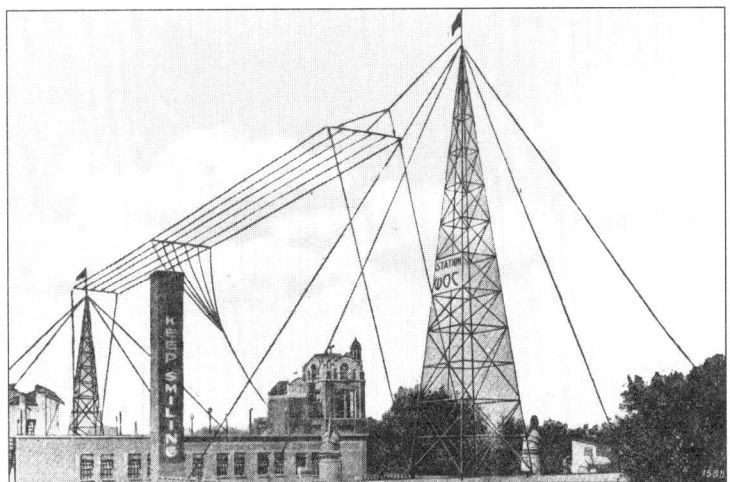

Figure 5-1: Photo appeared on a postcard distributed by the Palmer School of Chiropractic; caption read: "The Highest Point in Davenport, Ia. The Aerial Tower of Broadcasting Station WOC on top of Palmer School 300 feet above Mississippi River."

student body size that was not again to be seen in chiropractic education until the 1990s and the growth of Life College in Marietta, Georgia. The tuition dollars provided by veterans benefits enabled not only this spectacular expansion of the PSC, but also B.J.'s purchase and development of Radiophone Station WOC (Keating, 1995), which perched atop the PSC's buildings (see Figure 5-1).

The postwar years also brought an influx of foreign students, perhaps attributable to the broader geographic exposure that the profession had received during the conflict (Keating, 1994a, 1995). The PSC's 1925 yearbook depicted several dozen international students, who organized an International Chiropractors' Association (no relation to today's ICA; see Figure 9-1) (The Recoil, 1925, p. 129):

INTERNATIONAL CHIROPRACTORS' ASSOCIATION

This organization was founded in 1921 to consolidate and advance the interests of the students of foreign birth, not only at The Fountain Head of Chiropractic, but also when in the field abroad. The chief aims of the association are:

1. To unite chiropractors of foreign birth, and graduates of recognized schools, aspiring to practice in countries outside the boundaries of the United States.

2. To disseminate and uphold the principles and practice of Chiropractic, as defined in the UCA Model Bill, both among foreigners in the United States and in foreign countries.

3. To develop and maintain a bureau of information wherein students at school, or chiropractors in the field, may obtain information and data relative to the Chiropractic outlook in foreign countries.

HONORARY PRESIDENTS

A.E. Hunt-King...............England

J.J. Gillett............Belgium

OFFICERS

President..................................W.R. Carson, Canada

Vice-President.................... H.C. Lawrence, Canada

Secretary................................T.C. Halstein, Norway

Treasurer.....................................G.J. Webb, Canada

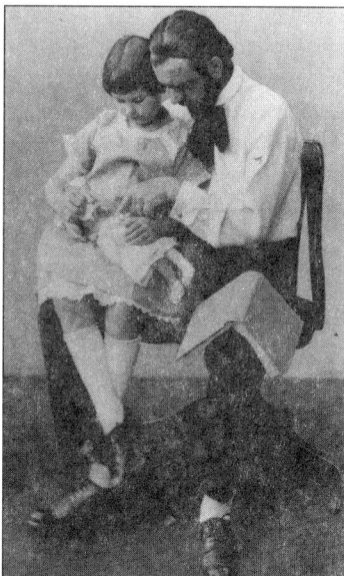

Figure 5-2: B.J. Palmer and young patient, circa 1925

This growth in enrollments and in numbers of chiropractic training institutes was short-lived. Many of the schools were "not viable" (Ferguson & Wiese, 1988), and soon folded once government-funded, tuition dollars dried up. Palmer (see Figure 5-2) noted his pleasure that these many fly-by-night schools had soon failed, although his opinion seems to have been at variance with many in the profession and with many veterans. When the Veterans Bureau's changing policies began to impact the Palmer School by disallowing enrollment of students who did not have two years of pre-chiropractic college training, B.J. apparently changed his strategy. His *Fountain Head News* echoed the sentiments of the Minneapolis chapter of the Disabled American Veterans:

...Be it therefore resolved that this Chapter go on record as being opposed to the above mentioned ruling of the United Sates Veterans Bureau that requires two years premedical schooling for entrance into the study of Chiropractic, and we therefore urge our legislative committee to immediately draft a bill to be presented before the congress of the United States at this session to repeal this ruling so that the requirements of the United Sates Veterans Bureau will be in accordance with the various state laws and the requirements of the recognized schools of Chiropractic... (Resolution, 1924a).

There were still some 60 chiropractic schools operating by the end of the decade, when the stock market crashed and economic depression engulfed the nation. The quality of these institutions ranged from correspondence programs, to the 18-month curriculum offered at the Palmer School and perhaps a majority of institutions in that period, to the four-year courses in chiropractic and naturopathy offered at schools such as the National College in Chicago, the Metropolitan Chiropractic College in Cleveland, Ohio, the Los Angeles College of Chiropractic (LACC) and the College of Chiropractic Physicians & Surgeons in Los Angeles. Ferguson and Wiese's (1988) research suggests that the loss of chiropractic educational institutions continued until the 1970s.

The 1920s saw the further growth and founding of several of the most significant colleges in the profession's history, including the zenith of the Palmer School's early development; the births of the Cleveland Chiropractic College of Kansas City (Keating & Cleveland, 1996) and the Lincoln Chiropractic College in Indianapolis (Stowell, 1984); the chartering of the Colorado Chiropractic University (forerunner of the University of Natural Healing Arts); the professionalization of the National College of Chiropractic and its purchase of the Lindlahr School of Natural Therapeutics (Keating & Rehm, 1995a&b; Kirchfeld & Boyle, 1994); and the evolution of the several schools that eventually merged to form today's non-profit LACC, including the Cale College of Chiropractic and the Cale College of Naturopathy (Keating et al., 1993).

Punctuated by the spurt of new blood that the veterans of the Great War provided, the philosophical, theoretical and technical divisions within the profession blossomed into formal institutions and organizational structures. Many if not most college aligned themselves politically with one of the two major societies (e.g., ACA vs. UCA), yet still attempted to steer a median course. Even in the face of their common antagonist, organized medicine, chiropractors' differences often prevented a united front in the growing legal wars. The colleges could not help but reflect these internal and external stresses.

Chapter 6

MEDICAL CRITICISM
OF CHIROPRACTIC EDUCATION

Chiropractic education evidently fascinated the AMA, which repeatedly "inspected" the Palmer School of Chiropractic (PSC) throughout the post-war decade. A 1920 evaluation by the AMA's Council on Medical Education found a 16-month course involving formal instruction in quackery (advertising) and leading to degrees such as the D.C. and the Ph.C. (Philosopher of Chiropractic); a 12-month short-course was also available (Gibbons, 1993). A "common school education," interpreted to mean the ability to read and write, was required for admission to Palmer, in contrast to the two years of college education then customary for admission to medical school. Students could enroll at any time during a term, and would graduate 18 months later, or whenever they had completed the required hours. The AMA inspector was also disapproving of Mabel Palmer's textbook of anatomy and the published works of other faculty members, apparently on the grounds that they were educationally under-qualified to have authored such material. The AMA likened the work of the Palmer faculty to "the blind leading the blind," and described the school's instructors as "largely uneducated louts" (Gibbons, 1993). In many, but not all chiropractic schools, such evaluation was factually incorrect (see Table 6-1).

The Palmer School was surreptitiously inspected in 1921 by George Dock, M.D., professor of medicine at Washington University (Dock, 1922; Martin, 1994). Dock was an 1884 graduate of the University of Pennsylvania's medical school, protege of William Osler, M.D. and a former professor of clinical medicine at the University of Michigan medical school (Davenport, 1987). He was known for his sense of humor and critical attitude toward medicine. Brennan (1983) noted of Dock's visit to the Palmer School that he:

> ...was prepared to dislike the school, given his experiences with former chiropractic patients and his earlier opinions on the subject, but instead discovered a fine osteological collection, many and spacious classrooms, and a student body of over 3000 persons, endowed with "friendliness, earnestness, and conviction." Dr. Dock felt compelled to add that the students would be more at home as cooks or barbers. He found that the lectures by B.J. were always presented to a full house. Mabel Palmer's lectures were judged to be correct in content, although replete with anatomical terms given unusual pronunciations. The clinic was a booming proposition, serving 1700 people daily.

> Dr. Dock's report generally expressed more a sense of curiosity than of hostility. His chief criticism was that political statements from and about the Palmer School were exaggerated. He also thought that the training in areas other than technic was not rigorous enough to allow chiropractors to treat infectious conditions or malignant tumors. The question of chiropractic licensing was relegated to the legal arena, and the matter was "not to be settled by physicians."

Despite any gentle tendencies, Dock also wrote that he "went from class-room to class-room, and from these one would never realize that the chiropractor had anything to do with medicine as a biologic science" (Dock, 1922). Chiropractors' ideas about science were very much at odds with those common in medicine and elsewhere (Keating et al., 1995).

A 1925 inspection of the PSC by A.W. Meyer, M.D. yielded a report which described:

> ...a confused place bedecked in epigrams and cluttered with Buddhas, busts and every manner of memorabilia. One suspects that his article may have served as a template for the later writings of Ralph Lee Smith and others...

The osteological studios were judged to contain a large collection of anomalous skeletons, but Dr. Meyer found many to be mislabeled. Wormian bones were called "osseous tumors," and an acromegalic skeleton was a "giant," (which, of course, it would be). The writer thought Mabel Palmer's anatomical ideas to be not completely accurate, especially concerning the famous "Duct of Palmer," connecting the spleen with the stomach. Her textbook was described as "garbled." Dr. Meyer was kindest to the students, calling them "unusually friendly, good-natured and ...quite ignorant of the sham in which they were playing a part." He was not pleased with the idea of coccygeal adjustments (Brennan, 1983).

Faculty Member	Years on Faculty:	Education & Scholarly Works
B.J. Palmer, D.C., Ph.C., *President*	1902-1961	10th grade; DC (PSC '02); author of dozens of books
Mabel H. Palmer, D.C. (owner)	1905? - 1949?	DC (PSC '05); studied anatomy at uncertain medical school in Chicago; author, *Chiropractic Anatomy* and *Stepping Stones*
Alfred B. Hender, M.D., D.C., Ph.C., *Dean*	1910-1943	pre-medical studies, Cornell College; MD, College of Medicine of the Iowa State University; DC (PSC' '10)
Frank W. Elliott, D.C., Ph.C., *Registrar*	1911?-1937	studied, Southwestern College; DC (PSC '11)
W.L. Heath, D.C., Ph.C.	1908? - ???	graduate, Cornell College (1870); DC (PSC '07)
James N. Firth, D.C., Ph.C.	1911-1925	graduate, Arenac County Normal College ('06); studied, Ferris Institute; DC (PSC '10), author, *Textbook on Chiropractic Symptomatology* and *Chiropractic Diagnosis*
Harry E. Vedder, D.C., Ph.C.	1913-1926	DC (PSC '12), author, *Textbook on Chiropractic Physiology, Textbook on Chiropractic Gynecology* and *Chiropractic Advertising*
Steven J. Burich, D.C., Ph.C.	1913-1926	graduate, Beloit College ('13); DC (PSC '13); author, *Textbook of Chiropractic Chemistry*
John H. Craven, D.D., D.C., Ph.C.	1913-1935	graduate, Kansas Wesleyan University; DC (PSC '12); author, *Chiropractic Orthopedy* and *Hygiene & Pediatrics*
E.A. Thompson, D.C., Ph.C., *Director, Palmer X-Ray Laboratories*	1914-1925	DC (PSC '14), author, *Text of Chiropractic Spinography*
Henri L. Gaddis, D.C., Ph.C.	1919-???	DC (PSC '16)
L.G. DeArmand, D.D.S.	???	DDS, Chicago College of Dental Surgery
Roy G. Maybach, D.C.	1920-???	DC (PSC '15)
K.G. Stephan, D.C., Ph.C.	1920-???	studied, Culver Military Academy and Purdue University; DC (PSC)
H.L. Vinkemeyer, D.C., Ph.C.	???	DC
C.C. Hall, D.C., Ph.C.	1919-???	graduate pharmacist, University of Michigan; DC (PSC)
Arthur G. Hinrichs, D.C., Ph.C.	1920-1925	studied, Butler University; DC (PSC '20), co-author, *X-Ray Technique & Spinal Misalignment Interpretation*
Ray R. Richardson, D.C., Ph.C., *Director, Palmer X-ray Laboratories*	1919?- 1932	DC (PSC '19)
Clyde G. Kern, D.C., Ph.C.	1916-1925	B.P.Ed., Ohio Northern University ('09); DC (PSC '16)
Ralph W. Stephenson, D.C., Ph.C.	1921-???	graduate, Iowa State University; DC (PSC '21); author, *Art of Chiropractic, Chiropractic Textbook* and *Traction System of Adjusting the Spine*
Earl I. Nott, D.C.	1921-???	DC (PSC)
L.V. Willes, D.C., Ph.C.	1921-1925	studied, University of Utah; DC (PSC '21)
C.A. Russell, D.C., Ph.C.	1922-???	studied, University of Illinois
W.L. Heath, Jr., D.C., Ph.C.	1922-???	DC (PSC '17)
Arleigh L. Willis, D.C., Ph.C.	1922-???	studied, Kansas State Agricultural College; DC (PSC '22)
C.F. Stoddard, D.C., Ph.C.	1922-???	graduate, Iowa Wesleyan College ('02); DC (PSC '22)
C.C. Flanagan, D.C., Ph.C.	1922-???	graduate, Grinnell College; DC (PSC '22)
Herbert C. Hender, D.C., Ph.C.	1924-???	DC (PSC '24)
Donald Kern, D.C., Ph.C.	1924-1926; 1946-1961	DC (PSC '21)

Table 6-1: Faculty of the Palmer School of Chiropractic in 1925; based on information from Gibbons (1993), Peters & Chance (1993), Rehm (1980), the *Bulletin of the ACA* (With, 1926) and *The Recoil* (1925).

Chiropractic education came in for further harsh review in the previously mentioned AMA report in 1928. A number of chiropractic and naturopathic institutions were inspected and uniformly found wanting (Schools, 1928), among them the Palmer, National, LACC, First National (Mecca) and American (Lust's New York City institution) schools. This was a period which saw two major claims against the chiropractic profession: firstly that adjustments were dangerous, and secondly that "educational standards, admissions requirements and faculty credentials" were inadequate (Cooper, 1985). One chiropractor of the period reported that in 1924 the AMA had "met in secret conclave in Chicago and adopted the slogan, 'Chiropractic must die.' They gave themselves ten years in which to exterminate it" (Reed, 1932, p. 35). Wardwell (1992, p. 162) notes that this report was not denied, and Cooper (1985) indicates that the campaign against chiropractic by means of attacks on its educational standards greatly increased in the 1920s.

Table 6-2: A 1927 pamphlet published by American College of Chiropractors, headquartered in New York City; the pamphlet was entitled "Medical Education versus Chiropractic Education, National Publicity Series No. 3" (Ratledge papers, Stockton Foundation for Chiropractic Research)

CHIROPRACTIC EDUCATION VERSUS MEDICAL EDUCATION
A Scientific Comparison Based on the Latest Available Authorities

The Practice of Medicine is regulated by law in 48 states	Hours	The Practice of Chiropractic is regulated by law in 38 states	Hours
Pre-Requisite education: Four years of high school or equivalent and two years of college.		Pre-Requisite education: Four years of high school or the equivalent	
Minimum course of study necessary for medical schools to be registered or accredited by the Board of Regents of New York State, consists of 3600 class hours, distributed as follows:		Minimum course of study necessary for chiropractic schools to be rated as Class A Schools by the American College of Chiropractors, consists of 3528 class hours, distributed as follows:	
ANATOMY, including gross anatomy histology, and embryology	648	ANATOMY, including gross anatomy, embryology, neurology, histology and orthopedy.	955
PHYSIOLOGY and Chemistry	432	PHYSIOLOGY and CHEMISTRY, including physiology, biological and physiological chemistry, toxicology, urinalysis and dietetics.	380
PATHOLOGY, including gross pathology, pathological histology and Bacteriology.	432	PATHOLOGY, including gross pathology, pathological histology and Bacteriology.	300
HYGIENE	108	HYGIENE, including public health and public health service	100
PHARMACOLOGY and THERAPEUTICS	216	DIAGNOSIS or ANALYSIS, including spinography (x-ray).	430
OBSTETRICS and GYNECOLOGY.	252	OBSTETRICS and GYNECOLOGY.	100
MEDICINE, including pediatrics, nervous and mental diseases, dermatology and syphilis, medical jurisprudence.	900	CHIROPRACTIC, including Chiropractic symptomatology, Chiropractic principles and practice. Chiropractic palpation and adjusting. Chiropractic jurisprudence. Contagious and infectious diseases. Eye, ear, nose and throat. Dermatology.	1147
SURGERY, including orthopedics, genito-urinary, ophthalmology, otology, laryngology, rhinology, roentgenology.	612	ELECTIVE SUBJECT or SUBJECTS	116
Total class hours, all subjects	3600	Total class hours, all subjects	3528

The medical curriculum shown above is reproduced from page 59 of the University of the State of New York's Handbook No. 9, Laws and Rules of Higher Education in Medicine, June, 1926. 73 medical schools in the United States are registered under these Rules. (Hospital internship is not a requirement of these Rules.)

For their part, the chiropractors attempted to create favorable comparisons between chiropractic and medical education. Patterned after comparative analyses prepared by organized medicine (Brennan, 1983), such contrasts compared hours and subjects studied in chiropractic vs. medical schools (see Table 6-2). Brennan noted that medicine's attempts at such comparisons, typically based upon the curriculum of the Palmer School of Chiropractic (PSC), proved arithmetically futile:

> The earlier medical papers made a point of calculating the hours of instruction per week necessary to achieve the certified 4103.5 hours of education. It was estimated at 59 hours per week in the sixteen-month course and 53 hours per week in the eighteen-month course. This would restrict the hours available for outside study and class preparation. Once the fact was known that each clock hour at PSC equaled only thirty minutes, the other calculations were dropped (Brennan, 1983).

Chiropractors' comparisons of medical vs. chiropractic education were not troubled by the use of 30-minute hours. Neither was the extended clinical training (hospital-based internship) required for medical graduates to qualify for licensure taken into account in chiropractors' published contrasts. These public relations efforts by chiropractors appear to have been most frequently initiated by marketing groups, although the comparison noted in Table 6-2 was prepared by the American

---

Table 6-3: Administration, faculty and staff of the National School of Chiropractic, from the school's 1918 catalogue; a majority of the instructors held both chiropractic and medical doctorates.

JOHN F. ALAN HOWARD, D.C., President, Professor Principles and Practice of Chiropractic. Former Director of Salt Lake Sanitarium; Author of the *Encyclopedia of Chiropractic*; Three Years' Post-Graduate Study in France and Switzerland; Honorary Member California, Pennsylvania and Ohio Chiropractors Societies; Licentiate of Illinois.

WILLIAM CHARLES SCHULZE, M.D., D.C., Dean, Professor of Gynecology and Obstetrics. Graduate Rush Medical College, the Medical Department of the University of Chicago; Author of *Clinical Lectures* and *A Text Book of the Diseases of Women*; Formerly Physician in Charge of The Institute of Physiological Therapeutics; Licentiate States of Illinois, Minnesota and Wisconsin.

ARTHUR LEOPOLD FORSTER, M.D., D.C., Secretary-Manager, Professor of Symptomatology and Diagnosis. Graduate Medical Department University of Illinois; Ex-Interne St. Elizabeth Hospital, Chicago; Formerly Attending Physician St. Francis Hospital, Evanston, Ill.; Author *Spinal Adjustment*; Editor-in-Chief *National Journal of Chiropractic*; Licentiate of Illinois.

ERIK JUHL, B.Sc., M.D., D.C., Professor of Anatomy and Dissection. Member Royal College, Flensburg, Denmark; Graduate Loyola University Medical Department; Attendant Polyclinic, Berlin, Germany; Licentiate State of Illinois.

EDWARD BUCKLEY RISPIN, M.D., D.C., Professor of Chemistry and Pathology. Graduate Bennett Medical College, Chicago; Formerly Pathologist McKellar General Hospital, Fort Williams, Canada; Formerly Bacteriologist, P. & S. Laboratory, Chicago; Licentiate of Illinois.

C. BERNHARD HERRMANN, B.Sc., M.D., D.C., Professor of Physiology. Active Member and Ex-Secretary Chicago Anatomical Society; Instructor Chicago Hospital College of Medicine; Formerly Professor of Physiology, Barnes School of Sanitary Science; First Lieut. M.R.C., U.S. Army; Licentiate of Illinois.

RICHARD JOHN MORRISON, M.D., D.C., Professor of Histology. Graduate Chicago College of Medicine and Surgery; Graduate University of London, England; Lecturer of State Board Review Course for Chiropractors; Licentiate State of Illinois.

ROSEMARY ROONEY, D.C., Dean of Women Students, Professor of Hygiene and Sanitation. Graduate Ohio Hospital for Women and Children; Attendant Cincinnati University; Graduate National School of Chiropractic; Formerly Lecturer on Hygiene and Public Health, Cincinnati Board of Health.

WINFIELD SCOTT WHITMAN, D.C., Professor of Chiropractic Technique, Post-Graduate Department. Graduate Linthicum Institute and National School of Chiropractic; Associate Editor *National Journal of Chiropractic*.

EUGENE P. HEINZE, D.C., Instructor "First Aid to the Injured." Graduate National School of Chiropractic; Lecturer for The National First Aid Association of America, Clara Barton, President; Licentiate State of Illinois.

NELS MOODY LUNDBERG, Professor of X-Ray and Spinography. Roentgenologist West Suburban Hospital, Oak Park, 3 1/2 Years; Roentgenologist Cook County Hospital 3 1/2 Years; Roentgenologist National Pathological Laboratories, Chicago.

College of Chiropractors (ACC), an honors society that continues to this day. The ACC claimed that its tally of the hours in the typical chiropractic curriculum were based on 45-minute instructional periods, and emphasized that:

> IMPORTANT: as the Chiropractor studies the basic science subjects more from a mechanical viewpoint rather than the chemical, and adjusting the cause of disease rather than the effect of disease; it absolutely precludes the possibility of any but a Chiropractic Board of Examiners to pass FAIRLY upon the competence of the Chiropractor (ACC, 1927).

The National College's strong faculty (see Table 6-3) and broader curriculum did not spare it from organized medicine's rebuke. The AMA's 1928 report suggested that:

NATIONAL COLLEGE OF CHIROPRACTIC

(Inspected, Feb. 25, 1927)

...The school is located at 20 North Ashland Boulevard, Chicago, in a brick building...by no means fitted for its present use; ventilation and lighting are poor, and the arrangement for clinical and laboratory work is abominable...the basement contains the chemistry laboratory and the dissecting room; with the exception of these four rooms, the school activities and all clinical work are confined to the first floor.

2. Institutions. - This one floor and the four other rooms accommodate several institutions of learning. These are: (1) The National College of Chiropractic, giving an eighteen months' course, tuition $600; (2) The National Academy, giving a six months' preparatory (high school) course, tuition $45; (3) The Hygieia College of Sanitary Science, giving a three months' course in personal and public hygiene, tuition $100; (4) The Lindlahr College of Natural Therapeutics, recently purchased, giving a three months' course in physiotherapy, tuition $100; (5) The National School of Obstetrics, giving a six months' course of lectures with privilege of observing a few deliveries (but not assisting) at the West End Hospital, tuition $150; and (6) a six months' Night School quiz course in preparation for the Illinois examination, tuition $200. There are also a three-month postgraduate course, tuition $150, with privilege of continuing indefinitely at $30 for each additional month; a two-week intensive review course offered twice a year, tuition $100; a six-month professional course, tuition $250; a roentgen-ray course; a dissection course; a first-aid course, and a variety of combinations of courses at fancy prices. All these courses, with anything else available, are thrown together into a cum laude course running through thirty-two months and "lumped off" to the student for the round sum of $1,000. These various colleges and courses, with all their associated clinics, are conducted on this one floor and in the four additional rooms mentioned...

...There is no endowment, but expenses are paid out of the income from tuitions, laboratory fees, graduation fees, and fees from examinations and semiprivate clinic treatments...

...This school claimed "approximately 350 students" in 1926. It now reports about 200, and this number doubtless includes post-graduates. These students lack enthusiasm. A large percentage of the school's recent graduates failed to pass the state board examinations. The students seen in laboratory, classroom and clinics move slowly, as if neither busy nor deeply interested; one of them, when asked, "How do you like it here?" replied, "Pretty well," but with an indifference that reflected doubt on even that mild statement.

...A small chemical laboratory on the first floor is used by interns only (that is, for work on clinic patients by graduate students). In this laboratory were seen the usual paraphernalia, including a microscope and a four-tube centrifuge. In the basement, in a large but poorly lighted room, were desks capable of accommodating about fifty students in chemistry. This laboratory was clean and in good order, with a profusion of reagent bottles and a number of Bunsen burners arranged on the desks. The equipment seen, however, was all for elementary work. No microscopes, distillation flasks, Kjeldahl apparatus, kymographs, nor anything else indicating even the occasional doing of advanced work in chemistry or physiology was seen either here or anywhere else in the building, though there was an evident desire to impress the visitor favorably. In cases near the entrance to this laboratory were a number of jars containing well mounted and well preserved pathologic specimens.

8. Dissection Room. - This room, also in the basement, was small, poorly lighted and poorly ventilated. It contained six tables, each holding a cadaver or the remains of one, and covered with a white cloth. Permission was given to examine this material. All of it had been allowed to deteriorate quite markedly from dehydration. None of it presented any carefully dissected structures. The bodies had been skinned and an attempt made to work out a few muscles, but no blood vessels had been followed and no nerves traced...

9. Roentgen-Ray Room. - In this room was roentgen-ray equipment of the most modern type, such as any high-grade technician might be justly proud of. The visitor was told that "it cost thousands of dollars and was hard to get because the medical men had a corner on it, but the school was able to get it for the students"...

11. Library. - When it was intimated that the tour of inspection was finished, the visitor requested that he be shown the library. The school catalogue contains a picture of this room, with the subscription, "The only one of its kind in the country, this library contains over 1,000 volumes." But his request elicited the astounding reply: "There ain't no library." Half doubting this statement, he inquired of a graduate student later, and was told the library was in the private office of one of the faculty members; no willingness to show it was manifested, and the visitor considered it unwise to insist.

12. Matriculation Requirements. - The visitor...was told that high school graduation or its equivalent was required of all students, but that one who had had no high school work whatever could easily gain the equivalent certificate by attending a quiz course two evenings weekly during the first six months of his chiropractic study and then passing an examination. "It isn't hard," said the registrar. "Nobody fails, and you don't need to worry about that at all."

13. Course. - The course is eighteen months long, and is so arranged that one may begin any day. "No matter what day you begin," said the registrar, "you will come round to that same point again at the end of eighteen months"...

Conclusions. - The conclusions are self-evident. 1. This school receives students who have no educational foundation. 2. It gives a course of training (a) under instructors not qualified to teach, (b) with equipment hopelessly inadequate, (c) with an all too meager supply of clinical material, and (d) reaching over a period entirely too short to qualify the most brilliant mind or the most skilful hand for the work of a physician. 3. It charges an exorbitant price for the service it claims to render. 4. Its graduates are not and cannot be healers of the sick, though they are taught to pose as such and so become a menace to the public health. 5. Such an institution is a disgrace, and it can best serve the public interest by quietly going out of existence (Schools, 1928).

Chapter 7

BASIC SCIENCE LAWS AND THEIR IMPACT

The American College of Chiropractors' (1927) emphasis on the impropriety of having medical doctors examine chiropractors for licensure was intended to ward off not only the threat of composite boards of examiners (e.g., those composed of M.D.s, D.O.s and D.C.s), but also to counteract the budding threat of basic science legislation. Political medicine had been unsuccessful in stemming the tide of legalized chiropractic; Turner (1931, pp. 292-3) noted that:

> By 1922 eleven supreme courts had upheld the legality of chiropractic boards....By October 1922, 22 states had established chiropractic examining boards and their legality had been upheld by eleven supreme courts. Other supreme court decisions had declared that the practice of chiropractic was not the practice of medicine....More than 15,000 prosecutions against chiropractors are said to have occurred in the United States during the first thirty years of chiropractic.

Table 7-1: Passage and revocation of basic science laws in the USA; jurisdictions are listed in chronological order of passage of the legislation (see also Table 19-1)

Passage & Revocation	Jurisdiction
1925-1975	Wisconsin
1925-1975	Connecticut
1927-1974	Minnesota
1927-1975	Nebraska
1927-1979	Washington
1929-1977	Arkansas
1929-1978	District of Columbia
1933-1973	Oregon
1935-1973	Iowa
1936-1968	Arizona
1937-1973	Oklahoma
1937-1976	Colorado
1937-1972	Michigan
1939-1967	Florida
1939-1975	South Dakota
1940-1971	Rhode Island
1941-1968	New Mexico
1943-1976	Tennessee
1946-1970	Alaska
1949-1979	Texas
1951-1975	Nevada
1957-1969	Kansas
1959-1979	Utah
1959-1975	Alabama

Unsuccessful in blocking chiropractic legislation, the medical community sought new strategies to prevent the licensing of doctors whom they considered "quacks." The expanded criticisms of chiropractic schools in the 1920s (Brennan, 1983; Cooper, 1985) coincided with the introduction of basic science laws (see Table 7-1), beginning in Connecticut and Wisconsin in 1925 (Gevitz, 1988; Keating & Rehm, 1993; Sauer, 1932). These regulations required that applicants for licensure in any of the healing arts (chiropractic, naturopathy, osteopathy, medicine) must first pass examinations in such fundamental topics as anatomy, bacteriology, hygiene, physiology, pathology, public health, and, in at least two states (Connecticut and Wisconsin), diagnosis (Adams, 1957). Although organized medicine was often successful in convincing state legislatures that such tests were intended only to raise the quality of health care and were common subjects for all healers, the irregular practitioners (i.e., D.C.s, D.O.s, N.D.s) complained bitterly that political medicine's specific and stated intent was to eliminate all competition (Gevitz, 1988; Sauer, 1932). Indeed, this intent and its effects were acknowledged later by elements within the medical community:

> ...The evident original purpose of enacting basic science laws as a prerequisite for licensure in the healing arts was to exclude chiropractors and other inadequately trained practitioners from being admitted to licensure. The number of chiropractors before basic science boards is decreasing each year (Bierring, 1948).

Ironically, the medical community's campaign to introduce a basic science barrier to chiropractic licensing received public support as a consequence of a medical "diploma-selling ring in Missouri" (Gevitz, 1988). The scam, which was exposed through the undercover investigations by *St. Louis Star* reporter Harry Brundidge and was featured in his newspaper and nationally in *Collier's Magazine*, had resulted in the licensing of hundreds of educationally unqualified medical practitioners, especially in Connecticut (Gevitz, 1988; Ring, 1923). Repeal of basic science legislation in those states which implemented it came about only when the medical community itself became frustrated with the system (Gevitz, 1988).

In some states the basic science examinations covered subjects that were directly related to the practice of medicine and surgery, and therefore not appropriate for practitioners of the "drugless" healing arts. Further, an equitable administration of the exams was often lacking (Sauer, 1932). Although the particular discipline of the basic science examinee was supposed to remain concealed from the test administrators, applicants from "unorthodox" professions were known to the examiners, who were themselves often medically trained or were Ph.D. biologists recruited from the medical schools of state universities. This sentiment was expressed by broad-scope professional leader Benjamin A. Sauer, D.C., of New York in a confidential report to leaders of the National Chiropractic Association:

> ....if the Basic Sciences are Basic Sciences, as the medical profession contends, and if all should be equally grounded in them and have the same viewpoint regarding them, why the fear of who should conduct the examination? Likewise, if the medical profession fears to take an examination in the Basic Sciences conducted by anyone other than themselves, haven't members of any other profession an equal right to fear discrimination at the hands of examiners made up of or influenced by physicians? If it is unfair for a Chiropractor or Osteopath to examine a medical practitioners, it is likewise unfair for a medical practitioner to examine an Osteopath or Chiropractor, whose science they are not familiar with.... (Sauer, 1932).

Sylva Ashworth, a 1910 Palmer graduate and president of the Nebraska Board of Chiropractic Examiners, was no less furious about the intent and effects of basic science legislation:

> ...the basic science law in Nebraska has been very detrimental to chiropractic. We have not had a single new chiropractor in the state since the basic science law went into effect. There have been five applicants for admission, but all failed, which was nothing more than we expected. I have been told that one member of the board said that no chiropractor should pass the board while he was on it. Of course that is the intention of the law. Any teacher knows that they can fail anyone. It is not a question of qualification or training (Ashworth, 1928).

While the intent of organized medicine in introducing basic science legislation was to exclude chiropractors and other "irregular" practitioners from legal practice, criticisms of the education of drugless doctors were often valid. The shortcomings of chiropractic schools in teaching the basic sciences, even those with obvious relevance to the D.C., were numerous. As late as 1933, graduates of the PSC lost the right to sit for the examination as drugless practitioners in the Canadian province of Ontario because of their lack of training in anatomy by dissection at the Davenport institution (Biggs, 1989, section 5.4).

Basic science examinations wrought havoc on the chiropractic profession and its schools. As noted earlier, Metz (1965, p. 100) reported that not a single chiropractor passed the basic science barrier in Nebraska from the time of the law's implementation in 1929 until 1950; accordingly, no examinations in chiropractic could be administered by the state's Board of Chiropractic Examiners, and no new chiropractic licenses could be issued. New chiropractic licenses in Minnesota dropped from an average of 39 during 1922-1926 to 1.4 during 1927-1937, a direct consequence of Minnesota's basic science law (Gevitz, 1988). Similar figures were found in other states; chiropractors were distinctly disadvantaged relative to allopaths and osteopaths (see Table 7-2).

Health Care Discipline	# Taking Examination	# Passed	% Passed
Chiropractic	135	36	26.6
Osteopathy	229	145	63.4
Medicine	3697	3313	89.6

Table 7-2: Success in passing basic science examinations in seven states during 1927-1932; from Gevitz (1988).

However, in the mid-1920s the basic science threat was still new, and in many states the legal struggle between chiropractors and medicine continued to center around the passage of licensing legislation. Chiropractic leaders, several of whom had questioned the utility of seeking any chiropractic licensing (e.g., Palmer, 1918), had since come out squarely for legislation. Ironically, the compromise which gave rise to the first chiropractic law in Connecticut was based on the passage of a basic science examination requirement as a stipulation. John J. Nugent, D.C. (see Figure 7-1), a 1922 Palmer graduate and future Director of Education for the broad-scope National Chiropractic Association (Gibbons, 1985), repeatedly scrapped with leaders of the straight chiropractic schools. He was no stranger to chiropractic orthodoxy, having been expelled by B.J. from the PSC in 1922, and reinstated by "faculty action" (PSC, 1921-22). Nugent noted in later years that it was his intervention at the state house which had created the first chiropractic statute in Connecticut, and that he had written the draft of the state's basic science law that was eventually enacted. Not surprisingly, this claim brought him much grief; speaking at a Cleveland Chiropractic College homecoming in Kansas City in 1949 he noted that:

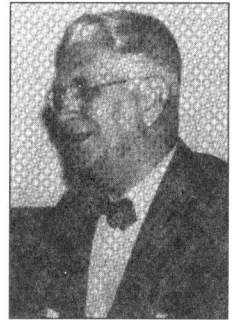

Figure 7-1: John J. Nugent, D.C.

> I'm not for Basic Science Boards. I've been accused in this State of being for Basic Science Boards, and my words have been distorted — twisted — taken out of context...I made that statement before Congress, I said that I had written the Basic Science act in Connecticut. And I did. I wrote it. I wrote it on my own little typewriter. Why? Because there had been a terrific scandal in the eclectic profession and a man had been killed on an operating table and the whole state of Conn. was in furor, and nineteen ?prefectors? in the State demanded some sort of qualifications for all practitioners, and Liberty magazine and Colliers were writing articles about Conn. and when I saw the powers that be they said, "Now look Doctor, we're supposed to be political leaders in this state but we can't stem this tide. There's got to be some sort of device. The State Chamber of Commerce, Kiwanis Club and all the Civic Clubs were up in arms about it and we were going to get a Basic Science Law. So I said to Mr. Roarback, who was the political boss of the State who was a Chiropractic patient — I said to him, "Well, if we have to have the damn thing then let's have a fair one." He said, "Can you write such a bill," and I said "yes." And I wrote that bill. I put it in my pocket and that's the Bill that came out. Yes I wrote that thing — and I wish that I'd had an opportunity to write every other one of the Basic Science bills too (Cleveland, 1949).

Within the chiropractic profession opposition to basic science laws was almost but not quite universal, and the most vocal critics were the leaders of the professional associations and the owners of the for-profit schools. Basic science laws threatened to shrivel the ranks of the profession, to dry up student enrollments and to force costly curricular changes that the proprietary training institutions were not prepared to make. The basic science laws also seemed to mandate instruction in topics that many straight chiropractic college and professional leaders considered anti-chiropractic or "medical" in character, such as diagnosis, chemistry and microbiology. Occasionally (e.g., in Arkansas), the chiropractic board of examiners ignored the basic science act and licensed chiropractors who had not taken the examination (Gevitz, 1988).

Not all leaders in the chiropractic community were as strongly opposed to the basic science laws as were B.J. Palmer and the straight chiropractic community. Chiropractor Julius A. Acquaviva suggested that "inadequate training in fundamental science, combined with lack of standardization of chiropractic courses, retards progress in the science of chiropractic" (Acquaviva, 1934). C.O. Watkins, D.C., founder in 1935 of the National Chiropractic Association's (NCA's) Committee on Education, initially referred to the "damnatory Basic Science laws" (Watkins, 1934), but his attitude softened in future years as basic science legislation increasingly aided the educational reform efforts of the NCA. Similarly, school presidents such as Homer G. Beatty of the University of Natural Healing Arts in Denver, Ralph J. Martin of the Southern California College of Chiropractic and later the LACC, and W.A. Budden of Western States (see Figure 7-2)

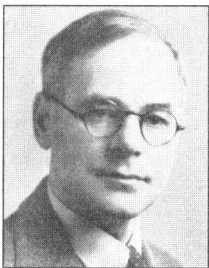

Figure 7-2: W.A. Budden, D.C., N.D., dean of the National College of Chiropractic, 1926-29

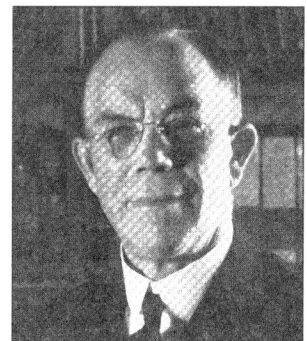

Figure 7-3: W.C. Schulze, M.D., D.C., president of the National College from 1918 to 1936

eventually relaxed as their institutions succeeded in preparing chiropractors to master the required fundamental subjects (Beatty, 1940; Gatterman, 1982; Martin, 1986). William C. Schulze, president of the National College in Chicago (see Figure 7-3), and National's dean during 1926-1929, William A. Budden, were of similar minds. The National College formula for dealing with the basic science threat was expressed in the school's journal:

FOUR WAYS TO BEAT THE BASIC SCIENCE LAW

1. Study Basic Scienc

2. Study Basic Science

3. Study Basic Science

and

4. Study Basic Science (National, 1928)

Chapter 8

SCOPE OF PRACTICE DISPUTES

Organized medicine's introduction of the basic science barrier to licensure for chiropractors commenced during a period of intense in-fighting among the D.C.s. At the end of the first World War the Universal Chiropractors' Association (UCA), at B.J. Palmer's direction, had begun to alienate a significant segment of the profession through the vehicle of its "Model Bill" and its 1921 creation of a National Board of Chiropractic Examiners (NBCE). The NBCE sought to enforce Palmer's ideas for the chiropractic curriculum (see Chapter 4), such as limiting coursework to 18 months (Keating & Rehm, 1993). These actions were at variance with the ideas of a growing number of chiropractic educators. For example, G.A. Fisk, D.C., editor of the LACC's journal, *The Chirogram*, noted his misgivings about Palmer's resistance to improving chiropractic educational standards:

> One of the finest articles it has been our pleasure to read for many a day was contained in the N.C.C. Journal recently, the author Dr. A.L. Forster. The subject was the necessity of raising the standards of chiropractic education, particularly the pre-chiropractic educational requirements. Some oppose this step. We shall try to believe that their motives are sincere.
>
> That the early pioneers in Chiropractic did not possess a high-school education or its equivalent is no argument to be applied to the present situation. As Dr. Forster aptly states, in those days it was chiropractic that was subjected to a test. Because of its inherent merit, that method has won the public confidence to an extent that assures it a place in the healing art for all time. Now, however, it is not chiropractic but chiropractors who are under examination by the public.
>
> The fact that Chiropractic has won recognition in many states of the Union, instead of assuring it a protected future, as so many seem to assume, is, in fact, the greatest menace to its perpetuation. Herein Dr. BJ Palmer concurs, for he has consistently displayed in his utterances and writings a note of doubt as to the ultimate value of legal recognition to chiropractic. However, we believe his reason for believing so is incorrect. He is against raising the pre-chiropractic educational requirements because he evidently fears it will cut down the output of chiropractors, thereby permitting the opposition to maintain an eternal numerical supremacy. We believe there are enough chiropractors in the country to safeguard the privileges so far won. A sufficient number of people are believers in chiropractic to help defend those rights (Fisk, 1923).

The broad-scope element within the profession was also dissatisfied with the UCA's "cleaning house" policies (see Chapter 4), which sought to enforce "straight" standards of clinical practice. Rehm (1980, p. 279) has suggested that the UCA sought "absolute control of chiropractic's destiny" according to B.J.'s vision for the profession, and had become an "instrument of intimidation to chiropractors and the various state associations." Accordingly, in 1922 a new national membership organization was created, the American Chiropractic Association (ACA). Palmer's attitude toward the new group was predictable:

> ...The ACA, therefore, was born of opposition to the UCA and all it stood for. It was a playground for mixers who wanted the fruit of Chiropractic without earning the right to Chiropractic by helping to sustain it (Palmer, 1931a, p. 5).

Recent Palmer graduate Carl S. Cleveland, Sr. (see Figure 8-1) expressed his sentiments towards the UCA's house cleaning policies in a letter to L.S. Hunter, D.C., founder and president of the Hunter School of Chiropractic in Springfield, Missouri, and a fellow member of the Missouri State Chiropractic Association (MSCA):

> I am indeed glad to find that you have joined the M.S.C.A. Being President of an Institution, teaching Chiropractic, you are thrown into closer touch with Chiropractic problems than the ordinary practitioner. This knowledge, in itself, goes a long way toward the solution of those problems. I am glad to hear you say you stand for Straight Chiropractic. You further say that many schools and Chiropractors do not advocate straight Chiropractic, because B.J. is for it. I know this is true.
>
> However, this "Cleaning House" Campaign is too vital to the welfare of Chiropractic, not to be aided simply because a few individuals don't happen to like B.J. Palmer, who leads the movement. I am glad that you are with him. I feel that we should be with him as he stands for those principles for which you and I stand. I want to see the Chiropractic schools do well (Cleveland, 1922).

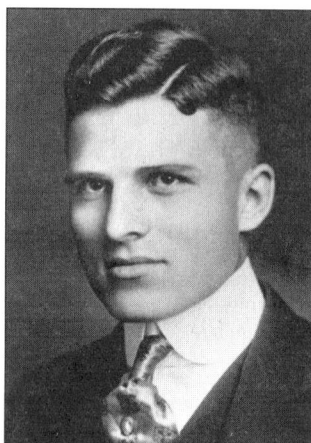

Figure 8-1: Carl S. Cleveland, D.C. in 1917

The viability of the new organization was based upon two issues: firstly, its tolerance for both "straight and "mixer" chiropractors within its ranks, and secondly, the ACA's dissociation from any particular school. Although ACA's longest serving president (1923-1929), Frank R. Margetts, LL.B., D.C., was a former instructor at the National College, the organization prided itself for its freedom from "school control":

A STATEMENT OF FACT

> Attention is called to the fact that in order to establish and keep the American Chiropractic Association as a pure democracy and safeguard it from any possible undue influence by any particular school group, it was provided in the by-laws that no officer should be a member of any Chiropractic school faculty.
>
> The officers of the American Chiropractic Association, including the President and Secretary-Treasurer, have not, since becoming officers of the A.C.A., been members of the faculty of any Chiropractic college or school, and are not now members of any such faculty (Sauer, 1925).

Apparently in response to the ACA's 1922 formation, the UCA renewed its commitment in 1923 to "support none but straight chiropractors" (Hayes, 1931b), and in so doing, reportedly lost some 1,500 members. While the ACA began to press for higher educational standards for chiropractors, a further depletion of UCA's ranks followed Palmer's 1924 introduction of the neurocalometer (NCM) (Palmer, 1924a). Palmer heralded the paraspinal, heat-sensing, subluxation-detection device as the central feature of a "BACK-TO-CHIROPRACTIC-NEUROCALOMETER-MOVEMENT" (Keating, 1991a), and predicted it would force mixer chiropractors to adhere to B.J.'s notion of straight chiropractic. The president of the PSC justified the $2,200 cost for a 10-year lease on the NCM by noting that he could have kept the instrument an exclusive selling point for his own school:

> ....keep it as a school trade secret, and make the world come to us...We knew that we could keep this a ONE-SCHOOL-DAVENPORT-IOWA-P.S.C.-SEVENTEEN-COUNTRY-MONOPOLY....We knew that would destroy confidence in you, because we would be here the sole purveyors of that service to 17 countries....Why, I could have built a hospital here.....That would have meant millions to me, but it would have meant total ruination to you (applause), for which I have been everywhere cursed as a grafter... (Palmer, 1924a, pp. 8-9).

Instead, he suggested, his leasing plan for the NCM was going to eliminate incompetent (i.e., "mixer") doctors from the profession, that is, the majority of the profession who were not practicing subluxation-only and adjustment-only chiropractic:

...the LEASE PLAN. This plan restricts the leases exclusively to chiropractors. It limits the number of sales to our profession. It limits it to but a limited percentage of our profession, for all are not competent or qualified....This will cull about 5,000 good out of 20,000, and lease a substantial number of competent and qualified chiropractors to construct a professional house that would be worth living in (applause), where we think and talk the same language and feel acquainted on the same subject... (Palmer, 1924a, p. 10-11).

Palmer likened the chiropractic profession to a cow. He suggested that he had been feeding the cow for many years, while the "mixers" had been working the other end of the beast and skimming all the cream. He asked whether he could not now have a glass of milk, and denied charges that the NCM program was merely a ruse to increase his wealth. His was a campaign to "save chiropractic," and what was good for B.J. and the Palmer School, he suggested, was good for chiropractic:

You know we will make money on the Neurocalometer. I will be absolutely frank with you. We will make money on the Neurocalometer, but I promise you here and now to continue doing just what I have always done, to put every dollar we make on the Neurocalometer back into Chiropractic to feed the cow. Make me rich and Chiropractic profits. We will but make it all over into a better, bigger, busier Chiropractic and safer and saner chiropractors (Palmer, 1924a, p. 35).

The ACA president's reaction to the PSC/UCA/NCM program was swift, and revealed the indignation felt by many:

Does Chiropractic Need a Saviour?

In all generations in every worthwhile movement there have been well meaning individuals who have constituted themselves saviours of something which they deemed needed saving. Much of the misunderstanding that has arisen in the profession of chiropractic has come about through the misdirected zeal of those who believed that chiropractic needed to be saved, and that it could survive only in the event that they did the heroic thing of playing the role of saviour.

Chiropractic needs neither a saviour, a guardian, nor a nurse....

Chiropractic leaders may come and they may go, but chiropractic will survive them all. If we need decisive, conclusive evidence of its vitality, all we need to do is to remember the fanaticism, bigotry, intolerance and malignancy that has existed in chiropractic circles almost from its birth, and yet today it is stronger than ever...

So let us eliminate one of the prolific causes of factionalism and animosity in our profession, by discontinuing the assertions that we are doing this thing or that thing with the motive of saving chiropractic (Margetts, 1924).

For his part, B.J. seems not to have fully appreciated at first the depth of dissatisfaction that his NCM campaign created in the field. He preferred to interpret the reaction his marketing program precipitated as another example of chiropractors being slow to appreciate the significance of his technological innovations:

TIMES CHANGE MEN

How well and vividly do I remember, a few years back, when the X-Ray was introduced to detect the correct POSITION of vertebrae, both normal and abnormal, in alignment and in subluxations.

The field split on the question. A few saw its value and began to take it up at once. Some of THE FIELD held off and waited "to see." Today - some 13 years later - it is an accepted form of technique by the entire field. Few chiropractors but what are for it.

The schools split. On one side - THE PSC. On the other side - ALL OTHER schools. Loban became bitterly opposed, and wrote much against this 'form of mixing.' Forster wrote much and said much more against its use. Other schools took much the same attitude, all trying to stem the tide of the new movement, not because the movement was wrong, BUT BECAUSE ONE B.J. PALMER ADVOCATED IT. Today - some 13 years later - Loban writes for Spinography, teaches it, uses it, advocates it. Today - some 13 years later - Forster puts it first in value to detect subluxations.

> Now comes the Neurocalometer idea. Loban is neither for nor forninst, he is riding both waves, ready to jump either way that proves to be the most popular. Forster will come too on this the same as they did on Spinography. They move upward only as the field forces them to come in.
>
> Times certainly do change men, but with some it takes a long, long time! (Palmer, 1924b)

With the advantage of hindsight, the reaction to Palmer's NCM program seems predictable. Membership in the UCA was further depleted, while the ACA grew correspondingly. Student enrollments at the PSC plummeted, and Palmer was encouraged to resign as secretary of the UCA at the organization's 1925 meeting in Chicago, which he did (Turner, 1931, pp. 177-80). The ACA renewed its commitment to remain "free from school strings" and free from the "rule or ruin policy of the Palmer-UCA combination" (Lee, 1927). Disaffection was also soon apparent from the non-PSC leaders of the UCA, such as Craig M. Kightlinger (1925), president of the Eastern Chiropractic Institute in New York City, and vice-president of the UCA. Kightlinger resigned in protest from his office and from membership in the organization, and elected to join the ACA. His letter of resignation was published in the ACA's *Bulletin*:

> After due consideration and weighing of all the facts I find it necessary that I tender my resignation as Vice-President of the UCA for the following reasons:-
>
> First - That I cannot longer agree with nor follow the policies of the Association.
>
> Second - That I feel it best for any chiropractic organization, that an officer of a school should not hold an executive office.
>
> Third - That Chiropractic should be organized along entirely different lines, making the State Associations the unit and calling at some different point each year a general convention of delegates selected from the unit membership.
>
> Fourth - That Chiropractic be placed in a more favorable position before the public, by adhering to the basic principles of the science, by discarding all mechanical devices that tend to lessen the efficiency of the palpater (Kightlinger, 1925).

Kightlinger played no formal role in the governance of the ACA, but he did serve as a spokesperson for those former Palmer followers who had fallen away from B.J., the self-styled "Developer" of the profession:

> ....We cannot forget the many trying times that the developer of our science went through to keep it alive and to bring it to a point where it could stand on its feet. To him we owe more than we can ever repay and to him is due the fact that the Science of Chiropractic is where it is today. He took us through the Dark Ages of the development, but now the time has come when once again the Natural Law must be taken into account and the leader of old must either sit at the council table and consult with the minds of the many or take his place on the side lines and let the march of Progress pass. We need him but we need as much and more the ideas that result from the clear thinking of the interested members of our profession. We must have the cool logic of the best minds and the greatest brains of the entire profession. The dictates of the one, no matter how sincere and honest they may be, can serve no more....It is not the nicest spectacle to see the old leader of the herd beaten and his leadership taken by a younger and stronger opponent and it is not the most pleasant thought to know that, sooner or later, the old leader must place his mantle on the shoulders of the best minds of the many. It is a fact and facts must be faced....
>
> There is nothing the matter with Chiropractic. There is a great deal the matter with Chiropractors. They have never been used to thinking for themselves. The time has arrived when they must think for themselves and must lead themselves, or they will go the way of all who oppose the progress of Natural Law and be forced into oblivion.... (Kightlinger, 1928).

The NCM debacle also hurt Palmer at home, when five of the school's faculty men departed the PSC during 1925-26: Drs. James N. Firth, Harry E. Vedder, Stephen J. Burich, Arthur E. Hinrichs [later renamed Hendricks] and Ernest A. Thompson (Keating & Rehm, 1993; Stowell, 1983). Although it has been suggested that the principal reason for their departure was dissatisfaction that B.J. had not more thoroughly informed them about the NCM's development (Quigley, 1989), there appears to be some agreement that the schism had more to do with Palmer's restrictions on academic freedom at the school (Keating, 1990b, 1992b; Marsh, 1991; Peters, 1992), restrictions involving NCM instruction at the PSC. In 1926 four of the above five organized the Lincoln Chiropractic College of Indianapolis (Stowell, 1983).

Although Palmer's insistence on the use of his instrument alienated many straight chiropractors, it did not lessen the passionate disagreements among straights and mixers. By the early 1930s, as Palmer introduced further practice and training dicta (e.g., instruction in Hole-in-One technique, later renamed Upper Cervical Specific), these disputes reached a new level of intensity. Stanley Hayes, D.C., editor of the *Bulletin of the West Virginia Chiropractors' Society*, suggested that "The schools have spoken. The radically straight chiropractor is doomed to extinction. The profession is definitely committed to broader drugless practice" (Hayes, 1931a). Hayes' editorial was reprinted in the LACC's house organ, the *Chirogram*, and served to fuel the already ferocious antagonisms between the straights and mixers, especially between the LACC and the Ratledge School of Los Angeles.

Chapter 9

THE INTERNATIONAL CHIROPRACTIC CONGRESS

With Palmer's departure from the UCA and formation of the Chiropractic Health Bureau, many anticipated a quick amalgamation of the UCA and the ACA. However, the old politics would not die quietly, and not until late in 1930 did the NCA, product of the union of these two membership organizations, make its debut. Part of the impetus for this merger was the successful operations of the International Chiropractic Congress (ICC), a federation of chiropractic organizations. The ICC had begun as the International Congress of Chiropractic Examining Boards (ICCEB) at a meeting called by Harry Gallaher, D.C., of the Oklahoma board, and held in Kansas City in 1926 (Carver, 1936, p. 156; Sauer, 1927; The International, 1927; Turner, 1931). Like the ACA, the Congress prided itself upon its independence from the influence of any particular chiropractic school, and may have been interested in regulating the colleges through licensing requirements (Turner, 1931, p. 168). The second meeting of the ICCEB, held in September 1927 in Memphis, attracted seven school leaders and several state association presidents, and called for state boards to seek licensing reciprocity among the states (Crider, 1936; Keating & Rehm, 1993). Meanwhile, the ACA created a "Board of Counselors to be composed of the Deans of the Chiropractic Schools and Colleges" during its 1927 convention (Bulletin, 1927). The third meeting of the ICCEB, held in Chicago in 1928, produced the expanded ICC, consisting of three divisions: licensing boards, state associations and schools (Metz, 1965, pp. 54-5).

When the ACA and UCA merged in 1930 to form the National Chiropractic Association (NCA) (see Figure 9-1), it became affiliated with the ICC, and the two organizations co-sponsored Loran M. Rogers' *Journal of the International Chiropractic Congress* (*JICC*; 1931-32) and its successor, NCA's *The Chiropractic Journal* (1933-63). However, by this time, the good works of the Congress were widely acknowledged, and NCA's involvement in the Congress was not a liability. Indeed, despite the long history of feuding among school leaders and alumni, the ICC schools division had, by 1932, involved college leaders from all corners of the chiropractic educational landscape (see Table 9-1). The PSC was represented at the ICC's 1932 convention in Kansas City by A.B. Hender, its dean. For a few years, T.F. Ratledge of Los Angeles attended ICC meetings and advertised his school in the *JICC* and *The Chiropractic Journal*. Carl S. Cleveland, Sr., president of the straight college in Kansas City which carries his name, served during 1931-32 as president of the ICC's Division Three: the International Congress of Chiropractic Educational Institutions (ICCEI; Keating & Cleveland, 1996). Henry C. Harring of the Missouri Chiropractic College served as secretary of the ICCEI during Cleveland's presidency. When Willard Carver succeeded Cleveland as president of the ICCEI, he noted that the ICC had created "a greater fraternal feeling among school and college heads, state examiners and the officers of state associations" (Turner, 1931, pp. 264-5). Such fraternal sentiments existed despite the ICC's avowed intention to:

> ....investigate all institutions teaching chiropractic and to maintain supervision over their work. Since many of the leading educators are active in the congress and its subsidiary organizations, this standardizing experiment is expected to bring notable results....The ICC has found it expedient to give temporary recognition to all schools having adequate courses, pending personal inspection by representatives of the congress....This open-mindedness has been demonstrated in numerous ways, particularly in extending membership to the National School of Chiropractic of Chicago despite the fact of its doctors being admitted to the county hospital under the medical banner... (Turner, 1931, pp. 216-7).

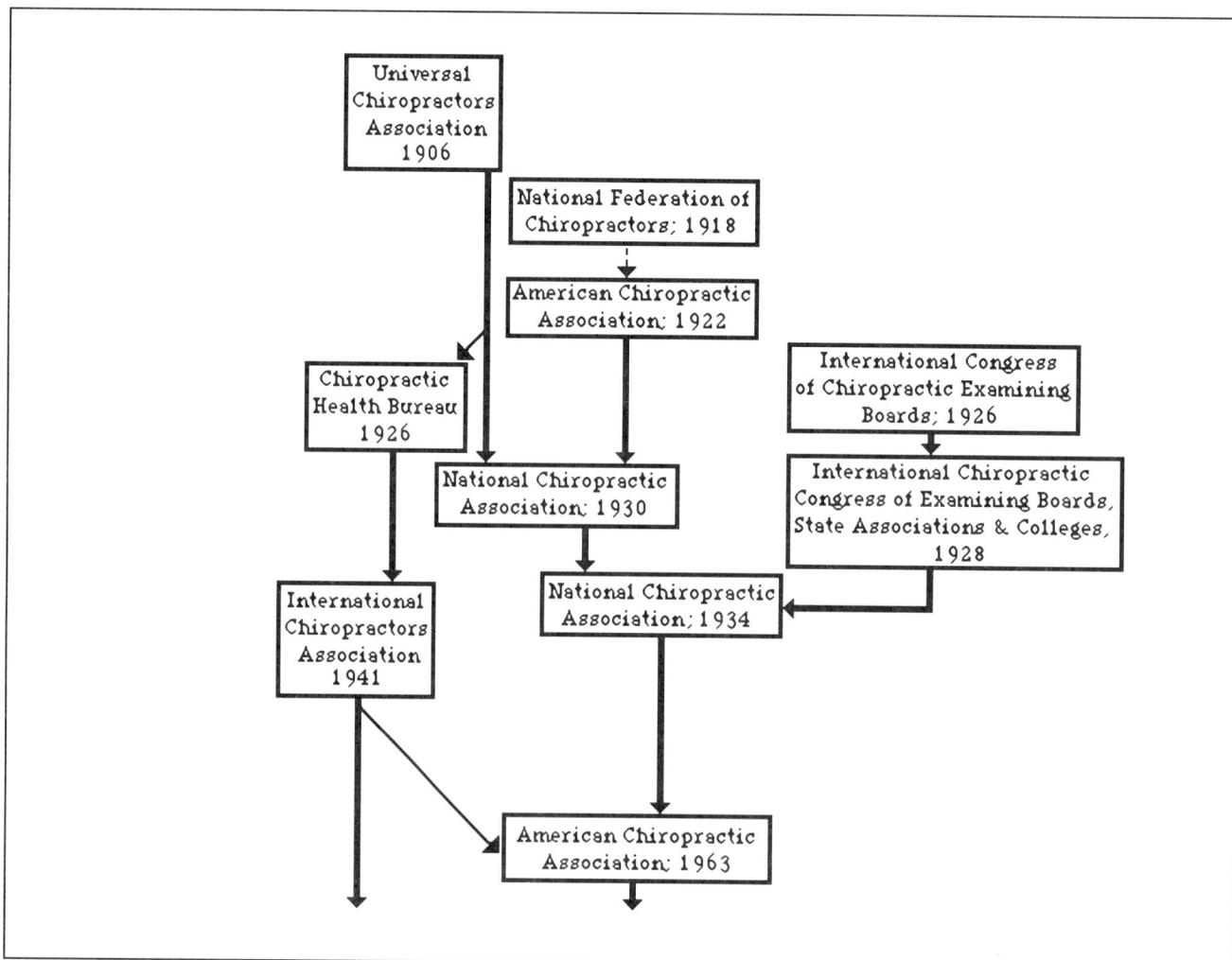

Figure 9-1: Mergers and developments that produced the ICA and today's ACA. Dates indicate founding, merging and re-organization; question marks indicate uncertain dates; diagonal arrows suggest splinter groups. The broken line between the National Federation of Chiropractors and the ACA suggests the tenuous continuity between these two organizations. Adapted from Keating & Rehm (1993) by permission of the *Journal of the Canadian Chiropractic Association.*

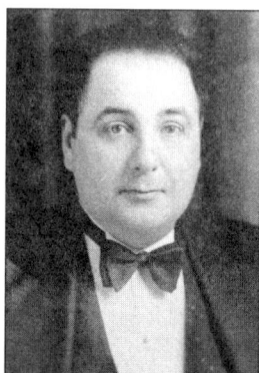

Figure 9-2: James E. Slocum, D.C., c1933

Loran Rogers, D.C., who took over from Sauer as executive secretary of the NCA in 1932, was responsible for part of the good will that the Congress generated. His periodical, the *JICC*, was impressive for its time, and created a sense of pride among chiropractors. By early 1932 the *JICC*'s circulation had reached 12,000, and presumably reached every D.C. in the country. The journal's headquarters were located in Webster City, Iowa, where Rogers had purchased (circa 1918) the practice of Carl Cleveland. Webster City was also home to James E. Slocum, D.C., president of the ICC (see Figure 9-2). The Iowa hamlet became the national home of the NCA for all of its remaining years (i.e., until the formation of today's ACA in 1963).

As the NCA became ever more active and gradually attracted a larger membership, the ICC receded in importance. Many of the Congress' leaders were also officers and representatives in the NCA; Ernest J. Smith, D.C., president of the Metropolitan Chiropractic College in Cleveland, Ohio, expressed the sentiments many felt when he recommended amalgamation of NCA and ICC in order to avoid "reduplication of effort and expense" (Smith, 1932). With the

American School of Chiropractic, New York NY	Missouri Chiropractic College, St. Louis MO
Carver College of Chiropractic, Oklahoma City OK	National College of Chiropractic, Chicago IL
Cleveland Chiropractic College, Kansas City MO	O'Neil-Ross Chiropractic College, Fort Wayne IN
Colorado Chiropractic University, Denver CO	Pacific Chiropractic College, Portland OR
Columbia Institute of Chiropractic, New York NY	Palmer School of Chiropractic, Davenport IA
Denver Chiropractic Institute, Denver CO	Ratledge System of
Eastern Chiropractic Institute, New York NY	Chiropractic Schools, Los Angeles CA
Institute of the Science of Chiropractic, New York NY	Standard School of Chiropractic, New York NY
Lincoln Chiropractic College, Indianapolis IN	Texas Chiropractic College, San Antonio TX
Mecca College of Chiropractic, Newark NJ	Universal Chiropractic College, Pittsburgh PA
Metropolitan Chiropractic College, Cleveland OH	

Table 9-1: Member institutions of Division Three of the International Chiropractic Congress: the International Congress of Chiropractic Educational Institutions, 1932 (Journal, 1932)

1932 formation of the National Board of Chiropractic Examiners (NBCE; the second so-named organization, and not related to today's NBCE), many of the activities of the ICC were further eclipsed or duplicated. Like the ICC itself, the new NBCE was independent of any school, and seemed to fulfill the need for organization among the various state boards of chiropractic examiners. Although this second NBCE did not survive, it probably hastened the dissolution of the ICC into the NCA. By January, 1935, the ICC was no longer listed as a sponsor for Rogers' *Chiropractic Journal*. The Council of State Chiropractic Examining Boards (forerunner of today's Federation of Chiropractic Licensing Boards), organized circa 1934-35 and ostensibly independent of the NCA, continued to function in the role first established by the ICCEB. Hariman (1970, p. 35) noted that this NBCE was still operating in 1940.

Chapter 10

THE THIRD WAVE
OF CHIROPRACTIC SCHOOLS

The second quarter of the chiropractic century saw the birth, development and, in some cases, the demise of a number of schools (see Figure 10-1). Among these were the Cleveland Chiropractic College of Kansas City; Metropolitan Chiropractic College in Cleveland, Ohio; Northwestern College of Chiropractic in Minneapolis; Lincoln Chiropractic College of Indianapolis; the Cale College of Chiropractic and Cale College of Naturopathy in Los Angeles; and the re-organization of the Pacific Chiropractic College of Portland, Oregon as the non-profit Western States College, School of Chiropractic and School of Naturopathy.

Figure 10-1: Frequency distribution of chiropractic schools, 1895-1988 (Ferguson & Wiese, 1988), by permission of *Chiropractic History*

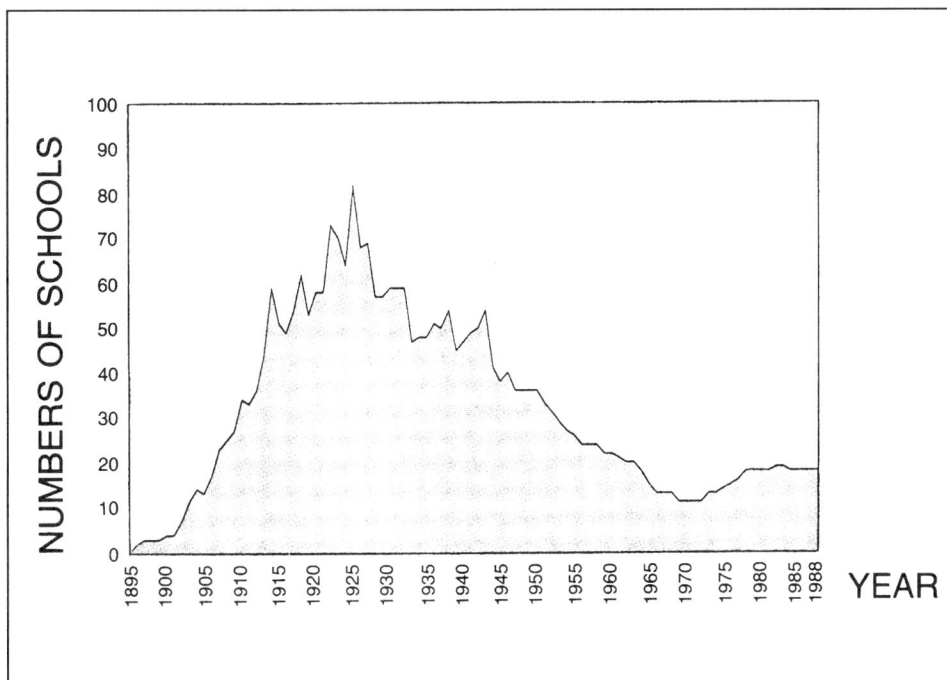

The Cale Colleges

Charles A. Cale, D.C., N.D. (see Figure 10-2) is perhaps best remembered for his 1911 founding of the LACC. However, by 1923 Cale and his wife and business partner, Linnie A. Cale, D.C., D.O., N.D., had separated, and the LACC was purchased by Charles H. Wood, D.C., N.D. in 1924. In 1925 and 1927 respectively, the former Indiana school teacher established at least two additional schools: the Cale College of Chiropractic and the Cale College of Naturopathy (Keating,

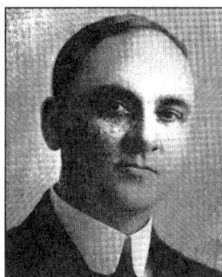

Figure 10-2: Charles A. Cale, circa 1920

Dishman et al., 1993), both of which eventually merged with the LACC. The larger of these two later additions, the Cale College of Chiropractic, earned a distinctive niche in the history of chiropractic education for its very broad scope, as suggested by its 1931-1938 renaming: the College of Chiropractic Physicians and Surgeons (see Figure 10-3).

Charles Cale earned his chiropractic degree through apprenticeship to 1901 Palmer graduate, Thomas H. Storey, D.C. In 1908 or 1909 Cale was licensed under California's naturopathic law by virtue of his membership in the state's naturopathic society. During 1914-1916 he and Linnie Cale suspended operations of the LACC to study at the College of Osteopathic Physicians and Surgeons in Los Angeles. Despite his early rhetoric to the contrary (Keating, Jackson et al., 1994), Cale was a broad-scope practitioner. His Cale College of Chiropractic, opened on April 11, 1925, in Los Angeles, reflected this "mixer" perspective, and was joined in 1927 by the Cale College of Naturopathy. An advertisement (Advertisement, 1928a) from that period indicates that both schools were intended to prepare students for licensure as chiropractors:

Cale Chiropractic Naturopathic College

One tuition pays for the entire Chiropractic Course and the entire Naturopathic Course and includes class work until you pass the Chiropractic State Board Examination and receive a license to practice. Tuition $700 in installments of $20 per month, or $600 cash.

A chance to earn your full tuition by doing office work. Free clinic day and evening.
DR. CHARLES A. CALE, D.C., N.D., President
1406 West 7th St., Los Angeles

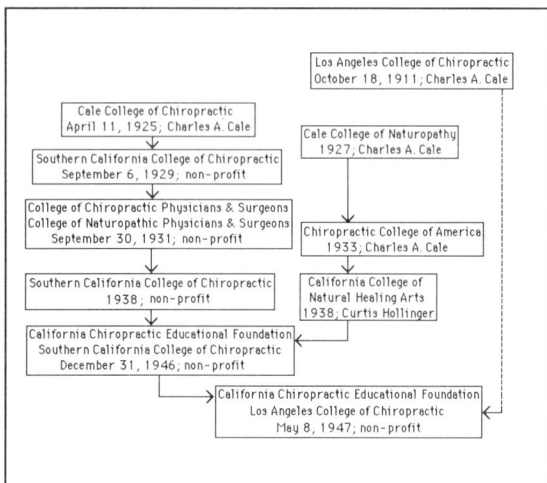

Figure 10-3: Genealogy of the three branches of today's LACC which were founded by Charles A. Cale. Broken line indicated Cale's discontinuance as president and owner after 1924.

In 1929, at about the same time that Cale acquired his chiropractic license under the terms of the 1922 Chiropractic Act he had helped to create, he re-incorporated the proprietary Cale College of Chiropractic as the non-profit Southern California College of Chiropractic (SCCC). So far as is known, the SCCC was the first non-profit chiropractic school in the state. For unknown reasons, Cale separated from the SCCC circa 1931, but continued to operate the apparently still for-profit Cale College of Naturopathy (Keating, Dishman et al., 1993); in 1933 this school was renamed the Chiropractic College of America. Following Charles Cale's death in 1938, the institution became the property of Curtis Hollinger, D.C., a 1923 graduate of the LACC.

On 30 September 1931, the SCCC was renamed the College of Chiropractic Physicians and Surgeons (CCP&S), and proceeded to train D.C.s for an even broader scope of practice than seemingly was allowed under California law. By 1933 Rangnar C. Bertheau, D.C., N.D. had assumed the presidency of the CCP&S (see Table 10-1), and served under a board of directors (see Table 10-2) who were intimately involved in the extensive political battles between straights and mixers in the state (Keating, Dishman et al., 1993). Indeed, historian Russell W. Gibbons has described California as "long a battleground for scope of practice test cases by advocates of both camps" (Gibbons, 1982). Chittenden Turner (1931, p. 143) noted the broad-scope Progressive Chiropractic Association's efforts to expand educational requirements so as to include "electro-therapy, hydro-therapy, biology, physics, minor surgery, optometry, obstetrics (including 25 bedside deliveries) and general hospital work." The International Chiropractic Congress, outraged at the state Board of Chiropractic Examiner's (BCE's) parallel efforts to expand the scope of practice, expelled the California BCE from its membership in 1930 (Brief, 1930).

In 1933, with Bertheau at the helm, the CCP&S offered a "Physicians and Surgeons Post Graduate Course" (see Table 10-3). Instruction was supplemented by training at Bellevue Hospital, a maternity facility (Gibbons, 1983). Watkins

Year*	School Name	President
1925-29	Cale College of Chiropractic	Charles A. Cale, N.D., D.C.
1929-31	Southern California College of Chiropractic	Charles A. Cale, N.D., D.C.
1933-37	College of Chiropractic Physicians & Surgeons;	R.C. Bertheau, D.C., N.D.
	College of Naturopathic Physicians & Surgeons	
1938-44?	Southern California College of Chiropractic;	Clifford B. Eacrett, D.C., N.D.
1944?-45?	Southern California College of Naturopathy	Lyle Holland, D.C., N.D.
	Southern California College of Chiropractic	
1944-46	College of Naturopathic Physicians & Surgeons/SCCC	Patrick Lackey, N.D., D.C.
1945?-47	Southern California College of Chiropractic	Ralph J. Martin, D.C., N.D.
1947	Los Angeles College of Chiropractic	Ralph J. Martin, D.C., N.D.

*Years with question marks refer to unconfirmed dates

Table 10-1: Presidents (and their terms of office) of the Cale College of Chiropractic and its descendants: Southern California College of Chiropractic, the College of Chiropractic Physicians and Surgeons, and the College of Naturopathic Physicians and Surgeons, 1925-1947. Reprinted by permission from the *Journal of Chiropractic Humanities* (1993; 3: 21-41). Years with question marks refer to unconfirmed dates.

Board of Directors
Joseph W. Gannon, D.C., N.D., Chairman
Gordon M. Goodfellow, D.C., N.D., Vice-Chairman
R. Clarke Howe, D.C., N.D., Secretary
R.C. Bertheau, D.C., N.D.
Robert J. Clayton, D.C., N.D.
E.P. Webb, D.C., N.D.
N.F. Jensen, D.C., N.D.
A.W. Jensen, D.C., N.D.
Paul F. Lasoway, D.C., N.D.
Clifford B. Eacrett, D.C., N.D.
Vinton F. Logan, D.C.
Faculty
Clyde F. Gillett, D.C., N.D.
H.A. Houde, D.C., N.D.
M.L. Hovey, D.C., N.D.
N.F. Jensen, D.C., N.D.
I.S. Kiehm, A.B., D.C., N.D.
S.M. Livingston, D.C., N.D.
Vinton F. Logan, D.C.
Alice Papa, D.C., N.D.
M.K. Shaw, D.C., N.D.
Helen Tilbury, D.C., N.D.
Paul D. VanDegrift, D.C., N.D.
L.A. von Rosenberg, D.C., N.D.

D.P. Webb, D.O.
G.N. Bartlett, O.D., D.C., N.D.
R.H. Swift, D.C., N.D.
A.F. Blair, D.C., N.D.
Floyd Cregger, D.C., N.D.
W.C. Dickson, O.D., D.C., N.D.
M.R. Mackintosh, D.C., N.D.
Administration
R.C. Bertheau, D.C., N.D., President
J.P. Mason, D.C., Dean
R.C. Howe, D.C., N.D., Comptroller
H.A. Houde, D.C., N.D., Director of Clinics
Visiting Faculty
A.J. Balkins, M.D.
Webster J. Daly, D.O.
A.R.M. Gordon, D.O.
Chas. J. Pflueger, M.D.
W.W. Sherer, M.D.
C.L. Taylor, D.O.
J.B. VanGelder, O.D., D.C., N.D.
R.C. Weiersbach, D.O.
L. Bigelman, M.D.
Ralph D. Hoard, D.O.
Lee Douglas, D.O.
R.D. Pope, M.D.

Table 10-2: Directors, faculty and administrators of the College of Chiropractic Physicians and Surgeons, according to the school's 1933-34 *Announcement* (College, 1934)

(1932a) noted that the post-graduate curriculum of the CCP&S involved four class hours per day, thereby allowing practicing doctors to care for their patients. The post-graduate program's purpose may have involved the expectation that the California Chiropractic Act could be modified or amended to approach a physician-surgeon role for the chiropractor. The school's 1934 Announcement described the post-graduate program:

> An advanced course in medicine and surgery extending over a period of two years is open to graduate Chiropractors, who desire to increase their knowledge of therapeutics and who can present to the College Credential Committee proper credentials of having completed a one-year course of college grade physics, chemistry and biology.

> At the completion of this course, the Chiropractor is in a position to intelligently give advice when called upon to do so. Surgery and surgical specialties are taught in such a manner that the student learns to distinguish cases which do and which do not require surgical care. The general management of surgical cases with the possibilities and disadvantages of surgical methods are made clear, but students are not expected, during the regular course, to become qualified as surgical specialists.

By 1938 (see Figure 10-4) the CCP&S had returned to its earlier name, the SCCC, and was located at Ninth and Union in Los Angeles. Robert W. Dishman, D.C., N.D., M.A. (SCCC 1942) recalls that:

...The "campus" was the second floor of a two-story building; the first floor was taken up by a one-pharmacist drugstore. The clinic, he recalls, was "equipped with standard physical therapy as well as surgical diathermy, cautery, dessication and hyfrecation devices. Examination rooms included obstetrical and gynecologic tables with all the appropriate instruments." However, lecture facilities were rather more limited. One main classroom accommodated all students, freshmen through seniors, and everyone sat through the same lectures, regardless of progress through the curriculum. Several small laboratories for chemistry and dissection filled the building with unsavory aromas (Keating, Dishman et al., 1993).

Table 10-3: Courses comprising the 2,060 hour curriculum of the CCP&S' post-graduate course for chiropractic "physicians and surgeons" (College, 1934)

Subjects	Hours
Biochemistry	180
Advanced Pathology, Bacteriology, Immunology	220
Surgery:	
First Aid	11
Principles of Surgery	55
General Surgery and Surgical Diagnosis	121
Urology	52
Otorhinolaryngology	44
Ophthalmology	44
Laboratory Surgery	64
Surgery Orthopedics	33
Surgery Fractures and Dislocations	22
Surgery Neoplasms	11
Clinical Chiropractic Surgery	154
Bone and Joint Surgery	39
Anesthesiology	50
Pharmacology	200
General Medicine:	
Nervous and Mental, Neurology, Psychiatry	90
Dermatology, Syphilology	69
Pediatrics	133
Gastroenterology and Proctology	140
Heart Diseases	25
Respiratory and Circulatory Diseases	55
Communicable Diseases	55
Endocrinology, Metabolic and Blood Diseases	60
Radiographic X-ray and Diagnosis	33
Advanced Obstetrics and Gynecology	100
Total	2,060

Table 10-3: Courses comprising the 2060 hour curriculum of the CCP&S post-graduate course for chiropractic "physicians and surgeons" (College, 1934)

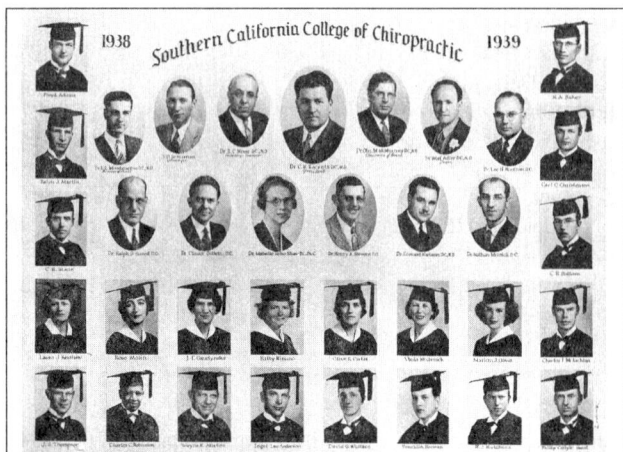

Figure 10-4: Faculty, administration and graduating class of the Southern California College of Chiropractic in 1938-39

Among the better remembered faculty and board members of the CCP&S were Floyd Cregger, D.C., N.D., Gordon M. Goodfellow, D.C., N.D. and Vinton F. Logan, D.C. Cregger became a political leader in the state, and served as president of the NCA during 1946-47. Goodfellow, who was elected vice-president of the NCA at its historic 1935 meeting in Hollywood and as president the following year, served for many years on the board of directors of the LACC following the 1947 merger of the LACC and the SCCC. He was also a central player in the NCA's mid-1930s efforts to upgrade chiropractic training (Keating, 1993a), and in 1944 was a co-founder of the Chiropractic Research Foundation, earliest ancestor of today's Foundation for Chiropractic Education and Research. Vinton Logan, son of 1915 Universal Chiropractic College (UCC) graduate Hugh B. Logan and himself a graduate of the UCC, served as dean of his father's St. Louis school (1935-1944), and later as president (1944-1961). The father-son team, who had practiced together in Los Angeles in the late 1920s, became well known for their Basic Technique, and for the school they founded in Missouri in 1935. At the CCP&S Logan headed the department of "Chiropractic Theory and Technic," where he taught chiropractic philosophy, palpation, spinal analysis, "chiropractic technic, professional ethics and clinic" (College, 1934). He was the only member of the board of directors who did not hold a naturopathic degree. Some 15 years later he wrote of the "Naturopathic parasitic growth," and called for "the immediate cessation of the N.D. degree issued from Chiropractic colleges" (Logan, 1949).

Less well remembered now, but an important player in California chiropractic politics in the 1930s, was Raymond Clarke Howe, D.C., N.D. (see Figure 10-5). Howe, a 1923 LACC graduate, played multiple roles: as an administrator and faculty member at the CCP&S, as a leader in the National-Affiliated Chiropractors of California (NACC), and as editor and editorialist for the NACC's journal, *The Scientific Chiropractor*. Also worthy of mention was CCP&S instructor Clyde F. Gillett, D.C., N.D., who earned a nationwide reputation within the profession for his many appearances at state and national professional conventions, and for his numerous published works on the conservative care of eye, ear, nose and throat disorders (e.g., Gillett, 1928a&b, 1929, 1938). Gillett continued his teachings in conservative health care as a private seminar instructor after his separation from the CCP&S.

Perhaps the best remembered alumnus of the CCP&S is Ralph J. Martin, D.C., N.D. (Keating, Dishman et al., 1993; Keating & Dishman, 1994). The CCP&S had been renamed the SCCC by the time that Martin graduated in the 22 member class of 1938-39; his instructors had included Wolf Adler, D.O., D.C., N.D., LL.B., then dean of the College. Martin joined the faculty of the SCCC in 1940, and after earning his N.D. in 1941 from SCCC's sister institution, the College of Naturopathic Physicians and Surgeons, also taught naturopathic courses. He was active with Henry G. Higley, D.C., M.S. and Dan Nash, D.C. in the campaign to defeat basic science legislation in California in 1942, and by the end of World War II had assumed the presidency of his alma mater. Martin (see Figure 10-6) collaborated with the NCA's director of education, John J. Nugent, to bring about the 1947 merger of the non-profit SCCC and the for-profit LACC, and served as one of the first presidents of the resulting non-profit LACC. In later years he also served the new school on its board of directors. In the early 1950s Martin was appointed to the NCA's Committee on Accreditation for chiropractic schools. He contributed to the creation of the ACA in 1963, and by 1968 had been elected to the ACA Board of Governors. He earned a reputation in later years for his many published papers on educational issues, research and physiotherapy (see Table 10-4), and for his teachings of Bennett's Neurovascular Dynamics (Martin, 1977).

Among the most fondly remembered of faculty members at the CCP&S/SCCC was Wolf Adler, a 1917 graduate of the Philadelphia College of Osteopathy, who earned a chiropractic degree from the New York School of Chiropractic (no relationship to today's New York Chiropractic College) in 1920, and later a naturopathic diploma from Benedict Lust's American School of Naturopathy. In the 1920s he taught at a variety of institutions on the East Coast, including the New York School of Chiropractic, the New York School of Philosophy, the New York School of Mortuary Science, the School of Modern Art, the American School of Chiropractic and Naturopathy, the School of Drugless Physicians, and earned a reputation for various political and clinical lectures and papers in periodicals such as *Psychology Magazine* and *The Thinker* (Editorial, 1970; Keating, Dishman et al., 1993). He was also a central player in the battles between organized medicine and chiropractic in the empire state in the 1920s and 1930s.

In 1936 Adler relocated to Southern California, and over a period of four decades taught and held administrative positions at the SCCC, Cleveland Chiropractic College of Los Angeles, the LACC and the Pasadena College of Chiropractic. Along the way he also earned

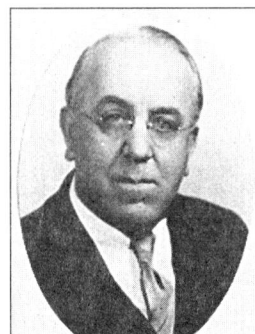

Figure 10-5: R.C. Howe, D.C., N.D., c1935

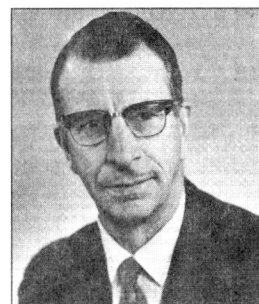

Figure 10-6: Ralph J. Martin, D.C., N.D., c1970

Table 10-4: Selected published papers of Ralph J. Martin, D.C., N.D.

Martin RJ. Study of ultrasonics. *Journal of the National Chiropractic Association* 1952; 22(7):24-

Martin RJ. Modern chiropractic education. *Journal of the National Chiropractic Association* 1954; 24(7): 24-5

Martin RJ. Neurophysiology and ultrasonics. *Journal of the National Chiropractic Association* 1956a; 26(2):15-

Martin RJ. Specialized diathermy technic. *Official Bulletin of the National Council on Chiropractic Physiotherapy* 1956b; 3(1): 20, 21, 23

Martin RJ. Specialized diathermy technic. *Official Bulletin of the National Council on Chiropractic Physiotherapy* 1956c; 3(1): 20, 21, 23

Martin RJ. New horizons. *Journal of the National Chiropractic Association* 1956d; 26(11):11-

Martin RJ. Field program in clinical research in ultrasonics. *Official Bulletin of the National Council on Chiropractic Physiotherapy* 1957; 3(4): 16, 20, 21

Martin RJ. Council research project. *Journal of the National Chiropractic Association* 1958; 28(4):29-

Martin RJ. Vasomotor reflexes. *Journal of the National Chiropractic Association* 1959; 29(7):21-

Martin RJ. Rational use of ultrasonics. *Official Bulletin of the National Council on Chiropractic Physiotherapy* 1960; 6(4): 3, 21

Martin RJ. Accreditation must come first. *Chirogram* 1966; 33(1): 16-7

Martin RJ. Chiropractic doctors must be primary providers. *Chirogram* 1974); 41(9): 11-5

a law degree from American University and an M.D. from a Mexican college. Adler developed a reputation as an anatomic illustrator, and eventually taught most of the courses in the chiropractic curriculum, including "physiology, gross anatomy, dissection, pathology, technic, x-ray, diagnosis, bacteriology and public health" (Editorial, 1970). When Dishman first arrived at the SCCC in 1939 after earning an academic degree from U.C.L.A., he had second thoughts about the wisdom of his career choice, given the very limited facilities of the school. However, he was invited to sit in on one of Dr. Adler's lectures, of which he recalls that:

> On this particular day Dr. Wolf Adler, N.D., D.C., D.O. was instructing osteology. I was invited to listen. By this time in my life I had graduated Junior College and had two semesters at U.C.L.A. listening to professors, some with exceptional reputations for classroom presentation. After a very short time listening to Dr. Adler I realized he was the best I had seen or heard. It was like watching Fred Astaire dance. It was extraordinary! Every facial expression, gesture, nuance of phrase was captivating and entertaining. His blackboard illustrations in colored chalk were clearly a work of art. I learned more in 30 minutes than I could ever imagine. Dr. Adler was warm, helpful and very supportive and I felt completely at ease (Keating, Dishman et al., 1993).

Table 10-5: Faculty of the Southern California College of Chiropractic in 1944-45

Clifford B. Eacrett, D.C., N.D., President
Otis M. McMurtrey, N.D., D.C.,
    Vice-President
Leo Montenegro, D.C., N.D.,
    Secretary-Treasurer
Patrick Lackey, N.D., D.C., Dean
George H. Haynes, A.B., N.D., D.C.
Wolf Adler, D.O., N.D., D.C., LL.B., D.D.
Mabelle Kelso Shaw, D.C.
Lee H. Norcross, D.C., N.D.
Ralph J. Martin, D.C., Ph.C., N.D.
H. Rainford Guest, D.C., N.D.

The SCCC's traditions were perpetuated in the new LACC, following the merger of 1947. Several of the SCCC's faculty (see Table 10-5) became members of the new LACC faculty, most notably Lee H. Norcross, D.C., N.D., George Haynes, D.C., N.D., M.A. and Ralph Martin.

Cleveland Chiropractic College

The Central Chiropractic College was chartered in December 1922 by Palmer graduates Carl S. Cleveland (president), his wife, Ruth R. Cleveland (secretary-treasurer), and his brother-in-law, Perl B. Griffin (dean) (see Figure 10-7a,b&c). The school was renamed Cleveland Chiropractic College (CCC) at the request of the student body in 1924, who did not wish any confusion between their alma mater and a nearby vocational training center of similar name. The CCC was incorporated as a non-profit, "benevolent association" (Becker, 1922), which may qualify it for distinction as the oldest surviving non-profit chiropractic college. Its first campus (see Figure 10-8) was a converted residence which doubled as college facility and home for Carl, Ruth and their young son, Carl Cleveland Jr. The turret windows at the front of the structure allowed the occupants to observe anyone who came to the front door, a precaution deemed essential given the many arrests of chiropractors for unlicensed practice prior to the 1927 passage of Missouri's chiropractic law.

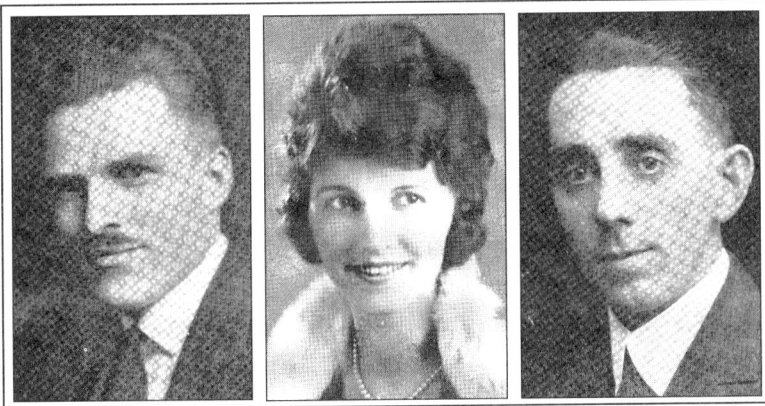

Figures 10-7a,b&c: Advertisement for Cleveland Chiropractic College includes photographs circa 1928 of (from left to right): Carl S. Cleveland, Sr., Ruth Cleveland, and Perl B. Griffin; from page 9 of a *Souvenir Program*, Seventeenth Annual Convention, Missouri State Chiropractors' Association, June 1-3, 1930, Kansas City, Missouri (Cleveland papers, Cleveland Chiropractic College of Kansas City)

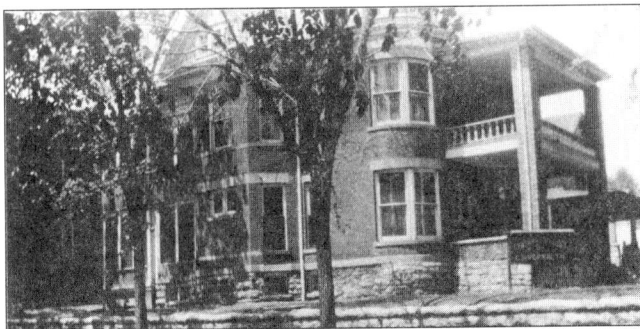

Figure 10-8: The first campus of the Central College of Chiropractic at 436 Prospect Avenue, Kansas City, Missouri, circa 1924. Founded by Carl S. Cleveland, D.C., Ruth R. Cleveland, D.C. and Perl B. Griffin, D.C., the school was renamed the non-profit Cleveland Chiropractic College in 1924

Kansas City was a competitive environment for a new chiropractic school in 1922. Since 1907 the Chiropractic University had been operated in Kansas City by A.E. Field, M.D., D.C. (Carver, 1936, p. 66; Ferguson & Wiese, 1988; Miscellany, 1988; Seventh, 1914-15), and had offered a 21 month curriculum since 1914-1915, which included hospital-based clinical training (Seventh, 1914-15; Eighth, 1915-16). W. Finis Sawrey, D.O., D.C., Ph.C., N.D. relocated his school "from the Black Hills of South Dakota" to 1855 Independence Avenue, Kansas City at about the same time that the CCC began operations. Sawrey's school, the Mo-Kan College of Chiropractic, offered a broad-scope curriculum taught by its president, his wife Bertha (a chiropractor-naturopath), H.A. Watson (a chiropractor-medical physician), and E.L. Taylor (a chiropractor-optometrist). The CCC would also have to compete for students with the Kansas City College of Osteopathy and Surgery, in operation in the city since 1916. The Cleveland school prided and projected itself on its straight chiropractic curriculum and its ties to the Palmer School in Davenport:

On December 28, 1922, the Great State of Missouri saw fit to grant Central College of Chiropractic a Charter, endowing them with the legal right to give standard courses in Chiropractic, to so equip men and women that they may be a credit to this land and our Profession...

We feel that there are many reasons why you should be a Central Chiropractor...:

1. The State of Missouri has authorized Central Chiropractic College to give Chiropractic instruction, grant diplomas, confer degrees, etc.

2. They offer Standard Courses only, including X-Ray.

3. The State of Missouri gives them the right to teach dissection (not given to some schools).

4. Central Chiropractic College has the Clinical advantages of a big City.

5. Central Chiropractic College teaches Palmer Method Chiropractic out of Palmer Text Books.

6. Central Chiropractic College has a Faculty composed of men and women who are all graduates of, and know Chiropractic as it is taught at, the Palmer School of Chiropractic, men and women who have had years of practical experience in the Chiropractic field... (Griffin, 1923).

Consistent with the UCA's and the PSC's scope of practice, adjustive instruction within the early CCC curriculum (see Table 10-6) focused exclusively on the spine. C.S. Cleveland came in for criticism from many in the profession for this, including James Slocum, the Clevelands' former classmate at PSC and future president of the International Chiropractic Congress, who insisted upon the appropriateness of adjustments to any joint in the body (Slocum, 1932). The Cleveland version of straight chiropractic would limit the interventions taught to students to spinal adjusting, but also provided greater-than-Palmer instruction in diagnosis. "Clinic" was usually held twice daily for an hour in the morning and again during the afternoon (Cleveland, 1986). The Clevelands took pride in their courses in anatomy and radiography; in the 1930s they developed a reputation for their "refresher" programs for graduates. Tuition was competitive: $360 for the 18-month day program, and $450 for the evening course. A husband and wife could complete the program for $100 more than the single tuition cost. In August 1929, the CCC opened at its new campus at 3724 Troost Avenue, where it remained until its 1977 relocation to the present campus at Meyer and Rockhill Road in Kansas City (Beginning, 1987; Scrapbook, undated).

Soon after the College's move to Troost the Depression struck; the institution's viability was sorely tested. Other external pressures upon the profession in Missouri also occupied the CCC's leaders. The threat of prosecution for unlicensed practice was replaced after Missouri's 1927 passage of a chiropractic act by the threat of a basic science barrier in the state. C.S. Cleveland Sr. intervened with political boss Thomas J. Pendergast to block passage of a basic science law. His persuasive argument was that to require basic science testing of D.C.s by M.D.s was "like telling a Catholic priest that he couldn't function as a priest until he took an examination from a rabbi" (Cleveland, 1986). Missouri did not enact basic science legislation. However, the bleak economics of the Depression years were followed by a severe student shortage produced by the military drafts of the 1940s.

Instructor	Alma Mater	Subjects
Carl S. Cleveland, Sr., D.C., President	Palmer School of Chiropractic	Symptomatology, Orthopedy, Chiropractic Analysis, Philosophy, Technique, Spinography
Perl B. Griffin, D.C., Dean	Palmer School of Chiropractic	Physiology, Histology, Technique, Physiology, Gynecology, Orthopedy, Clinic
Ruth R. Cleveland, D.C., Secretary-Treasurer	Palmer School of Chiropractic	Anatomy, Gynecology, Palpation, Nerve Tracing, Brain and Nervous System, Clinic
Corinne Abney, D.C.	Cleveland Chiropractic College	Anatomy, Hygiene and Public Health, Terminology
Marion E. Huscher, D.C.	Cleveland Chiropractic College	Splanchnology, Word Analysis
R.C. Jackson, D.C.	?	X-Ray and Spinography
A.E. Miller, D.C.	?	Chiropractic Philosophy
H.L. Poole, D.C.	Palmer School of Chiropractic	Philosophy of Chiropractic
Dr. W.E. Sanderson	St. Louis University	Chemistry & Urinalysis
Loren H. Trotter, D.C.	Palmer School of Chiropractic	Osteology, Syndesmology, and Myology

Table 10-6: Instructors and subjects taught at the Central College of Chiropractic, 1923-25

As noted earlier, Carl Cleveland, Sr. was an active participant in the ICC, and served as president of the Congress' schools division during 1931-32 (Keating & Cleveland, 1996). However, with the dissolution of the ICC in 1934 and the growing efforts of the NCA to regulate the colleges through standardization and a rating system (Gibbons, 1985; Keating, 1993a), Cleveland became progressively more distanced from his broad-scope colleagues. By the late 1930s he had joined with straight chiropractic school presidents James R. Drain, Craig M. Kightlinger, and T.F. Ratledge in the formation of the Associated Chiropractic Colleges of America (ACCA), an organization which stood in formal opposition to the NCA's positions on school accreditation and scope of practice (Keating, Brown & Smallie, 1991, 1992).

Metropolitan College of Chiropractic

The name of the earliest forerunner of the Metropolitan College of Chiropractic (MCC) is a mystery. However, sometime in the mid-1920s Ernest John Smith, A.B., D.C., a 1921 graduate of Western Reserve University (Budden, 1951) and a 1922 graduate of the National College of Chiropractic (Dzaman et al., 1980, pp. 223-4), purchased this "small chiropractic college" and created the MCC of Cleveland, Ohio (Association, 1988; Ferguson & Wiese, 1988). The school was apparently renamed the Metropolitan College of Chiropractic and Mechano-Therapy circa 1943 (Ferguson & Wiese, 1988), perhaps to accommodate the mechano-therapy licensing laws in Ohio. Under Smith, the MCC became the first chiropractic college (circa 1927) to offer a four-year program (Budden, 1951).

By 1941 the MCC's curriculum had so evolved that NCA college inspector Wayne F. Crider, D.C., who was surprised to find that a

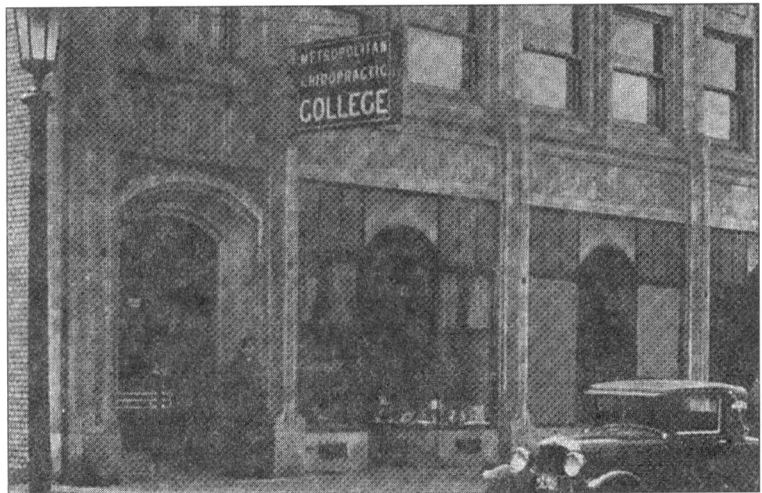

Figure 10-9: Metropolitan College of Chiropractic and Mechano-therapy, located at 3400 Euclid Avenue, Cleveland, Ohio, circa 1938. This school was first to offer a four-year curriculum in chiropractic, and offered degrees in chiropractic, mechanotherapy and naturopathy. Its president during 1927-1947 was Ernest J. Smith.

class hour at MCC actually equaled 60 minutes, wondered whether the 5,040 hour curriculum at MCC, which was 40% longer than the 3,600 required for NCA-approved schools, was too much (Crider, 1941). Other NCA inspections in the 1939-41 period noted a functional library of as many as 2,000 volumes which were readily accessible to students, well equipped "Chemical and Bacteriological Laboratory," "large class rooms...with ample ventilation and lighting," and extensive physiotherapy equipment. The school offered instruction in chiropractic, electrotherapy, mechanotherapy and naturopathy, and granted three types of doctorates: D.C., D.M. (mechanotherapy) and N.D. (naturopathy) . The MCC was chartered as a non-profit institution on December 16, 1937 (Application, 1941b), and was located at 3400 Euclid Avenue (see Figure 10-9).

Also exceptional in this time frame was the MCC's insistence on verifying the high school credentials of applicants; by contrast, high school "equivalency" was still accepted at the National College in Chicago in the late 1920s. New students were enrolled only twice per year (February and September), in contrast with the open enrollment policies of many other chiropractic schools at that time. The school's vice-president and dean, Paul C. Moyer, Mt.D. (doctor of mechano-therapy), was active in the NCA's college reform efforts in the 1930s. As early as 1938, at the NCA's convention in Toronto, he had proposed a four-year curriculum with emphasis in the basic sciences and a two-year college pre-requisite for chiropractic schools (Moyer, 1943); his ideas quickly ran afoul of those college leaders offering 18-month curricula.

The MCC may also have been unusual in this period for its strong faculty (see Table 10-7). Like his mentor at National College, William C. Schulze, (Keating & Rehm, 1995a&b), President Smith set a scholarly tone for the institution, as exemplified by a number of his publications (see Table 10-8). He also advocated a very broad scope of chiropractic. Smith joined

Full-Time Faculty	Alma Mater	Courses & Duties
Ernest J. Smith, A.B., D.C., Ph.C., Mt.D., N.D., *President*	Western Reserve University; National College of Chiropractic	Administration, diagnosis
Paul C. Moyer, Mt.D., *Vice-President & Dean*	Metropolitan Chiropractic College; post-grad at National College of Chiropractic	Chair, Department of Anatomy, Clinic Director, diagnosis
Mary C. Hibbard, A.B., D.C., Ph.C., Mt.D., N.D., *Secretary-Treasurer*	Buchtel College; Palmer School of Chiropractic	Chair, Department of X-ray, philosophy, orthopedy
Robert C. Mangle, D.C., E.T., Mt.D., N.D.	Metropolitan College of Chiropractic; post-grad at Cleveland Chiropractic College	Physiology
John E. Rupert, A.B., D.C., Mt.D., N.D.	Western Reserve University; Universal Chiropractic College; Metropolitan College of Chiropractic	Chair, Department of Chemistry & Bacteriology, pathology, embryology, histology
Florence Franck, D.C.	Metropolitan College of Chiropractic	Chemistry, anatomy
Louis E. Edwards, D.C., E.T., Mt.D., N.D.	Metropolitan College of Chiropractic	Chiropractic (palpation)
Part-Time Faculty		
Ben Levy, B.S., D.C., E.T., Mt.D., Ph.C., N.D.	Ohio State University; Metropolitan College of Chiropractic	Physiotherapy
Paul Lederman, D.D.S.	Miami University; Western Reserve University	Dentistry
Charles J. Bucknell, D.C., Ph.C., Mt.D., N.D.	John Marshall College; Metropolitan College of Chiropractic; post-grad at National College of Chiropractic	Chiropractic (technique), diagnosis
Harry Riley Spitler, N.D., D.C., Mt.D.	McFadden Sanitarium	Mechanotherapy
Dr. Carlisle H. Snell	?	Dissection
Dr. Joseph F. Borta	?	Orthopedy

Table 10-7: Full-time and part-time faculty of the Metropolitan College of Chiropractic in Cleveland, Ohio, circa 1939-41 (information based on records in the archives of the Council on Chiropractic Education)

with Budden of Western States, Beatty of the University of Natural Healing Arts in Denver and others in forming the apparently short-lived Affiliated Universities of Natural Healing in 1935 (Advertisement, 1935), an agency which seems to have been organized in reaction to the limitations on physiotherapy (particularly electro-cautery and fulguration for tonsils and hemorrhoids) suggested by the NCA at its convention that year in Los Angeles (Keating, 1993a). By 1947, Smith had departed the institution for private practice in California, and Moyer became the MCC's president. The school lost its rented campus circa 1949 (Key, 1943a&b), and by 1950 had closed its doors. Its corporate records and alumni were later transferred to the National College (Association, 1988).

Table 10-8: Selected titles of Ernest J. Smith, D.C., published in the NCA's *Chiropractic Journal.*

A questionnaire. 1933 (Mar); 1(3): ??
Change is demanded. 1934 (Aug); 3(8): 5
Gynecological therapy. 1939 (Feb); 8(2): 13
The problem case. 1942 (Apr); 11(4): 14
Rational diagnosis. 1942 (May); 11(5): 10
Wartime needs. 1942 (June); 11(6): 10
Drugless therapy (with M. Tennant). 1942 (July); 11(7): 17
Industrial health (a 10 part series). 1942-1943.
Women in industry. 1942 (Nov); 11(11): 17
Our public education program (with others).1954 (Aug); 24(7): 18

Lincoln Chiropractic College

In the earliest available issue of its school *Bulletin*, the founders of the Lincoln Chiropractic College described their view of the straight/mixer controversy which then plagued the profession and its educational institutions:

The Lincoln Chiropractic College assumes the position that the continuance of strife between the straight Chiropractor and the mixer so effectively saps our energy, depletes our resources and scatters our forces that if long continued it will lead to the obliteration of the profession as a movement (Tolerance, 1927).

It was characteristic of the school's leaders to find a moderate position on many contentious issues. Rejecting the restrictions on academic freedom introduced by B.J. Palmer following his announcement of the neurocalometer, the "Big Four" of the future Lincoln College departed the PSC in 1925-26. These men were James N. Firth, Harry E. Vedder, Stephen J. Burich, and Arthur E. Hendricks (Keating & Rehm, 1993; Stowell, 1983). Their curriculum at the Indianapolis school was noted for the strength of its commitment to basic science and diagnostic instruction. The Lincoln's early emphasis on diagnostic training was not surprising, given its founders' published works (see Table 10-9). A former pupil and fellow school leader, Carl S. Cleveland, Sr., predicted that Lincoln's founders "will run a good school, with

Table 10-9: The founders of the Lincoln Chiropractic College, their education, and several of their published works (from Chiropractic, 1929, Stowell, 1983 and Wiese & Lykins, 1986)

Harry E. Vedder, D.C., Ph.C., PSC 1912. *A Textbook on Chiropractic Physiology* (1916); *A Textbook on Chiropractic Gynecology* (1919); *Chiropractic Advertising* (1924)

James N. Firth, D.C., Ph.C., Arenac County Normal College, 1906; Ferris Institute; PSC, 1910. *A Textbook on Chiropractic Symptomatology* (1914); *Chiropractic Diagnosis* (1929)

Stephen J. Burich, D.C., Ph.C., Beloit College, 1913; PSC, 1913. *A Textbook of Chiropractic Chemistry* (1919)

Arthur G. Hendricks, D.C., Butler University; PSC, 1920. co-author, *X-Ray Technique and Spinal Misalignment Interpretation*

just a little too much tendency toward analyzing effects rather than causes" (Cleveland, 1926a). Theirs was not a Palmer-straight curriculum, although the mainstay of the therapeutic armamentarium at Lincoln was the adjustment, and physiotherapy was not part of the instructional program (Foreword, 1928). However, dietetics were included in the training. The first students graduated on March 16, 1928 (Our, 1928).

Classes at the newly chartered, "tax-exempt" school commenced on September 20, 1926, on the second floor of the Lumber Insurance Building at 518 North Delaware Street in Indianapolis (Lincoln, 1927, 1929; Stowell, 1983). The initial curriculum required 18 months to complete the 2,210 hours (see Table 10-10), but by 1929 an elective, four-year program was also available, and in 1942, in accordance with the NCA's new standards (Gibbons, 1985; Nugent, 1941), the four-year program became mandatory (Stowell, 1983). The Lincoln school also quickly developed a well-received post-graduate program, and was proud of the international enrollment it attracted, including visitors from Belgium, Canada, Australia, New Zealand, Europe and South Africa (Foreign, 1929; Post, 1929). Saskatchewan chiropractor Joshua N. Haldeman's "Six Weeks Post Graduate Certificate," dated August 21, 1936, and signed by the "Big Four," noted instruction in "Physical

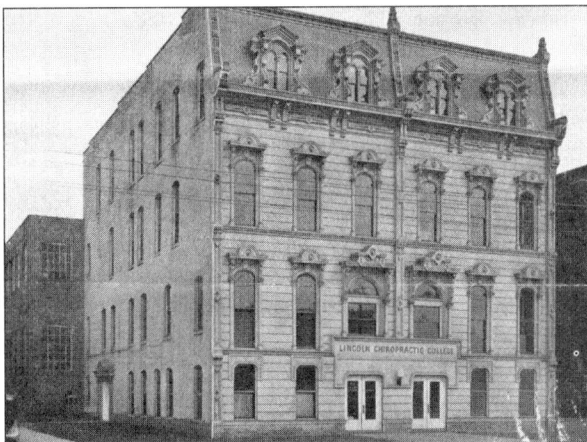

Figure 10-10: Lincoln Chiropractic College purchased this campus, the former Dental College of Indiana University in 1935, during the presidency of Harry Vedder.

Courses	Hours
Anatomy	650.00
Physiology	97.50
Pathology & bacteriology	146.25
Chemistry & urinalysis	71.25
Hygiene & public health	48.75
Symptomatology (including x-ray)	536.25
Principles & practice	487.50
Dietetics	75.00
Office conduct & jurisprudence	48.75
Ethics & first aid	48.75
Total	**2,210.00**

Table 10-10: Initial curriculum of the Lincoln Chiropractic College of Indianapolis, 1926 (based on Stowell, 1983)

Faculty	Department
James N. Firth, D.C., Ph.C., President	Chiropractic
Stephen J. Burich, D.C., Ph.C., Vice-President & Secretary	Anatomy
Arthur G. Hendricks, D.C., Ph.C., Treasurer	Diagnosis
L.M. King, D.C., Ph.C., Dean	Bacteriology, Pathology
Rudy O. Mueller, D.C., Ph.C.	Physiology
B.E. Pitzer, D.C., Ph.C.	Clinical Laboratories
W.A. Watkinson, D.C., Ph.C.	Chemistry

Table 10-11: Faculty of the Lincoln Chiropractic College, according to the school's *Catalogue*, 1943-1944

Diagnosis, Dietetics, Transillumination, Urinalysis and the Technic of Scientific Spinal Correction."

Like many chiropractic schools, the college published its *Lincoln Bulletin*, which featured authors such as Stanley Hayes, editor of the *Bulletin of the West Virginia Chiropractors' Society* (e.g., Hayes, 1928), John Monroe, A.M., D.C., chairman of the ACA's Bureau of Research (e.g., Monroe, 1929) and former PSC radiologist, E.A. Thompson of Baltimore (Thompson, 1929), in addition to the school's faculty. The *Lincoln Bulletin* also provided school announcements, national and state professional and legislative news, anecdotes from alumni, and a chiropractic directory. By the end of 1929, the *Lincoln Bulletin* boasted a circulation of 6,000, or about half of the population of chiropractors in the United States.

The former campus of the Dental College of Indiana University (see Figure 10-10) became the new home of the Lincoln Chiropractic College in 1935 (Catalogue, 1943-1944, Stowell, 1983). In 1940 the school's first president, Harry Vedder, retired, and J.N. Firth. assumed the office. By 1943, despite the military draft of World War II, student enrollment still supported a faculty of seven (see Table 10-11), and Lincoln was one of the few schools to receive the NCA Committee on Educational Standards' early rating as "fully approved" (Stowell, 1983). However, as the war dragged on, enrollments at all chiropractic schools fell precipitously. In 1944, the Universal Chiropractic College (UCC) of Pittsburgh, founded by Joy M. Loban in Davenport, Iowa, in 1910, merged with the Lincoln College. The merger brought Leo J. Steinbach, former director of research for the ACA in the late 1920s (Keating et al., 1995) and past president of the UCC, to the Lincoln College as professor of "Universal Technique" (Stowell, 1983).

Logan Basic College of Chiropractic

Hugh B. Logan, D.C., a graduate of the Universal Chiropractic College (UCC) in 1915, was the founder of the Logan Basic College of Chiropractic in St. Louis, Missouri, in 1935. He was assisted in this effort by his son, Vinton F. Logan, a 1926 UCC graduate. The pair had practiced together in Loew's State Building at 707 South Broadway in Los Angeles in the late 1920s (Advertisement, 1928b; Logan, 1928a&b), and promoted their practice as "X-Ray Diagnosis, Anatomical Adjustors, Nerve Release Specialists" (Advertisement, 1928c). However, H.B. Logan lost his license to practice chiropractic in California in 1929 (State, 1929), apparently a victim (along with Charles Cale, James Compton, and others) of intra-professional political intrigue among the warring factions of chiropractors in the state (CCA, 1931; Ratledge, 1934). The elder Logan had gained a reputation by this time as a guest lecturer at the LACC (Chirogram, 1925), and Vinton Logan taught technique and served on the board of directors of the College of Chiropractic Physicians and Surgeons in the early 1930s (College, 1934).

The senior Logan became a traveling seminar instructor for "Aquarian Age Healing" (AAH) circa 1932 (Hurley, undated; Ratledge, 1934). Aquarian Age Healing (Hurley & Sanders, 1932), a novel chiropractic theory and technique created by Hollywood chiropractors (husband and wife) John Hurley and Helen Sanders (Aquarian, 1933), eventually gave rise to several brand name and generic "technics," including Logan's "Basic," John M. Bauer's "Orthodynamics" (Bauer, 1937), Terrence J. Bennett's "Neurovascular Dynamics" (Martin, 1977; Nelson, 1991), and perhaps aspects of M.B. DeJarnette's "Sacro-Occipital Technique" (Hurley, undated a&b). Aquarian Age Healing also formed the basis for NCA Director of Research James E. Slocum's "Bio-Mechanics=Bio-Engineering" seminars for the NCA (Announcing, 1938; Rogers, 1938a; Slocum, 1942a&b). In some ways mimicking the dispute between D.D. Palmer and the osteopathic community at the turn of the century, the originality and uniqueness of Logan Basic Technique (LBT) vs. AAH became the basis for lengthy legal battles between the two founders, Logan vs. Hurley (Hurley, undateda&b, 1942), and the source of considerable turmoil in the field (Sauer, 1934; Watkins, 1944). Unwitting writers about technique sometimes felt the wrath of those who claimed originality for their proprietary methods, as Clarence Weiant, dean of the Eastern Chiropractic Institute, learned in 1938:

Dear Dr. Rogers:

I am in receipt of a letter from Dr. John L. Hurley, of the Aquarian-Age Healing Institute, Denver, Colorado, in which he takes exception to a paragraph in my article "Spinal Analysis," which appeared in your January issue. This paragraph read as follows:

"I should not like to leave the subject of DeJarnette, however, without a word of admiration and praise for the refinements of method which he has introduced for the examination of the patient in the upright posture. The combination of plumb line, fixed foot plates, and uprights with adjustable cross-pieces makes possible a very complete record of the patient's posture."

It is Dr. Hurley's contention that the essential features of this method originated with him, and that my failure to credit him with the discovery was an injustice.

The purpose of my article was not primarily to record the history of the various methods of examination, but to analyze their principles. Inasmuch as I was not familiar with Aquarian-Age Healing (an unfortunate and perhaps, even an inexcusable circumstance), I could not include this method in my discussion, nor ascribe to it the priority which, according to Dr. Hurley, belongs to it. To correct any injustice which may have been done, unwittingly, by myself, I hope that you will print this communication at an early date (Weiant, 1938).

By 1932 Logan was teaching LBT as an original contribution to chiropractors around the nation (Sausser, 1933). Like Hurley's AAH, instruction in LBT was proprietary, and seminar attendees were required to agree to keep the content of their learning secret (Holmes, 1934; Watkins, 1944; Keating, 1992a, p. 397-400). Logan's ideas captured the imagination of many chiropractors. Among the more prominent of these were John H. Craven, (Annual, 1934), former faculty member of the PSC, Thomas F. Maher, member of the Missouri Board of Chiropractic Examiners (Maher, 1934), Benjamin A. Sauer, former secretary of the ACA and the original secretary of the NCA and editor of the original *Journal of the National Chiropractic Association* (1931), William H. Werner, organizer of the American Bureau of Chiropractic (Lombardo, 1990), and Sylva L. Ashworth, president of the Nebraska Board of Chiropractic Examiners. (Certificate, 1935; Keating & Cleveland, 1992). Warren L. Sausser credited his creation of the first 14x36" full-spine, weight-bearing x-ray to his interest in H.B. Logan's theories (Sausser, 1933). Logan's followers established a research foundation to further his concepts (Tegren, 1934); in January 1934, the NCA's *The Chiropractic Journal* reported that:

On November 18, 1933, there met at the Statler Hotel, Buffalo, N.Y., approximately 100 chiropractors who are users of Basic Technique. During this two day session there was organized the International Chiropractic Research Foundation which is to be purely a scientific research society. Its members are to be selected by invitation only. It appears to be a move in the right direction. A splendid set of By-Laws was adopted and the first official family elected.

The new officers follow: Directors: Dr. Wm. H. Werner, Dr. W.A. Collinson, Dr. A.B. Cochrane, Dr. J.K. Cheney, Dr. T.F. Maher, Dr. J.H. Craven and Dr. E.A. Thompson. President, Dr. H.E. Warren of Rochester, N.Y.; first vice-president, Dr. E.W. Ferguson, New Haven, Conn.; second vice-president, Dr. Charles R. Bunn, Denver, Colo; sec'y-treas., B.A. Sauer, Syracuse (Research, 1934).

Considered "one of the most colorful and dynamic characters within the profession" (National, 1934), Hugh Logan was a featured speaker at several NCA conventions, and his theories and methods were considered a scientific breakthrough by many D.C.s. The first meeting of the newly formed International Chiropractic Research Foundation (ICRF) was held in conjunction with the NCA's 1934 convention in Pittsburgh (Annual, 1934). At its 1935 convention in Syracuse, New York, the ICRF decided to "sponsor" a non-profit, professionally controlled, chiropractic college wherein the LBT would be the featured centerpiece of the curriculum. Organized by H.B. Logan, the Logan Basic College of Chiropractic (LBCC):

...enrolled its first class, a small group of seven young men and women, the first of September, 1935, in a converted residence at 4490 Lindell Boulevard, St. Louis. Five more students were added to the class in February of the following year, and thus the college began its early struggle for survival and growth. The next September a larger group of Chiropractic students found their way to its doors, and by December of 1936 the college had outgrown its quarters and Dr. Hugh B. Logan, the founder, was surveying St. Louis county for a new and permanent location for the growing school. He found and chose a huge residence atop a beautifully wooded hilly tract just outside Normandy (see Figure 10-11), and there it was that the Logan Basic College of Chiropractic "took root."

Dr. Hugh B. Logan dreamed and planned the new Chiropractic college because of the need he had realized through extensive travel and teaching in the field for more intensive and more thorough training for chiropractors. He dreamed of the time when Chiropractic would be accepted for the true and advanced healing science that it is, and withal he saw the need for raising the standards of both the science and its practitioners through better education. With this firm conviction he instituted the longer course of four school years of 9 months each, and a required clinic internship for each student before graduation. During these early years the four years of study seemed a barrier to some, and classes were small, too small to support the hungry financial needs of a new school. Dr. Logan poured his energies and finances into the college, and although many times disheartened by opposition even within the profession itself, he clung tenaciously to his ideals and hopes for the future.

Thus the Logan Basic College became the first non-profit, tax-exempt Chiropractic educational institution, and the pioneer in instituting the four-year of nine months, or 36-month resident course of training (Logan, 1952-1953, p. 8).

Viola Nickson, D.C., a member of the first graduating class, recalls that the first class was actually composed of eight students, rather than the seven noted in the above account (personal communication).

The LBCC was "Chartered under Pro-Forma Decree 1936 (revised 1938) by State of Missouri as a Non-Profit Educational Institution" (Logan, 1952-1953). Despite its non-profit status, the school soon ran afoul of its board of directors, who resigned in protest in 1937. Faculty and student unrest were also apparent early on, and the school apparently suspended operations temporarily when at least four of its faculty, John M. Bauer, Robert E. Colyer, J.W. Grostoeler and J. Dalton Craven, and "twenty-three of the school's fifty-nine students resigned" (Bauer, 1937; Dr. Hugh, 1937). NCA *Journal* editor Loran M. Rogers (1937) commented on the transfer of 40 students from LBCC to Missouri Chiropractic College and the Lincoln School, and reprinted the sentiments of the LBCC's former board:

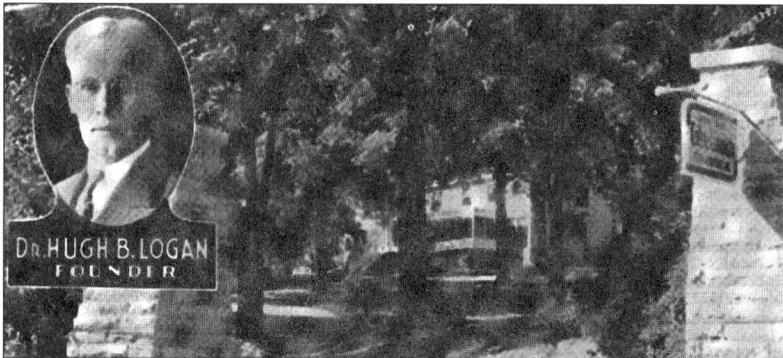

Figure 10-11: The second campus of the Logan Basic College of Chiropractic at 7701 Florissant Road, St. Louis, Missouri, c1938.

To the Members of the International Chiropractic Research Foundation:

On account of existing conditions, placed before the Board of Directors of the College of Chiropractic, and the Board of Directors of the Chiropractic Research Foundation, at a specially called Board meeting in St. Louis, Missouri, Sunday, Sept. 12, 1937.

Conditions proving that the Logan Basic College of Chiropractic is not a professionally owned and operated College of Chiropractic, such as was proposed to be sponsored at the 3rd Annual Assembly of the I.C.R.F. held at Syracuse, N.Y., in the year 1935.

In view of the existing conditions, we the undersigned members of the Board of directors of the Logan Basic College of Chiropractic or Logan College of Chiropractic, Inc., do hereby tender our resignation to take effect immediately, we wish to be relieved of the responsibilities of all duties imposed upon this Board by the members of the Chiropractic Research Foundation, and we further wish to be fully relieved of all moral and financial responsibilities connected with this Board.

Respectfully submitted,

Signed: J.B. Wedge, Chairman; C.S. Brandon; F.A. Black, D.C.; Walter L. Vaughan; J. Fred Brewer; J.F. Fallot, D.C.; John H. Craven, D.C.; Thos. L. Reese, D.C.; W.A. Collinson; H.W. Lavender

John M. Bauer, D.C., an original faculty member at the LBCC, wrote to Carl S. Cleveland, Sr., to offer to teach a LBT-derivative called "Orthodynamics," and noted:

> I resigned as I did not wish to be a party to his undertakings as I did not approve of the manner in which he was presenting his school as a professionally owned school....we are not only capable of teaching B.T. but we have added to it considerably and are teaching it under the name of "Orthodynamics". There is no secrecy attached to our course, there are no silly contracts to be signed and the doctors are under no obligation of any kind to us. Notes are not only permitted but are suggested and our tuition is One Hundred Dollars (Bauer, 1937).

The Logans were undeterred by this turn of events, and the college grew slowly. The eight members of the first graduating class in 1939 included Viola and Art Nickson, co-founders of the Association for the History of Chiropractic in 1980, and assemblers of an extensive collection of chiropractic historical artifacts: the Logan Archives. The 1940 graduating class included Beatrice Hagen, future president (1981-1993) of the institution. A "one-year course for Chiropractic office assistants" was established also in 1940 (Logan, 1952-1953). Like most other schools of the period, the USA's entry into World War II "took a major portion of the Logan male student body" and "there arose the fear that this hardship would be overwhelming to Logan" (Logan, 1952-1953). The college encouraged enrollment by females (Logan, 1943), and later noted that the size of the student body had actually grown very modestly throughout the war (Logan, 1952-1953, p. 9).

By the middle of the war years the curriculum included 4,760 class periods of 45 minutes each, and the school advertised that the program included instruction in "Marlowe Office Procedure" (Logan, 1943), presumably the practice-building work of PSC graduate R.S. Marlowe of San Antonio, Texas (Cleveland, 1932). The LBCC noted an enrollment of 60 students in 1943, this despite the loss of 40 students to the military draft (Logan, 1943). The following year, on May 31, H.B. Logan died, and his son assumed the presidency of the school. Vinton F. Logan presided over the college until his death in 1961.

Western States College, School of Chiropractic and School of Naturopathy

The Pacific Chiropractic College (PCC) evolved from several of the earliest schools formed by chiropractors in Oregon, including the Fountain Head School, transferred by Old Dad Chiro in 1908 from Oklahoma City to Portland (see Figure 1-6). The school was purchased by Oscar W. Elliott, D.C., Ph.C., M.C. in 1917, who operated the institution until his death in December 1926 (Gatterman, 1982; Ritter, 1991). The PCC's catalog described the school as a "Class A School," and reported that its training program "prepares you for any Chiropractic State Board in the United States" (Pacific, 1922). Three curricula were offered in 1922: a 2,400 hour program (two years of nine months each) leading to the D.C. degree (see Table 10-12) and meeting the requirements for licensure in Oregon, a three year program (of seven months each) involving 3,900 hours, and a four year course (of seven months each) leading to the Ph.C. degree. It seems likely that course hours would have involved less than 60 minutes each, since a 21-month program could not be expected to include 3,900 hours; moreover, the hours listed in the College's catalog for the 18-month program totaled to 3,140 hours. The school claimed "hospital privileges," although these were not described in the college catalog (Pacific, 1922). Tuition for the "standard course" was $450; if a husband and wife took the training together, the second tuition was $275. Students could opt for the day or evening program.

With Oscar Elliott's death, his wife, Lenore, became owner of the college, and appointed N.S. Checkos, M.D. to be dean. To accommodate Oregon's 1927 revised statutes regulating chiropractic, which required instruction in physiotherapeutic modalities, an

Table 10-12: The "Standard Course" offered by the Pacific Chiropractic College in 1922 (Pacific, 1922)	
	Hours
Anatomy	510
Histology	135
Physiology	260
Chiropractic Theory and Practice	1000
Chemistry	120
Pathology	270
Gynecology	105
Obstetrics	195
Hygiene and Sanitation	125
Diagnosis	340
Toxicology	40
Minor Surgery	40
Total:	**3,140**

Table 10-13: Some writings of W.A. Budden, D.C., N.D.

A pocket guide to physiotherapy technique and treatment. Chicago: the authors, 1928

Visceral pathology in relation to spinal subluxations. *Journal of the International Chiropractic Congress* 1932; 1(7): 9

Oregon fights for healing arts amendment to constitution! *The Chiropractic Journal (NCA)* 1934; 3(9): 17

Medical propaganda, aided by BJ Palmer, defeats healing arts amendment. *The Chiropractic Journal* (NCA) 1935; 4(2): 9-10, 38

Place of college in association affairs. *The Oregon Chiropractor* 1937; 1(1): 1, 3

Spinal subluxations usually result in visceral pathology. *National Chiropractic Journal* 1943; 12(3): 9-10, 46

The scope of chiropractic obstetrics. *National Chiropractic Journal* 1944; 14(4): 9, 46

Russian research supports chiropractic. *National Chiropractic Journal* 1945; 15(1): 9-10, 60-1

Cervical trauma from car accidents. *National Chiropractic Journal* 1945; 15(4): 9, 56-8

An approach to mental hygiene. *National Chiropractic Journal* 1946; 16(3): 8-9, 55

Economic rivalry vs. public health. *National Chiropractic Journal* 1946; 16(4): 7, 8, 46

Scope of chiropractic. *National Chiropractic Journal* 1946; 16(12): 26-7, 54

Educational standards at conventions. *National Chiropractic Journal* 1947; 17(2): 29

An outline for research projects. *National Chiropractic Journal* 1947; 17(10): 11-2

Public health and public relations. *Journal of the National Chiropractic Association* 1950; 20(4): 16-7

Aspects of juvenile delinquency. *Journal of the National Chiropractic Association* 1950; 20(7): 12-3, 66, 68, 70

What next in school development! *Journal of the National Chiropractic Association* 1951; 21(1): 9-10

Don't neglect your kidneys. *Journal of the National Chiropractic Association* 1951; 21(3): 39

The halogens in drinking water. *Journal of the National Chiropractic Association* 1951; 21(4): 11-2, 70, 72

An analysis of recent chiropractic history and its meaning. *Journal of the National Chiropractic Association* 1951; 21(6): 9-10

Another important victory! *Journal of the National Chiropractic Association* 1951; 21(9): 56

---

expanded course of "three years of nine months each" was offered (Ritter, 1991). On January 17, 1929. William A. Budden, D.C., N.D., purchased the PCC for $20,000 (Gatterman, 1982), just months before the stock market crash and the onset of the Great Depression. Budden, a former faculty member in economics at the University of Alberta (Rehm, 1980, pp. 318-9), had graduated from the National College of Chiropractic in 1924, joined the faculty during William C. Schulze's administration, and succeeded Arthur L. Forster as dean of his alma mater. His writings as editor of the *National (College) Journal of Chiropractic* had brought him to prominence in the profession before his relocation to Oregon. He subsequently served as editor of the *Bulletin of the Oregon Association of Chiropractic Physicians* (National, 1933), and continued his writing throughout his career (see Table 10-13).

The college struggled to avoid bankruptcy, and had to suspend operations in July 1932. However, by the end of that year the institution was reorganized (Ritter, 1991) as the non-profit Western States College (WSC), which included schools of chiropractic and naturopathy. The formation of the WSC coincided with the passage of a basic science law in the state, and Budden determined that his students would meet the challenge. However, his attempt to have chiropractic and naturopathic applicants for licensure be examined by their own boards rather than a basic science board was thwarted by B.J. Palmer, whom Budden accused of "stabbing one of the contestants in a battle in the back" Budden described the situation in the NCA's *Journal*:

> Two days before the election the state newspapers carried large advertisements advising the people that "America's Leading Chiropractor, B.J. Palmer - agrees with the entire medical profession of Oregon" in urging people to vote against the amendment and for the strengthening of medical monopoly...

> It is also laughable to note the reaction on the part of the medics. They do not hail their newfound ally with any degree of enthusiasm. Two years ago the Senate of the Oregon Legislature was treated to a mordant and bitter attack on the Palmer school by the medical senators, in fact, by the very gentlemen who now find themselves cheek by jowl with innate intelligence and the Ductus Palmer!!! Ah, well, there must be some fun to every battle, and certainly we are all enjoying a hearty laugh over the above (Budden, 1935a).

In later years Budden expressed his belief that the basic science examinations in Oregon were administered fairly. He became an active participant in the NCA's campaign to raise educational standards throughout the profession, and one of the early members of the joint committee of state examining boards and school leaders who organized for this purpose in 1935 (Crider, 1936). By this time the WSC was offering a curriculum of 36 months, and contemplated an alliance with other schools offering broad-scope chiropractic and naturopathic instruction (Advertisement, 1935). His presentation at the NCA's convention that year in Hollywood, California, enumerated the basic and diagnostic subjects he felt essential in the training of chiropractors:

1. A knowledge of human morphology and embryology and the ability to apply such knowledge to the problems of human disease.

2. A clear grasp of the segmental arrangements of the human body and the interaction of visceral upon somatic segments, together with an appreciation of the appearance of same under careful examination.

3. A definite understanding of the significance of the fact that man belongs to the biological order of the orthograde vertebrates.

4. A working acquaintance with modern neurology.

5. The ability to successfully arrange the conclusions arising from the use of the above sciences and add up such conclusions so as to arrive at the correct answer.

This may seem to be a hard and difficult road to follow, yet the successful doctor, or at least diagnostician, must be prepared to devote the whole of his time and effort thereto, if he wishes to stand at the head of his profession, and I take it that such an ambition should be the goal of all who have the interests of humanity at heart (Budden, quoted in Slocum, 1935).

To further his vision of chiropractic and the chiropractic physician, Budden and co-workers organized the non-profit Health Research Foundation (HRF) in 1937 (see Figure 10-12), the stated purposes for which were:

...to provide, without profit, for the advancement of human healing arts and science; to improve the mental and physical well-being of its members and others; to provide proper facilities and equipment for the conduct of scientific research and experimentation in human health and healing; and to collect or originate and publish data concerning the methods of combating and preventing human disease (Gatterman, 1982).

The new facilities for the HRF were dedicated on November 15, 1938, and the state journal described the institute's further plans:

The first unit of the Foundation will house the Western States College, where research laboratories will be maintained for research work not only for the student body but for any member of the profession that may have something to offer to our science...

The second unit of the Foundation will be a three story building joining unit No. 1 and will be the home of the Free Drugless Child Clinic

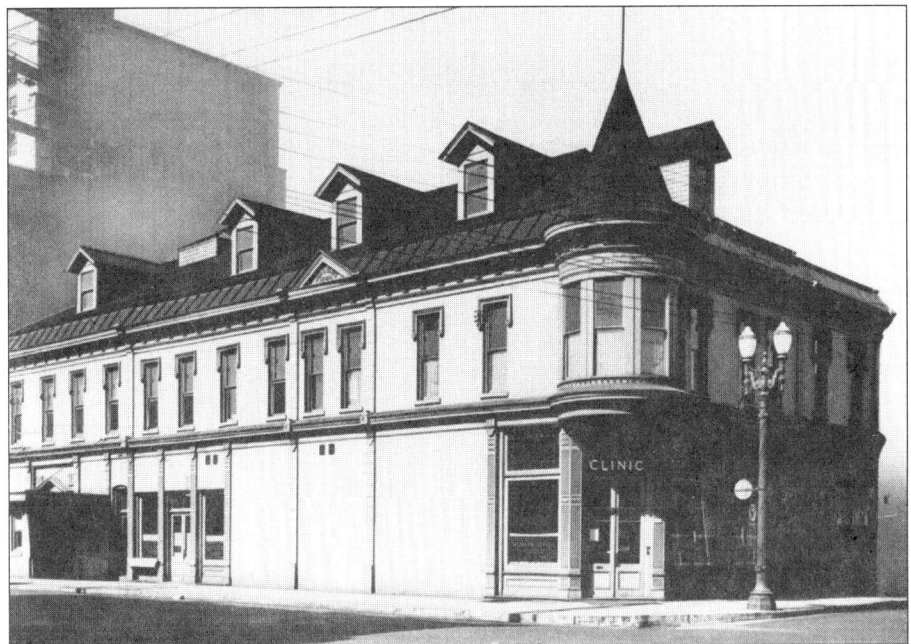

Figure 10-12: Western States College, School of Chiropractic and School of Naturopathy, circa 1938; the facility also housed the non-profit Health Research Foundation, Inc.

for Oregon, where worthy and needy children can obtain drugless service free of cost.

The third unit will rise on the lot willed to chiropractic a short time ago. What a worthy cause!...

Dr. Budden, the founder of the Foundation, along with Dr. Ross Elliott, Dr. P.G. Strapran and others have given of their time, their money for two years in the organization of this Foundation, and now it is time others come forward, express their willingness to do a little toward the success and completion of the Health Research Foundation program... (Dedication, 1938).

Although the HRF did not achieve its goals, it did create a model that was imitated in the 1940s by the NCA, which created a Chiropractic Research Foundation in 1944. Ironically, despite his concern for the scientific bases of chiropractic, Budden disputed former NCA board chairman C.O. Watkins's (1948) call for training chiropractic students in the philosophy of science and in clinical research methods. Budden argued instead that instruction in the basic sciences was sufficient to create a scientific attitude among chiropractors (Budden, 1948; Gatterman, 1982). Ironically, as longtime chairman of the NCA's National Council of Public Health and its Committee on Research, he assumed an advisory role relative to the investigations of the Chiropractic Research Foundation (Weiant, 1946). His reputation was further enhanced by his many speaking engagements for chiropractic groups throughout the nation (e.g., Convention, 1939; Nelson, 1938; Nugent, 1954). Budden was also a strong voice among the 1947 founders of the NCA's Council on Education, predecessor to today's Council on Chiropractic Education (Chirogram, 1974). He envisioned the chiropractic physician as a conservative alternative to allopathy, which included obstetrics and minor surgery. He repeatedly defended this broad scope of practice in Oregon (Gatterman, 1982), and earned strong condemnation from Palmer and other straight chiropractic educators

Chapter 11

NUGENT AND THE BIRTH OF THE ACCREDITATION MOVEMENT

As chiropractic approached its fortieth anniversary, 41 American states had enacted laws to license the profession (Whitten, 1935). However, by 1935 these politico-legal achievements were mitigated in nine jurisdictions (Arkansas, Connecticut, District of Columbia, Iowa, Minnesota, Nebraska, Oregon, Wisconsin and Washington) by basic science laws, and the threat of basic science battles loomed large in others. Between 1936 and the end of World War II an additional eight states (Arizona, Colorado, Florida, Michigan, Oklahoma, Rhode Island, South Dakota and Tennessee) erected basic science barriers to licensure. California's chiropractors waged a successful but wearying struggle against basic science laws in 1942 (Gevitz, 1988; Keating, Dishman et al., 1993), and similar confrontations taxed the profession in other locales. Basic science legislation not only threatened the licensing of D.C.s, but the viability of the colleges themselves (Beatty, 1935b; Cooley, 1935a; Cooper, 1985), and therefore, the future of the profession. Gibbons (1985) estimates that the total enrollment at all chiropractic schools in 1935 was barely 1,500, a mere shadow of the student bodies in the post-war era a decade before.

Chiropractors' considerations of the basic science threat were embedded in their ongoing internal dispute over scope of practice (e.g., Budden, 1935a, 1951; Keating, 1993a; Liberal, 1933; Rodgers, 1935; Steele, 1935; Turner, 1931, p. 143), or what Gibbons (1985) has described as "bitter internecine warfare." Many who had broken with the "Developer" in the 1920s felt that the profession had waited long enough to improve the training of chiropractors, and believed that B.J. Palmer's reluctance to expand the chiropractic curriculum beyond the PSC's standard 18-month program must be confronted. Chiropractic students, they believed, could not be adequately prepared in basic and diagnostic subjects within the traditional "3 years of 6 months." A higher standard was called for (Acquaviva, 1934; Beatty, 1935c; Bonham, 1932; Schulze, 1933; Steinbach, 1936; Watkins, 1932b, 1934). Straight chiropractors, on the other hand, often viewed efforts to lengthen chiropractic training not as a means of battling the basic science threat, but as a ploy to introduce and/or legitimize quasi-medical (or frankly medical) physiotherapeutic and naturopathic subject matter to the educational program (e.g., Drain, 1935a&b; Ratledge, 1935a). James R. Drain, (see Figure 11-1), president of the Texas Chiropractic College, sought to keep the duration of the "standard" chiropractic curriculum to a minimum length, perhaps at the average duration required by existing state boards, i.e., 23 months (Drain, 1935a).

Figure 11-1: James R. Drain, D.C., circa 1937

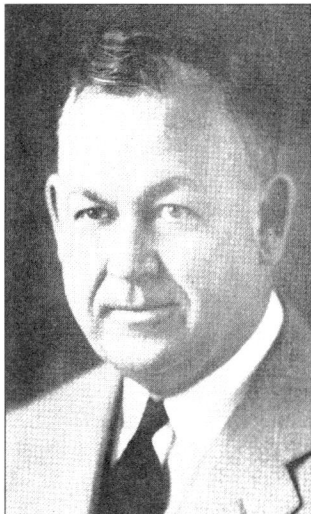

However, the point was becoming increasingly moot; in February 1935, S.E. Julander, D.C., legislative chairman for the Chiropractic Society of Iowa, wrote to college president Carl S. Cleveland to ask his opinion about the Iowa Chiropractors' Association's introduction of a bill to raise the educational requirements for licensure to "4 years of 9 months each with High School preliminary" (Julander, 1935). Ontario had been requiring a four year course for drugless healers for a decade (Biggs, 1989). A 1931 survey of curricular lengths, which included 24 of 27 schools then identified (not including the Palmer, Cleveland and Ratledge schools) had revealed that a minority of the chiropractic colleges still held to the 18-month standard (Hayes, 1931a).

Homer G. Beatty, D.C., N.D., president of the University of Natural Healing Arts in Denver, prepared his own list of some 38 chiropractic colleges (see Table 11-1), and summed up the school problems in 1931:

Schools Need Improvement

Under present conditions, and in general, our Chiropractic schools are not properly housed, equipped or financed. Student bodies are not as large as they should be and the personnel of the teaching staffs might well be improved. There is no standardization of curricula, and proper research work is almost impossible. There are wasted efforts and expense by more than one school serving an area. It is the most wasteful, and the most inefficient system one could imagine. There is even little chance for transfer of ideas and methods of real value...

Schools Not Dictators

We now recognize that in the past the powers in Chiropractic were not properly placed. They should be in the hands of the individual practitioners. The schools should be subservient to the needs and wishes of the practitioners, rather than the dictators.

The schools can be of greater service to the practitioners and the practitioners can be of greater help to the schools. The forming of one strong, central Chiropractic organization, with every Chiropractor a member, will make this possible, for if the central organization has an educational department of a board of regents or governors that are elected by a vote of the practitioners, then that department would have the support and co-operation of the entire field and it is the field that sends the schools the new students.

The board of regents would have such problems as standardization of requirements and curricula, placement of schools, financing, text books, methods, adjuncts and many other problems... (Beatty, 1931a).

It was into this turmoil, set within the context of the nation's economic depression, that the NCA determined that educational improvements and standardization could not be delayed any longer. Beatty, who was serving as president of the NCA Council of Educational Institutions in 1935, called upon all school leaders to attend or send representatives to the NCA's annual convention, scheduled for August in Hollywood, California (Beatty, 1935c). Wayne F. Crider, D.C., president of the NCA-allied (but officially unaffiliated) Council of Chiropractic Examining Boards, successor to the ICCEB, requested the input of all state boards. The Council attempted to do what the school leaders had been unable or unwilling to do themselves:

> Plans will be presented whereby our schools may be rated according to EXACTLY WHAT THEY HAVE AND ARE DOING - BY MERIT ALONE. This scale, when perfected, can be tied in with any state laws now existing.

Table 11-1: Schools of chiropractic, according to a 1931 list prepared by Homer Beatty (Beatty, 1931b)

Akron College of Chiropractic, Akron, Ohio
American School of Chiropractic, New York, N.Y.
Berkeley College of Chiropractic, Berkeley, Calif.
Blodgett Chiropractic College, Cleveland, Ohio
Carver College of Chiropractic, Oklahoma City, Okla.
Cleveland Chiropractic College, Kansas City, Mo.
Colorado Chiropractic University, Denver, Colorado
Columbia Institute of Chiropractic, New York, N.Y.
Colvin College of Chiropractic, Wichita, Kansas
Doty-Marsh College of Chiropractic, Philadelphia, Pa.
Eastern Chiropractic Institute, New York, N.Y.
Indianapolis College of Chiropractic, Indianapolis, Ind.
Lincoln Chiropractic College, Indianapolis, Ind.
Los Angeles College of Chiropractic, Los Angeles, Calif.
Marchand College of Chiropractic, Philadelphia, Pa.
Mecca College of Chiropractic, Newark, N.J.
Metropolitan Chiropractic College, Cleveland, Ohio
Missouri Chiropractic College, St. Louis, Mo.
National Eclectic Institute, New York, N.Y.
National College of Chiropractic, Chicago, Ill.
New York School of Chiropractic, New York, N.Y.
Pacific College of Chiropractic, Portland, Ore.
Palmer School of Chiropractic, Davenport, Iowa
Pasadena College of Chiropractic, Pasadena, California
Peerless College of Chiropractic, Chicago, Ill.
Ramsay College of Chiropractic, Minneapolis, Minn.
Ratledge College of Chiropractic, Los Angeles, Calif.
Ross College of Chiropractic, Fort Wayne, Ind.
San Francisco College of Chiropractic & Drugless Therapy, San Francisco, California
Seattle College of Chiropractic, Seattle, Wash.
Standard School of Chiropractic, New York, N.Y.
Texas Chiropractic College, San Antonio, Texas
Toronto College of Chiropractic, Toronto, Canada
Universal College of Chiropractic, Pittsburg, Pa.
Washington School of Chiropractic, Washington, D.C.
West Coast College of Chiropractic, Oakland, California
Western Chiropractic College, Kansas City, Mo.
Denver Chiropractic Institute, Denver, Colorado

Further, the legislative committee will have a draft of proposed legislation embodying within it the corrections of errors that are only too evident in many of the present acts.

Many have been wondering just how it is possible to combat the pro-medical, Basic Science campaign being waged during the past ten years. One answer is - to present a program that has superior merit. This is the duty of the State Examining Boards - to lead the way to formulating and adopting such a program to hand down to our profession for concerted action. Unfortunately in this we have been grossly negligent. Lethargy for years has been the rule and for which many states have paid a very dear price. Shall we accept this assignment? There can be only one answer - yes!

The council officers take this opportunity of inviting every State Chiropractic Examining Board to send either an official delegate or observer to the Hollywood meeting. It is imperative that concerted action be achieved in the future (Crider, 1935a).

A number of college leaders did attend (see Table 11-2); however, conspicuously absent were B.J. Palmer and T.F. Ratledge. Like his straight chiropractic colleague, James Drain (1935b), Ratledge (1935b) was already considering the formation of a rival school group opposed to the NCA's educational endeavors. But a formal confrontation between

College leader	Affiliation
Omer C. Bader, D.C., N.D.	National College of Chiropractic, Chicago
Homer G. Beatty, D.C., N.D.	University of Natural Healing Arts, Denver
Rangnar C. Bertheau, D.C., N.D.	College of Chiropractic Physicians & Surgeons, Los Angeles
William A. Budden, D.C., N.D.	Western States College, Portland
Charles A. Cale, D.C., N.D.	Chiropractic College of America, Los Angeles
James R. Drain, D.C., Ph.C.	Texas Chiropractic College, San Antonio
Robert Ramsay, D.C.	Minnesota Chiropractic College
Charles H. Wood, D.C., N.D.	Los Angeles College of Chiropractic, Los Angeles

Table 11-2: Some of the college leaders who attended the 1935 NCA convention in Hollywood

straight and mixer factions of the educational community was still a few years in the future. In the meanwhile, the NCA's Hollywood convention created a benchmark in chiropractic history, for it was here that Montana practitioner C.O. Watkins, D.C. introduced a resolution to create the Committee on Education (Keating, 1993a; Martin, 1974), and became the first chairman of this newly formed NCA group (Chirogram, 1974; Keating, 1988).

The issue of "straights" vs. "mixers" in the 1930s significantly revolved around the use of "modalities," which were considered aspects of physiotherapy by many D.C.s. A 1928 survey of 500 chiropractors by the ACA Bureau of Research yielded a 60% return, or 302 replies. The survey suggested that a substantive majority (78%) of D.C.s employed some form of non-adjustive or physiotherapeutic methods, and 80% reported that they had received some form of instruction in "drugless methods" at the chiropractic school from which they had graduated (Survey, 1928). However, the ACA's report, prepared by then ACA Director of Research Leo J. Steinbach of the Universal Chiropractic College, had significantly over-represented UCC graduates and under-represented Palmer graduates. A 1930 survey published by the Lincoln Chiropractic College revealed some important variations among chiropractors (see Table 11-3). Although the composition of the sample from which more than 1,800 responses were drawn is not known, the Lincoln College did not teach physiotherapy modalities, and its respondents therefore might be expected to under-represent the sentiments of mixers. Nonetheless, a general consensus of opinion was apparent, and suggested a fairly firm middle ground wherein many non-adjustive procedures were endorsed by the overwhelming majority. Slightly less than a third of the sample reported using "electro-therapy," and 48% endorsed instruction in these methods at chiropractic colleges.

Both "straight" and "mixer" standards of accreditation were at first considered by the NCA (Crider, 1936). The organization also officially decried the continuing movement toward "physician and surgeon" status by some schools, and announced that the NCA would no longer insure chiropractors who practiced "coagulation of tonsils and dehydration of hemorrhoids, which practice has been construed to be the practice of surgery" (NCA, 1935). Budden of Western States College responded:

The current issue of the *Chiropractic Journal* contains the following item:

"In view of the fact that this practice has been construed to be surgery, the N.C.A. will not afford any legal defense in mal-practice cases arising from the coagulation of tonsils or the dehydration of hemorrhoids."

Regarding the above, we wish to call your attention to the fact that the Western States College stands foursquare behind the members of the profession who are engaged in the practice of electrotherapy as a part of chiropractic.

There is no reason to back down or to retreat from the position we have already established. It has been supported by judicial interpretation and by public sentiment. Let us stand by our guns.

The college has developed the legal status of this phase of our art and will gladly assist any chiropractor who finds himself attacked along this line.

Very truly yours,

WESTERN STATES COLLEGE

Dr. A. Budden, Director (Budden, 1935b)

Perhaps in further reaction to what they perceived as a retreat from broad-scope chiropractic, the Hollywood convention was followed by the creation of an independent organization of mixer schools, known as the Affiliated Universities of Natural Healing:

We wish to encourage the profession in efforts toward reasonable, higher and broader standards; and wish to help blaze the way to greater progress and development in conformity with the great merits of chiropractic.

A regular standard, four years of nine months each, course in Chiropractic and allied subjects is warranted by our profession and offered by the following school members of this affiliation:

Table 11-3: Results of a survey conducted by the Lincoln Chiropractic College in 1930 (Turner, 1931, pp. 208-11)

Survey Questions	% Yes	Total
1. Is your examination confined to the spine?	18	1883
2. Do you question your patients about subjective symptoms (abnormal symptoms)?	95	1861
3. Do you investigate objective symptoms (through inspection, palpation, percussion, auscultation, etc., other than the spine)?	86	1869
4. Do you examine the heart and pulse?	86	1838
5. Do you employ a spinal meter instrument (either resistance type or thermocouple type)?	35	1862
6. Do you use any of the various types of "radionics" equipment?	16	1859
7. Do you take the blood pressure?	77	1871
8. Do you use the clinical thermometer?	78	1873
9. Do you employ urinalysis?	78	1884
10. Do you advise your patients as to diet?	89	1867
11. Do you advise as to exercise, habits, etc.?	88	1867
12. Do you employ massage?	55	1821
13. Do you use a vibrator?	28	1893
14. Do you employ a heat lamp?	48	1861
15. Do you employ radionics?	16	1864
16. Do you use "light therapy"?	37	1858
17. Do you employ any form of "electro-therapy"?	32	1860
18. Do you employ any form of "hydro-therapy" (baths, enemas, colonic irrigation, etc.)?	40	1876
19. Do you practice "foot correction"?	49	1856
20. Do you give spinal adjustments to every case?	82	1893
21. Do you favor chiropractic schools teaching diagnostic methods	90	1883
22. Do you favor chiropractic schools teaching "light therapy"?	54	1806
23. Do you favor chiropractic schools teaching "hydro-therapy"?	56	1779
24. Do you favor chiropractic schools teaching "electro-therapy"?	48	1786
25. Do you favor chiropractic schools teaching "radionics"?	30	1642
26. Do you favor chiropractic schools teaching massage?	63	1805
27. Do you favor chiropractic schools teaching "foot correction"?	74	1800
28. Do you favor chiropractic schools teaching diet?	90	1861

(Membership open to qualifying schools)
WESTERN STATES COLLEGE
438 SE Elder, Portland, Oregon
METROPOLITAN COLLEGE OF CHIROPRACTIC AND PHYSIOTHERAPY
3400 Euclid Ave., Cleveland, Ohio
UNIVERSITY OF THE HEALING ARTS
840 Asylum Ave., Hartford, Conn.
UNIVERSITY OF NATURAL HEALING ARTS
1631 Glenarm St., Denver, Colorado

Write direct for catalogs or further information. Your support of the above educational standards
through new students, is solicited (Advertisement, 1935).

Little more is known about the Affiliated Universities of Natural Healing, except that their initiative greatly alarmed straight chiropractic college leaders (Kightlinger, 1936), and may have led to the formation of the rival body, the Associated Chiropractic Colleges of America (ACCA). The ACCA was the precursor to the Allied Chiropractic Educational Institutions, an affiliate of B.J. Palmer's International Chiropractors' Association.

W.A. Budden later recalled events leading up to and surrounding the birth of the NCA's accreditation movement:

> That the private ownership of the institutions in a measure militated against a generous and whole-sale upsurge to finance this idea is true and must be taken into account in appraising the situation prevailing at that time. Only an optimist, however, and one quite unfamiliar with the economics of chiropractic schools and colleges would suggest that, by advancing scholastic requirements, more money could be made. The facts being quite the contrary, as we have intimated, the "school men" as a group hesitated. Some suggested that while the idea was a good one, the time was not yet. Nevertheless, Dr. E.J. Smith, young graduate of the National College and of Western Reserve University in 1921, gave the first real impetus toward what is now so far developed by establishing a four- year school in Cleveland, Ohio. The Metropolitan College of Chiropractic opened its doors to the first four-year students and the new era had begun. Shortly after this pioneer effort, the National College proclaimed that it would issue certificates of graduation "cum laude" to those who successfully negotiated its thirty-two months course. The writer of this article initiated this action and signed as "Dean" the first diplomas. It should be stated here, and with no sense of derogation of those who took a leading part in this advance, in the case of the N.C.C. certainly, the fact that a medical board of examiners held sway over chiropractic activities in Illinois, and to some extent in Ohio, tended powerfully to fertilize the soil in which the actual four-year course took root.
>
> Almost simultaneously with these events, the new idea appeared in Colorado. The late Homer Beatty, head of the college in Denver and author of the well-known text, "Anatomical Adjustive Technique," now began to raise his voice calling for thirty-six months training. A vigorous advocate of any cause he espoused, the impact of his personality and propaganda soon began to make itself felt. Dr. Beatty, however, was not alone. Associated with him in this crusade were several of the teachers of the school, notably Dr. Niel Bishop, as well as a number of men "in the field." Behind them all, however, and adding powerfully to the growth of the movement, loomed the figure of Professor Jones, dean emeritus of Northwestern University, School of Psychology, and doctor of chiropractic of National College.
>
> Now another voice from the far west was added to the growing debate. The pages of the National Journal began to reflect the views of C.O. Watkins of Montana. Logical, incisive persistent "C.O." hammered away at the bulwarks of the short-course school of thought. There can be no doubt that his rapid rise to a leading place in the councils of the NCA brought powerful aid and comfort to the four-year idea (Budden, 1951).

Parallel efforts were initiated by the NCA Committee on Education and the Joint Committee (of Examining Boards and School Heads). Crider (1936) reported that the preliminary rating scheme, which distinguished between straight and mixer schools,

> ...was adopted in principle, specific details and minor changes to be considered later. The final draft by mutual consent to be approved by a joint Committee of State Examining Boards and School heads.

The joint committee is composed as follows: Drs. HG Beatty, A. Budden and Jas. Drain for the Schools and Drs. WF Crider of Maryland, CO Hunt of California and FO Logic of Michigan for the State Boards. The recommendations as to inclusions, rejections and modifications were incorporated.

Visits were made to Chicago and Indianapolis, following the convention, consulting Drs. Schulze, Bader and Golden of the National, and Drs. Vedder, Firth and associates of the Lincoln, thus ironing out more of the scales' faults, and obtaining the general reaction after these groups had time to study copies of the scale. It has not been heretofore mentioned that similar tactics were practiced on the journey to the meeting. Universal of Pittsburgh and Metropolitan of Cleveland were given copies and they forwarded their approval, in principle, of the proposal. Dr. BJ Palmer was also contacted with similar intent. However, the astute qualities usually ascribed to him were evidently lacking upon this occasion as he was unwilling to even listen 'to anything that smacked of NCA' - in spite of repeated declarations that the Council of State Examining Boards on the contrary was separate and distinct from any and all other organizations....

The revised draft was completed and forwarded to members of the joint committee. Other incorporations and modifications were listed. However, it was not possible to incorporate all suggestions.

It is interesting to note that the schools' opinions were still sharply defined and divergent - while the State Boards were unanimously in favor of higher standards.

A synopsis of the Joint Committee's findings is as follows:

1.It will be necessary to rate schools teaching the orthodox methods and those teaching the more liberal methods in separate categories as regards list of class hours and equipment.

2.All authorities agree, two thousand sixty-minute hours is the maximum that can be taught in three years of six months. This basis, although somewhat less intent, is used in compiling the scale and setting it as regards to curriculum.

3.It must be comparable with other professions' standards.

4.The Schools being commercial in character (with very few exceptions) it is necessary to give due consideration to financial stability of the Institution.

5.In accordance with the tendency of all state laws, wherever amended, the trend being upward from the three years of six months level, it became obvious the scale minimum for grade A probationary rating must be twenty-four months for the fundamental course and four years of eight months for the liberal course.

6.In order that all schools may have an opportunity to meet the final requirement of fundamental (three years of nine months) and the liberal (four years of nine), one calendar year - until January 1, 1937, is given for probationary rating of all Chiropractic Schools and colleges.

7.The scale must be so constructed as to include from the minimum of set requirements to the maximum as taught by any Chiropractic school of today.

The Council of State Boards will not enter into a discussion of the definition of chiropractic. Suffice it to say that each type of thought is recognized and given opportunities to develop. We, therefore, have divided the schools into two groups - the Basic or Fundamental Schools (teaching only Chiropractic) and the Liberal or Physical Therapy Schools (teaching Chiropractic and Physical Therapy)... (Crider, 1936).

These early initiatives also involved an attempt to "raise chiropractic standards through uniform examinations" (Nugent, quoted by Gibbons, 1985), a tactic which was later abandoned. Accreditation eventually became the vehicle for improving the education of the chiropractor, and it required the combined efforts of the Committee on Education and the Council of State Examining Boards. A preliminary commitment to establishing standards of education was voted upon at the NCA's 1938 convention in Toronto, when it was decided that:

...the NCA approve a standard of education of four years of twenty-seven weeks each, effective September 1, 1938, and that a course of four years of thirty-two weeks each, of not less than 3600 hours, be effective September 1, 1941, and that students already enrolled may be graduated (quoted in Rogers, 1938b).

The chair of the Committee on Education passed from Watkins to Gordon Goodfellow in 1938, when Watkins was elected to the NCA's board of directors (Chirogram, 1974). Goodfellow moved to combine the two groups, thereby creating the Committee on Educational Standards:

> The Council of State Examining Boards had a similar program going on at the same time - one was offsetting the other.
>
> In 1938 Dr. K.C. Robinson, president of the NCA, appointed Dr. Gordon Goodfellow as chairman of the committee and allowed him to appoint the rest of the members. He appointed Drs. Wayne Crider, John J. Nugent, L.F. Downs and F.A. Baker; thus combining the two groups as the Committee on Educational Standards. The self-evaluation request was sent to all of the then 37 chiropractic colleges in the United States, fifteen colleges responded and requested approval.
>
> In 1939 the Committee adopted the first criteria for the approval of chiropractic colleges, which has often been modified and brought up to date.
>
> In 1940 Dr John J. Nugent was hired as the Director of Education to inspect the colleges. In 1941 the first list of provisional approved colleges was issued (Chirogram, 1974).

The appointees to the Committee on Educational Standards for 1939-40 are presented in Table 11-4. Some confusion existed in the very earliest years of NCA accreditation, owing to the premature release of lists of NCA-accredited schools by Crider and Goodfellow (Cheatham, 1939; Goodfellow, 1940, Palmer, 1941). However, with Nugent at the helm as Director of Research in 1941, the long journey toward federal recognition proceeded in a more orderly fashion. The first compilation of accreditation criteria were adopted by the NCA at its 1939 convention (Nugent, 1953), and were published in Nugent's (1941) *Chiropractic Education: Outline of a Standard Course*. The *Outline* set out the areas (see

Table 11-4: Members of the NCA's Committee on Educational Standards for 1939-40 (Schnick, 1939)
Gordon M. Goodfellow, D.C., N.D., Chairman, Los Angeles Wayne F. Crider, D.C., Hagerstown, Maryland John J. Nugent, D.C., New Haven, Connecticut John K. Couch, D.C., Oklahoma City F.A. Baker, D.C., Mankato, Minnesota

Table 11-5) with which any school would have to comply in order to receive a favorable rating; this booklet is generally acknowledged as the first substantive educational accreditation guidelines for the chiropractic profession. Nugent had clearly relied heavily upon AMA standards in devising his recommendations (Nugent, 1941, p. 22), a fact that surely served to antagonize straight chiropractic college leaders. The NCA leader's preamble described the chiropractor as a "physician," a term which was anathema to straight chiropractors.

Also by 1941, any idea of separate criteria for straight vs. mixer schools had been abandoned, and a minimum of "four years of eight months each," involving not less than 3,600 hours of training, was mandated (Nugent, 1941, p. 20). The NCA's curriculum approximated the "minimum medical course" recommended by the AMA's educational accrediting body. Nugent claimed that with the exclusion of instruction time for general surgery, the number of required hours for chiropractic and medical training were equivalent (see Table 11-6). W.A. Budden later recalled events surrounding the NCA's commitment to the four year curriculum:

> It was, however, to Dr. R.D. Ketchum, of Bend, Oregon, that credit must go for giving final impulse toward definite action by the NCA. The doctor was at that time state delegate for Oregon, and was generally admitted to be one of the most influential and respected members of the then House of Counselors. It was as such that he issued his call to arms. Said he at the close of a short but powerful exhortation, "We have talked a lot about the four-year course, let us get busy and do something about it."
>
> Some time previous to this event, however, a committee appointed by the NCA had been at work attempting to evaluate the status of the schools. The outline of an accreditation system already had emerged. The groundwork was being laid for what was to come. The challenge from the West then was caught up and echoed by this committee and the wheels began to turn. At this point there strode into the forefront of the picture a stalwart figure. Already a leading member of the committee, he now took a commanding position. From that moment on, the incisive logic, the mordant sarcasm, the merciless dialectic, coupled with a calm, rock-like resistance to criticism and opposition that is J.J. Nugent, served as a rallying point in the conflict which surged and eddied around the four-year idea.

Table 11-5: Table of contents from Nugent's (1941, pp. 6-8) *Chiropractic Education: Outline of a Standard Course*

Introduction
School Code of N.C.A.
  Physical Equipment
  Equipment
  Faculty
  Prerequisites for Admission
    Age
    Education
    Character
  Curriculum
    Preclinical Subjects
    Clinical Subjects
  Length of Course
  Admission to Advanced Standing
  Financial Ability
The Essential Elements
The Student
  Preliminary Requirements
The Faculty
The Curriculum
Length of Course
  Minimum Medical Course Percentages
  Minimum Chiropractic Course
    Percentages
  Table I, Comparison of Medical and
    Chiropractic Courses
Synopsis of Medical Course
Table II, First-Fourth Years
Table III, Suggested Curriculum for
Chiropractic Schools

Curriculum Building
The Quarter System
The Sixty-Minute Hour
Buildings and Equipment
Organization and Administration
  Organization
  Administration
    Supervision
    Records
    Credentials
    Advanced Standing
    Degrees Conferred
    Publications
The Library
Textbooks
Anatomy, Histology and Embryology
  Gross Anatomy
  Dissection
  Embryology
  Histology
Physiology and Physiological Chemistry
  Physiology
  Physiological Chemistry
Pathology and Bacteriology
  Pathology
    General Pathology
    Systemic Pathology
  Bacteriology
Clinical Studies
  Physical Diagnosis & Clinical Laboratory

    Methods
    History Taking
    Physical Examination
    Physical Diagnosis
    Laboratory Diagnosis
  Clinical Training
    Outpatient Departments
    Lecture Clinics
  Clinical Chiropractic
    Study of Medical Diagnosis
    (Demands on General Practitioners)
    Grouping of Medical Diagnosis
    Office Visits
    Home Visits
    Opinions of Graduates of Medical Course,
      Table of
    Osteopathic School, Table of Subject
      Hours
  Principles of Chiropractic, The
    Physiology of the Nervous System
  History of Chiropractic, The
  Chiropractic Technique
  Physical Therapy
  Pediatrics
  Gynecology and Obstetrics
  Hygiene, Sanitation and Public Health
  Roentgenology
  Psychiatry
  Jurisprudence

Subject	Minimum Chiropractic Course	AMA Minimum Medical Course	Typical Medical School, No. 1	Typical Medical School, No. 2	AMA Maximum Medical Course
Anatomy, including Embryology and Histology	666	666	663	663	814
Physiology	216	216	225	229	264
Biochemistry	162	162	180	203	198
Pathology & Bacteriology	468	468	487	524	572
Basic Sciences - Total	1,512	1,512	1,555	1,619	1,848
Public Health & Sanitation	144	144	92	132	176
Obstetrics & Gynecology	180	180	245	296	220
Principles & Practice	1,764	1,134	1,876	1,620	1,386
Common Subjects - Total	3,600	2,970	3,668	3,667	3,622
General Surgery	not taught	630	841	521	778
Total Hours in Course	3,600	3,600	4,509	4,288	4,400

Table 11-6: Comparison of NCA educational criteria with those of the AMA (Nugent 1941, p.22).

Powerful aid now also came from members of the Executive Committee. The secretary, Dr. L.M. Rogers, as an executive, long a silent sympathizer, became effectively articulate on the affirmative side. Drs. Gordon M. Goodfellow, of California, Downs, of Montana, Harriman, of North Dakota; men from Iowa, from Illinois, from Minnesota, from Wisconsin, stood up to be counted for the new day in education. Thus ended phase one (Budden, 1951).

Although it is not certain, it seems likely that the NCA's decision to commit to a single criterion of four academic years of training for all schools wishing accreditation was influenced by the activities of the previously mentioned Allied Chiropractic Educational Institutions (ACEI). The ACEI was the successor to the Associated Chiropractic College of America, which had been formed at Carl S. Cleveland's suggestion by disaffected straight college presidents Cleveland, Drain of the Texas College, Kightlinger of the Eastern Institute in New York, and Ratledge (Ratledge, 1935c). Cleveland, it may be recalled, had served as president of the International Chiropractic Congress' Division of Schools in 1931-33; he protested the NCA's educational policies on behalf of the straight schools at the NCA's 1940 convention in Minneapolis (Ratledge, 1940b). The Kansas City school leader was therefore in a good position to contrast the NCA's new standards with the ICC's older, laissez-faire policies. Although he initially continued to advertise his school in the NCA's *Journal* [e.g., Advertisement, 1936], the seeds of discontent had been sown. Ratledge expressed the sentiments of the proprietary and straight school leaders in a letter to Willard Carver:

....I have agreed already with Cleveland, Texas and Eastern colleges to form such an organization of CHIROPRACTIC schools to offset the menace of the N.C.A. and those naturopathic schools with it now seems to be in league as against real chiropractic schools....I believe that Lincoln will join in the movement as I know that they are disgusted with the N.C.A.'s policy and apparent purposes in relation to forcing chiropractic schools to engage in medical and other foreign instruction.

Also, I believe that Universal will join in such a movement and that Palmer will at least be friendly or at least not adverse to us in such a movement. If all the schools mentioned, except Palmer, would get together on a policy of adhering to chiropractic instruction exclusively, I believe that we could direct the trends in chiropractic instruction even if Palmer remained aloof or even opposed to us....I believe that there are thousands of chiropractors who would rally to the support of any group which would come out strongly for chiropractic and who appeared to be strong enough to uphold their position.... (Ratledge, 1938b).

Adding to the dissatisfaction produced by NCA's longer, "mixer" standards for chiropractic training was the national society's imperious attitude toward the rating of schools. The NCA did not initially construe its accreditation program as voluntary, and sought to force reluctant schools to upgrade. Fiery straight school leader T.F. Ratledge reacted with outrage, and sent the following note to Loran M. Rogers, executive secretary of the NCA:

Gentlemen:

Your affiliate council, the 'Council of State Chiropractic Examining Boards,' through it's [sic] President, Dr. Wayne F. Crider of Hagerstown, Maryland, has notified me in writing of it's [sic] avowed purpose of classifying the Ratledge Chiropractic College in spite of our previous written objection thereto.

On July 9th, we notified Dr. Crider that we would not consent to any classification whatsoever by the N.C.A. or any of it's [sic] affiliates and definitely warned that in case he or the Council does attempt to so classify our institution among Chiropractic teaching institutions we will resort to the courts to recover any damages which we believe to have resulted to said Ratledge Chiropractic College by such classification....

....We regret to feel it necessary to call your attention to this matter but in view of the very arbitrary position assumed by the Council of State Boards of Chiropractic Examiners, whose purpose and ability are both highly questionable, from our point of view, we feel that we would not be fair with you if we did not advise you in advance of Dr. Crider's threat and of our defiance to same (Ratledge, 1937).

The NCA apparently took the hint, for in May 1940, Gordon M. Goodfellow, chairman of the NCA's Committee on Educational Standards, indicated to Ratledge that the Committee intended to publish a vocational guidance booklet in March of the following year, and that the booklet would list only NCA-accredited institutions (Goodfellow, 1940). In other words, schools that did not apply to the NCA for review were to be ignored. Ratledge wrote back to express his contempt for the NCA's "drugless" and "naturopathic" policies, and again indicated his refusal to cooperate with the NCA's educational reforms (Ratledge, 1940a).

The ACCA was reorganized as the ACEI in 1939 (Ratledge, 1939). The Cleveland, Eastern, Ratledge and Texas colleges were formally joined in their opposition to the NCA under the ACEI banner by B.J. Palmer, the PSC and the soon to be renamed Chiropractic Health Bureau [renamed ICA/International Chiropractors' Association in 1941 (Metz, 1965, p. 55)], Willard Carver's Oklahoma school, Frank Dean's Columbia Institute in New York City (today's New York Chiropractic College), and by the O'Neil-Ross College in Fort Wayne, Indiana (ACEI, 1940, 1941; ICA, 1986; Palmer, 1941). The Cleveland College of Kansas City and Kightlinger's Eastern Chiropractic Institute (ECI) were apparently unswayed in their opposition to the NCA's educational reform efforts by the fact that they had been included on the broad-scope organization's initial lists of approved schools. Although the Lincoln Chiropractic College had been expected to join with the straight college leaders in the ICA's rival school organization (Ratledge, 1938b), the Indianapolis school had already committed itself to a curricular length acceptable to the NCA (Firth, 1941). The ACEI threw down the gauntlet before the NCA in mid-1940:

> The Allied Chiropractic Educational Institutions in convention assembled at Kansas City, Missouri, this the 20th day of July, A.D. 1940....recommends as its unswerving policy that Chiropractic in its simplicity and purity shall be protected and carried on without being encroached upon by any entangling alliances.....this organization of educational institutions demands that any national organization within the Chiropractic profession that expects to....maintain the friendly cooperation of the educational institutions this organization represents.... must advocate that Chiropractic educational institutions shall teach maintain only a specific course in Chiropractic education....
>
> ....all branches of medicine are particularly declared to be not a part or not a possible part of a course of study in Chiropractic. The prohibited subjects, it will thus appear, are the prescription and administration of drugs, the practice of surgery by instrumental and intervention or use of instruments in any surgical effort, and this includes radionics, diathermy in any of its aspects, and all other allied machines generally classified as auxiliaries and professing any aspect of cure or relief. This also includes hydrotherapy, and all phases of naturopathy and all allied subjects thereto, which includes water cure and all so-called natural therapeutic methods....
>
> To the National Chiropractic Association ....and all allied organizations, the Allied Chiropractic Educational Institutions goes on record and states that unless a reorganized plan of your bodies, association, or by whatever name known, reorganized, amend and change said organizations in such way as to be in conformity with the suggestions and demands of allied educational institutions.... we shall withdraw all support that has ever come from the members of this organization to your organization....and we say to you now in all kindness and truth that unless reorganization, amendments, etc., are accomplishments by you within a reasonable time, the members of the Allied Chiropractic Educational Institutions shall feel free to organize a separate national organization that will be strictly Chiropractic....
>
> Signed....Per TF Ratledge, D.C., Secretary, Jas. R. Drain, Acting President (ACEI, 1940).

The die had been cast, and the two factions, straights and mixers, struggled for more than three decades over the accreditation process. The feud created some unexpected allies. For instance, Willard Carver, LL.B., D.C., who had battled with Palmer for decades, accepted C.S. Cleveland's nomination to the ICA Board of Control in 1941 (ACEI, 1941), where he was joined by his former pupil T.F. Ratledge, nominated to the same board that year by H.E. Weiser, D.C., of the Texas Chiropractic College. Although Hugh B. Logan, founder of the St. Louis school which bears his name, did not serve on the ICA governing body, his son Vinton became a staunch Palmer ally. Gibbons has noted that "The senior Logan was a bitter opponent of Nugent's role in obtaining basic science legislation"; Logan remained "in the limbo" of NCA and ICA. At one point, Vinton Logan accused Nugent, the NCA's director of education from 1941 to 1961, of "misstatements of fact and expressions of animus" (Gibbons, 1985).

Craig Kightlinger's role in the ACEI seems somewhat contradictory, inasmuch as he continued to play an active role in the NCA. However, his views may exemplify a few straight chiropractic college leaders who objected not so much to the lengthier course that NCA called for, but more especially to broad-scope instruction. Indeed, in November of 1940 this founder of the ECI authored an article that appeared in the *National Chiropractic Journal,* and called for lengthening of the standard curriculum. He explained his reasoning:

During our legislative session in New Jersey a year or so ago, one of the State legislators made this statement, "You presume to tell me that my son who graduates from high school this June, at the age of 18, can be so educated in a year and a half that he will be able to take life and death in his hands and understand it thoroughly so that he can efficiently administer to the sick at the age of 19 years and 6 months. If you have the presumption to assume this attitude on education, then I for one will vote against your Bill every time it comes up..."

We are for the longer course and have a 4 year course of 9 months each. We also maintain a 3 year course of 10 months each. We wish to give them more. We desire to teach in detail the following subjects: bacteriology, philosophy, psychology, neurology, orthopedy, pathology, symptomatology and diagnosis, anatomy, histology, physiology, hygiene, chemistry, gynecology, obstetrics, analysis, palpation, technique of adjusting, adjusting service, spinography, nerve tracing, first aid, dietetics, toxicology, jurisprudence, ethics, public health and we feel that even 3 years of 10 months each is not sufficient to teach them as thoroughly as we would like to in order that they may graduate as properly qualified Doctors of Chiropractic (Kightlinger, 1940).

Nugent's strategy for standardization involved voluntary application for review, completion of a written self-report concerning admission criteria, facilities, curriculum and personnel, and inspection for any institution that wished to comply with the NCA standards (Nugent, 1941). Several schools were turned down, including the Nashville College of Drugless Therapy (Cheatham, 1943), and many more did not apply. The education director's first official list of NCA-approved schools, issued shortly after America's entry into World War II, included "National, New York School, Eastern, Detroit College, Lincoln, Southern California, Metropolitan (Cleveland), Minnesota, Universal, Missouri, Western States and the University of Natural Healing Arts" (Gibbons, 1985). Though admirable as a beginning, Nugent and the NCA proceeded in an occasionally fumbling pattern towards accreditation categories, procedures and policies.

A subsequent NCA list established "provisional" accreditation status; only the Lincoln, National and Western States Colleges maintained a "fully approved" rating. The reduced status could not have come at a worse moment for the Universal Chiropractic College (UCC), which was already beginning to feel the effects of the military draft. By 1944 Leo J. Steinbach, dean of the non-profit UCC, had come to accept the need for merging smaller schools into larger institutions, and in May 1944, Nugent announced the merger of UCC with the Lincoln College in Indianapolis (Nugent, 1944). Steinbach was appointed to the board of trustees of the amalgamated school, and served as chairman of the technique department. Nugent used the occasion to explain his plan for school amalgamations:

Our survey of the schools indicated that there were too many schools in the same general area competing for the limited number of students available. Further, with few exceptions these schools were "proprietary," or privately owned schools...

As in other professions, most of the ills to which our profession is heir lies in the fact that many of our schools are privately owned. We, then, must follow the example of other professions and as fastly [sic] as possible make the change from "proprietary" schools to professionally controlled schools. To this the NCA is committed...

With a standard curriculum; four years of training; a higher grade of instructors; with additional teaching and laboratory facilities and increased income, the remaining schools will be sounder and stronger. If in addition these schools are controlled and directed by boards of trustees representing the public and the profession our educational institutions will be on a par with other professions (Nugent, 1944).

The Eastern Chiropractic Institute (ECI) reacted strongly but professionally to its reduced status. Kightlinger wrote to Nugent and the NCA "to protest the PUBLICATION of this accrediting at this time" (Kightlinger, 1943). With the wartime draft siphoning off potential students, none of the chiropractic schools could afford to lose prospects because of the NCA's less than favorable ratings, no matter how loyal to NCA a college might hope to be. In New York, he noted, where chiropractors were still unlicensed, the law prevented the Eastern Institute from meeting all of NCA's educational standards. Clarence W. Weiant, D.C., who had earned a Ph.D. in anthropology from Columbia University in 1943 and served as dean of the ECI, echoed Kightlinger's sentiments and added a plea for "straight chiropractic" in a letter to Loran M. Rogers:

We concur with Dr. Kightlinger on the following three points:

(1) We should have been presented with a bill of particulars concerning our deficiencies before any public action was taken in order that we might determine to what extent we could comply with

the prescribed conditions.

(2) Schools which have declined to cooperate in any way or, which are outside the NCA have not been penalized by having the fact published that they are not approved.

(3) There has been no disposition on the part of the NCA to strengthen schools financially in some way so that they might attain the desired standard, as, for example, by the creation of scholarships, publicity campaigns for students, endowments, etc.

...If one must decide between, on the one hand, putting out of business schools that cannot, for financial reasons, come up to an ideal standard and, on the other handd, letting such schools live (provided they do the best they can), then we, as a group vote for the second alternative. We do this not out of selfish motivation, (the Lord only knows we get little enough out of the venture) but because, unless the schools survive, straight chiropractic cannot survive... (Weiant, 1943).

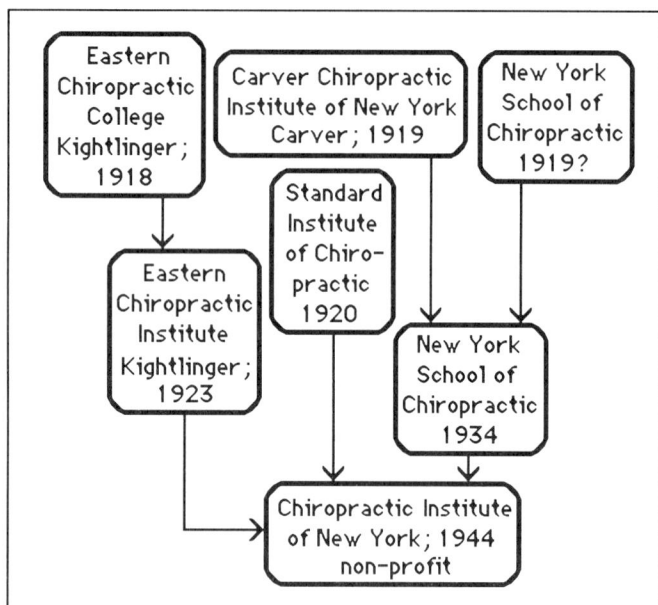

Figure 11-2: Institutional genealogy of the Chiropractic Institute of New York (CINY); dates refer to earliest known operations of the school; reprinted by permission from the *Chiropractic Journal of Australia*

Nugent mentioned the idea of merging ECI and several other New York City schools in a memorandum to the NCA's executive board and members of the Committee on Educational Standards (Nugent, 1943). The NCA education director had befriended the head of the New York State Board of Regents' committee on professional education, and sought his expertise in uniting the several chiropractic schools located in New York City into a fiscally sounder, non-profit, professionally-controlled institution. Nugent, with the assistance of Stephen E. Owens, D.C. (Wardwell, 1992, p. 94), persuaded Kightlinger of the necessity of higher standards in chiropractic education, and the ECI founder approved of Nugent's testimony before a state legislative committee on chiropractic, wherein the provisional rating of ECI was offered as part of a rationale for licensing D.C.s in New York (Kightlinger, 1944). By the end of 1944 Nugent had merged three of the four New York schools into the non-profit Institute of the Science and Art of Chiropractic (Ebrall, 1995; Rogers, 1944), which was soon renamed the Chiropractic Institute of New York (CINY) (see Figure 11-2). Kightlinger served as president, Weiant as dean, and Thure C. Peterson, D.C., former dean of the Carver Institute and the New York School of Chiropractic (Rehm, 1980, p. 307; Wardwell, 1992, p. 94), served as executive director of CINY (see Table 11-7). The Columbia Institute of Chiropractic (today's New York Chiropractic College), under Frank Dean, chose to remain outside the NCA's orbit. He served instead on the ICA's Board of Control (ICA, 1949).

Part of Nugent's early success in merging small schools into larger non-profit corporations resulted from the severe student shortage caused by the war. The pinch had begun to be felt at some schools even before the bombing of Pearl Harbor and Franklin Roosevelt's official declaration of war, because a "peace time draft" had been established in 1940 (Parker, 1992; Ratledge, 1940b). The war not only discouraged prospective students from enrolling, but also removed students from their studies. The Lincoln College's bulletin listed some 148 "Lincoln men in the armed service" (Lincoln, 1942) in October 1942, although this number probably included graduates as well as students. The LACC noted 36 students had entered military service in 1942, and this number rose to 90 the following year (LACC, 1986). By 1944 the LACC could count only 29 new students (LACC, 1986), but this decline may be attributable not only to the draft but to expansion of the required hours in the curriculum to 4,000. Although California law required only 2,400 hours of instruction under the 1922 Chiropractic Act, the state Board of Chiropractic Examiners (BCE) had raised the standard by administrative action (Keating et al., 1991). Already severely depleted of students by the war (Ratledge, 1943b), Ratledge's Los Angeles school eventually brought suit against the BCE on the grounds that it lacked the authority to raise educational requirements for licensure (Gingerich, 1948).

Table 11-7: Faculty and administration of the Chiropractic Institute of New York in 1949 (TraCoil, 1949)

However, by April 1945, the Ratledge College had also "lost its contract with the Veterans Administration for veteran training" (Ratledge, 1951). The school was forced to suspend operations in 1949, and in 1951 negotiated a sale to Carl S. Cleveland, Sr.

Severe loss of students was not universal (Ratledge, 1943b), and a few schools actually managed to hold constant or increase the number of students graduated during the war (see Figure 11-3). The Logan Basic College of Chiropractic vigorously recruited women, and was relatively undamaged by the wartime shortage of students. However, most chiropractic colleges suffered considerable enrollment shortfalls, and their weakened fiscal conditions made them ripe for Nugent's and the NCA's reform and consolidation efforts. Nugent and NCA legislative representative Emmett J. Murphy, D.C. had petitioned unsuccessfully for commissions for chiropractors in the armed forces (Gibbons, 1985; Murphy & Smith, 1940; Vedder, 1940). Straight chiropractic colleges leaders, particularly those outside of NCA's influence, instead sought to have chiropractors and chiropractic students granted exemptions (by presidential order) from the draft as "essential personnel" on the home front (Cleveland, 1942, 1944; Ratledge, 1943a), along the lines that had been suggested by Harry E. Vedder of the Lincoln College (Vedder, 1940). They were joined in these sentiments by George F. Kelley, D.C., president in 1943 of the Minnesota Chiropractic Association (Freedom, 1943). Kelley served as president of the NCA in 1951-52, and for many years as a trustee of the Northwestern College of Chiropractic (Rehm, 1980, p. 317).

Chiropractors were united in their outrage that medical doctors and medical students were either exempted from the draft or commissioned in the Medical Corps (Hopkins, 1942; Mighton, 1942). Like the chiropractors, the osteopathic community was similarly unsuccessful in its pursuit of commissioned status for osteopaths during World War II (Gevitz, 1982), but this was not at first certain (Extract, 1943). However, the chiropractors, recognizing their failure to coordinate their petitions to the federal government on matters of the draft, commissioning of chiropractors and post-war veterans' educational benefits, reached a surprising consensus of thought at the Interstate Chiropractic Congress held in Kansas City during June 28-30, 1943. The group, which included such divergent opinion leaders as Willard Carver, Carl S. Cleveland, Sr., Ruth Cleveland, Grace Edwards, George Kelley, Hugh B. Logan, John J. Nugent, B.J. Palmer, and Warren Roepke, offered a resolution which called upon the NCA and the ICA to work in harmony for these common goals:

> Recommendation No. 2 War Recognition. WHEREAS, the Chiropractic profession has offered the services of its members in the capacity for which our men have been trained in both World War No. 1 and World War No. 2; and such specialized professional services have been rejected on the grounds that not sufficient practitioners were available within the age limits qualifying them for War Service,
>
> THEREFORE, BE IT RECOMMENDED: That the Army follow their usual procedure as in cases where manpower in certain specialized services are necessary and desired; that being the training of additional men at Government expense.
>
> Recommendation No. 3. Rehabilitation. WHEREAS, At the close of World War No. 2 there will undoubtedly be many ex-service men who will request to study Chiropractic as a rehabilitation occupation,
>
> THEREFORE, BE IT RECOMMENDED: That all such request be allowed by the National Rehabilitation Committee without interference of choice of Chiropractic school or college, that being left entirely to the decision of the ex-service man or woman, himself or herself,

Recommendation No. 4. NOW THEREFORE, be it recommended that in the interest of unity, the science and art of Chiropractic shall be considered to be the adjustment of vertebral subluxations of the human spinal column.

Recommendation No. 5. WHEREAS, The National Chiropractic Association and the International Chiropractors Association filed separately appeal briefs with the War Manpower Commission and did otherwise separately approach the Commission in efforts to secure recognition on the War Essential Activity List, and

WHEREAS, Such Briefs and appeals to the War Manpower Commission were not one and the same and resulted in considerable confusion within the Commission and in the profession as to actual needs and desires, and

WHEREAS, At other times different Government Agencies have been separately approached by the N.C.A. and I.C.A. on matters vital to the welfare of the profession, and

WHEREAS, Such different approaches to Government Departments have not at times been in accord resulting in some confusion as the desires of the profession and much controversy within the profession over the differences, and

WHEREAS, The present emergency demands united action on the part of our profession if we are to properly meet the problems confronting us and attain our proper place in the field of healing arts and all differences and controversy must be eliminated so that such unity may be brought about, So,

BE IT RECOMMENDED, that The Council of Chiropractic Schools, National and State Organizations, appeal to the National Chiropractic Association and the International Chiropractors Association to name a joint committee of the strongest men in each association and that such committee be charged with working out united appeals and approaches on all major problems and efforts of the profession for the duration of the present war emergency. And be it,

FURTHER RECOMMENDED, That: A copy of this resolution be forwarded to the President and the Secretary of the N.C.A. and to the President and the Secretary of the I.C.A.

Respectfully submitted, Dr. Julius W. Bechtold, Chairman, Dr. C.S. Cleveland, Secretary, Dr. Wm. Hugh Warden, Dr. George F. Kelley and Dr. Max C. Hintz (Edited, 1943).

With his initial success in merging three of the four New York schools, Nugent set his sights on California (Martin, 1986; News, 1946). Ralph J. Martin, D.C., N.D., who served as the last president of the non-profit Southern California College of Chiropractic (SCCC) and one of the first presidents of the newly non-profit (in 1947) LACC, recalled in later years that:

It was at about the time of the end of World War II that the LA Metropolitan District of the CCA had the Initiation Banquet, and Dr. John J. Nugent, Director of Education for the National Chiropractic Association, was present, and announced to the doctors present that he had come to California to amalgamate the Chiropractic Colleges of the state into one professionally owned non-profit college. I had a long talk with him after the meeting, and assured him that, as president of the Southern California College and of the Metropolitan District, he could count on my full cooperation.

Dr Nugent immediately began negotiations with Dr Wilma Churchill, owner of LACC, and it soon developed that she refused to sell to the So. California College, so we began setting up a new holding non-profit corporation, the California Chiropractic Educational Foundation... (Martin, 1986).

It required several years for Nugent to accomplish his goals in the Golden State. A non-profit holding corporation was set up (known as the California Chiropractic Education Foundation or CCEF), under the control of the California Chiropractic Association (an NCA-state affiliate organization) and the California chapter of the Chiropractic Research Foundation (CRF). In mid-1947 the CCEF, having already acquired the SCCC, closed a deal by Nugent and Martin for the purchase of the still proprietary LACC, thus creating today's non-profit LACC.

A decade after it had been born in Hollywood, the accreditation movement revisited the West Coast. Nugent and his Committee on Educational Standards were soon aided by the end of the world war and the influx of tuition dollars that returning veterans' GI benefits provided. However, there already was recognition that tuition dollars alone could not sustain the educational innovations that the NCA envisioned. Support from the profession, government and from private philanthropy must be sought if chiropractic education was to develop to its maximum potential.

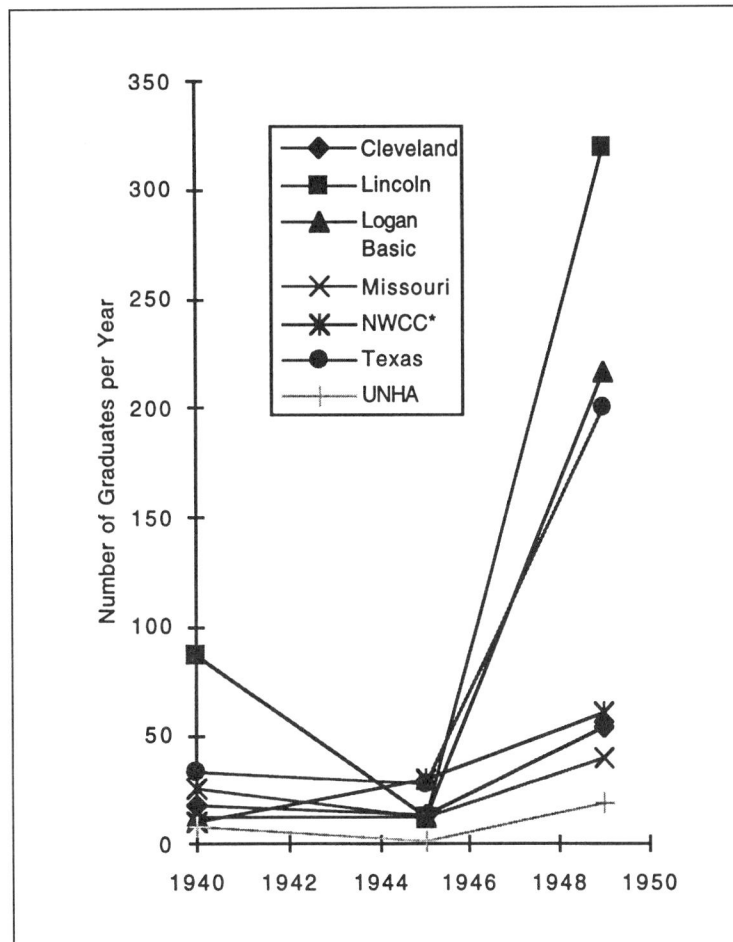

Figure 11-3: Number of students graduated in each of three years at seven chiropractic colleges (Archives of the Council on Chiropractic Education, #35-02-1956); *NWCC: Northwestern College of Chiropractic

Chapter 12

THE CHIROPRACTIC RESEARCH FOUNDATION

As the war years drew to a close the leadership of the NCA (see Figure 12-1), perhaps buoyed by the sense of purpose which permeated Americans' consciousness, chose to heed the many repeated calls for the establishment of a research organization. The idea of a "National Foundation" for research, education and fundraising had been discussed as early the NCA's 1938 Toronto convention (Schierholz, 1986, p. 2). The profession had missed an opportunity for infusion of private philanthropy a decade before, when the Rockefeller Foundation had refused to donate to chiropractic science because of the lack of a non-profit, research conducting body in the profession (Hariman, 1970, p. 29-30; Lerner, 1954, p. 758). Further impetus was provided by the donation of a million dollars to research in physical medicine (including chiropractic, osteopathy and naturopathy) by philanthropist Bernard M. Baruch (McCall, 1945; Watkins, 1944). Although Baruch's commission apparently had little lasting influence within organized medicine (Wardwell, 1992, p. 253), despite the influence of AMA past president R.L. Wilbur, M.D. (Wilbur, 1946), the NCA's immediate past chairman of the board, C.O. Watkins, D.C., was furious at his peers' complacency:

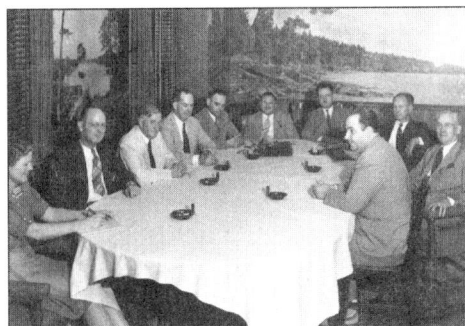

Figure 12-1: 1940 meeting of the NCA's Board of Directors, in Minneapolis; C.O. Watkins and F.O. Logic are seated fifth and sixth from the left, respectively

...Recently, Mr. Bernard Baruch, a layman, gave a large sum of money to the medical profession to test and find the specific facts concerning chiropractic methods. The fact that it has become necessary for a layman to ask organized medicine to do clinical research upon our methods in order to determine their scientific worth should cause every chiropractic leader who has opposed the development of a scientific organization and the organization of profession-wide clinical research to hang his head in shame. If we will not develop a scientific organization to test our own methods, organized medicine will usurp our privilege. When it discovers a method of value, medical science will adopt it and incorporate it into scientific medical practice. One would think that the mere mention of these facts to chiropractic leaders would be sufficient to persuade them to develop a scientific organization to organize our science. However, these facts have been called to their attention again and again in the past few years with meagre results. Chiropractic government of yesterday was dominated by the philosopher who believed a sound, philosophical argument was sufficient basis for chiropractic methods. Cultism developed and thrived under this leadership. Chiropractic government of today is dominated by those who feel that good, basic theory is sufficient of substantiate chiropractic methods of practice. But recognized sciences base their methods not upon philosophy or theory but upon specific facts demonstrated in practice through clinical research. By its failure to build a scientific organization to organize profession-wide clinical research to scientifically test our methods, chiropractic leadership has throughout the years failed to give chiropractic methods of practice a scientific foundation.

The present situation is critical, and unless something definite is done to provide an organization such as will establish chiropractic upon a scientific basis, chiropractic as such will soon cease to exist. In such an event, we should not blame medicine for stealing our methods but rather, we must blame our own leaders whose imprudent leadership has failed to provide the scientific organization essential to the development of an organized science of chiropractic... (Keating, 1992a, pp. 381-2; Watkins, 1944).

Now the leadership, influenced by the repeated prompting of men like Watkins and C.W. Weiant, D.C., Ph.D. (who became NCA Director of Research in 1943), took action. In 1943 Earl Liss, D.C., NCA delegate from Michigan, introduced a resolution to the House of Delegates which called for the creation of a non-profit research corporation. On 26 July 1944, NCA board chairman Gordon M. Goodfellow (see Figure 12-2) offered articles of incorporation for the Chiropractic Research Foundation (CRF) to the NCA Council of Past Executives, a body composed of former presidents and vice-president of the UCA, ACA and NCA, who served as the incorporators of the Foundation. The following day the Articles were notarized in Chicago and filed with Delaware's secretary of state (Schierholz, 1986, p. 3). The Articles specified:

1. The name of the Corporation is Chiropractic Research Foundation, Incorporated.
2. The objects or purposes to be promoted or carried on are:
   a) To receive gifts for the use and benefit of chiropractic education, research, sanitarium, hospitals, and to administer said gifts according to its discretion, except as to gifts subject to a condition of the donor, which gifts are to be administered according to said conditions.
   b) To promote the science of chiropractic, particularly in the research of all the scientific aspects of chiropractic.
   c) To promote adequate facilities and equipment for the full and complete education of students in chiropractic colleges. .
   d) To promote chiropractic sanitariums, hospitals and clinics.
   e) To gather and disseminate reliable information concerning the science of chiropractic, and to generally promote the science of chiropractic (Schierholz, 1986, p. 4).

It is helpful to keep in mind that several of the organizers and early officials (see Table 12-1) of the CRF were best known for their marketing efforts on behalf of chiropractic. Few of the NCA's leaders had any experience in chiropractic education, none had any formal training in scientific research, and a few had decidedly anti-scientific conceptions of research. Their purposes had as much to do with public relations and fund-raising as anything else (Keating et al., 1995). Well intentioned though they were, the CRF was ill prepared to accomplish the academic missions it set for itself. Despite the determined, guiding hand of its first president, Arthur W. Schwietert, D.C. (see Figure 12-3), whose passionate commitment to the CRF became legendary, confusion about the new agency's priorities was quickly apparent. Co-founder Sylva Ashworth believed that raising money for the schools was the foundation's primary function (Ashworth, 1944), but this was not a universal sentiment. News releases at times emphasized research as the CRF's primary goal (e.g., McIlroy, 1945), but on other occasions suggested that support and development of the colleges were the first priority:

...The Foundation has received official exemption from Federal taxation and all contributions to the Foundation are allowable as deductions from your individual Federal Income Taxes.

The object of the Foundation is to endow accredited chiropractic colleges teaching a minimum standard of four years of not less than 3600 hours; to establish extensive laboratories for scientific research in the principles of chiropractic; to establish and promote chiropractic hospitals sanitaria and clinics; to explore new fields of scientific research in the interests of public health (CRF, 1945).

A quarter century later George Hariman, D.C. (1970, pp. 30-1) listed college funding as the CRF's original priority, and noted the formation of a Student Loan Fund (which actually preceded formation of the CRF by several years). Goodfellow suggested that there was a commitment to an equitable distribution of CRF funds among the chiropractic schools:

If it should, at some future time appear necessary to acquire or construct an institution for pure research, that can be done. For the present it is contemplated that the Research Foundation shall work through those educational institutions of the profession already existing and which have met the highest standards which the profession has found it necessary to establish.

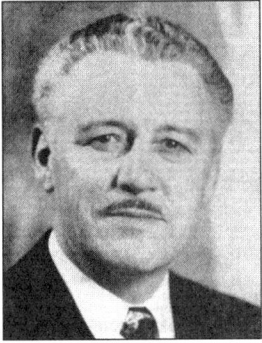

Figure 12-2: Gordon M. Goodfellow, D.C., N.D.

It will be a flexible endowment, to be apportioned to these institutions according to their needs, and not designed to help one to flourish while others starve, but to keep the best in Chiropractic alive through difficult periods, to encourage them to hold to the highest of standards, and to insure a future membership of our ranks to which we can point with pride and which will command public respect... (Goodfellow, 1945).

The CRF stumbled repeatedly in its earliest efforts to raise funds, develop research programs and support the schools (Keating, 1992a, pp. 65-6; Keating et al., 1995; Schierholz, 1986). A decade later, however, when the CRF was renamed the Foundation for the Advancement of Chiropractic Education and re-committed itself to improving the chiropractic colleges, it became a significant factor in the bootstrapping of chiropractic education (Schierholz, 1986).

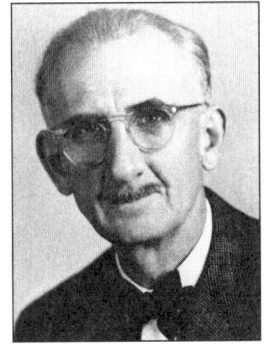

Figure 12-3: Arthur W. Schwietert, D.C.; first president of the Chiropractic Research Foundation, 1944

Table 12-1: Members of the first board of trustees and officers of the Chiropractic Research Foundation (Hariman, 1970, pp. 30-1; Schierholz, 1986, pp. 5-6)

Arthur W. Schwietert, D.C., President
Frank O. Logic, D.C., Vice-President
Charles C. Lemly, D.C., Secretary-Treasurer
George E. Hariman, D.C.
Harry K. McIlroy, D.C.

Chapter 13

THE REFORMATION SCHOOLS

The end of the second quarter of the chiropractic century saw the birth of several schools which pioneered new standards for the training of doctors. Several of these have already been mentioned, including the birth of CINY, brought to term through Nugent's effort to merge smaller, proprietary schools in New York City (significantly including the straight-oriented Eastern Chiropractic Institute). Nugent's efforts were paralleled by those internal to the National College of Chiropractic in Chicago, which in 1941 had become a non-profit corporation, and in 1945 appointed Joseph Janse, D.D.T., D.C., N.D., its president (see Figure 13-1). Janse eventually led the profession into its first federally recognized accreditation. In 1945, as the profession enjoyed its fiftieth anniversary, Nugent had just begun down the trail that led to government recognition, and was involved in a campaign that would make the very broad-scope, merged LACC/SCCC into a model for other chiropractic institutions. Also deserving of consideration in this period were the arrivals of the Canadian Memorial Chiropractic College and the Northwestern College of Chiropractic.

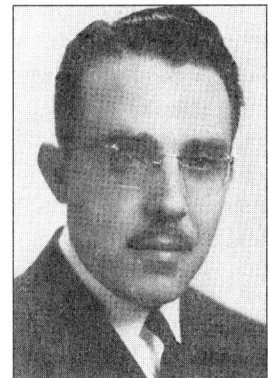

Figure 13-1: Joseph Janse, D.D.T., D.C., N.D., 1945

Canadian Memorial Chiropractic College

As noted in Chapter 3, at least four schools of chiropractic functioned in Canada prior to 1945 (Biggs, 1989: Chapter 6; 1991; Lee, 1981). The Robbins School of Chiropractic in Sault Ste. Marie, Ontario, was a straight chiropractic institution operated during 1909-1914 by several M.D.-D.C.s (Biggs, 1986). The Canadian Chiropractic College (CCC) was founded in Hamilton, Ontario. in 1914 by former PSC faculty member Ernest G. DuVal who involved his family (A.R. DuVal, D.C., E. Robert DuVal, D.C., Becky DuVal, T.E. Patterson, D.C.) in the institution's operations. The school continued to train chiropractors at its Toronto location through 1928 (Biggs, 1989). DuVal's perspectives on chiropractic closely paralleled those of B.J. Palmer (Forster, 1923), and he played a pivotal role in the Royal Commission investigation of chiropractic during World War I (Sutherland, 1985). DuVal had also participated in the 1917 formation of the International Association of Chiropractic Schools and Colleges (see Table 4-2). Lee (1981) noted the operation of the Imperial Chiropractic College in Toronto in 1922. The Toronto College of Chiropractic was founded in 1922 by John S. Clubine, a CCC graduate who played an even more significant role in the profession several decades later. The Toronto College closed its doors in 1928. For the next 17 years, all new D.C.s in the nation would have to be American-trained.

The creation of the Canadian Memorial Chiropractic College (CMCC) was a noble experiment. Prompted by concern that the federal parliament's wartime consideration of a national health plan for Canadians might exclude chiropractic, and by the desire to see chiropractors commissioned in the armed forces (News, 1943), representatives from most of the country's provinces met in Ottawa early in 1943 to create the Dominion Council of Canadian Chiropractors (DCCC; see Figure 13-2). This national organization, forerunner of today's Canadian Chiropractic Association, soon added to its mission the establishment of a college to provide the new practitioners that the nation required. Despite considerable but gentlemanly disagreement within the Council about the character of the school (Keating & Haldeman, 1995), the CMCC became the profession's first truly professionally-owned and non-profit educational institution. Although Nugent was successful in creating

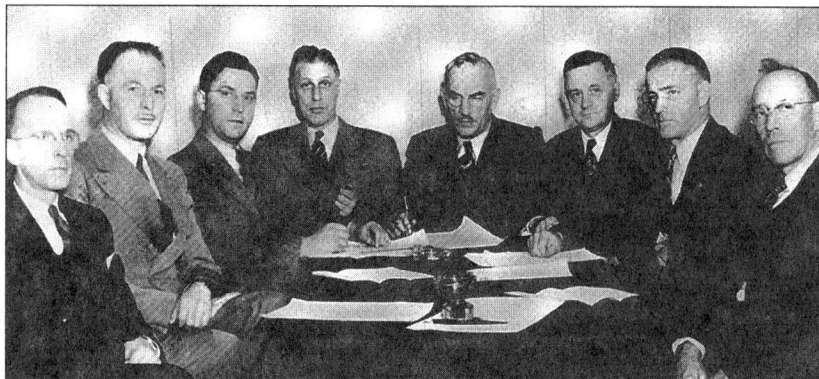

Figure 13-2: photo taken in Ottawa on January 11, 1943, and appearing in the *National Chiropractic Journal* 1943 (March); 12(3): 27; original caption read: "Pictured above are Directors of the recently organized Dominion Chiropractic council, representing all Provinces in Canada. (Left to Right) Dr. Gaudet, Montreal; Dr. Haldeman, Regina; J.S. Burton, Vancouver; Dr. J.A. Schnick, Hamilton; Dr. Sturdy, Vancouver; Dr. J.S. Clubine, Toronto; Dr. McElrea, Winnipeg; Dr. Messenger, Calgary."

many non-profit chiropractic schools in the U.S., the CMCC had the added distinction of a corporate board of trustees who represented the chiropractic professional societies of most Canadian provinces.

The DCCC's disagreements concerning the college were several. Should the school be proprietary or non-profit? Ontario representative John Schnick, D.C., former president of the NCA, insisted that non-profit status was essential if the school wished to be the beneficiary of philanthropic gifts and endowments from government and private sources. How much control should the DCCC exercise over the college? Saskatchewan representative to the DCCC, Joshua N. Haldeman, D.C., saw the Council as the school's overseer, but Clubine and Walter T. Sturdy, D.C. felt that if politics were introduced to school operations, the college might suffer or fail (Keating & Haldeman, 1995), a notion that was borne out in later years (Biggs, 1989, Chapter 6). How should chiropractic be defined (Schnick, 1943), and should the school teach physiotherapeutic methods, or offer a strictly "straight" chiropractic program of instruction? Representatives from the western provinces (Drs. Haldeman, McElrea, Messenger and Sturdy) held out for a straight college, while eastern provincial interests, including Quebec representative, chiropractor-naturopath Jean Maurice Gaudet, argued for a broad scope of instruction. How long should the curriculum be? Wouldn't a straight chiropractic curriculum require less training than a broad-scope program? The noble experiment required experience and competence in areas that few members (e.g., Clubine) of the Dominion Council could claim.

To aid in its deliberations, the Council enlisted the expert advice of NCA educational director, John J. Nugent (Lee, undated). A number of the thorny issues confronting the group were decided upon at several meetings of the DCCC in Toronto in March and October of 1944, wherein several compromises were reached (Minutes, 1944a&b). Although the DCCC held a federal charter, the laws regulating educational institutions required a provincial charter. Since the school was to be located in Toronto, a legally distinct and independent charter from Ontario, initially known as the Canadian Association of Chiropractors, had to be obtained. This gave the college corporation a certain degree of autonomy from the national organization, although representatives to the DCCC also frequently served as college trustees. A 12-member board, including one representative each from British Columbia, Alberta, Saskatchewan, Manitoba and the Maritimes, two from Quebec and five delegates from Ontario, was accepted.

Several curricula were proposed (e.g., Gauthier, 1943), but a final product involving four years of eight months each was agreed upon, and the program emphasized the basic and diagnostic sciences. The school would be non-profit, and the DCCC agreed, by simple majority vote, that physiotherapy would not at first be taught. However, to accommodate the requirements for licensure in Ontario under the drugless healers' act, a four month post-graduate program in physiotherapeutics was offered to those students requesting it. An eclectic technique program gave students the opportunity to "specialize" in their fourth year in one or more "major techniques" (Carver, Logan Basic, Meric or Upper Cervical Specific Technique) after they had mastered full spine adjusting (Biggs, 1989, Section 6.2.3).

The Dominion Council's deliberations relative to a straight vs. mixer curriculum provides an interesting example of B.J. Palmer's continuing if diminished influence in the profession. Provincial representatives Walter T. Sturdy of British Columbia, C.E. Messenger of Alberta, Joshua N. Haldeman of Saskatchewan and F. B. McIlrea of Manitoba were all Palmer loyalists, and objected strongly to introducing non-adjustive (i.e., physiotherapeutic and naturopathic) interventions to the educational program. However, when Messenger indicated that he had been in communication with Palmer, and had asked the ICA president to encourage Sturdy to insist upon a straight curriculum for the CMCC, 1926 PSC graduate Haldeman objected to any "influence from the United States in running Chiropractic affairs in Canada" (Minutes, 1944b). The

Saskatchewan doctor also indicated that he did not expect that the western provincial societies, comprised primarily of Palmer graduates, could support the college if mixer methods were taught. Nonetheless, Haldeman agreed to abide by the majority's will, and accepted the Council's vote in favor of an optional course in physiotherapy. The curriculum they finally agreed upon, comprised of eight semesters, approximated that which was recommended by Nugent and the NCA Committee on Educational Standards (see Table 13-1).

Under the direction of John A. Henderson, D.C., who was already actively engaged in soliciting financial support from chiropractors across Canada and soon served as the school's first registrar, the college corporation purchased the former Medonia Hotel at 252 Bloor Street in Toronto for its first campus at a cost of $51,000 (Lee, undated). A committee of five members of the college organizing committee, including Clubine and Lee, toured the United States to visit various chiropractic schools. Lee recalls that:

Table 13-1: Four Year Schedule at the Canadian Memorial Chiropractic College (Dedicatory, 1947).

Freshman Year - First Semester   Hours
Anatomy I. (Osteology and Arthrology)................90
Embryology (Development Anatomy)....................90
Chemistry I. (Inorganic-general)............................90
Physiology I. (Nerve and Muscle)..........................90
Lexicology 45
Principles and Theory of Chiropractic...................<u>45</u>
                                                                          450

Second Semester
Anatomy II. (Myology)...90
Histology..90
Chemistry II. (Organic)...90
Physiology II. (Digestion and Metabolism.............90
Palpation I..45
Principles and Theory of Chiropractic...................<u>45</u>
                                                                          450

Sophomore Year - Third Semester
Anatomy III. (Splanchnology)...............................90
Chemistry III. (Physiological)...............................90
Physiology III. (Special Senses)............................90
Bacteriology I. (General)..90
Palpation II..45
X-Ray Physics and Technique..............................<u>45</u>
                                                                          450

Fourth Semester
Anatomy IV. (Angiology).......................................90
Chemistry IV. (Pathological)..................................90
Physiology IV. (Neurological)...............................90
Bacteriology II. (Special)..45
Pathology I. (General)..45
Technique (Chiropractic).......................................<u>90</u>
                                                                          450

Junior Year - Fifth Semester
Anatomy V. (Central Nervous System)................90
Pathology II. (Systemic)..90
Hygiene, Sanitation and Public Health I................90
Diagnosis I. 90
Physical Diagnosis 45
Dietetics 45

First Aid and Toxicology.......................................45
Technique (Chiropractic).......................................<u>45</u>
                                                                          540

Sixth Semester   Hours
Anatomy VI. (Peripheral Nervous System)..........90
Pathology III. (Systemic).......................................90
Diagnosis II...90
Hygiene and Public Health II 45
Laboratory Diagnosis & X-Ray Interpretation......45
Technique (Chiropractic).......................................90
Clinic..<u>132</u>
                                                                          582

Senior Year - Seventh Semester
Anatomy VII. (Dissection)...................................180
Pathology IV. (Systemic).......................................90
Diagnosis III..90
Gynecology I...90
Pediatrics...90
X-Ray Interpretation (Soft Tissue).......................45
Technique (Chiropractic).......................................45
Clinic..<u>180</u>
                                                                          810

Eighth Semester
Diagnosis IV..90
E.E.N.T..45
Dermatology..45
Psychiatry..90
Gynecology II..45
Obstetrics...45
Technique (Chiropractic) Provincial and
     State Board Review..45
Chiropractic Jurisprudence, Ethics, Economics
     and Public Speaking.......................................45
Clinic..<u>180</u>
                                                                          630

Total (50-minute) hours for eight semesters of eighteen weeks each
                                                4,362.
Drugless Therapy optional the last two years - Total Hours, 360

...the group first visited National College. Dr. Janse cut short a holiday to meet with the committee. He gave valuable advice on faculty, course content, clinic and financing. They then proceeded to Davenport and spent a very profitable day with "B.J." First it was a conducted tour by "B.J." through his private Clinic, the College classrooms and laboratories, the printing department, the radio studio...and the beautifully kept grounds... He discussed different aspects and problems of owning and managing a school.

The next day it was off to St. Louis to visit the Logan College...

The last College visited was the Lincoln College in Indianapolis. Dr. Jim Firth spent most of the afternoon with the visitors and spoke of various aspects of Lincoln and answered many questions put to him.

The information, advice and opinions were compiled and a detailed report was given to the Board of Governors... (Lee, undated).

The school's organizers worked frantically throughout the summer of 1945 to prepare the new campus for its opening. Enrollment began on 7 September 1945, and a class of 96 students "made up mainly of veterans recently discharged" was assembled (Lee, undated). On 18 September 1945 at 8 a.m. the first class was taught by Herbert K. Lee, D.C., a National College graduate who continues on the CMCC's faculty to this day. Nugent (see Figure 13-3) reported the CMCC's initial activities in the NCA's *Journal*:

A vigorous campaign to raise $100,000 was initiated and the profession's response was immediate and generous. The greater part of this sum is now raised and the balance will shortly be forthcoming. A $50,000 building has been purchased in the heart of the University of Toronto district, and teaching equipment, school, dormitory and office furniture have been bought and paid for.

The school will operate as a non-profit, professionally owned institution under a charter obtained from the Ontario government, and under the direction of a Board of Directors elected by the Canadian Association of Chiropractors, Inc. The Board of Directors will appoint a Board of Governors, consisting of prominent chiropractors and laymen.

The course of study will consist of 4,200 to 4,600 hours over a period of four years of eight to nine months in each calendar year. The minimum entrance requirement is junior matriculation or its equivalent - high school graduation.

The curriculum includes all of the basic science subjects and a thorough training in "straight" chiropractic. For those wishing to qualify under the Province of Ontario Drugless Therapeutists Act, there will be a separate course in physiotherapy.

The tuition fee is $300.00 per year....

The school has been accredited by the Department of Veterans Affairs and a number of Canadian veterans are enrolled (Nugent, 1945).

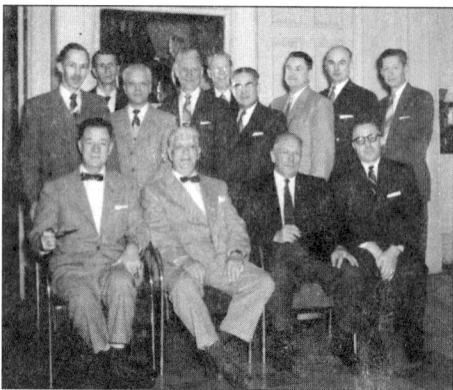

Figure 13-3: John J. Nugent (seated second from left) meets with the NCA Council on Education in Toronto in 1956 (photo courtesy of Herbert K. Lee, D.C.)

Among the earliest matriculants, and a graduate of the school's first class (in 1949), was Herbert J. Vear (see Figure 13-4), who later served as dean of his alma mater, as a co-founder (in 1975) of the College of Chiropractic Sciences (Canada), as president of Western States Chiropractic College, and as president of the Council on Chiropractic Education (Canada). Vear was typical of many of the first CMCC students, in that he was a veteran of the war, and somewhat more mature when he matriculated at CMCC than was typical of some chiropractic students. Many early CMCC graduates believe that the high quality of instruction provided in the first years of the institution is attributable to the expectations that they brought to the school as veterans: there was a "no nonsense" attitude characteristic of men who had fought for their country and now wished to get on with their lives.

The CMCC's board turned first to John J. Nugent in their search for a dean. The NCA leader declined, but was influential in bringing Rudy O.

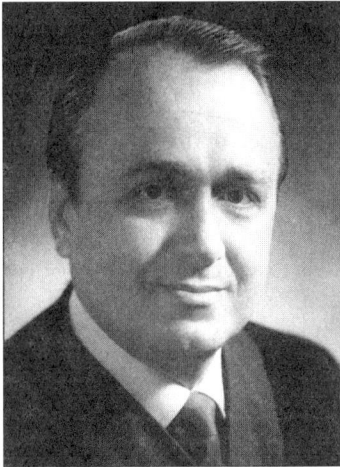

Figure 13-4: Herbert J. Vear, D.C., graduate in 1949 of the first class at CMCC

Muller, D.C. (see Table 13-2 and Figure 13-5), a graduate of and longtime faculty member at the Lincoln Chiropractic College, to the campus to succeed John Clubine, who served as the College's first dean (Lee, undated). Duncan Allan "was the first full-time faculty member hired," and A. Earl Homewood, D.C., N.D., a 1942 graduate of Western States College and future president of the CMCC, served as a part-time instructor (Lee, undated). Homewood later served as president of the College, and supervised the CMCC's 1968 move to its present campus.

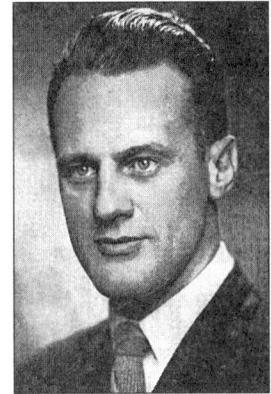

Figure 13-5: Rudy O. Muller, D.C., Ph.C., second dean of the CMCC

Table 13-2: Some of the published works of Rudy O. Muller, D.C., Ph.C.

Lincoln organizes ball club!!! *Lincoln College Yearbook*. Indianapolis: the College, 1938

The eternal question - why aren't chiropractors organization-minded? *National Chiropractic Journal* 1941; 10(5): 8, 46

Chiropractic rights vs. duties. *National Chiropractic Journal* 1947; 17(3): 10

Professional aptitude testing. *National Chiropractic Journal* 1947 ; 17(8): 26

A survey on spinal balance. *National Chiropractic Journal* 1948; 18(1): 23

Analysis of chiropractic education. *Journal of the National Chiropractic Association* 1950; 20(6): 24, 66

An analytic approach to your problem cases is presented. *Journal of the National Chiropractic Association* 1952; 22(12): 17

Autonomics in chiropractic: the control of autonomic imbalance. Toronto: Chiro Publishing Company, 1954

Care of patients suffering from acute barbiturate poisoning. *Journal of the National Chiropractic Association* 1955; 25(4): 11-2

A presentation of a new measurement in chiropractic diagnosis. *Journal of the National Chiropractic Association* 1955; 25(10): 11-2

Northwestern College of Chiropractic

In contrast to the Logan Basic College, whose organization was fostered by a particular set of clinical procedures, the Northwestern College of Chiropractic (NWCC) has always prided itself for its independence from any brand name technique. The NWCC was chartered on June 2, 1941, and began operations on the sixth floor of the W.T. Grant department store building in downtown Minneapolis (Hinz, 1987). The principal founder of the college, and 50% share-holder in the proprietary institution, was second-generation chiropractor John B. Wolfe (see Figure 13-6). Wolfe had earned his bachelor's degree in civil engineering from the University of Minnesota in 1936, and then took his first chiropractic doctorate in the 18-month program at the PSC in 1938, graduating in the same class as B.J. Palmer's son, Dave, with whom he developed a friendship. Unable to qualify for the basic science examination in Minnesota based on his training at Palmer, he enrolled at the Minnesota Chiropractic College (MnCC), an institution originally established as the Minnesota College of Non-Medicinal Therapy circa 1909-12 (Hinz, 1987; Wardwell, 1992, p. 97). Wolfe earned his second doctorate of chiropractic in 1940 (Fay, 1986), and taught the basic sciences at the MnCC. Dissatisfied with the standards of his second alma mater, he

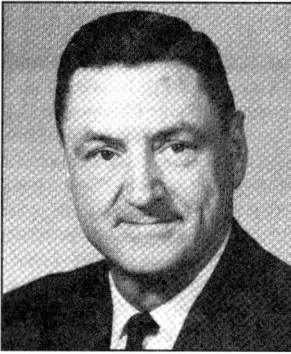

Figure 13-6: John B. Wolfe, D.C. served as president of NWCC during 1941-1984

joined with Jennings Wilson, D.C. and three MnCC students to found the NWCC. Thirty-five students enrolled in the first class, most of whom were transfers from MnCC. The first diplomas were awarded in December 1941 (Hinz, 1987), just as the United States entered the war.

Volunteer instructors and student tutors kept the NWCC open during the war years, although the program was reduced to an evening division only. The student body "slowly climbed to 19 by the end of the war," and the first student to graduate, Thomas Hove, earned his doctorate in 1944 (Hinz, 1987). However, the new school had already been deprived of its leader, for Wolfe was called from the officers' reserve corps into active military duty; he served on General Douglas MacArthur's staff as a lieutenant colonel, and helped to survey the effects of the nuclear weapons dropped on Japan (Fay, 1986; Hinz, 1987). He did not return to Minnesota until 1946, and it was not until then that the remarkable journey of this small, deliberately provincial institution, began its winding way toward innovation and accreditation.

Chapter 14

THE EARLY POST-WAR PERIOD

At the end of World War II chiropractic was poised for major changes. The overwhelming majority of states licensed chiropractors in 1946, and although basic science laws prevented new licensure in a number of them, there was a growing confidence among the graduates of some chiropractic schools that basic science examinations could be passed. Those schools which survived the fiscally demanding years of the depression and the war could now look forward to relief in the form of the G.I. Bill, which provided federal funding for veterans who wished to study chiropractic. Indeed, the first few years of the post-war period saw a rapid expansion in student bodies (School, 1949), although the glut was short-lived (see Figure 14-1).

Perhaps not surprisingly, confidence that students could meet the basic science barrier was considerably less among ICA-affiliated schools and those which continued to offer 18-month curricula, most notably the PSC (Basic, 1948; Berch, 1949; Frankly, 1949; Texans, 1949; Virginia, 1949; We, 1949). The conflict between ICA and NCA intensified, and each side warned prospective students about the consequences of choosing the wrong school:

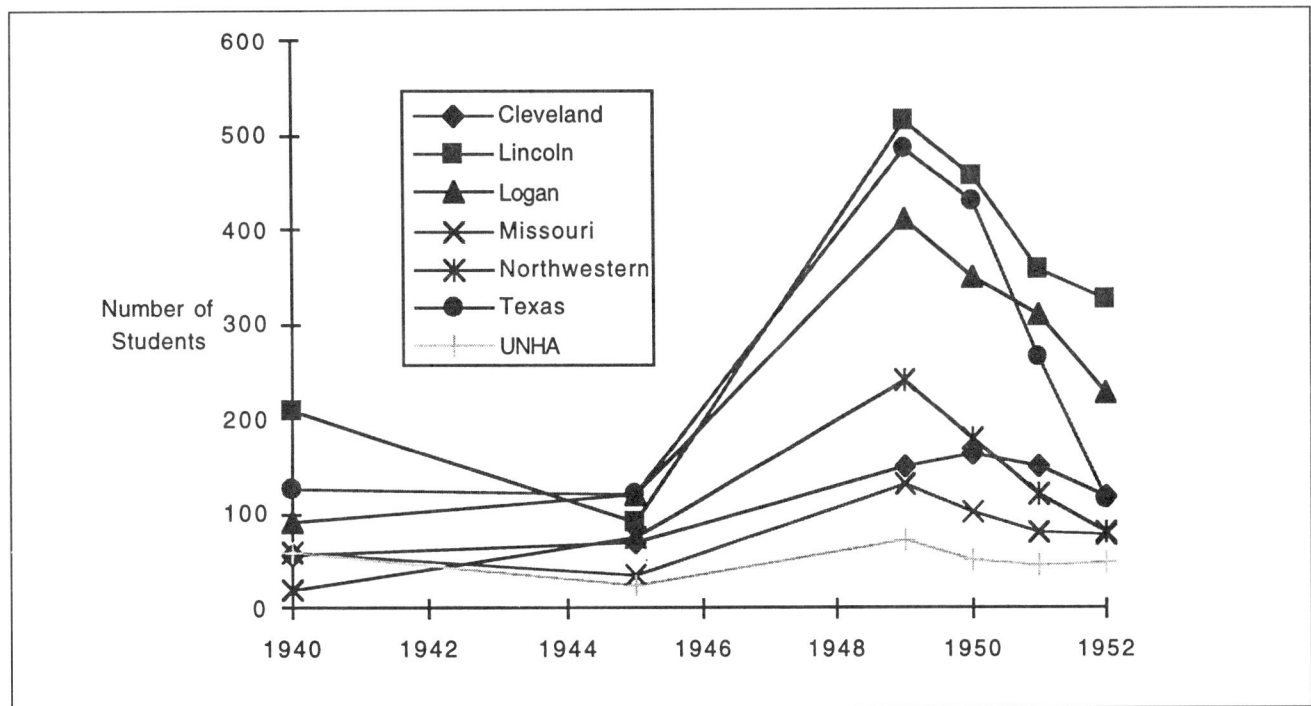

Figure 14-1: Student enrollments during 1940-1952, based on a survey by the National Chiropractic Association; data were prepared by the registrar, dean or president of seven schools (Archives of the Council on Chiropractic Education, #35-02-1956)

IMPORTANT

Warning to GI Students of Chiropractic

Dr. J.J. Nugent, director of education of the National Chiropractic Association, issued a note of warning to chiropractic students now enrolled in low-standard, unapproved schools giving courses of less than four years. He pointed out that of the forty-six states recognizing the practice of chiropractic, thirty-two states require four years of education for licensure; that of the remainder, ten states have basic science, medical or mixed examining boards whose examinations are of such a character as to require four years of education to qualify. The remaining four states, he warned, may quite likely raise their requirements while these students are still in school.

Dr. Nugent urged all students, particularly GI students, now enrolled in courses of less than four years to carefully consider the tragic predicament they may find themselves in later on when they attempt to qualify for licensure.

He cited many incidents of disillusioned and embittered GI's, graduates of short courses, wandering from state to state futilely trying to obtain a license to practice.

A vocational pamphlet giving information on state requirements can be obtained by writing the National Chiropractic Association, National Building, Webster City, Iowa (Important, 1948).

and:

WARNING to Chiropractic Students

Enroll in schools recognized by International Chiropractors Ass'n. Be certain that the school of your choice teaches an adequate Chiropractic course.

Unfortunately a few so-called "Chiropractic" schools teach quasi-medical methods. These methods cannot be practiced legally in most jurisdictions under a Chiropractic license.

Better investigate before you enroll. Consult members of International Chiropractors Ass'n., or write direct to International Chiropractors Ass'n., Education Division, 838 Brady Street, Davenport, Iowa. Vocational guidance booklet, list of approved schools on request (Warning, 1949).

Los Angeles College of Chiropractic

As World War II drew near to its end, Nugent enjoyed two dramatic successes in his educational reform campaign. The first was the 1944 merger of the Lincoln and Universal colleges, and the second was the 1944 formation of the Chiropractic Institute of New York (see Chapter 2). Gardner (1946), an NCA delegate from California, related that another of Nugent's victories took shape in California in 1946, when the education director commenced a campaign in conjunction with the California branch of the Chiropractic Research Foundation (CRF):

CALIFORNIA: DR. NUGENT STRESSES EDUCATION.

To the many pre-arranged meetings held throughout the length and breadth of California have come hundreds of members of our profession to hear the educational aims and objects of the NCA, as revealed by its Educational Director, Dr. John J. Nugent, New Haven, Conn. Having arrived in this state just five weeks ago, his message of chiropractic education has already been heard all over the state.

Public school teachers, city, county and state officials in the department of education have already heard his message and though they came primarily to scoff and chide many stayed to congratulate and encourage this educator who represents us even in this Nation's Capitol...

The CRF has been one of the major subjects of Dr. Nugent's many talks out here and in all of them he has praised highly the work done by the John's committee in behalf of the CRF, and most highly has he offered his praise to its fine and able leader, Dr. John. Nugent (Gardner, 1946).

By the end of 1946 the CRF and the NCA established a non-profit holding company which acquired all of the assets and the charter of the non-profit Southern California College of Chiropractic (SCCC), and commenced negotiations for the purchase of the Los Angeles College of Chiropractic (LACC) from its owner, Wilma Churchill Wood, D.C., N.D. (Keating, Dishman et al., 1993). The arrangements were finalized on 8 May 1947 (see Figure 2-11), and the expanded and newly non-profit LACC began operations immediately. This new school's structure, non-profit status and professional control created a model for others to emulate. Among the new institution's innovations was an attempt to create a "graduate school," which became a vehicle for license renewal coursework, naturopathic education, and instruction in subjects considered too esoteric for the regular curriculum (e.g., hypnoanalysis; Journal, 1951). New laboratories for anatomy, pathology and x-ray were built (LACC, 1986). However, the LACC stopped awarding naturopathic degrees in 1948 (Homola, 1963, p. 75). Subjects such as herbology were discontinued, but radionics continued to be taught in so-called "research courses" (Journal, 1949; Naturopathic, 1957). Naturopathic doctorates were awarded at the National College until the early 1950s, and similar training continued at the Western States College in Portland, Oregon until a few years after W.A. Budden's death in 1954.

Soon after its merger with the SCCC, the LACC began a search for a larger campus, which was accomplished in 1950 (see Figure 14-2). Arthur V. Nilsson, D.C., who had taught anatomy at the LACC since 1930 (Gruber, 1984), reflected on the transition to the new non-profit status and the re-location to Glendale, California:

> At that time [1929] the College was privately owned as were all Chiropractic schools in those early years, and the practitioners had too little time to spare toward professional organization. As the years passed the enrollment of new students increased, until after World War II, it was necessary to add a sprawling one-story building to accommodate the heavy post-war enrollments. By then, the practitioners out in the field had organized into a growing group which became known as the California Chiropractic Association. Among the members of this organization, a smaller group was formed, which, on behalf of leading Chiropractors, purchased the College from its principal owner, the late Dr. Wilma Churchill. She placed a very strong emphasis on academic qualities although because of economical necessities, she had to accept students with only a High School diploma (or the equivalent). The period of those years between 1948 and 1952 were especially rewarding because of the physical and academic transformation the College was subjected to. Everybody was busy, schedules were reorganized, subjects were revised and improved, and a system of audio-visual methods were added to aid in the teaching procedures. How did all of us react to this change? Did it upset our former routines? No, indeed! It was exciting, interesting, gratifying! It was as if our College was undergoing growing pains. And then came Glendale! It was quite a change to leave the smaller class rooms as they were on Venice Boulevard and Ninth and Union Streets in Los Angeles to move up to the beautiful premises on Broadway in Glendale. No one complained. All of us were thrilled and happy! (Nilsson, 1975).

Despite the satisfaction these early developments in the new LACC produced, the school's new president soon ran afoul of his board of trustees; Ralph Martin, D.C., N.D. related that:

> The school was moved to 920 E Broadway in Glendale in 1950, which was the former Harrower Laboratory property. I had put in a tremendous amount of effort to secure non-profit status for the Foundation and the school, and as elected President of the LACC, I no longer had a vote on the Board of Regents of the Foundation. When the regents agreed in the purchase of the property, to pay Cecil DeMille's taxes, I resigned as president in protest. I was immediately thereafter appointed to the Committee on Accreditation of the Council on Chiropractic Education of the National Chiropractic Association, in which capacity I served for nine years until 1960. This position involved meeting twice a year with the Council on Education, and evaluating the schools we had visited, and providing accreditation recognition as our standards were met (Martin, 1986).

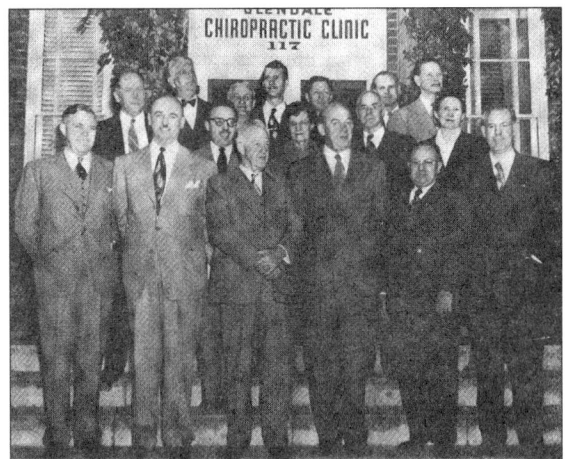

Figure 14-2: NCA Council on Education met in Glendale in early 1951 (National, 1951)

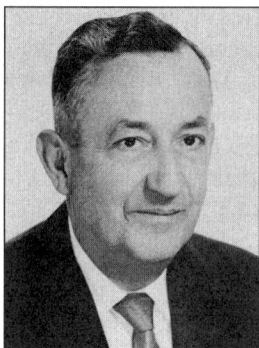

Figure 14-3: Henry G. Higley, D.C., M.A.

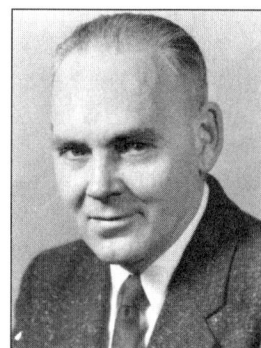

Figure 14-4: C.O. Watkins, D.C., circa 1955

Two important 1936 graduates of the Ratledge Chiropractic College grew to increasing prominence within the profession while serving the LACC in the late 1940s and early 1950s. Henry G. Higley, D.C., M.A. (see Figure 14-2), who earned a graduate degree in mathematics and statistics (Rehm, 1980, p. 329), co-authored *General Chemistry* with George H. Haynes in 1939 (Smallie, 1990), a text created expressly for chiropractic students. The pair had also been active in pro-chiropractic politics in the state, and probably played minor roles in the merger of the SCCC and the LACC while serving on the faculty of the former institution. Higley served as the first editor, in 1941, of the NCA's patient magazine, *Healthways*, and in 1948 was named chairman of LACC's Department of Physiology (Rehm, 1980, p. 329). In the wake of the CRF's expensive failure to raise funds for chiropractic research from outside the profession and the bad taste this left in the mouths of many chiropractors who contributed (Keating et al, 1995; Schierholz, 1986), Higley collaborated with C.O. Watkins, D.C. (Watkins, 1951) (see Figure 14-3) and John B. Wolfe, D.C. (president of Northwestern College of Chiropractic and secretary of the NCA Council on Education) in the early1950s' activities of NCA's Committee on Research, and in 1958 was named Director of Research and Statistics for the NCA (Rehm, 1980).

Higley was seemingly influenced by Watkins' repeated calls (Budden, 1947; Watkins, 1944, 1951) for clinical research in practice; at the NCA's 1953 convention in Los Angeles he proposed to the NCA Council on Education that honors students be recruited to interpret, under the NCA Research Director's supervision, clinical data collected by field practitioners (Higley, 1953). Apparently, nothing came of this suggestion. In 1959 Higley received the first research grant, from the Foundation for the Advancement of Chiropractic Education (FACE) (Schierholz, 1986, p. 18; Timmins, 1976), which was the old CRF revamped, and with a substantially increased commitment of resources from the NCA/ACA (Martin, 1974). The project, essentially a literature review entitled "Intervertebral Disc Syndrome" (Higley, 1960), was conducted at the LACC and also involved an institutional self-study (Schierholz, 1986, p. 18) which was somewhat more involved than was then the custom for chiropractic schools. The LACC's self-analysis and research funding became something of a model for other colleges to follow. Soon, similar small research grants were made to the Lincoln Chiropractic College (1962), the National College (1964) and the Texas Chiropractic College (1966) (Timmins, 1976). In 1965 FACE awarded LACC more than $10,000 for a "Study, Analysis and Evaluation of Chiropractic Education in the United States" (Schierholz, 1986).

George Haynes, D.C., N.D. (see Figure 14-4), who had earned a master's degree from the University of Southern California in 1938, joined the faculty of the SCCC not later than 1941. When the LACC and the SCCC merged in 1947, Haynes was appointed professor of chemistry at the amalgamated institution. The Ratledge graduate was appointed assistant dean at the new LACC in 1950, and became administrative dean (chief executive officer of the college) in 1953 (Rehm, 1980, p. 329). His scholarly contributions included

Table 14-1: "TOPICS FOR DISCUSSION AT THE MID-YEAR MEETING OF THE NATIONAL COUNCIL ON EDUCATION," January 11-14, 1951, Santa Monica, California (Peterson, 1950); see Appendix B

1. Further consideration of the effect of Selective Service on college enrollments and discussion of steps to be taken to achieve parity with other professions on deferments and postponements.
2. Discussion of Veteran Administration rulings, changes as they effect the chiropractic colleges.
3. Discussion of economic problems of the chiropractic colleges in view of changing national picture.
4. Consideration and discussion of rearrangement of accrediting system.
5. Discussion of scholarship arrangements and grants.
6. Consideration of new teaching methods and report from Dr. Muller on progress of plan started at the Canadian Memorial Chiropractic College a year ago.
7. Discussion of legal reports for N.C.A. Journal.
8. Advertising of schools (accredited) on single page of N.C.A. Journal.
9. Analysis of costs of student preparation with view to increased tuition charges.
10. Discussion of case history - final form approval.
11. Discussion of national contest on research for Council on Psychology.
12. Report on Pennsylvania discussion.
13. Discussion of formation of Danish School of Chiropractic

serving as editor of the LACC's *Chirogram*, and author of a number of papers in the NCA's and ACA's periodicals (Hicks & Keating, 1988; Rehm, 1980). He continued as LACC's CEO until 1976, and was officially named president of the LACC in 1974. In 1954 he was appointed president of the NCA's Council on Education, and is acknowledged as a major influence in the early and continuing efforts of the NCA and ACA to establish federal recognition of chiropractic schools (Martin, 1986; Rehm, 1980, p. 329). During the 1950s and early 1960s Haynes struggled to keep his school afloat during a decade of declining enrollments (Martin, 1986), a phenomenon of increasing concern throughout the educational system as the Korean War first took prospective students, and later as GI educational benefits became more restricted and eventually came to an end (see Table 14-1). Haynes worked with John Nugent as the NCA leader tirelessly continued his reform work. Martin (1974) suggests that following Nugent's retirement in 1961, George Haynes:

> ...gradually assumed much of the leadership which had been carried by Dr. John Nugent. It was particularly necessary at that time that a member of the profession develop the vision, the motivation and the initiative toward our accreditation goals since the office of Director of Education had become rather fluid after Dr. Nugent stepped out of the position. Dr. Haynes provided these factors...

Accrediting Bodies

Nugent's educational/organizational program was formalized on 4 August 1947 when the NCA House of Delegates created its Council on Education by merging the Committee on Educational Standards and the National Council of Educational Institutions (CCE, 1984; Chirogram, 1974; Hariman, 1970, p. 28). The first members of the new agency included the chief administrators (presidents or deans) of participating schools, the former members of the standards committee, plus Nugent as Director of Education (see Table 14-2). The Council included a five-person Committee on Accreditation (CCE, 1984). In later years it was considered unorthodox to have the NCA's administrative officer (Nugent) serve on the governing Council, but in the early period the Director's influence was formidable. Nugent even advertised to recruit faculty for NCA-accredited schools (Advertisement, 1948). By 1951 Nugent had logged some 180,000 air miles in his campaign to upgrade the schools (NCA, 1951). Among his first major accomplishments was his successful collaboration with Emmett J. Murphy, D.C., Director of Public Relations for the NCA, in obtaining draft exempt status for chiropractic students (Chiropractic, 1951; Murphy, 1951a&b; Nugent, 1951).

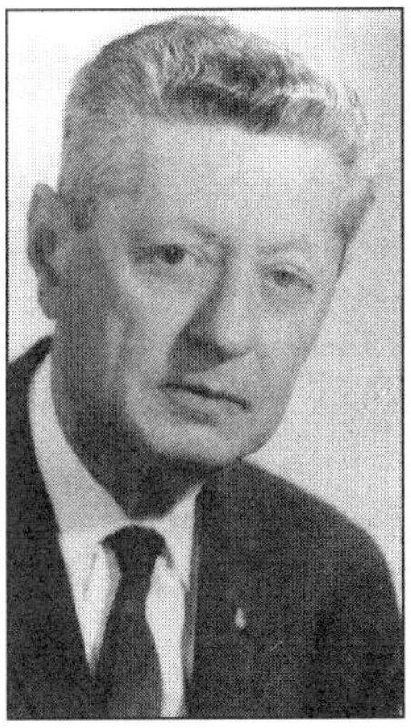

Figure 14-5: George H. Haynes, D.C., N.D., M.S.

Palmer graduate Earl R. Bebout, who had operated the Central States College in Indianapolis in the 1920s and opened the Bebout College of Chiropractic (BCC) circa 1946 (Miscellany, 1983), was passionately opposed to Nugent's reform efforts (Bebout, 1952). The BCC may deserve "the dubious distinction" (Miscellany, 1983) of offering the last 18-month chiropractic curriculum (until 1959), and outlasted even the PSC in this respect. The iconoclastic Bebout criticized Palmer and the International Chiropractors' Association (ICA) for not having done more to curtail the NCA Director of Education's activities at the outset. Bebout felt that ICA had abdicated its authority by turning accreditation matters for ICA-affiliated colleges over to the North American Association of Chiropractic Schools and Colleges (NAACSC).

Homer G. Beatty, D.C., N.D., University of Natural Healing Arts	Rudy O. Muller, D.C., Canadian Memorial Chiropractic College
T. Boner, D.C.	John J. Nugent, D.C., NCA Director of Education
W.A. Budden, D.C., N.D., Western States College, School of Chiropractic and School of Naturopathy	Paul O. Parr, D.C., Carver Chiropractic College
	John A. Schnick, D.C.
E.H. Gardner, D.C.	Clarence W. Weiant, D.C., Ph.D., Chiropractic Institute of New York
Henry C. Harring, D.C., M.D., Missouri Chiropractic College	
Arthur G. Hendricks, D.C., Lincoln College of Chiropractic	John B. Wolfe, D.C., Northwestern College of Chiropractic
Joseph Janse, D.C., N.D., National College of Chiropractic	Justin C. Wood, D.C.

Table 14-2: Original members of the National Chiropractic Association's Council on Education, 1947 (Chirogram, 1974)

The NAACSC was chartered in Oklahoma on 1 March 1952 by Paul O. Parr, D.C. (whose Carver College had by then reconsidered its role within the NCA), Vinton Logan of the Logan Basic College of Chiropractic and Carl S. Cleveland Jr. of the Cleveland Chiropractic College of Kansas City (Articles, 1952; Parr, 1952c). The organization had been formed despite the explicit disapproval of the NCA's Council on Education (Peterson, 1952), which saw the new body as a competitive threat. George Hariman, D.C., then serving as chairman of the board of the NCA and a long-time supporter of higher standards for chiropractic education, wrote to Vinton Logan to encourage him to reconsider his participation in the NAACSC:

> Dear Doctor Vinton:-
>
> The North American Association of Chiropractic Schools and Colleges was organized and your name appears as one of its members.
>
> This flank movement is a medium of "protection" to the schools rather than a guarantee that they will give the profession a high quality of instruction befitting a professional school.
>
> As individuals they have every right to "protect" their investment. What more prestige could such an association give them than that which they already enjoyed by being recognized by the ICA? Or is this just a smoke screen behind which they are attempting to hide in their effort to "accredit their own schools"; and achieve a measure of respectability equal to that accorded the accrediting agency of the National Chiropractic Association?
>
> The question in my mind Vinton is this, why did YOU associate your school with this group which has standards and facilities inferior to yours? I cannot blame some of those schools for some of them will never meet any standards other than their own, and others cannot meet even that.
>
> Your school is a non-profit institution. It has the qualifications of a professional school. It has the following and promise of a permanent Chiropractic College; therefore for you to be associated with schools of lesser stature will not, in my estimation and belief, enhance your position.
>
> Perhaps they wanted color, standing and physical equipment to back up their association claims. However, I am thinking Vinton, why did you not seek "a mail order education" for your degree? Because, you wanted your degree to mean something after your received your diploma! Likewise, those boys of ours who graduate from our schools would like to have a good diploma which has a meaning behind it. An approval and recognition of a college of their choice — not a profit bearing institution that may not exist a few years from now.
>
> I do not mind telling you that the entire field looks toward the day when, like the medical profession, we will count our schools with sufficient laboratories, staffs and equipment to constitute a profession.
>
> Your school with the PSC is among those that will carry on the educational work of the Chiropractic world. As a friend, and as one who has always spoken to you frankly and from the heart, I say to you, regardless of where the student graduates, Chiropractors at large are tired of divisions and pretense. They want the profession united as chiropractors, their schools operating as educational units, and they as the electors of their destiny.
>
> They want control of the situation and the time is not far distant when this will come to pass. When selfishness and profit motives will no longer divide and conquer, when slander and vilification will not prevail, and when Chiropractic will enter its own era of UNITY in matters of national importance, instead of personal differences.
>
> When that time comes, your school should be among the permanent institutions. So I say again to you Vinton, steer your ship to a straight course regardless of the little vexations. Like Farragut say with earnestness and vigor "Damn the torpedoes, full steam ahead!" for progress and better Chiropractic world.
>
> You have attended the Schools Council long enough now to know that they are trying to pattern their course of accreditation after the recognized schools and colleges of our country. Upon that day our Colleges must have enough standards to be admitted among the various accredited colleges of the country. We MUST have the institutions with the physical equipment and staffs comparable to those colleges that accord degrees of highest merit. All must take their place in this council and with equal standing. I say to you, YOURS can easily be one of those schools! Why not work toward this goal. Do not let us down in our expectations of you.

> All this is written from the heart and in a most sincere and friendly spirit. I am sincere and interested in you. You are valuable to our profession and its growth. We need fine leadership. Don't let others use you to accomplish their own ends to the detriment of your profession. Sincerely,...
> (Hariman, 1952)

Carl Cleveland, Jr. had written to Thure C. Peterson, chairman of the NCA Council on Education, to assure the NCA that the purpose of the NAACSC was to provide a forum for discussion of the school men's problems which would be independent of the professional association. The Kansas City school leader indicated that he could "not be a party to anything that would tend to destroy the National Council on Education" (Cleveland, 1952a). Carl Cleveland, Sr. expressed similar sentiments (Cleveland, 1952b). Bebout, however, believed that the purpose of the proposed NAACSC was "to offset the accrediting program of the N.C.A.," and felt the plan was "doomed to failure":

> ...Just what will be the ultimate effect on the I.C.A. when its accrediting baby fizzels [sic] out and the whole idea becomes a good laugh for Chiropractors everywhere.
>
> The N.C.A. = 4 years of 9 - mixer or straight
>
> The I.C.A. = 4 years of 9 - mixer or straight
>
> Things equal to the same thing are equal to each other. Even the P.S.C. now advertises the teaching of 4,485 hours only 1723 of which are in "non-medical subjects" (Bebout, 1951a).

Bebout, who had withdrawn from the NAACSC by the end of 1952 (Logan, 1952) owing to his dispute over length of curriculum, believed that Nugent's work would destroy the profession by shrinking the ranks of practitioners:

> ...Nugent and his like seem to do everything in their power to reduce still further the number practicing in the U.S. and Canada. Sad to relate some schools, school men, and leaders of other factions, men associated with International Chiropractors Association, are talking of following closely in footsteps of Nugentism, largely because of political, economic and personal ambitions. All because of selfishness that looks to expediency, rather than principle (Bebout, 1951b).

Although the NAACSC was undoubtedly a response to the growing threat of broad-scope chiropractic education posed by Nugent's campaign, the organization publicly and privately (Cleveland, 1952b) denied that its purposes included opposition to the NCA Council on Education. In a letter to Robert O. McClintock, D.C., owner and president of the broad-scope California Chiropractic College in Oakland, NAACSC's first president, Paul O. Parr, D.C., indicated that:

> ...I should like to personally, as a member, and officially, as President of the new Association, invite you to write me a letter applying to be considered for membership.
>
> I personally assure you that we are not forming for the purpose of combat, debate or argument with any other organization, but only to further those points upon which we agree for the mutual advancement of our profession and our institutions, and urge you to join us in these laudable endeavors.
>
> I feel quite sure that if you submit a letter of request to be considered a member, we can circulate the request among the members and obtain full consent of membership. I am sure it will enthuse those of us who are already members to have you join us and I feel quite sure that your counsel and advice would be of great aid to us. It is altogether possible that this strength, prestige and support can be of considerable moral and material aid to us (Parr, 1952b).

McClintock's response was affirmative (Cleveland, 1952b). His California Chiropractic College was one of several schools outside the orbits of NCA and ICA who were interested in a school organization established by school leaders (e.g., Parr, 1952c). The NAACSC's initial public communication was issued by Paul O. Parr, D.C., the organization's first president:

NEWS RELEASE TO ALL CHIROPRACTORS, CHIROPRACTIC ORGANIZATIONS AND CHIROPRACTIC PUBLICATIONS

At a meeting in Chicago on March 1st the NORTH AMERICAN ASSOCIATION OF CHIRO-PRACTIC SCHOOLS AND COLLEGES was formed. Eleven of our chiropractic colleges were represented. Dr. Paul O. Parr, President, Carver Chiropractic College, was elected President; Dr. Carl S. Cleveland, Jr., President, Cleveland Chiropractic College, was elected Vice-President; and Dr. Vinton F. Logan, President, Logan Basic College of Chiropractic, was elected Secretary-Treasurer.

The deliberations took two days. The purposes of the organization are: (1) Perpetuation and advancement of chiropractic; (2) The advancement of chiropractic colleges and chiropractic education; (3) To make our cooperation available to state associations and others to further the interest of chiropractic; (4) To cooperate with state boards in meeting our mutual problems in their various states.

The representatives attending the Association, including the above officers, were as follows:

Dr. E.R. Bebout   Dr. Frank E. Dean

Dr. P.J. Cerasoli   Dr. Herbert C. Hender

Dr. C.S. Cleveland, Jr.   Dr. Vinton F. Logan

Dr. William N. Coggins   Dr. Fannie R. McCoy

Dr. Kenneth H. Cronk   Dr. Paul O. Parr

Dr. A.J. Darling

Colleges participating in the initial organization meeting were: Atlantic States Chiropractic Institute, Bebout Chiropractic College, Carver Chiropractic College, Cleveland Chiropractic College, Columbia Institute of Chiropractic, Kansas State Chiropractic College, Logan Basic College of Chiropractic, Palmer School of Chiropractic, Ratledge Chiropractic College, Rest View University of Chiropractic.

This new organization meets the need of an independent organization of schools and colleges whereby deliberations and organized action can purposefully accomplish the aims and objectives of our great profession. Such an organization has been thought of by many and requested by some, and will be acclaimed by the profession as an opportunity for unity of action among all chiropractic colleges for better unity of action in the profession.

The North American Association of Chiropractic Schools and Colleges earnestly solicits the cooperation and suggestions of any and all organizations and individuals interested in its noble objectives. We sincerely want to make our organization, its facilities, its deliberation chambers and mechanism available for consideration of any and all problems that may affect these objectives. This is an organization dedicated to unity of action in the things upon which we all agree. We should like to see all chiropractic organizations and institutions prosper and flourish to the aggrandizement of our profession and to the enhancement of health services for the troubled citizens of a troubled world (Parr, 1952a).

The formation of the NAACSC coincided with the 1952 formation of the ICA's Chiropractic Education Commission (CEC), which involved many of the same schools that constituted the membership of the NAACSC. Part of the impetus for the CEC's formation was a 1949 study of chiropractic education by O.D. Adams, Ed.D., then Assistant Superintendent of Schools for the City of San Francisco, whom the ICA had recruited as an educational consultant. When the CEC was estab-

Table 14-3: Schools accredited by the ICA's Chiropractic Education Commission in 1956

School Name	President or Dean	Location
Atlantic States Chiropractic Institute	Martin I. Phillips, D.C.	Brooklyn, New York
Carver Chiropractic College	Paul O. Parr, D.C.	Oklahoma City, Oklahoma
Cleveland Chiropractic College	Carl S. Cleveland, Jr., D.C.	Kansas City, Missouri
Cleveland Chiropractic College	Carl S. Cleveland, Sr., D.C.	Los Angeles, California
Columbia Institute of Chiropractic	Frank E. Dean, M.B., D.C.	New York, New York
International Chiropractic College	A.M. Valdiserri, D.C., D.M.	Dayton, Ohio
Logan Basic College of Chiropractic	Vinton F. Logan, D.C.	St. Louis, Missouri
Palmer School of Chiropractic	B.J. Palmer, D.C., Ph.C.	Davenport, Iowa

lished, Adams was hired as ICA's Education Director, and in this capacity visited and inspected many of the ICA schools. The ICA's standards for college accreditation did not require the school to adopt non-profit status, but emphasized the need for faculty (almost exclusively D.C.s) to provide a curriculum, including the basic sciences, with a strong chiropractic orientation. By 1956 the ICA's CEC had accredited eight schools (see Table 14-3), and had applications from several more.

The existence of ICA's Commission created some unlikely bedfellows. Apparently unable or unwilling to meet the NCA Council's standards, the Hollywood College, School of Chiropractic (but presumably not its sister organization, the Hollywood College, School of Naturopathy) applied for CEC recognition. According to the Stanford Research Institute (Stanford, 1960, p. 101), the Hollywood Chiropractic College (HCC) was "organized along the lines of a typical sole proprietorship"; that alone was sufficient to exclude it from consideration for recognition by the NCA Council on Education. The Stanford report further noted that:

> ...On October 26, 1956, WE Thomas DC, wrote a letter to the ICA requesting that HCC be inspected for purposes of becoming an accredited school. (copy of letter obtained from the files of the Research and Education Corporation, San Francisco, consultants to ICA.) HCC's unsuccessful efforts to gain approval have extended over a period of more than two years. ICA still has not accredited the school, although in a letter dated February 27, 1957, OD Adams Ph.D., President of the Education and Research Corporation, San Francisco, recommended that HCC be accredited by the ICA (Stanford, 1960, p. 98).

By late 1962 the HCC had closed, and its records were sent to LACC (Homewood, 1975; LACC, 1986).

Bebout (1951), Palmer and others continued to direct special animosity at Nugent, whom B.J. referred to as the "Anti-Christ of Chiropractic" (Gibbons, 1985; Strauss, 1994, p. 187). However, when the NCA leader's publicly expressed attitudes towards basic science legislation at a Cleveland Chiropractic College homecoming in Kansas City were misstated, Carl S. Cleveland, Jr. (see Figure 14-6), dean of the school his parents had established and a founding member of the NAACSC, circulated the following correction:

> Quoting—-Dr. John Nugent at Cleveland Chiropractic College
>
> "Homecoming" —- 1949
>
> I'm not for Basic Science Boards. I've been accused in this State of being for Basic Science Boards, and my words have been distorted — twisted — taken out of context. When you don't answer a man you ballywack him. You lie about it — you haven't got the real answer.
>
> The real answer was — I made that statement before Congress, I said that I had written the Basic Science act in Connecticut. And I did. I wrote it. I wrote it on my own little typewriter. Why? Because there had been a terrific scandal in the eclectic profession and a man had been killed on an operating table and the whole state of Conn. was in furor, and nineteen prefectors in the State demanded some sort of qualifications for all practitioners, and Liberty magazine and Colliers were writing articles about Conn. and when I saw the powers that be they said, "Now look Doctor, we're supposed to be political leaders in this state but we can't stem this tide. There's got to be some sort of device. The State Chamber of Commerce, Kiwanis Club and all the Civic Clubs were up in arms about it and we were going to get a Basic Science Law." So I said to Mr. Roarback, who was the political boss of the State who was a Chiropractic patient — I said to him, "Well, if we have to have the damn thing then let's have a fair one." He said, "Can you write such a bill," and I said "yes." And I wrote that bill. I put it in my pocket and that's the Bill that came out. Yes I wrote that thing — and I wish that I'd had an opportunity to write every other one of the Basic Science bills too (Nugent, 1949).

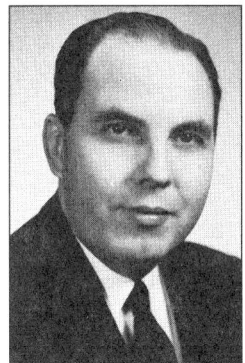

Figure 14-6: Carl S. Cleveland, Jr., D.C., c1954

Cleveland Chiropractic Colleges

The younger Cleveland, who earned a bachelor's degree in physiology from the University of Nebraska and his doctorate from his parents' school in 1942, assumed the leadership of his chiropractic alma mater in the early 1950s, when Carl Cleveland Sr. relocated to Los Angeles to take over the Ratledge College (Keating et al., 1991, 1992). Although father and son both served with B.J. Palmer on the ICA's Board of Control, their correspondence from the early 1950s reveals their regular communication with the NCA education director, John Nugent. The Cleveland schools attempted to find a middle ground within the profession, and promoted what they considered:

> A PRO-CHIROPRACTIC POLICY: The Policy which we try to maintain at Cleveland College is not anti-medical, anti-mixing or anti-anything but a PRO-CHIROPRACTIC Policy. This helps all Chiropractors, mixers and straights...

By 1950 the Cleveland schools had broken with B.J.'s position, and were reconciled to a four-year curriculum (Cleveland, 1950). The Cleveland College of Los Angeles had no choice in this matter, since voters revised the state law in 1948 to mandate in excess of 4,000 hours of instruction to qualify for licensure. Indeed, the increase in required curriculum, including coursework in physiotherapy and diagnosis, had been part of Ratledge's motivation for offering in 1950 to sell his California institution to Cleveland (Keating et al., 1991, 1992; Ratledge, 1950). Although the Cleveland schools embraced the four year curriculum, they resisted the growing movement to increase pre-chiropractic education as a condition for admission to professional training. The Los Angeles branch also sought ways to thwart the state law's mandate to qualify students in the use of physiotherapeutics. Reports of inspections of the new Cleveland College during its earliest years of operation noted that:

> At no time during the course of approximately thirty visits to Cleveland Chiropractic College was the room containing physiotherapy equipment found in use. The administrators at that college, while accepting the edict of the Board ruling, openly disclaimed the value of training in physiotherapy for "straight" chiropractic students. A similar observation was made by Morris Jerlow, D.C., Commissioner on College Inspection, in a report on the Ratledge College of Chiropractic (now CCC) in 1952: "Physiotherapy is not given sufficient prominence on the curriculum. Though it is relatively well presented in lecture and demonstration in the classroom, this is not sufficient application and operative experience and clinical practice to assure a sound and stable appreciation of the place of physiotherapy in the field of chiropractic or to adequately guard against improper use of standard modalities or even to protect himself from imposition by salesmen of various types of gadgets (Stanford, 1960, p. 98).

The senior Cleveland's strong commitment to straight chiropractic was in evidence in 1955, when he organized a state organization known as Chiropractors for Chiropractic, a group characterized as "the most conservative of all California chiropractic associations" (Stanford, 1960, p. 29). His continuing concerns about preventing the introduction of physiotherapeutics to the curricula of straight chiropractic were still in evidence more than a decade later (Rutherford, 1968).

The sale of the Ratledge Chiropractic College (RCC) and its re-birth as the Cleveland Chiropractic College of Los Angeles marked the end of T.F. Ratledge's 43-year career in straight chiropractic education. Ratledge, who had been a central player in acquiring the state's Chiropractic Act in 1922, had battled the broad-scope chiropractors of California throughout most of his 40 years in the Golden State. In the late 1940s, however, he experienced a number of defeats from which he could not recover. A lawsuit brought against the Board of Chiropractic Examiners (BCE) to block an increase, by administrative ruling, in the number of instructional hours required for licensure, was lost (Keating et al., 1991, 1992). In 1948 the BCE's administrative rulings were replaced by the above-mentioned change in the state law mandating more than 4,000 hours of education (the RCC curriculum had been 2,400 hours since 1922). Moreover, the new state law required that students learn subjects that Ratledge considered "medical," such as diagnosis and physiotherapies. Additionally, the Veterans Administration had ruled that the RCC curriculum did not meet the federal government's standards, and veterans were therefore not eligible for tuition support if they attended the Ratledge school.

By 1948 the student body at RCC was so depleted that the school suspended all but post-graduate instruction. At the end of 1950 Ratledge, the "missionary of straight chiropractic in California," offered to sell his school to Carl S. Cleveland, Sr. for $40,000. Transfer of all stock interest was delayed until 9 April 1955, owing to the death of Ratledge's wife (who owned one third of the corporation), and in the interim the school operated as the Ratledge College "under Cleveland management" (Keating et al., 1991, 1992). Ratledge retired to Arkansas, where he was honored by the state legislature by the granting of a special license to practice chiropractic, despite his unwillingness to sit for the basic science examinations.

Raising Standards

Admissions standards were an especially difficult matter for all chiropractic colleges, and a source of contention within the profession (Barad, 1948; Hariman, 1970, p. 39). Watkins, the first chairman of the NCA Committee on Education, had noted as early as 1938 that over half of all medical schools then required a four-year college degree for admission (Watkins, n.d., circa 1938). Perhaps the most vocal advocate of increased pre-chiropractic education was W.A. Budden of Western States College (e.g., Budden, 1954). Three schools (Columbia/Baltimore, LACC and Western States) later claimed to be first (circa 1952-53) in implementing a two-year, liberal arts training as a condition for admission to chiropractic college (Homola, 1963, pp. 71-2; LACC, 1986; Rehm, 1992a). The Columbia College in Baltimore (1946-1954), a branch of Frank Dean's New York school, put the two-year, pre-professional requirements in place so as to meet new standards mandated by the state of Maryland in 1951. The Baltimore branch closed in 1954 owing to a severe decline in enrollment, and the other three institutions rescinded the two-year college requirement at about the same time.

Table 14-4: "Entrance Requirements" derived from a survey conducted at a meeting of the "General Committee of the Profession on Education," in Detroit, June 24, 1962 (Haynes, 1961)

	ASCI	CMCC	CINY	CCC-K	CIC	LCC	LBCC	LACC	NCC	NoCC	PCC	TCC
Application form	Y	Y	Y	Y	Y	Y	Y	Y	Y	Y	Y	Y
Age limit	18+	17	18	No	No	No	No	17+	No	No	No	No
Student Rate Sheet	No	No	Y	Y	Y	No	Y	Y	Y	Y	No	Y
High School Equivalence	Y	No	Y	Y	Y	Y	Y	Y	Y	Y	Y	Y
High School Diploma	Y	No	Y	Y	Y	Y	Y	Y	Y	No	Y	Y
Require Transcript	Y	Y	Y	Y	Y	Y	Y	Y	Y	No	Y	Y
Grade Average (High School)	C	60%	C	No	No	No	No	C	C	No	No	Pass
Require Sp. H.S. Subjects	No	Y	No	No	No	No	No	No	No	No	No	Y
Require College Credits	No		1*	No	No	No	No	No	1*	Y	No	No
Entrance Test	No	No	Y	No	No	No	No	Y	No	Y	No	Y
Entrance Test Type	-	-	SAT	-	-	-	-	ACT	-	SAT	-	ACT
Finger Prints	No	No	No	No	No	No	No	Y	No	No	No	No
Picture	Y	Y	Y	Y	Y	Y	Y	Y	Y	Y	Y	Y
Advanced Standing from: College Arts & Sciences	No	Y	Y	No	Y	Y	Y	Y	Y	Y	No	Y
Grade Req.	C	60%	C	-	C	Pass	C	C	Pass	Pass	-	C
D.O. or M.D. College	Y	Y	Y	No	Y	Y	Y	2*		Y	No	Y
All D.C. Colleges	No	No	No	No	No	No	No	No		No	No	No
Grade Req.	C	60%	C	Pass	C	Pass	C	C		C	Pass	C
Other Schools	No	No	No	No	Y	Y	Y	No		No	No	No

1* For States with college requirements.
2* Limited to not over 1,200 hours - Basic Sciences only.

ASCI	Atlantic States Chiropractic College		LBCC	Logan Basic College of Chiropractic
CMCC	Canadian Memorial Chiropractic College		LACC	Los Angeles College of Chiropractic
CINY	Chiropractic Institute of New York		NCC	National College of Chiropractic
CCC-K	Cleveland Chiropractic College-Kansas City		NoCC	Northwestern College of Chiropractic
CIC	Columbia Institute of Chiropractic		PCC	Palmer College of Chiropractic
LCC	Lincoln Chiropractic College		TCC	Texas College of Chiropractic

Martin (1974) suggested that "Budden was too eager to initiate the new standards; he had them incorporated into the state law and the results nearly destroyed the college" when prospective students apparently elected to matriculate elsewhere. Although Haynes (1962) reported to the NCA in 1962 that 9 of 12 schools surveyed required some pre-chiropractic college education (see Table 14-4), Homola (1963, p. 71) reported that Western States College was the only chiropractic school which mandated at least two years of pre-professional training. Even this requirement could be waived if the student intended to practice in a state where such college preparation was not legally mandated.

An unsuccessful attempt was made in 1962 to bring about "uniform certification of credits for all State Boards of Examiners" and standardized admissions criteria among straight and mixer schools. At a meeting in Detroit on 24 June 1962 of the "General Committee of the Profession on Education" leaders from NCA and ICA schools did reach a series of understandings and agreements about entrance and graduation requirements. Led by George Haynes, D.C., president of the NCA's National Council on Education and dean of the LACC, and William Coggins, D.C. of the NAACSC, the group considered:

> Age limit - agreed that students must be over 21 to graduate
> Grade average - The I.C.A. schools will consider the "C" grade requirement for entrance.
>
> Entrance test - The I.C.A. will consider the institution of a college entrance test, conducted and graded by an outside agency.
>
> Finger prints - was recommended for use by all schools - action pending.
>
> College of Arts & Science - on a limited basis of subject per subject.
>
> D.O. or M.D. school - limited as above and only applicable to basic science subjects (Haynes, 1962).

Table 14-5: *Comparison Between Class Hours Approved Medical School and the Palmer School of Chiropractic.* Davenport, IA: Palmer School of Chiropractic, c1950 (Cleveland & Keating, 1995)

Subject	Johns Hopkins Class Hours	Johns Hopkins % of Total	PSC Class Hours	PSC % of Total
Anatomy	508	15.0	520	11.6
Physiology	256	7.3	520	11.6
Pathology	401	11.8	195	4.4
Chemistry	200	5.9	325	7.2
Bacteriology	114	3.4	130	3.0
Diagnosis	224	6.6	520	11.6
Neurology	112	3.3	130	3.0
X-Ray	48	1.4	292	6.5
Psychiatry	144	4.3	65	1.4
OB/GYN	198	5.8	65	1.4
Pharmacology	80	2.4	0	
Psychology	16	.5	0	
Medicine	656	19.3	0	
Pediatrics	72	2.1	0	
Surgery	352	10.4	0	
Therapeutics	16	.5	0	
Clinic	0		585	13.0
Hygiene	0		65	1.4
Chiropractic Technic	0		553	12.3
Chiropractic Philosophy	0		195	4.4
Public Speaking	0		65	1.4
NCM and NCGH	0		65	1.4
Principle/ Practice	0		130	3.0
Ethics and Jurisprudence	0		65	1.4
TOTAL	3397	100%	4485	100%

However, a highly competitive spirit among the schools amplified the philosophical and theoretical differences that had long divided chiropractic educational institutions. Hayes (1962) noted that recruitment abuses such as enticing students from one school to another with inducements of scholarships, continued to hinder harmonious relations among the colleges. With such competitiveness, many schools continued to be reluctant to raise admissions standards and risk a decrease in student applicants. However, in 1969 the Foundation for Chiropractic Education and Research (FCER), formerly FACE, provided added incentive to raise admissions standards:

> In January 1969, the FCER Trustees informed each college that Grant-in-Aid funds would be withheld and placed in escrow by FCER until the Foundation receives word from the Council on Chiropractic Education to the effect that the college had instituted the two-year pre-professional requirement for entrance or had given satisfactory evidence that it is phasing into the two-year pre-professional requirement (Schierholz, 1986, p. 28).

Admissions standards were only one of the continuing weaknesses in the standards for chiropractic colleges. In the early 1950s a few hold-out schools, such as Palmer and Bebout, still offered 18-month programs leading to the doctor of chiropractic degree. Yet by this time, most jurisdictions that licensed chiropractors moved to require much longer curricula, and the PSC bowed to the practical reality of the licensing laws. The PSC's expanded program seemed to compare favorably with medical school curricula (see Table 14-5).

Palmer School of Chiropractic

The postwar years brought many changes to the Palmer School of Chiropractic. Although the PSC had weathered the war years as well or better than most chiropractic colleges, enrollments had suffered and the once glorious campus (see Figure 14-7) seemed somewhat deteriorated to alumni (Ashworth, 1944). As the profession emerged from the worldwide conflagration, the PSC enjoyed the same new prosperity that other schools experienced, and was better prepared, by virtue of its facilities, to cope with the influx of new students. However, licensing laws were changing in many states, including the continued introduction of basic science laws and lengthening of the curricula required for licensure. Palmer and the PSC abandoned the 18-month curriculum when it became clear that the overwhelming majority of states insisted on a lengthier education, and that to persist meant that PSC graduates would generally be unable to be licensed (Quigley, 1989; Strauss, 1994). This was a prudent move; by the end of the decade, all but two of the U.S. and Canadian jurisdictions that licensed chiropractors required a four year degree, and

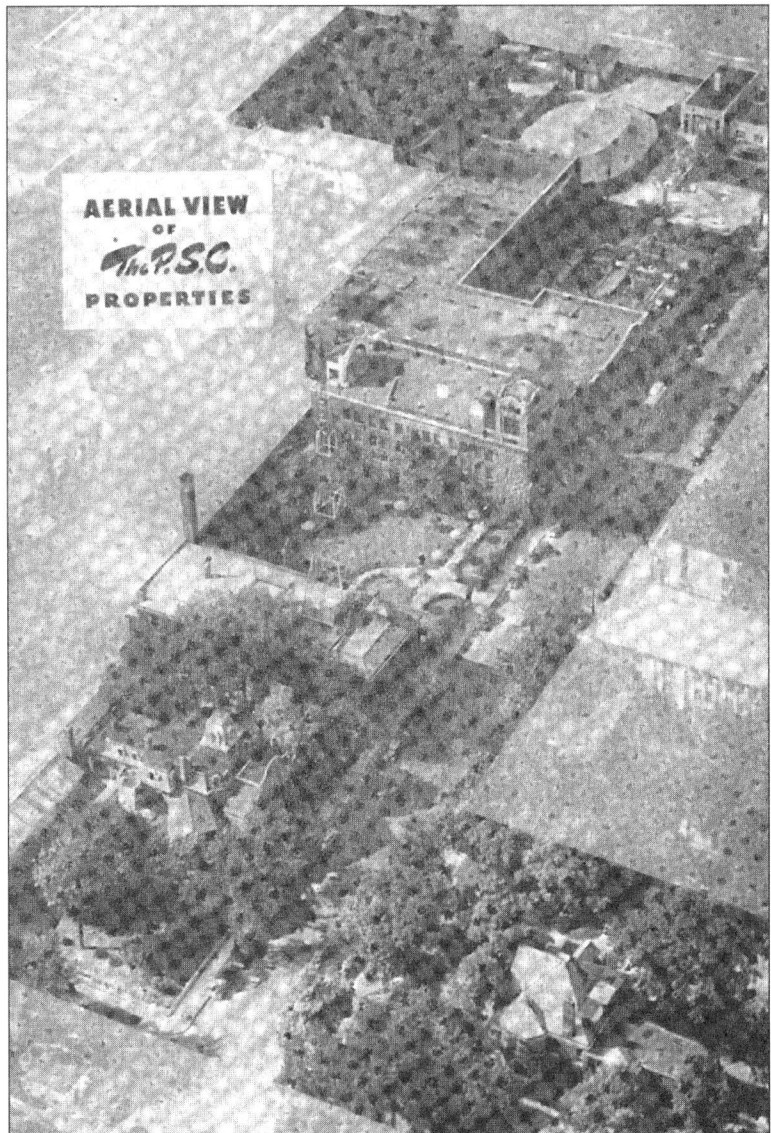

Figure 14-7: campus of the Palmer School, 1956

Table 14-6: Education Requirements for Licensure, as of March 20, 1961, from the catalog of the Chiropractic Institute of New York (Chiropractic, 1962, pp.24-5)

UNITED STATES State or Province	Preliminary Education Required	Statutory Requirement Prof. Education	Type of Examining Board
Alabama	High School*	4 yrs. of 9 mo. Each	C-B
Alaska	H.S. & 2 yrs. College	4 yrs. of 9 mo. Each	C-B
Arizona	High School	4 yrs. of 9 mo. Each	C-B
Arkansas	High School	4 yrs. of 9 mo. Each	C-B
California	H.S. & 2 yrs. College	4 yrs. of 9 mo. Each	C
Colorado	High School	4 yrs. - 4,000 hrs.	C-B
Connecticut	H.S. & 2 yrs. College	4 yrs. of 8 mo. each - 4,000 hrs.	C-B
Delaware	H.S. & 2 yrs. College	4 yrs. of 8 mo. Each	C-B
District of Columbia	H.S. & 2 yrs. College	4 yrs. of 9 mo. Each	C-B
Florida	High School	4 yrs. - 4,000 hrs.	C-B
Georgia (4)	H.S. & 1 yr. College	4 yrs. of 9 mo. each	C
Hawaii	H.S. & 2 yr. College	4 yrs. of 9 mo. each	C
Idaho	H.S. & 2 yr. College	4 yrs. of 8 mo. each	C
Illinois	High School	4 yrs. of 8 mo. each	MX
Indiana	H.S. & 2 yr. College	4 yrs. - 4,000 hrs.	MX
Iowa	High School	4 yrs. - 4,000 hrs.	C-B
Kansas	High School	4 yrs. of 9 mo. each	MX-B
Kentucky	High School	4 yrs. of 9 mo. each - 4,000 hrs.	C
Louisiana	not regulated		
Maine	H.S. & 2 yrs. College	4 yrs. - 4,000 hrs.	C
Maryland	H.S. & 2 yrs. College	4 yrs. - 4,000 hrs.	C
Massachusetts	not regulated		
Michigan	High School	4 yrs. - 4,000 hrs.	C-B
Minnesota	High School	4 yrs. of 8 mo. each - 4,000 hrs.	C-B
Mississippi	not regulated		
Missouri	High School	3 yrs. of 9 mo. each	C
Montana	H.S. & 2 yrs. College	4 yrs. of 9 mo. each	C
Nebraska	High School	4 yrs. - 4,000 hrs.	C-B
Nevada	High School	4 yrs. - 4,000 hrs.	C-B
New Hampshire	High School	4 yrs. - 4,000 hrs.	C
New Jersey	H.S. & 2 yrs. College	4 yrs. of 9 mo. each	MX
New Mexico	High School	4 yrs. - 4,000 hrs.	C-B
New York	not regulated		
North Carolina	H.S. & 2 yrs. College	4 yrs. of 9 mo. each	C
North Dakota	H.S. & 2 yrs. College	3 yrs. of 8 mo. each	C
Ohio	H.S. & 2 yrs. College	4 yrs. of 6 mo. each	MX
Oklahoma	H.S. & 2 yrs. College	4 yrs. of 9 mo. each - 4,150 hrs.	C-B
Oregon	H.S. & 2 yrs. College	4 yrs. of 9 mo. each	C-B
Pennsylvania (1)	H.S. & College credits	4 yrs. of 9 mo. each	C
Puerto Rico	H.S. & 2 yrs. College	4 yrs. of 9 mo. each	C
Rhode Island	H.S. & 1 yr. College	4 yrs. of 8 mo. each	MX-B
South Carolina	High School	4 yrs. of 9 mo. each	C
South Dakota	High School	4 yrs. of 9 mo. each	C-B
Tennessee	High School	4 yrs. of 9 mo. each	C-B
Texas	H.S. & 2 yrs. College	4 yrs. of 8 mo. each	C-B
Utah	H.S. & 1 yr. College	4 yrs. of 8.5 mo. each	C-B
Vermont	High School	4 yrs. - 3,600 hrs.	C
Virginia	H.S. & 2 yrs. College	4 yrs. of 8 mo. each	MX-B
Washington	High School	4,000 hrs.	C-B
West Virginia	H.S. & 2 yrs. College	4 yrs. of 9 mo. each	MX
Wisconsin	H.S. & 2 yrs. College	4 yrs. of 9 mo. each	C-B
Wyoming	H.S. & 2 yrs. College	4 yrs. of 9 mo. each	C

CANADA State or Province	Preliminary Education Required	Statutory Requirement Prof. Education	Type of Examining Board
Alberta (2)	Junior Matriculation	4 yrs. of 8 mo. each	C
British Columbia	Junior Matriculation	4 yrs. of 8 mo. each	C
Manitoba	Junior Matriculation	4 academic years	C
New Brunswick (2)	Junior Matriculation	4 yrs. of 9 mo. each	C
Ontario	Junior Matriculation	4 yrs. of 9 mo. each - 4,200 hrs.	DP
Saskatchewan (3)	Junior Matriculation	4 yrs. of 8 mo. each	C
Quebec	not regulated		
Other Maritime Prov.	not regulated		

Table 14-6, cont.

Explanation of Requirements:

Symbols designating Boards: C - Chiropractic; C-B - Chiropractic and Basic Science; MX - Mixed (composed of medical and chiropractic members); DP - Drugless Practitioners; MX-B - Mixed and Basic Science.

*High School or equivalent. The states of Florida, Illinois and Montana do not accept equivalents.

(1) High school or its equivalent and one year of college credits in biology, physics and chemistry are preliminary requirements.

(2) A Junior Matriculation Certificate or its equivalent is equal to a high school diploma or its equivalent.

(3) British citizenship is a requirement for licensure.

(4) Two years of additional college credits after 1964.

Table 14-7: "PSC Faculty and Executives," from *Lyceum and Homecoming, 1956 Program*

B.J. Palmer, D.C., Ph.C.	President, Head, Dept. of Philosophy
Ralph Evans	Executive Vice-President
D.D. Palmer, D.C., Ph.C.	Vice-President
H.C. Hender, D.C., Ph.C.	Dean, Head Dept. of Psychiatry, Symptomatology
H.C. Chance, D.C., Ph.C.	Director P.S.C. Student Clinic, Neurology
K.H. Cronk, D.C., Ph.C.	Head Dept. of Chemistry, Physiology, Bacteriology
P.A. Reimer, D.C., Ph.C.	Director of Spinograph & X-Ray Dept.
M.B. DeNio, D.C.	Ass't. Director of B.J. Palmer Chiropractic Clinic
Galen Price, D.C., Ph.C.	Ass't. Head Dept. of Philosophy
W. Heath Quigley, D.C., Ph.C.	Director of Clear View Sanitarium, Pathology
D.O. Pharaoh, D.C., Ph.C.	Head Dept. of Anatomy
L.E. Gosser, D.C.	Principles and Practice, Neurology, Neurophysiology
D.O. Kern, D.C., Ph.C.	Ass't. Director P.S.C. Student Clinic, Principles and Practice (X-Ray)
O.W. Murphy, D.C.	Anatomy, Physiology
H.M. Himes, D.C., Ph.C.	Head Technic Dept., Philosophy, Business Administration
J. Clay Thompson, D.C., Ph.C.	X-Ray, Hygiene, NCM-NCG
John R. Quigley, D.C.	Head Dept. of Principles and Practice, Anatomy, Physiology
Elmer L. Crowder, D.C.	Principles and Practice (Technic, NCM-NCG), Public Speaking
Marion Anger, D.C.	Principles and Practice (X-Ray)
Virgil Strang, D.C.	Anatomy
Sidney Cook, D.C.	Principles and Practice (Technic), Chemistry
H. Dale Evans, D.C.	Principles and Practice (Technic)
Arthur L. Manus, D.C.	Principles and Practice (Technic)
Richard Nelson, D.C.	Principles and Practice (Technic)
James Kern, D.C.	Principles and Practice (X-Ray, Technic)
Ray T. Kern, D.C.	Bacteriology, Chemistry
J. Millman, D.C.	Chemistry
George Kneisel, D.C.	Principles and Practice (X-Ray)
Harry Andrews, M.D.	Physiology
Levern Chance, D.C.	Student Clinic
Luther Tucker, D.C.	Principles and Practice (X-Ray)
Charles Smith, D.C.	Principles and Practice (Technic)
Sherman Allen, D.C.	Principles and Practice (Technic)
L.G. Fraser, D.C.	Technic and Research
Mary Hazel Pharaoh, D.C.	Technic and Research
Eleanor S. Ridgway, D.C.	Technic and Research
Ruth G. Kersten, D.C.	Technic and Research
Leita H. Kaufman, D.C.	Technic and Research
Richard L. Hall, D.C.	Technic and Research
John M. Carswell, D.C.	Technic and Research
Lyle J. Nagel, D.C.	Technic and Research
Hugh E. Chance	Ethics and Jurisprudence
Jack Crenshaw, D.C.	Ethics and Jurisprudence
Gordon L. Gunning	Registrar, Ethics, Business Administration
Ralph Volkmann	Assistant Registrar
Otto Schiernbeck	Head, Neurocalometer Dept.
Verne Link	Supt. Buildings and Grounds

none accepted the 18 month program (see Table 14-6).

Approaching his seventh decade as the 1950s dawned, B.J. Palmer was slowing down (Quigley, 1989), and was less willing to fight the battles required to maintain the status quo. Although he remained the president of the PSC, and survived an attempt to remove him from the presidency of the ICA in 1949 (Quigley, 1989), he was frustrated. In his final years he spent less and less time in Davenport, and directed the affairs of the school from his winter home in Sarasota, Florida.

Despite the wear and tear upon the "Fountainhead" and its president, the PSC remained the undisputed leader among chiropractic institutions in terms of size of the student body and faculty (see Table 14-7). The PSC's membership among straight chiropractic schools enabled the narrow-scope faction of the profession to argue that its accrediting bodies, rather than those of the NCA/ACA, were the most representative of the chiropractic educational institutions. This factor was a significant stumbling block for the CCE in its efforts to achieve recognition with the U.S. Department of Education in the early 1970s.

Changes in curricular content were also seen in the 1950s at this, the oldest of chiropractic colleges. On 4 January 1956 Herbert M. Himes, D.C., Ph.C., then chair of the Technic Department at the PSC (and later dean of the CMCC), announced to the student body that a 20 year old policy had been rescinded by B.J. (Himes, 1956). Henceforth, the Hole-in-One technique (renamed Upper Cervical Specific in 1946), would not be the sole type of adjustive instruction provided at the "Fountainhead." Once again PSC students learned to thrust into spinal segments below the atlas-axis complex, although they were not initially permitted to use these full-spine procedures in the student clinics. Himes' laborious and carefully worded declaration suggests the perceived significance of this curricular change, and that he anticipated that at least some practicing Palmer graduates would not be pleased. However, PSC-trained chiropractors had been experiencing increasing difficulties in passing state board examinations owing to their restricted adjustive training, and the policy change had become essential (Quigley, 1989).

Danish Chiropractors' School

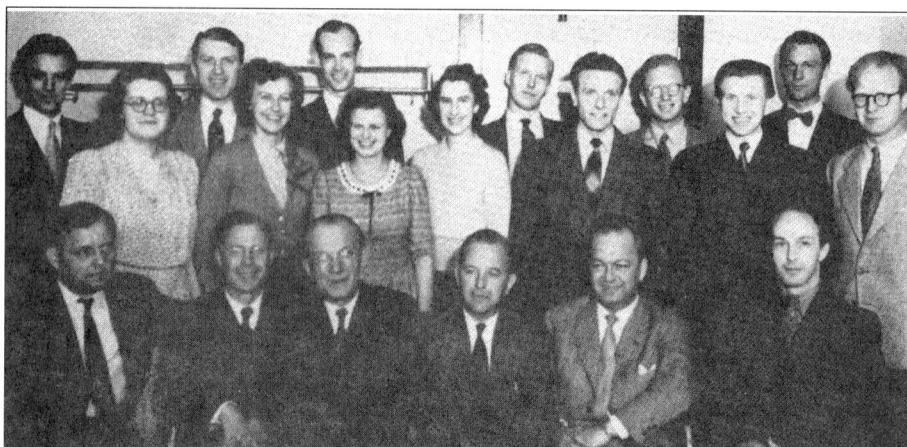

Figure 14-8: Faculty and students of the sole class of the Danish Chiropractors' School, Copenhagen, Denmark, 1948-1951 (Simonsen et al., 1989)

While the distinction of founding the first chiropractic college outside the United States probably belongs to the Robbins Chiropractic Institute of Sault Ste. Marie, Ontario (see Chapter 3), the first overseas school of chiropractic appeared in Denmark (see Figure 14-8). On 1 September 1948 the Danish Chiropractors School (DCS) opened in Copenhagen (Chance, 1986; Gautvig & Hviid, 1975; Hviid, 1990; Simonsen et al., 1989). Intended as a temporary means of meeting the need for chiropractors in the immediate post-war period, when currency exchange did not yet permit travel to North America, the DCS provided training to 15 students. Unbeknownst to the administrators and faculty at the medical school of the University of Copenhagen, the 15 enrolled simultaneously in the medical curriculum while studying chiropractic in the private offices of five American-trained practitioners: E.O. Rames, M.D., D.C. (a specialist in orthopedics and radiology), Aage Pedersen, D.C., Finn Christensen, D.C., H.A. Simonsen, D.C. and Hugo Dohn, D.C. These men constituted the faculty of the DCS, and all but Dohn, a graduate of the Lincoln Chiropractic College, had earned their chiropractic doctorates at the Palmer School. Not surprisingly, the medical school authorities were quite chagrined to learn they had been training future chiropractors. There seems to have been considerable redundancy in the training provided by the medical and chiropractic faculty (e.g., Simonsen et al., 1989).

The Danish Pro-Chiropractic Association, a patients' advocacy group, collaborated with the Danish Chiropractic Association to finance a clinic which provided free care to patients and offered clinical experience for the future doctors. After passing their final exams in chiropractic, an additional six months of supervised practical experience, an externship in today's parlance, was also required. Graduation exercises took place in Copenhagen on 4

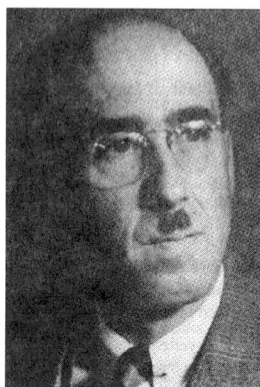

Figure 14-9: Fred Illi, D.C.

June 1951 in conjunction with the organizational meeting of the European Chiropractic Union, at which time Swiss chiropractor Fred W. Illi (see Figure 14-9) was elected the organization's first president (Simonsen et al., 1989). By this time, more favorable currency exchanges between North American countries and the European nations devastated by the war had been re-established, and the DCS was dissolved.

Canadian Memorial Chiropractic College

Newspapers in 1949 noted receipt of diplomas by "the first students of the only chiropractic college in the British Empire" (First, undated). In that year the CMCC graduated its first 75 students, including 52 veterans. Three women were in the graduating class. Dean Rudy O. Muller, D.C. conferred the degrees, and president S.F. Sommacal, D.C., administered the oath to the new chiropractors. Most of this first class (73%) had been able to complete their training

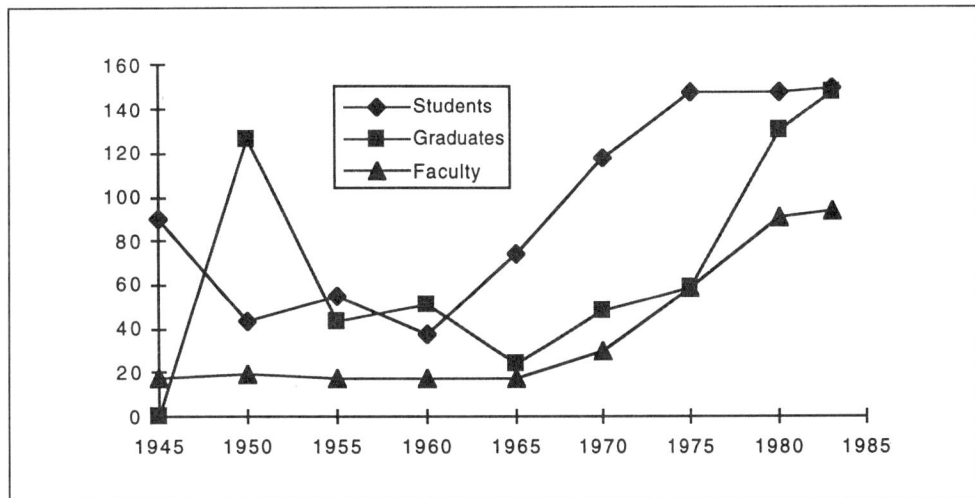

Figure 14-10: Student enrollment, graduation trends and faculty size at Canadian Memorial Chiropractic College, 1945-1983 (Biggs, 1991; reprinted by permission of the *Journal of Manipulative and Physiological Therapeutics*)

because of funding received from the Department of Veterans Affairs, but this tuition source lasted for only a few years. The College remained a fairly small institution for decades (see Figure 14-10), and struggled until the early 1970s to remain financially viable (Biggs, 1991). When entrance requirements were raised from a grade 12 education to grade 13 in 1957, admissions dipped to an all-time low of 21 (Brown, 1988). Historian Lesley Biggs has labeled the first decades of the CMCC its "black years" (Biggs, 1989: Chapter 6).

Complicating the difficulties brought about by the drop in enrollment in the 1950s was a complex governance structure which allowed national political divisions (i.e., the "straight" oriented western provinces vs. the "mixer" eastern provinces, particularly Ontario) to intrude upon the operation of the College. Although the broad-scope influence dominated the school by the late 1950s, thereby bringing greater stability to the composition of the faculty, external forces created a whole new set of seemingly insurmountable challenges. The school's financial viability was already stretched by its building programs, when in 1959 the City of Toronto decided to build a subway through the rear of CMCC's Bloor Street property (Brown, 1988). The construction seriously interfered with daily school operations for nearly three years, and consumed the energies of the College's president and dean, A. Earl Homewood, D.C., N.D. (see Figure 14-11). Homewood resigned as president in 1961, but returned to this office in 1967 after a stint as business manager of the Lincoln Chiropractic College and an unsuccessful effort to create a chiropractic school within Brandon University in Manitoba (Brown, 1989). During this interim he also earned a degree in law, and authored two significant books: *The Neurodynamics of the Vertebral Subluxation* (Homewood, 1961/1979) and *The Chiropractor and the Law* (Homewood, 1965).

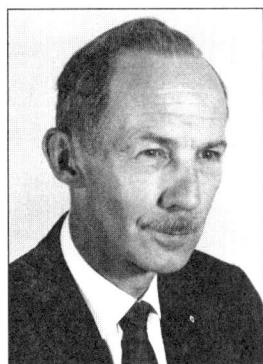

Figure 14-11: A. Earl Homewood, president of CMCC

Period	Chairman of the Board	President	Dean
1945-46	John S. Clubine, D.C.	John S. Clubine, D.C.	John S. Clubine, D.C.
1946-47	Walter T. Sturdy, D.C.	Walter T. Sturdy, D.C.	John S. Clubine, D.C.
1947-51	S.F. Sommacal, D.C.	S.F. Sommacal, D.C.	Rudy O. Müller, D.C., Ph.C.
1951-53	Keith Kennedy, D.C.	Keith Kennedy, D.C.	Rudy O. Müller, D.C., Ph.C.
1953-54	G.H. Young, D.C.	G.H. Young, D.C.	Rudy O. Müller, D.C., Ph.C.
1954-55	James A. Price, D.C.	James A. Price, D.C.	Major Colbeck
1955-56	James A. Price, D.C.	James A. Price, D.C.	A. Earl Homewood, D.P.T., D.C., N.D.
1956-57	Fred L. Clubine, D.C.	Fred L. Clubine, D.C.	A. Earl Homewood, D.P.T., D.C., N.D.
-1957-58	Colin A. Greenshields, D.C.	Colin A. Greenshields, D.C.	A. Earl Homewood, D.P.T., D.C., N.D.
1959-61	A. Earl Homewood, D.P.T., D.C., N.D.	A. Earl Homewood, D.P.T., D.C., N.D.	A. Earl Homewood, D.P.T., D.C., N.D.
1961	R.N. Thompson, D.C.	R.N. Thompson, D.C.	D.W. MacMillan, D.C.
1962-63	Neil Harris, D.C.	Neil Harris, D.C.	D.W. MacMillan, D.C.
1963-66	W.F. Trelford, D.C.	W.E. Trelford, D.C.	Herbert Marshall Himes, D.C.
1966-67	Donald H. Viggiani	A. Earl Homewood, D.C., N.D., LL.B.	Ronald J. Watkins, D.C., Ph.C.
1967-68	Howard L. Gauthier, D.C.	A. Earl Homewood, D.C., N.D., LL.B.	A. Earl Homewood, D.C., N.D., LL.B.
1969-70	Fred L. Clubine, D.C.	A. Earl Homewood, D.C., N.D., LL.B.	Herbert J. Vear, D.C.
1970-72	Fred L. Clubine, D.C.	Fred L. Clubine, D.C.	Herbert J. Vear, D.C.
1972-73	David A. Churchill, D.C.	David A. Churchill, D.C.	Herbert J. Vear, D.C.
1973-76	William S. Baird, D.C.	William S. Baird, D.C.	Herbert J. Vear, D.C.
1976	David I. West, D.C.	Donald C. Sutherland, D.C.	Tom Maxwell, D.C.
1976-77	David I. West, D.C.	Donald C. Sutherland, D.C.	Donald C. Sutherland, D.C.
1977-78	David I. West, D.C.	Donald C. Sutherland, D.C.	Terry Watkins
1978-80	J.G. Cochrane, D.C.	Donald C. Sutherland, D.C.	Alan H. Adams, D.C.
1980-82	Richard Luck, D.C.	Donald C. Sutherland, D.C.	Alan H. Adams, D.C.
1982-83	Douglas M. Brown, D.C.	Donald C. Sutherland, D.C.	Alan H. Adams, D.C.
1983-84	Douglas M. Brown, D.C.	Ian D. Coulter, Ph.D.	Alan H. Adams, D.C.
1984-85	Leonard Cunningham, D.C.	Ian D. Coulter, Ph.D.	Alan H. Adams, D.C.

Table 14-8: Leadership of the Canadian Memorial Chiropractic College during its first four decades (Kennedy, 1985; Moss, 1996; Vear, 1996)

After a strenuous legal battle that took the College's grievance against the city as far as Canada's Supreme Court, the school eventually abandoned its civil suit against Toronto's subway authority owing to the financial drain of the legal battle (Brown, 1988). This left the institution without satisfactory quarters, and an outstanding debt of half a million dollars. In 1966 Homewood commenced a successful nationwide tour to raise funds from the profession in Canada to settle this debt and to underwrite the building of a new home for CMCC. The following year, after his re-appointment as president of the College, Homewood, board chairman Howard L. Gauthier, D.C. and Donald C. Sutherland, D.C. (future CMCC president; see Table 14-8) negotiated with land developer Gerhard Moog for the acquisition of the CMCC's current campus at 1900 Bayview Avenue in Toronto. Brown (1988) credits Homewood as "the prime mover in designing the College's new physical facilities," which were dedicated on 21 September 1968.

Homewood's years as a faculty member, and later as president and dean of the CMCC, were marked by a strong curricular commitment to training chiropractors as broad-scope, conservative, drugless physicians. Over the years, clinical training expanded relative to basic science instruction (see Table 14-9). Coburn (1991) suggests that in recent years the profession has sought increased legitimacy through a narrowing of the scope of practice. However, during his years as CMCC president, Homewood helped to sustain a holistic clinical orientation, and his papers (see Table 14-10) provided scholarly examples for faculty and students to emulate. Homewood was succeeded as CMCC dean by another chiropractic scholar, Herbert J. Vear, a graduate of the College's first class and the future president of Homewood's chiropractic alma mater, Western States College.

Table 14-9: Distribution of CMCC's curriculum by %-subject area, 1948 to 1988 (Biggs, 1991; reprinted by permission of the *Journal of Manipulative & Physiological Therapeutics*)

Subject Area	1948	1958	1968	1978	1988
Biological sciences	44.3	37.6	37.2	41.5	23.7
Chiropractic Sciences	20.8	24.7	22.9	18.2	19.4
Clinical Sciences:					
Diagnosis	9.4	4.8	4.3	6.2	10.2
X-ray	0.9	3.8	5.3	5.0	9.2
Nonchiropractic	14.2	8.2	8.1	7.0	6.2
Drugless therapy	-	2.1	2.1	2.2	2.0
Internship	9.4	17.8	18.3	18.5	26.8
Office management, jurisprudence, research	0.9	1.0	1.8	1.4	2.5

Table 14-10: Some published works of A. Earl Homewood, D.P.T., D.C., N.D., LL.B.

Naturopathic history in Ontario. *Journal of the Ontario Naturopathic Association* 1954 (Dec)
Muscles - the neglected system. *Journal of the National Chiropractic Association* 1955; 25(1): 9
Administrative dean's report. *Journal of the Canadian Chiropractic Association* 1957; 1(1): 5
Chiropractic jurisprudence. *Digest of Chiropractic Economics* 1958; 1(1): 9
Chiropractic. *University of Toronto Medical Journal* 1961; February: 168
The neurodynamics of the vertebral subluxation. 3rd Edition. Toronto: Chiropractic Publishers, 1961/1979
A posturometer survey. *Journal of the Canadian Chiropractic Association* 1964-65; 9(1): 9-10
The chiropractor and the law. Toronto: Chiropractic Publishers, 1965
Canada's contribution to chiropractic. *Digest of Chiropractic Economics* 1967; 10(1): 33-4
The question of professional stature. *Digest of Chiropractic Economics* 1967; 10(3): 26-9
With Martin RJ. Researching research: outline for the preparation and processing of research proposals as prepared by the ACA
        Department of Research and Statistics. *ACA Journal of Chiropractic* 1971; 8(1): 10-4
77 years of turning the other cheek. *Digest of Chiropractic Economics* 1973; 15(4): 26-9
With Bittner H, Harper WD, Janse J, and Weiant CW. Chiropractic of today. *ACA Journal of Chiropractic* 1973; 10(11): VII, S81-8
Cervical adjusting. *Digest of Chiropractic Economics* 1978; 20(6): 116
This I believe. *Digest of Chiropractic Economics* 1979; 12(2): 33
Twenty-five years of evolution. *Digest of Chiropractic Economics* 1982; 25(1): 11-2
Visceral vs. musculoskeletal. *Digest of Chiropractic Economics* 1983; 25(5): 46-137
Micro-manipulation. *Digest of Chiropractic Economics* 1985; 28(2): 45-6
The challenge of the future. *Digest of Chiropractic Economics* 1987; 29(6): 78, 81
What price research? *Dynamic Chiropractic*, March 15, 1988, pp. 32-3

Chapter 15

THE LEADERSHIP CHANGES

Profound changes in the educational leadership of chiropractic occurred in the 1950s and 1960s. W.A. Budden, president of the Western States College and longtime advocate of higher educational standards, died in August 1954 (Nugent, 1954), and Ralph M. Failor, D.C. was appointed in his place. By the end of 1956 the school was renamed Western States Chiropractic College (WSCC), and Robert E. Elliott, D.C. was appointed as its new president (see Table 15-1). At this time also the College abandoned its naturopathic program (which evolved into today's National College of Naturopathic Medicine), largely owing to the repeated promptings of the NCA to distance chiropractic institutions from the naturopathic profession (Minutes, 1950, 1954; Watkins, 1939). The National College announced in 1950 that it would no longer enroll students for naturopathic training (Naturopathy, 1950). Budden had resisted the NCA's pressure to the last (Minutes, 1954).

The abandonment of the ND degree at schools such as National, WSCC and LACC did not mean the end of instruction in all broad-scope, non-adjustive methods. Physiotherapeutics, obstetrics and minor surgery, dietetics and exercise prescriptions continued to form a part of the DC's clinical training (Gibbons, 1982, 1983); instruction in obstetrics and minor surgery continued at WSCC into the 1990s. Eventually, physical therapy modalities came to be thought of as "chiropractic physiological therapeutics" (Gerlt, 1965; Johnson, 1977) among a wide segment of the profession.

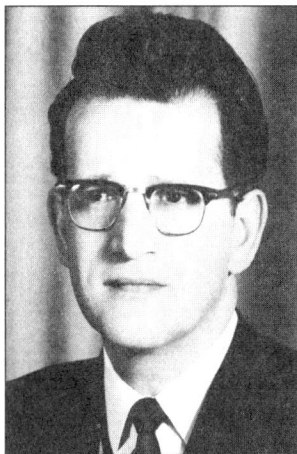

The year 1959 saw Ernest Napolitano, D.C. (see Figure 15-1), a 1942 graduate of the Palmer School of Chiropractic, assume the leadership of the Columbia Institute of Chiropractic in New York City. Frank Dean, the school's founder, died on May 12, 1958 (Rehm, 1980, p. 298), after nearly 40 years at the helm of the college. Napolitano, who initially maintained his school's alliance with the NAACSC, resigned from the ICA's Board of Control in April 1964 (Dr. Napolitano, 1964) and announced that his school sought accreditation from the Council on Education of the newly formed American Chiropractic Association (ACA). Later that same year Napolitano supervised the Columbia Institute's absorption of one of its rivals in the New York City school market, the Atlantic States Chiropractic Institute (ACA, 1964b). The former ICA leader also briefly considered the possibility, encouraged by the ACA, of merging the Columbia Institute of Chiropractic with Thure Peterson's non-profit Chiropractic Institute of New York (Future, 1965), perhaps in order to meet the provisions

Figure 15-1: Ernest Napolitano, D.C., president of the Columbia Institute of Chiropractic

Table 15-1: Chronology of the presidents of today's Western States Chiropractic College and its predecessor institutions, 1904 to present

Marsh School and Cure
John E. Marsh, 1904-09
Pacific College of Chiropractic
William O. Powell, 1909-13
D.D. Palmer College of Chiropractic
D.D. Palmer, 1908-1910
Oregon Peerless College of Chiropractic
John E. LaValley, 1911-1913
Pacific Chiropractic College
Oscar W. Elliott, 1913-1926
Lenore B. Elliott, 1926-29
William A. Budden, 1929-1932
Western States College, School of Chiropractic & School of Naturopathy
William A. Budden, 1932-1954
Ralph M. Failor, 1954-1956
Western States Chiropractic College
Robert E. Elliott, 1956-1974
Samuel G. Warren, 1974-76
Richard H. Timmins, 1976-79
Herbert J. Vear, 1979-86
William H. Dallas, 1986-

Table 15-2: John J. Nugent's accomplishments as NCA Director of Education during 1941-1961 (CCE, 1984; see Appendix A)

1. Conversion of a major number of the chiropractic colleges from proprietary status to that of an evolving eleemosynary status
2. Formation and on-going development of criteria for chiropractic colleges, which were eventually adopted as the requirements for accreditation by the CCE
3. Supervision of the NCA Council on Education's accreditation committee, and assistance to the colleges in meeting the criteria for accreditation
4. Liaison between the colleges, the accrediting agency and the state boards of chiropractic examiners
5. Upgrading of admissions criteria and pre-professional requirements for chiropractic education
6. Separation of chiropractic education from naturopathic education
7. Initial contacts with the U.S. Office of Education, and many contacts with state education, basic science and licensing boards (1953, 1960, 1961)
8. Encouragement of grants programs for chiropractic colleges by the National Chiropractic Association and the National Chiropractic Insurance Company

of New York State's first chiropractic act, which Governor Nelson Rockefeller had signed into law on April 26, 1963. Although the new law included a "grandfather" provision which authorized the licensing of D.C.s who had been in practice prior to the legislation's passage, future D.C.s were not eligible for license unless they had graduated from a chiropractic college accredited by an agency recognized by the U.S. Office of Education. There were no schools of chiropractic which held such recognition prior to 1971.

A number more milestones in the history of chiropractic education were achieved in 1961. John J. Nugent retired after 20 years as the NCA's director of education (Achenbach, 1961) with an impressive albeit contentious record of educational reforms (see Table 15-2) and consolidations which left just eight schools accredited by the NCA (see Table 15-3). Nugent was replaced during 1961-1964 (Hayes, 1965) by Dewey Anderson, Ph.D., former director of the Public Affairs Institute of Washington, D.C. Gibbons (1985) attributes Nugent's departure in 1961 to Emmett J. Murphy's introduction of Anderson, a Stanford University trained economist (In memoriam, 1975), as an alternative, and to the passing of strong Nugent supporters such as W.A. Budden and Thure Peterson. Martin (1974) attributes Anderson's replacement of Nugent as NCA Director of Research to the impression which Anderson's reports (Anderson, 1960, 1961), such as *Chiropractic in California - and the Nation*, had upon the NCA's board of directors. The reports, written in response to the Stanford Research Institute's scathing criticism of chiropractic education in California (Stanford, 1960), placed chiropractic education in a positive light. Anderson was also familiar with members of the U.S. Office of Education (USOE), the federal bureaucrats who regulated accreditation in higher education (Wolf, 1993). By this time, federally recognized accreditation was a goal that had come increasingly to the fore among the NCA/ACA leaders (Haynes, 1973), although the implications of a lack of federally approved accreditation had been recognized among college leaders for some time (Coggins, 1952). Indeed, the earliest contacts between Nugent and the USOE dated to 1952-1953 (Chiropractic, 1952; McMurrin, 1961; Nugent, 1961).

Anderson's term as Director of Education overlapped the 1963-64 transition in broad-scope organizations: from NCA to the ACA. In the process, the internal structure of the Council on Education and its relationship to the parent society, ACA, was altered:

> In 1963, at the annual convention of the National Chiropractic Association, significant and far-reaching conclusions were reached and changes made.
> 1. The old NCA and other groups were reorganized as the American Chiropractic Association.
> 2. The CCE [sic] was reorganized to the following extent:
> (a) While the director of education was assigned to serve both the accrediting agency and the colleges, he was held responsible directly to the ACA Board of Governors and the ACA executive director. His vote on institutional status was rescinded making him a neutral element, functioning only on an advisory, counseling and staff basis.
> (b) The accrediting committee of the CCE became officially known as the Accrediting Agency of the American Chiropractic Association and was provided with full authority to conclude upon the status of accreditation of any of the participating institutions of education. The membership of the Committee consisted of:
> Walter B. Wolf, Chairman - Eureka, South Dakota
> Orval L. Hidde, Secretary - Watertown, Wisconsin
> Herbert E. Hinton - Dania, Florida
> John Richard Quigley - Tacoma, Washington

Canadian Memorial Chiropractic College, 252 Bloor Street, Toronto, Ontario

Chiropractic Institute of New York, 325 E. 38th Street, New York, New York

Lincoln Chiropractic College, 3171 N. Meridian Street, Indianapolis, Indiana

Los Angeles College of Chiropractic, 920 E. Broadway, Glendale, California

National College of Chiropractic, 20 N. Ashland Boulevard, Chicago, Illinois

Northwestern College of Chiropractic, 2222 Park Avenue, Minneapolis, Minnesota

Texas Chiropractic College, San Pedro Park, San Antonio, Texas

Western States Chiropractic College, 4525 SE 63rd Avenue, Portland, Oregon

Table 15-3: NCA Council on Education's 1961 "Accredited Chiropractic Colleges in the United States and Canada" (*Journal of the National Chiropractic Association* 1961 [Dec]; 31[12]: 13)

(c) The CCE [sic] members representing the educational institutions did not have voting authority in relation to the accreditation status of any of the participating colleges; it was considered a conflict of interest for any school person to have a right to vote on the status of any other institution. Their voting authority in relation to all other CCE matters was retained. Actually, the accrediting agency gained full autonomy in the area of accreditation.

(d) To the membership of the CCE was added three appointees of the Council of Chiropractic Examining Boards (CCEB), namely the president, vice-president and the secretary. They were, however, only auditing members and did not possess voting authority in relation to any CCE affairs (CCE, 1984).

As NCA (later ACA) Director of Education, Anderson introduced more in-depth self-evaluations and inspections of the chiropractic schools (Wolf, 1993), thereby preparing them for the accreditation process common in higher education. He recognized the growing threat posed by AMA's renewed campaign to eliminate the chiropractic profession, in the form of its Committee on Quackery, and attempted to warn the profession (Digest, 1964). Formed in November, 1963, the Committee on Quackery sought to "contain and eliminate" the chiropractic profession (Trever, 1972, pp. 2-3), and the chiropractic colleges were an important target in their campaign.

Anderson made several additional but unsuccessful applications (Nugent had been first) to the USOE for recognition of the ACA's Council on Education as an accrediting body for chiropractic schools. He also put his influence behind a plan to "push one college ahead of all the rest as a sort of spear-head" (Martin, 1974). This policy was formalized by the FACE in 1960 (Schierholz, 1972). Not surprisingly, the singling out of one college for special investment created disgruntlement among the other schools, but may have enabled the National College of Chiropractic in 1971 to become the first federally recognized, regionally accredited school in the profession.

Significant investment in chiropractic education (see Table 15-4) became possible with the Chiropractic Research Foundation's 1959 re-organization as the Foundation for Accredited Chiropractic Education (FACE), and continued after FACE became the Foundation for Chiropractic Education and Research (FCER) in 1969 (Martin, 1974). The NCA, and later the ACA, "dedicated 40% of every member's dues for distribution through FACE and FCER among the accredited colleges and for research" (Kimmel, 1965). In 1964 these contributions may have amounted to as much as $350,000 in funding for the chiropractic schools (Kimmel, 1965). Schierholz (1986, p. 22) suggests that the ACA's 1964 commitment of 40% of its members dues was supplemented by an additional $100,000. The ACA's annual donation to chiropractic education, by way of its "grant-giving body," remained constant for decades. Additional significant funds were contributed to FACE by the

Table 15-4: "Total amount in dollars" given by the FACE/FCER to chiropractic colleges in grants during 1960-1972.

Year	Amount
1960	$38,400
1961	58,400
1962	153,300
1963	141,114
1964	238,500
1965	225,000
1966	243,000
1967	237,000
1968	182,917
1969	172,342
1970	193,544
1971	227,324
1972	228,810
*	72,500

* "An additional amount totaling $72,500 has been set aside for specific programs in some of the colleges" (Schierholz, 1972)

National Chiropractic Insurance Company, beginning in 1959 (NCIC, 1965; Schierholz, 1965b).

In the early 1970's, William Harris, D.C., set up a private foundation to support chiropractic education, through matching grants to the chiropractic colleges. His Foundation for the Advancement of Chiropractic Education, which has contributed just under five million dollars in challenge grants, has the same acronym as the earlier FACE (FCER), leading to some confusion (Harris, 1998).

As suggested earlier, strong leadership for the Council on Education came to rest with George Haynes of LACC, who became president of the Council in 1960 (Martin, 1974). The possibility of greater intra-professional unity and cooperation in educational matters seemed more likely in 1961, with the passing of two significant ICA college leaders: Vinton F. Logan and B.J. Palmer. Logan died on July 9, 1961 (Rogers, 1961a), just a few months after the passing of the Davenport leader. The St. Louis leader was succeeded as president of the Logan Basic College of College of Chiropractic by its dean, William N. Coggins, D.C., who moved the school into the ACA's orbit. B.J.'s death on May 27, 1961, and the transfer of the presidency of the Palmer School to his son, David D. Palmer, D.C. (see Figure 15-2), portended greater cooperation among school leaders and accelerated educational development (Griffin, 1988; Rogers, 1961b).

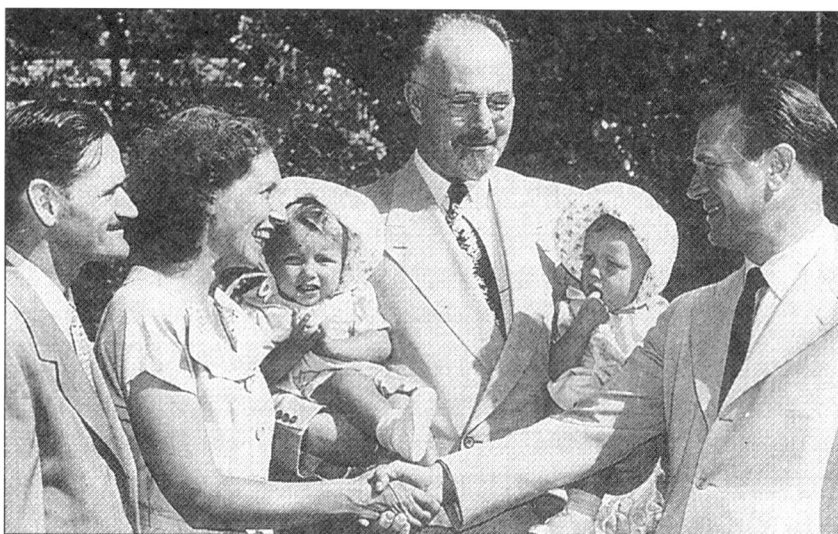

Figure 15-2: Dave Palmer, D.C. (far right), then vice-president of the Palmer School, greets ICA board members Leonard K. Griffin, D.C. (far left) and Joshua N. Haldeman, D.C., Mrs. Haldeman, and the Haldeman twins, during the 1949 homecoming of the Palmer School in Davenport. Dave Palmer would rename the institution the Palmer College of Chiropractic and assume the presidency following B.J. Palmer's death in 1961.

With the possibility of cooperation over educational issues among the warring factions of the profession, Devere E. Biser, D.C., who served in 1961 as president of the Council of State Chiropractic Examining Boards (CSCEB) and as vice-president of the ICA, announced a meeting (see Table 15-5) to bring the chiropractic colleges together for common goals and to establish standards:

> Considerable progress toward a united front in the educational field was made at a meeting of the General Committee on Chiropractic Education, in Chicago, November 11 and 12. Agreement on a basic minimum curriculum was regarded as something needed very much for many years by all chiropractic colleges. A standard form for transfer of class credits, grades and hours between colleges and the various state examining boards was worked out. Another important step was the agreement to create a National Board of Chiropractic Examiners.

> The Council of State Chiropractic Examining Boards was responsible for the conference. For some time the Council has felt it could be a strong factor in getting the NCA and ICA Educational Commissions together in an effort to iron out some of the problems. It was finally agreed that a committee of three men from the Council - in this case the officers - and three members of the other two Educational Commissions would be the best procedure to follow (Biser, 1961).

One beneficial effect of this conference was the formation in 1962 (Saunders, 1965) of the current National Board of Chiropractic Examiners (NBCE), the third such agency to be so named (Keating & Rehm, 1993), and a genuine forum for unified action in chiropractic licensing and educational matters. The NBCE may have played a small role in the eventual reversal of basic science laws (e.g., Holman, 1971), although it was predominantly the dissatisfaction with the basic science

Participant	Representing	Affiliation
William N. Coggins, D.C.	Logan Basic College of Chiropractic	ICA
Ernest G. Napolitano, D.C.	Columbia Institute of Chiropractic	ICA
Kenneth Cronk, D.C.	Palmer College of Chiropractic	ICA
George H. Haynes, D.C., M.S.	Los Angeles College of Chiropractic	NCA Council on Education
John B. Wolfe, D.C.	Northwestern College of Chiropractic	NCA Council on Education
Joseph Janse, D.C., N.D.	National College of Chiropractic	NCA Council on Education
Devere E. Biser, D.C.	Council of State Chiropractic Examining Boards	ICA
R. Dwayne Moulton, D.C.	Council of State Chiropractic Examining Boards	NCA
Gordon L. Holman, D.C.	Council of State Chiropractic Examining Boards	?

Table 15-5: Participants in the Council of State Chiropractic Examining Boards' 1961 meeting of the educational commission of the ICA and the NCA (Biser, 1961)

laws among medical physicians that eventually led to their reversal (Gevitz, 1988). Moreover, not all chiropractors were ready for unity. Gordon V. Pefley, D.C. of Portland, vice-president of the NCA's Council on Physiotherapy, cautioned against any attempt at a quick reconciliation, and cited recent efforts by straight chiropractors in Oregon to reduce educational standards and narrow the broad-scope of practice in that state. He also recited the sentiments of Dewey Anderson, soon to become NCA Director of Education, who had suggested at the NCA's 1957 convention that:

> It is better to have a single house of a few going in the same direction, shoulder to shoulder, than a house peopled with many, all of whom are going in different directions at once. I plead for a strong, central concept of chiropractic, broad in its definition to include all who seriously follow the profession, and a commitment to a growing body of science, as science increases the knowledge of mankind (Pefley, 1961).

The continuing schism within the profession was evident to all in 1963, when today's ACA was established (Griffin, 1988; Plamondon, 1993). Extensive discussions between representatives of the ICA and NCA produced a preliminary plan for the merger of the two membership societies. However, at an August 1962 meeting of the ICA in Davenport, which was attended by four NCA officials, the anti-amalgamation sentiments of a majority of the ICA's Board of Control became obvious. Fears raised by the California Medical Association's 1960-61 effort to eliminate osteopathy through absorption were cited as a likely outcome for straight chiropractors in any attempt to integrate the two chiropractic bodies. The first ACA executive body was formed by representatives of the NCA and five former ICA leaders: A.A. Adams, Devere Biser, Leonard K. Griffin, Harold F. Russell and Richard W. Tyer (Griffin, 1988). Each organization (ICA and the new ACA) maintained its own accrediting body for chiropractic education, and during the next decade competed with one another for status with the USOE.

A final change in the leadership within chiropractic education deserves mention here. Dewey Anderson retired as ACA Director of Education early in 1965, and in his place John A. Fisher, Ed.D. was appointed (Council, 1984; Schierholz, 1965a). Fisher steered the ACA's Council on Education toward independent incorporation as the Council on Chiropractic Education (CCE) in 1971, and facilitated the CCE's recognition by the USOE in 1974. He was unique as the first chiropractic Director of Education to have experience as a college administrator, and is credited with establishing standardized methods for auditing and reporting college finances and for the conduct of college visitations/inspections. Fisher served as a consultant to those ACA-allied schools which sought to bring their operations in line with other institutions of higher education in the U.S. in terms of departmentalization, faculty governance, personnel, admissions, records, curricula and planning (Council, 1984).

Fisher's initial assessment of the ACA-affiliated colleges was released in January 1965:

> National College is on the move — shows evidence of upgrading but still has problems. The "climate" is right and the "atmosphere" is good, yet there are areas needing considerable work.

Los Angeles College has a fine new laboratory — has come a long way developing a qualified faculty. The clinic is on the way but not as far along as other areas of the college.

Lincoln — facilities good — laboratory in process of improvement. The administrative procedures are good or in the process of correction. Clinic operation seems somewhat less than optimum.

Logan College has a campus — looks like a college. The library has overcome problems. Faculty and student qualifications need improvement.

Texas — has makings for good college but needs local support — and the leadership of a strong new president soon.

New York Colleges — some problems are not educational — problem in securing a charter and merging present schools.

Northwestern and Western States — not suitable upgrading — will require important studies and a great deal of money. There appears to be a fierce tenacity to exist (Schierholz, 1986, p. 23).

Chapter 16

CONTINUING STRUGGLES WITH MEDICINE

Organized medicine's efforts to ostracize and eliminate the chiropractic profession reached their maximum in the third quarter of the chiropractic century, and had significant effects upon chiropractic education. Chiropractors might have expected a respite after Morris Fishbein, M.D., editor since 1924 of the *Journal of the American Medical Association* and a long-time vocal opponent of chiropractic, was discharged from his office (Wardwell, 1992, p. 162). Such was not to be the case, however. In the immediate post-war years, as chiropractors once more pressed the legislatures in those states which still provided inadequate or no licensure (Louisiana, Massachusetts, Mississippi, New York, Texas), political medicine stepped up its anti-chiropractic rhetoric.

Exemplary was a 1953 pamphlet entitled *Science vs. Chiropractic* (Doyle, 1953), which was widely distributed by the Massachusetts Medical Society (Conlin, 1953). The author relied primarily upon the chiropractic literature, including the self-critical reports of NCA Director of Education John J. Nugent, to make a case that "chiropractic is still a shortcut for the would-be professional man who has the ambition but neither the time, the money, nor the ability to become a qualified doctor" (Doyle, 1953, pp. 10-11). While allowing that "Unquestionably there are sincere and zealous practitioners who are doing all in their power to raise the cult to a professional level," she believed that chiropractic schools had not achieved the standards set by Nugent and the NCA, and concluded that:

> Chiropractic education actually falls short of professional standards on three counts: (1) the length of training; (2) the quality of instruction; (3) the failure of chiropractic schools to give their students an opportunity to study disease in human beings.

Similarly damning praise was seen that same year in a pamphlet entitled *The Cult of Chiropractic* by C.E. Boyd, M.D., who, like Doyle (1953), added "charges of chicanery and invalid theoretical foundations" (Cooper, 1985) to his criticisms of chiropractic education:

> We can see that the more intelligent chiropractors, realizing the extremely low standards, have been trying to raise the standards to some extent. John J. Nugent, D.C. has even suggested that the State Boards raise their requirements to the standard of their "approved" schools. Assuming **Mr. Nugent's** good faith, and also assuming that chiropractors were chosen with an intellectual level average to other professions, and assuming further that the basic sciences taught in the chiropractic schools were as good as those taught in the medical schools, assuming all of these things which are certainly not all true, the end result would still be, even according to Mr. Nugent, a man who still believed that disease of the human body could be treated by manipulation of the vertebral column, by the "chiropractic thrust" (Boyd, quoted in Homola, 1963, p. 73). (boldface emphasis added)

An incredible amount of gall was apparent in the mid-1950s when the American Medical Association (AMA) Council on Medical Education and Hospitals sought private meetings with the NCA Council on Education for the purpose of gaining information on the conduct of chiropractic schools (Minutes, 1955; see Appendix B). Organized medicine's campaign against chiropractic was invigorated by the 1960 release of the Stanford Research Institute's *Chiropractic in California* by the Haynes Foundation of Los Angeles (Stanford, 1960). The report reviewed both the history and then contemporary function of chiropractic colleges in the state. Total tuition varied greatly among the three active schools: Cleveland Chiropractic College ($1,292), Hollywood College, School of Chiropractic and Naturopathy ($1,646) and LACC ($1,819). The LACC's library was considered exceptional, in that it subscribed to 38 periodicals and contained 4,000 volumes, although 92% of these were more than 10 years old (Stanford, 1960, pp. 115, 232). The report also criticized the corporate status, personnel policies and administrative structures of the California schools:

> Thirty-nine chiropractic schools have functioned in the state at one time or another since the opening of the first California chiropractic school in 1900. Today three remain, all three are located in the Los Angeles area...Instructors are paid an average of $3.00 per hour. Full-time teaching schedules average 27 hours of instruction per week...average total tuition cost of $1,250 (8 semesters).
>
> *California Chiropractic Educational Foundation.* This nonprofit, tax-exempt California corporation owns and operates the Los Angeles College of Chiropractic in Glendale, California. The five directors of the corporation, designated as regents, are chosen from the ranks of the CCA and the NCA...
>
> *Cleveland Chiropractic College.* CCC is organized as a profit corporation under the laws of the State of California. The board of directors consists of three persons, the president, vice-president, and secretary-treasurer of the corporation. The administration of CCC is centralized in the office of the president and principal stockholder, C.S. Cleveland, Sr., DC. Operational characteristics of the college, as shown in an accreditation report filed by the college with the Chiropractic Education Commission, suggest that there is no delegation of authority or administrative responsibility from the office of the president. Although one faculty member was introduced as an "associate dean," he had no assigned office space in the college or administrative duties outside his own classroom.
>
> Since the administration of CCC is not departmentalized, and since there appears to be little delegation of authority and responsibility, the organizational structure of the college would be characteristic of the sole proprietorship. In October 1958 the college had five regularly scheduled faculty members on the payroll plus one employee retained for part-time maintenance work...
>
> *Hollywood Chiropractic College.* HCC is presently organized as a nonprofit corporation under the laws of the State of California. The board of directors consists of the president, vice-president and secretary-treasurer of the corporation. The dean of the college assumes all responsibility for administrative functions. This institution is much the same as CCC in its organization structure in being organized along the lines of a typical sole proprietorship (Stanford Research Institute, 1960).

Whatever realistic fear that chiropractors in California may have harbored about the future of their profession was amplified by interactions between the medical and osteopathic communities in the Golden State during 1960-62. There the state medical society attempted to eradicate osteopathy by absorbing its practitioners, its teaching hospitals and the sole osteopathic college in the state (Gevitz, 1982, pp. 99-116). Eighty-five percent (about 2,000) of the state's D.O.s opted to relinquish their osteopathic credentials, attend several weekend seminars (Wardwell, 1992, p. 36), and receive MD degrees. The deal between the California Medical Association and the California Osteopathic Association, previously a division of the American Osteopathic Association (AOA), also called for the College of Osteopathic Physicians and Surgeons (COP&S) in Los Angeles to become an AMA-accredited institution and to cease instruction in osteopathy. (The former COP&S is today's University of California at Irvine, School of Medicine). When many former D.O.s became dissatisfied with their "second-class status" as M.D.s, efforts to absorb the osteopathic profession in other states wavered, and the AMA "adopted a series of new resolutions in the late 1960s aimed at destroying the AOA" (Gevitz, 1982, p. 124).

For chiropractors, a new and ominous specter emerged. Although there was probably never any likelihood that AMA would seek a similar resolution of the "chiropractic problem," many straight chiropractors likened the activities of the ACA's Council on Education relative to ICA's educational accrediting agency (ACC) to the actions of the AMA and the CMA. If the ACA Council were to be recognized by the USOE, its accredited schools would have a distinct advantage in recruitment, since its students would become eligible for federally guaranteed loans. Moreover, it seemed likely (and time bore this out) that state licensing regulations for chiropractors would be revised to permit only graduates of ACA Council-recognized institutions to sit for the licensing examinations. Capitulation to ACA seemed to threaten the demise of straight chiropractic; this theme permeated chiropractic educational politics for decades (e.g., Armstrong et al., 1979). Fears encouraged by the osteopathic situation in California seemed realistic to many in chiropractic, the more so owing to the 1963 creation of the ACA through merger of the NCA and a splinter group from the ICA:

American Chiropractic Association: the ICA Position

The attack against the principle, the straight chiropractor and ICA has been a possessing goal of certain NCA officials for decades.

Even the newest ruse, romantically called the American Chiropractic Association, is not new....

Selected NCA strategists and a quintet of defecting ICA Board members, under the false guise of unity, will try to lure unsuspecting ICA members into a trap. This trap is the American Chiropractic Association, a trap that is scheduled to be closed within 90 days through absorption of these doctors as second class citizens into the NCA.

The five defectors gave up their positions of trust as members of the ICA Board of Control to become membership chairmen for the NCA through the "puppet state" ACA... Such doctors will soon realize the truth, that the ACA is part of the NCA "master plan" to divide and conquer, to destroy the ICA, to weaken the Chiropractic principle, and to gain membership and control of the profession (American, 1963).

Attention to chiropractic educational issues was also focused on Louisiana in the early 1960s. Here, chiropractors' struggle against the medical monopoly provided part of the impetus for the final push for accreditation. In May, 1957, Jerry England, D.C. (see Figure 16-1) and fellow Louisiana D.C.s challenged the constitutionality of the state's medical practice act, which created a monopoly by requiring a medical education and licensure as a physician and surgeon as a pre-condition for the practice of chiropractic (Adams, 1961, 1965; Beideman, 1995, pp. 110-1; Collins, 1959; England, 1965; The England, 1965). The legal challenge, which was fought in state and federal courts, united the warring internal factions of chiropractors in a common cause, and both the ICA and the NCA "passed resolutions offering the Louisiana Chiropractic Association financial help. Each association has set aside $5,000 for expenses incurred by the Louisiana unit..." (Louisiana, 1959). In March, 1965, the continuing legal battle with medicine came to a head as the case was tried in New Orleans; the testimony of chiropractic educators Joseph Janse, D.C., N.D. (see Figure 16-2) of the National College and William D. Harper, D.C. of the Texas Chiropractic College were central to the chiropractors' argument that the Louisiana law was unreasonable. Counsel for plaintiff chiropractors, J. Minos Simon, recruited these college leaders to make the point that chiropractors practiced a rational, scientific form of healing:

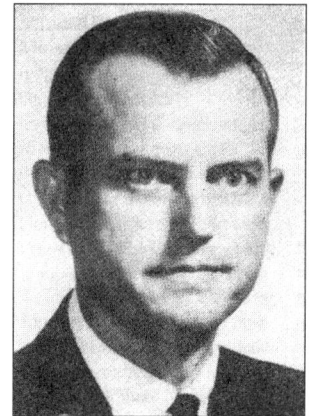

Figure 16-1: Jerry England, D.C.

When Mr. Simon learned at the pretrial conference that the book, Anything Can Cause Anything, by Dr. W.D. Harper, of the Texas College, would be used by the defense he called Dr. Harper and asked him to be present at the trial. Mr. Simon had read the book and was familiar with its contents. He placed Dr. Harper on the stand as rebuttal witness Wednesday morning. After direct questioning by Mr. Simon he was tendered for cross examination by the defense. Some of the subject matter covered was more or less repetitious of that submitted to Dr. Janse on Monday. The defense brought up the question of two schools of thought within the profession and attempted to identify the subject with some national organization. The attempt was not successful. Dr. Harper deftly fielded these questions and gave explanations that were theoretically inoffensive and legally satisfactory.

The questions concerning the book began with the title and ran to the last paragraph. This took several hours. All questions were answered without hesitation and with authoritative references from such texts as Boyd's Pathology, Iatrogenic Diseases, Best and Taylor and Grey. Dr. Harper never groped for an answer nor hesitated with an explanation. I have heard him lecture many times in a more friendly atmosphere. He was always impressive but I believe he was his greatest on this occasion.

The case concluded with his testimony. Mr. Simon described Dr. Harper's presentation as being the most dramatic court room scene he had ever witnessed....Another eight years of preparation could not have added anything (Adams, 1965).

Ironically, another six years produced a profound difference, for it brought recognition of the National College of Chiropractic as a regionally accredited institution (by the New York State Department of Education). The final motivation for National's accreditation campaign grew out of Janse's experience in the England case. Published accounts of Janse's testimony (e.g., Harper, 1965) painted a rosy picture of the occasion:

> Dr. Janse was our chief witness and occupied the stand most of Monday. His forthrightness and obvious sincerity coupled with his knowledge were most impressive. There was no evidence of evasiveness in his answers on cross examination. Some of the questions related to statements on principles, practice and concepts made by authors during the past twenty-five years. Accreditation of colleges prompted several questions. Etiology, diagnosis and treatment of most every disease problem came into the picture. Specific emphasis was placed on infectious and fatal disease processes, particularly those of great notoriety and fear-instilling quality, e.g., tetanus, polio, typhoid, cancer, etc. The subject of immunization was not ignored. Dr. Janse maintained his composure, forthrightness and dignity. We think his testimony was indeed an outstanding contribution (Adams, 1965).

The reality of the situation was something different (Beideman, 1995). Louisiana physician Joseph Sabatier, M.D., a member of the AMA's Committee on Quackery, was determined that the effort to legalize chiropractic should fail. Former ACA governor Robert B. Jackson, D.C., N.D. recalls:

> At the trial, Dr. J.J. was raked over the coals so badly by the medical attorneys over the issue that no DC college had any accreditation status with USOE or any regional accreditation agencies, that our education was therefore in fact inferior to medical schools and that we were all a bunch of uneducated so-and-so's. J.J. was so stimulated by his handling, he became the driving force, along with Geo. Haynes of LACC, to get an accreditation agency for the profession, and we know what happened. J.J. then went for regional accreditation and I believe was first to receive this type of status.... (Jackson, 1993).

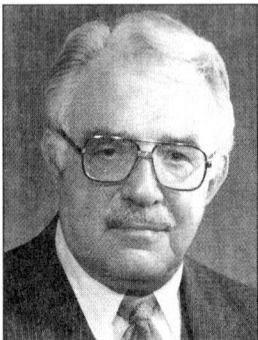

Figure 16-2: Joseph Janse, D.C., N.D.

Janse left Louisiana determined to establish federal recognition for chiropractic education "or leave the profession" (Beideman, 1995, p. 111). Between 1965 and 1971, when New York State accreditation was established, Janse and his school were single-minded in their resolve to make the improvements necessary to meet the state education department's requirements for accreditation. In this they were opposed by the medical lobby. After losing its 48 year campaign [1915-1963] to prevent the licensing of D.C.s in New York, organized medicine sought to "exert more control over the NYSED than they had been able to show in (their recent loss of) control of the New York State Legislature and its then governor, Nelson A. Rockefeller" (Beideman, 1995, pp. 262-4). National College historian Ronald P. Beideman also attributes part of the impetus for the college's accreditation drive to the "'adopted' sons and daughters from CINY [who] were prime movers in encouraging NCC to perpetuate the chiropractic profession in New York through accreditation" (Beideman, 1983).

Medical opposition to chiropractic involved efforts to block the profession's eligibility for Medicare reimbursement, to prevent recognition of the CCE by the USOE, to hinder accreditation of the National College by New York State, to encourage the continuance of the feud between ICA and NCA/ACA, to encourage anti-chiropractic policies by various health organizations, dissemination of

---

Table 16-1: Anti-chiropractic articles appearing in popular magazines during 1963-1970 (based on Moore, 1993, pp. 156-7)

Foot in the door. *Newsweek*, April 8, 1963

Smith M. If your back is out, you're in. *Life*, April 9, 1965

Smith RL. Chiropractic: science or swindle? *Today's Health*, May 1965

Fineberg H. Letter to the editor: chiropractic education. *Science*, June 3, 1966

Sabatier JA. Letter to the editor: chiropractic education. *Science*, June 3, 1966

The medical dispute about treatment by chiropractors. *Good Housekeeping*, May 1967

Smith RL. Golden touch for chiropractors. *Today's Health*, June 1968

Smith RL. Visit to a bizarre world - chiropractic alma maters. *Today's Health*, July 1968

HEW rejects chiropractic. *Today's Health*, April 1969

Smith RL, Sabatier JA. Chiropractic: issues and answers. *Today's Health*, January 1970

1963:	National College relocates to new campus in Lombard, Illinois		of Public Instruction to offer the B.S. and D.C. degrees
1963:	Faculty tenure plan established	1966:	Accredited under Chapter 36, Title 38, U.S. Code for Veterans' Benefits to offer the B.S. and D.C. degrees
1965:	Membership in the American Library Association established	1966:	Eligibility to be listed in State Directory of Schools and Colleges (Illinois) established
1966:	Membership in the Medical Library Association established	1966:	First contact with North Central Association of Colleges and Secondary Schools
1966:	Membership in the National Association of Collegiate Registrars and Admissions Officers established	1967:	Included in the Education Directory, Part 3: Higher Education published by the U.S. Office of Education
1966:	Membership in the Illinois Association of Student Financial Aid Administrators established	1967:	Federal funds for student housing received from U.S. Department of Housing and Urban Development
1966:	Recognized by Illinois' state teacher certification board to offer accredited courses in science and biology at the junior college level	1968:	Application for accreditation is made to the New York State Education Department under newly drafted guidelines
1966:	Accreditation by the ACA Council on Education to offer the D.C. degree	1970:	Application is made to the North Central Association of Colleges and Secondary Schools for correspondent status
1966:	Accredited by the Illinois' Office of the Superintendent		

Table 16-2: Educational achievements of the National College of Chiropractic, 1963-1970 (based on Beideman, 1995, pp. 262-273)

anti-chiropractic pamphlets to guidance counselors and members of the higher education community, and prevention of "a chiropractic chapter in a *Health Careers Guidebook* being prepared by the United States Department of Labor for distribution to guidance counselors and others" (Wardwell, 1992, pp. 161-4). The AMA encouraged a number of anti-chiropractic articles in the public media, and supported the preparation and dissemination of Ralph Lee Smith's *At Your Own Risk: the Case Against Chiropractic* (Smith, 1969). J. Stuart Moore (1993) has enumerated a number of derogatory magazine articles in the 1963-1970 period (see Table 16-1).

Despite the AMA's propaganda, the National College was granted status with Illinois' Office of the Superintendent of Public Instruction (OPSI) in 1966, and awarded its first bachelor of science degree. In fairly short order, the college achieved a number of other "firsts" in chiropractic education (see Table 16-2)

Chapter 17

FURTHER MERGERS AND ABSORPTIONS

The latter part of the third quarter of the chiropractic century saw a number of additional mergers and closures of chiropractic institutions. Several of these were supervised by Dewey Anderson, who had succeeded John J. Nugent in 1961 as NCA Director of Education, and who shared with Nugent the desire to merge the many small, for-profit chiropractic schools into 12 to 14 larger, non-profit colleges. Ralph G. Miller, Ed.D., former executive vice-president of the CCE, listed a number of institutional changes and amalgamations in the post-war years (see Table 17-1).

In 1962, the Hollywood Chiropractic College closed, and sent its records to the Los Angeles College of Chiropractic (LACC). Late in 1963, the last of the California Chiropractic Colleges (in Oakland), originally chartered in Long Beach in 1913 (see Figure 1-13), announced that it was going to merge with the LACC:

1944: Universal Chiropractic College of Pittsburgh merges with the Lincoln Chiropractic College of Indianapolis

1945: Eastern Chiropractic Institute, Standard School of Chiropractic and the New York School of Chiropractic amalgamate; become the Chiropractic Institute of New York

1946: Continental College of Chiropractic merges with the Southern California College of Chiropractic

1947: Southern California College of Chiropractic amalgamates with the Los Angeles College of Chiropractic

1948: Detroit College of Chiropractic ceases operations; in 1967 its registry and alumni were affiliated with the National College of Chiropractic

---: Metropolitan Chiropractic College of Cleveland, Ohio ceases operations and its registry and alumni were affiliated with the National College of Chiropractic

---: Ross-O'Neil Chiropractic College of Ft. Wayne, Indiana discontinues operations; affiliates with the National College of Chiropractic in 1970

1950: University of Natural Healing Arts in Denver ceases operations; in 1964 its registry and alumni become affiliated with the National College of Chiropractic

1951: Ratledge Chiropractic College comes under the management of Carl S. Cleveland, Sr., D.C.; becomes Cleveland Chiropractic College in 1955

1952: Kansas State Chiropractic College ceases operations; in 1967 its registry and alumni were affiliated with the National College of Chiropractic

1954: International College of Chiropractic in Dayton, Ohio terminates operations

1962: Hollywood College, School of Chiropractic and School of Naturopathy merges with the Los Angeles College of Chiropractic)

1963: California Chiropractic College ceases operations; records are sent to the Los Angeles College of Chiropractic

1964: Atlantic States College of Chiropractic amalgamates with the Columbia Institute of Chiropractic (today's New York Chiropractic College)

---: Carver Chiropractic College gives it registry to and affiliates its alumni with Logan College of Chiropractic

---: Missouri College of Chiropractic in St. Louis amalgamates with the Logan Basic College of Chiropractic to form the Logan Chiropractic College

1968: Chiropractic Institute of New York closes; registry and alumni are affiliated with the National College of Chiropractic

1971: Lincoln Chiropractic College ceases operations and its registry and alumni were affiliated with the National College of Chiropractic

Table 17-1: Chiropractic college closures, mergers and management changes in the postwar years (modified from Miller, 1981 and other sources)

CALIFORNIA CHIROPRACTIC COLLEGE AMALGAMATES WITH LACC

The Los Angeles College of Chiropractic proudly welcomes the graduates of the California Chiropractic College into the fold. The amalgamation of the CCC student records with those of the LACC took place on August 3, 1963.

Through the gracious cooperation of Dr. G. Stanley Hesse the dream of amalgamating the graduates of the different California schools under one protective roof has taken another step towards realization.

California Chiropractic College President Hesse, with a view to strengthen the educational development of our profession and desirous of protecting the graduates of his college, has transferred all his students' records to the LACC 'for that college to act as a permanent repository of records for the students of Chiropractic that graduated or attended the California Chiropractic College.' He also wishes that the CCC graduates be considered as part of the LACC alumni. The college is more than glad to accede to this request.

The LACC re-assures the graduates of the CCC of the fulfillment of all its obligations assumed by the amalgamation, including the certification of credits earned.

This amalgamation following that with the Hollywood College of Chiropractic, took place last November fifth. It is powerful evidence of the rapidly developing solidarity of Chiropractic in California. A great debt of gratitude is owed to Dr. Helen Sanders and Dr. Robert Gray of the former Hollywood College for their unselfish action in supporting Chiropractic educational progress and forcibly giving it added impetus (Chirogram, 1963).

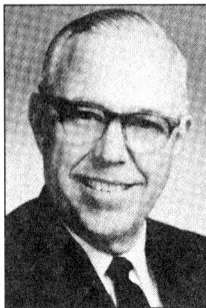

Figure 17-1: William N. Coggins, D.C.

In September of the following year the Missouri Chiropractic College (MCC) in St. Louis also closed its doors after 44 years, and amalgamated with the Logan Basic College of Chiropractic. Originally incorporated as a proprietary institution, the MCC had been rechartered as a non-profit school in 1962 under the leadership of its third president, Otto C. Reinert, D.C., a 1936 graduate of the college. The merger of MCC and Logan Basic College had been proposed by Dewey Anderson, who recommended that Reinert assume the chair of a "Diversified Technique" department of the merged institution, thereby broadening the technique offerings for the new school. However, Logan Basic's third president, William N. Coggins, D.C. (see Figure 17-1), and academic dean, D.P. Casey, D.C. (a nephew of college founder Hugh B. Logan) "resisted the extensive inclusion of dynamic thrust techniques, full-spine adjusting, and extra-spinal manipulations as we taught in the Missouri curriculum" (Reinert, 1992).

The deadlock was broken by the suggestion from National College of Chiropractic president, Joseph Janse, that if Logan Basic College did not wish to merge with MCC, then the National College (newly relocated in 1963 from Chicago to Lombard, Illinois) was willing to consider a merger, and thereby create a "National College of Missouri." This prospect apparently tipped the balance for the Logan Basic College, and:

> ...a merger agreement was signed by William N. Coggins for Logan and Otto C. Reinert for Missouri on September 24, 1964. Essentially all proposals recommended by Anderson were included in the merger agreement. Fifty-nine students from Missouri were accepted into the student body of Logan, with full credit and advanced standing into the respective classes attended. Those whose courses were to be completed within two years would be issued Missouri diplomas, which were acceptable in all licensing jurisdictions. The remainder, upon satisfying Logan requirements would be given Logan diplomas. All would be welcomed into the Logan Alumni Association without prejudice (Reinert, 1992).

The new school was known as the Logan College of Chiropractic, and although Basic Technique continued as a featured course offering, the term "Basic" was removed from the institution's name. The school was immediately recognized by the ACA's Council on Education as an accredited institution (ACA, 1964a). Reinert continued as technique department chair until 1970, and served as a research consultant in the 1980s (Reinert, 1992).

Logan College also acquired the records and alumni of the Carver Chiropractic College in 1964. The Carver school's final commencement had been held in September 1958, and the trustees of the 52-year old non-profit school had briefly considered a merger with the Texas Chiropractic College (Hearn, 1958). The school's closure was apparently prompted by a serious decline in enrollments following the end of federal educational benefits for veterans (Locklar, 1954). Unfortunately, little has been published about the five decade story of Willard Carver's first institution.

The school situation in New York had long been a concern among the leadership in the accreditation movement, and with the 1964 enactment of the state's first licensing law, the American Chiropractic Association renewed its consolidation campaign. The *ACA Journal* and the *Digest of Chiropractic Economics* reported on "the formalities of the merger of Atlantic States and Columbia Institute of Chiropractic" (ACA, 1964b; Columbia, 1964). All but forgotten now, the Columbia Institute of Chiropractic (CIC; now New York Chiropractic College) and the Chiropractic Institute of New York (CINY) also briefly considered a merger in the mid-1960s at the urging of the ACA. Clarence W. Weiant, dean of the CINY, wrote to Stanley Hayes, D.C., editor and publisher of the *Bulletin of Rational Chiropractic*, in February 1965:

> Some excellent news. There is now little doubt that fusion of the two schools in New York into one strong institution is in the works. With the best of will on both sides the details are being worked out. Each is opening up to the other its books, records, financial status, material assets, liabilities, etc. No one knows yet precisely when the merger will be in effect, but it could be as early as September. Dr. Napolitano is being very cooperative. He asks nothing for himself other than some kind of formal affiliation with the new school. Dr. Peterson has agreed to assume leadership during the formative years, and no faculty member of C.I.N.Y. will be sacrificed (Weiant, 1965).

The following month the *ACA Journal of Chiropractic* published an announcement by Ernest G. Napolitano and Thure C. Peterson, presidents of the two schools, entitled "Future plans for a school in New York":

> *Editor's note: The following article is a joint statement by the Presidents of the Chiropractic Institute of New York and the Columbia Institute of Chiropractic.*
>
> It has long been acknowledge that a single strong school of chiropractic in the State and City of New York is an ultimate goal for the advancement of the educational structure for the entire profession.
>
> At Des Moines, Iowa last month, where the American Chiropractic Association, its Council on Education, Board of Governors, and Trustees of the Foundation for Accredited Chiropractic Education held mid-year meetings, it was decided that an overall plan to support such a school should now be advanced.
>
> Discussions centered around a plan to institute a fund-raising project to provide one million dollars for the purchase or the building of an adequate physical plant for such a school, which would be eligible for a charter and registration by the State Education Department, and it is expected that the American Chiropractic Association will lend its financial support to the extent of more than one hundred thousand dollars on a matching basis.
>
> In view of this positive support, Dr. Thure C. Peterson, President of the Chiropractic Institute of New York, and Dr. Ernest G. Napolitano, President of the Columbia Institute of New York [sic] reached the decision that the time was now appropriate to discuss consolidation of the two schools. Talks were instituted in Des Moines which led to agreement on fundamental matters, and this was reported to the American Chiropractic Association.
>
> On Sunday, January 31, 1965, the faculty, trustees, and officers and directors of the Alumni Association of both schools were informed simultaneously of the new development, as was the student body the next day.
>
> Further discussions for exchange of pertinent information necessary to implement the consolidation will be held so that initial steps can be taken in the near future.
>
> It is evident that the chartering and registration of one fine school by the State Education Department of New York will be a giant step forward for the profession and will greatly enhance the acceptance of the Council on Education of the American Chiropractic Association by the Department of Health, Education and Welfare as the accrediting agency for the profession.
>
> The entire profession, especially along the Eastern Seaboard States, is urged to lend support to this constructive development (Napolitano & Peterson, 1965).

The consolidation of the CIC with the CINY did not take place. The ACA, which had been expressing its desire for one "Eastern Seaboard Regional College" (Columbia, 1964a), apparently "wrote off" the schools of New York, and CINY in particular, this despite the strength of the CINY faculty, the recent legislative successes enjoyed in New York, and the growing rapport between the leadership of CINY and officials with the state's Department of Education (Weiant, 1964). Block grants to CINY from the ACA's Foundation for Accredited Chiropractic Education (FACE), called "grants-in-aid" (Schierholz, 1986, pp. 18-20), had amounted to $14,000 in 1963-64, but were not forthcoming in 1964-65. According to Weiant, the ACA indicated that until greater progress in amalgamating CIC and CINY took place, such funds were to be held in reserve (Weiant, 1964). For their part, the CINY administration and faculty were reluctant to submit to an amalgamation with the Columbia Institute which might lower standards and submit them to a Napolitano presidency. Dintenfass (1995) notes that "There was a long period of negotiation between CINY and Columbia. Talks were broken off because Columbia refused to accept CINY's demand for equal representation on the Board of Trustees."

The withdrawal of ACA funding was probably a major factor in the demise of CINY:

> CINY itself was unable to obtain a charter from New York, largely because it could not meet the fiscal resource requirements stipulated by the regulations of the state education department.
>
> Unable to cope with the continued ineligibility of its modern graduates to practice in its home state, CINY's trustees considered a merger to be the only solution for preserving its heritage as well as providing its graduates with a legal repository for their records.
>
> In September of 1968 they chose NCC [National College of Chiropractic] to be the official, legal trustee and curator of their institutional records, including those from the three that had amalgamated to form CINY in 1944 - Carver's New York Institute and the Cosmopolitan school.
>
> Dr. Earl G. Liss and Dr. Thure C. Peterson, Chairmen of the Boards of Trustees of NCC and CINY respectively, published a glowing account of the affiliation as a consolidation of strengths and traditions which represented a forward step of significance to the progressive future of the chiropractic profession (*ACA Journal October 1968*).
>
> Little did they know just how important the merger would become to the perpetuation of chiropractic in the state of New York as well as a boon to chiropractic's educational sector in general.
>
> CINY's "adopted" sons and daughters would gain immediate representation on both NCC's college and alumni boards. This further stimulated many CINY graduates to provide transfer students and send more than one hundred matriculants per year as well as money and moral support for National's growth and development.
>
> They encouraged NCC to persist in its already vigorous pursuit of accreditation through registration with the Board of Regents of the State Education Department of the University of the State of New York. In 1971 NCC became the first, and for seven years the only, chiropractic institution to be accredited by New York State (Beideman, 1995, p. 132).

Table 17-2: Institutions recognized by the ACA Council on Education in 1968 (*ACA Journal of Chiropractic* 1968 [Oct]; 5[10]: 24)

Institution	Level of Recognition
Lincoln Chiropractic College	Accredited
Los Angeles College of Chiropractic	Accredited
National College of Chiropractic	Accredited
Logan College of Chiropractic	Provisionally Accredited
Northwestern College of Chiropractic	Provisionally Accredited
Texas Chiropractic College	Provisionally Accredited
Chiropractic Institute of New York	Approved Conditionally
Columbia Institute of Chiropractic	Approved Conditionally

Although the ACA Council on Education listed the CINY within its three-tier rating system (i.e., "Accredited," "Provisionally Accredited" and "Approved Conditionally"; see Table 17-2) in October 1968, the die had already been cast, and the CINY was absorbed by National College of Chiropractic (Rehm, 1980, pp. 298-9). The announcement of the CINY/NCC affiliation appeared that same month in the *ACA Journal*.

Another very significant amalgamation took place, when in 1971 the Lincoln Chiropractic College of Indianapolis closed its doors and affiliated with the National College of Chiropractic (Janse, 1971; National, 1971). This merger brought to a close the NCA/ACA consolidation efforts that had begun during John Nugent's reign as NCA Director of Education in the 1940s, and increased the resources of the National College.

Chapter 18

Toward a Scholarly Infrastructure

Scholarship, research and research training for chiropractors were sorry step-children of the profession in its third quarter. Nevertheless, there were a number of developments that merit mention either because they created a template for higher educational standards and research development in the last 25 years of the chiropractic saga, or because they provide examples of barriers to scholarly development during 1946-1970.

Many mistaken and/or anti-scientific ideas about the nature of science were common throughout the profession in its first 50 years. These included the notions that basic science instruction was sufficient to produce a "scientific chiropractor," that science meant perfect predictability, that scientific investigation served to reveal the will of God, that observation without experimentation was sufficient to determine cause/effect relationships, and that the main purposes of science and research in chiropractic were their role in marketing (Keating et al., 1995). When, at the end of World War II, the NCA created the Chiropractic Research Foundation (CRF), its organizers were predominantly NCA doctors with interests in public relations and marketing. Although the CRF earned high marks in later years for its financial support in upgrading chiropractic education (Schierholz, 1986), its earliest operations were remarkable for the amount of money lost in an unrealistic nationwide fund-raising campaign (Keating et al., 1995). By the early 1950s research had become something of a dirty word within the NCA, and continuing organizational interest came to reside within the NCA's Committee on Research, headed by C.O. Watkins. Henry Higley of the LACC attempted unsuccessfully to launch a field-based research program from his position within this committee (Higley, 1953). Watkins (1948) called upon the NCA colleges to provide clinical research training to students, but his proposal was rejected by W.A. Budden, president of the Western States College (Budden, 1948), who argued that training in the basic sciences had to suffice, and that clinical research and clinical research training were things the colleges could not afford.

The CRF did try to create centers for research and training. Noteworthy was a short-lived effort to take over Leo Spears' Denver hospital; although this did not happen, Spears Hospital did offer internship experience to many chiropractors (Rehm, 1984; Spears, undated). Perhaps the strongest CRF accomplishment in promoting scholarship during its early years resulted from the small grants it provided to Clarence W. Weiant, then dean of the Chiropractic Institute of New York (CINY) and the first NCA/CRF Director of Research. Weiant assembled a team of investigators at CINY which included Bruno Oetteking, Ph.D. (physical anthropologist and Weiant's former mentor at Columbia University) and H.M. Burry, D.C. This team collaborated with chiropractors Sol Goldschmidt, Joseph Janse, Doris Siebern and S.S. Ulrich in the production of more than seven dozen publications during 1945-1949. Few of these works were published in scholarly journals (most appeared in the NCA's *Journal*), but a special issue of *Revista Mexicana de Estudios Antropologicos* was devoted to the Oetteking's investigations while at CINY, and the German scientist produced a volume entitled *Human Craniology* while on staff (Rehm, 1980, p. 333). One can imagine that this level of scholarly activity must have had some beneficial influence upon the intellectual climate within CINY at that time.

The CRF became the Foundation for Accredited Chiropractic Education (FACE) in 1959, at which time Higley was appointed chairman of an FACE advisory committee. In this capacity he produced his celebrated study of the "Intervertebral Disc Syndrome," which involved an extensive review of then available literature on the topic. However, little other scholarly activity was readily apparent in the chiropractic colleges:

> In reporting to NCA and FACE on July 1, 1960, Dewey Anderson, Ph.D., Education consultant,
> said that the lack of research projects being conducted as part of the work of college teachers was
> most noticeable. Not even the nomenclature and conditions of controlled research techniques were

taught generally. Yet the unverified body of knowledge and practice in the field of chiropractic was enormous. Nothing would upgrade the colleges and improve the status of the profession more markedly than a well-conceived and administered program of research going on in the colleges of chiropractic, the findings published in the National Journal, and thus brought to the attention of those in active practice.

In a move to overcome the lack of research in chiropractic colleges, the Trustees in 1961 appointed Dr. Henry Higley, Director of a FACE Research Department located at the Los Angeles College with two defininte aims by the department. Objectives were to make studies related to the theoretical and practical application of chiropractic concepts, and to develop step-by-step a solid scientific foundation which would withstand any outside critical test and upon which the professional structure would continue to develop. For his preliminary work, the Trustees awarded Dr. Higley an honorarium of $1,000 and a grant not to exceed $6000 for honorarium and expenses from July 1, 1961 to June 30, 1962 (Schierholz, 1986, pp. 17-8).

FACE also commissioned the development of cineroentgenological equipment for use by chiropractors through grants made to the Lincoln Chiropractic College in Indianapolis in 1962. Here, Earl Rich, D.C. collaborated with the Picker X-ray Company to develop the new technology. An initial award of $32,000 was supplemented with payments for supplies as needed. Other small research awards were given to the National and Texas schools in the next few years (Schierholz, 1986; Timmins, 1976). However, most of the FACE's contributions in the 1960s were directed toward developing the ACA colleges' instructional programs, facilities and teaching faculty rather than research; as noted earlier, this involved raising ACA dues and committing 40% of membership dues to FACE (Kimmel, 1965; Schierholz, 1986, pp. 18-22).

The FACE became the Foundation for Chiropractic Education and Research (FCER) in 1969 (Martin, 1974). Arthur M. Schierholz, D.C., secretary-treasurer of the FCER, noted the organization's purposes and its role in the merger of CINY with the National College:

The primary purpose and objective of the foundation is "to receive gifts for the use and benefit of chiropractic education and research...to administer said gifts... to promote the science of chiropractic, particularly in the research of all the scientific aspects of chiropractic, to provide adequate facilities and equipment for the full and complete education of students in chiropractic colleges..."

A major effort by the foundation was assumed in agreeing to supporting the merger and moving of the Chiropractic Institute of New York to the National College of Chiropractic at Lombard in Illinois. This took place in the autumn months last year and involved the efforts of both colleges and a goodly number of people not directly associated with the two schools. The loading of two full vans with the official records and transcripts of CINY and the moving of the library and the useable physical equipment involved hard work and many hours of effort. The foundation underwrote the transfer of twelve students who wished to move from New York to Lombard. This meant paying transportation one way for the student, his family, and also a part of his personal property (Schierholz, 1969).

With the 1969 death of Henry Higley who had served for several years as ACA's Director of Research and Statistics (Chiropractic, 1969), the organization (i.e., ACA/FCER) paused to reconsider its mission and purposes (Martin, 1969). Ralph Pressman, Ph.D. was appointed Director of Research for the LACC and for the ACA (Chirogram, 1969b). Ralph J. Martin, D.C., N.D. (see Figure 10-6), former president of the LACC and then serving as ACA Research Coordinator, called upon the profession to meet the challenge presented by the U.S. Department of Health, Education and Welfare (which had advocated exclusion of chiropractors from Medicare reimbursement) through a renewed commitment to research. He suggested that:

...research has moved up to number one priority for our profession. Until we meet these tests of research sufficiently to satisfy the scientific community, we must expect our credibility to be questioned. This is reason enough for each and every one of us to involve ourselves in some meaningful phase of research which is relevant to our profession (Martin, 1970).

Martin's plan called for county societies to provide $500 scholarships to chiropractic students, who would work under the supervision of various research directors at the chiropractic colleges. The plan resembled Higley's (1953) earlier proposal, and little came of it. Martin listed a variety of projects then "in progress" at the ACA-affiliated institutions (see Table 18-

1), of which many were presumably stalled owing to personnel shortages. Taking a chapter from C.O. Watkins, who had been urging field and school-based programs of clinical studies for 30 years (Keating, 1987), Martin (1969) cautioned:

> The message that is important is that without acceptable research in adequate volume, we are not a profession. It is something that we just must not try to do without. Our ACA research programs must have general participation from the field in at least two important ways: The first is to support your state association in setting up annual research fellowships, and the second is to participate in the new Clinical Research Program directed by Dr. Edwin Kimmel...The discipline that you will acquire will improve the quality of your work in your office and also the satisfaction that your clinical experience will be vitally intensified.

A noteworthy contribution to scientific studies from the straight chiropractic educational community derived from the subluxation studies conducted by Carl S. Cleveland, Jr., D.C. Cleveland was serving as dean of the Kansas City school his parents had founded in 1922 when he published his animal analogue investigation of subluxation in rabbits (Cleveland, 1965). This work anticipated the later studies of DeBoer (1981) and others. A review of Cleveland's project appeared nearly two decades later in the first issue of the *Chiropractic Research Archives Collection* (CRAC, 1984):

> 2155 Cleveland CS, Jr. Researching the subluxation on the domestic rabbit. *Science Rev Chiro* 1965; 1(4): 5-28
>
> This report consists of a resume of a series of pilot experiments conducted to determine the advisability of conducting an extended series of complicated experiments on animals. For the experiments in researching spinal subluxation and nerve pressure, the large domestic rabbit was used. the relationships between the function of the nervous system and the cause of disease are explained. Case histories, the experimental procedures and final results comprise the bulk of the report.

Unfortunately, intra-professional politics often overwhelmed any scientific considerations in the 1960s. Cleveland was repeatedly denied permission to present

---

Table 18-1: Research projects "presently in progress" at ACA-affiliated chiropractic colleges in 1969 (Martin, 1969)

Lincoln Chiropractic College
1. Visceral diseases and their effect upon posture
2. Asymmetrical lumbosacral facet facings
3. Relationship of sacral position to low back symptoms
(Due to faculty limitations all of these studies are at a standstill)

Los Angeles College of Chiropractic
1. Dietary influences on urinary nitrogen output (work in progress)
2. Occipito-atlanto-axial relationship (work completed)
3. Consistency of palpation as a means of spinal diagnosis (work in progress)
4. Postural study of junior and senior high school students (work in progress)
5. Therapy for sub-deltoid calcific bursitis (report completed and is in manuscript form)
6. A study of orthopedic cases under chiropractic care (work in progress)
7. A study and evaluation of chiropractic education in the United States (work in progress)
8. Chiropractic population in the United States - a comparative study (report completed and is in manuscript form)
9. Why delinquency? A study of community judgment (preliminary report completed and in manuscript form - awaiting further development from LA County)
10. A study of dietary habits of arthritic patients (work in progress)
11. Effects of vitamin A on the sensitivity of rats to irradiation (work in progress)
12. Proposed project: The beneficial use of a fast as an important therapeutic approach in the treatment of assorted disease processes (work still in preparation form)

National College of Chiropractic
1. Vitamin C effects on bone matrix
2. Effect of vertebral fixations on ulnar nerve impulse velocities and the result of their correction
3. Neurological effects of artificially induced vertebral fixation (temporarily inactive)
4. Osteoarthritis managed by Vitamineral supplementation and spinal manipulation
(Progress on all projects requested)

Northwestern College of Chiropractic
1. Cineroentgenological studies of the cervical spine (Progress on project requested)

Table 18-2: Some of the members of the editorial board of the *Journal of Clinical Chiropractic*

William Coggins, D.C., President, Logan College of Chiropractic
Julius Dintenfass, D.C., Professor, Chiropractic Institute of New York
Henri Gillet, D.C., Private Practice, Belgium
Scott Haldeman, D.C., M.Sc., Doctoral student, University of British Columbia
William D. Harper, D.C., President, Texas Chiropractic College
Roy W. Hildebrandt, D.C., Chairman, Department of Roentgenology, Palmer
     College of Chiropractic
Joseph Howe, D.C., D.A.C.B.R., Professor, National College of Chiropractic
Edwin H. Kimmel, D.C., Professor, Chiropractic Institute of New York
Ernest G. Napolitano, D.C., President, Columbia Institute of Chiropractic
Herman Schwartz, D.C., Professor, Chiropractic Institute of New York
Chester C. Stowell, D.C., Dean, Lincoln Chiropractic College
Clarence W. Weiant, D.C., Ph.D., Dean, Chiropractic Institute of New York

his findings at meetings conducted by broad-scope leaders, owing to his and his father's participation in straight chiropractic educational affairs.

The third quarter of the chiropractic century also witnessed the birth of several of the earliest attempts to provide scholarly periodicals for the profession's knowledge base. Exemplary were the *Annals of the Swiss Chiropractors' Association* (begun circa 1961) and the *Journal of Clinical Chiropractic* (*JCC*; established 1968). Neither of these journals were published by the chiropractic colleges, but the *JCC* included a number of college leaders on its editorial board (see Table 18-2). The JCC's stated purpose was to "present basic research, educational information, scientific and technological data, and relevant tangential materials to the chiropractic profession. The *JCC* has no social or political design whatsoever..." (Keating, 1992, pp. 67-70). The *JCC* did not survive beyond 1981, but by that time the National College of Chiropractic had created its *Journal of Manipulative and Physiological Therapeutics*, which was accepted for inclusion in the National Library of Medicine's *Index Medicus* in 1981.

The *JCC* may be seen as an ancestor from which the *JMPT* eventually arose. The *JCC* provided preliminary editorial experience for the future founding editor of the *JMPT*, Roy W. Hildebrandt (see Figure 18-1). The 1949 PSC alumnus raised concerns at his alma mater, where he served as chair of the Department of Roentgenology, when in 1967 he authored an article in the *ACA Journal of Chiropractic* which questioned the traditional epistemologies within the profession, and called for substantive clinical research as a basis for chiropractic practice (Hildebrandt, 1967). Of particular interest was the response that Hildebrandt's article drew from another, earlier Palmer graduate, Frank W. Elliott. Elliott (see Figure 18-2) had been a faculty member and administrator at the Davenport institution in the early decades, serving at various times as Registrar and business officer of the PSC, and later as manger of Station WOC. His previously close association with B.J. Palmer therefore lent prominence to his call for greater unity based upon scientific principles:

> Dear Editor:
>
> Finally I have found time in my new capacity as the executive secretary-treasurer of our state association to read the October 1967 issue of the [ACA] Journal. Let me congratulate you on that issue...It is the best one that has appeared in print since I graduated in 1911!
>
> "World Chiropractic Conference Report"; 'Validity of Chiropractic Therapy Clearly Established'; and then the scholarly paper 'The Science of Chiropractic' by R.W. Hildebrandt, D.C.
>
> If the schools will unite and agree to Dr. Hildebrandt's methodology and the ACA and ICA get behind it, there is yet hope that chiropractic can be accepted by HEW and if the general membership of both associations let the colleges do the job along the lines that Dr. Hildebrandt outlined, we will be doing what D.D. Palmer said to me in 1911 when he lived next door to me in Los Angeles. I did not take much stock in what he said then as I was prejudiced by my close connection with B.J. and Mabel Palmer (She was my cousin). However, since being in the field, and having taken two semesters of general semantics at Denver University, I heartily agree with Dr. Hildebrandt and sincerely hope that something useful will develop (Elliott, 1968).

Unfortunately, as the third quarter of the chiropractic century drew to a close, there was still relatively little access to the *JCC* nor to other chiropractic periodicals outside the profession (Keating, 1992, pp. 307-10). For the most part, there was no interest in creating a scholarly literature; indeed, not until 1970 did the ACA consider establishing a library at its headquarters (ACA, 1970), and another 23 years passed before the ACA sponsored a blind-peer-reviewed periodical for distribution to its membership (Haldeman, 1993).

The LACC's *Chirogram* was exceptional among chiropractic journals in the 1960s for engaging in quality, critical reviews of submitted materials through a formal referee process (Chirogram, 1963b). No chiropractic journal was regularly reviewed in interdisciplinary indexes (Hildebrandt, 1978, 1981a&b), and the Chiropractic Library Consortium's (CLIBCON's) *Index to the Chiropractic Literature* was still more than a decade in the future (Whitehead, 1990). When the ACA decided to create a "Library Information Committee," its purposes were primarily political; the committee was apparently not interested in gathering scientific data that did not support "the chiropractic principle":

> The objectives of this committee are:
>
> 1. To serve as a collecting agency for all chiropractic information, especially in the legal, legislative, research, and news media fields.
>
> 2. To catalog, index, file, and safeguard all this literature.
>
> 3. To guarantee that somewhere in the nation there exists a total acquisition of the world's chiropractic literature and information.
>
> 4. To make the materials available to those who can use it. This is indeed, an ambitious undertaking; but if chiropractic is to meet its problems and the onslaughts of its adversaries with the greatest ease and confidence, then we must proceed with an accelerated pace to fulfill these objectives.
>
> Following is a list of material we should collect:
>
> *Copies of articles in newspapers, magazines, etc., which are favorable or unfavorable to chiropractic thought.
>
> *Copies of scientific papers in scientific journals which give support to the chiropractic principle (Bierman, 1969).

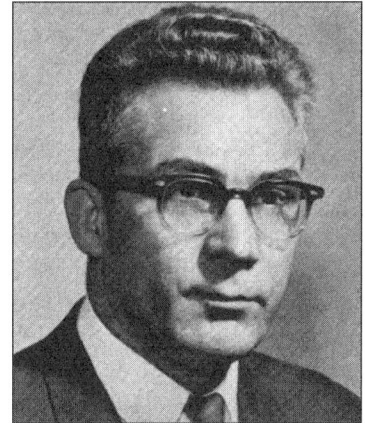

Figure 18-1: Roy W. Hildebrandt, D.C., circa 1970

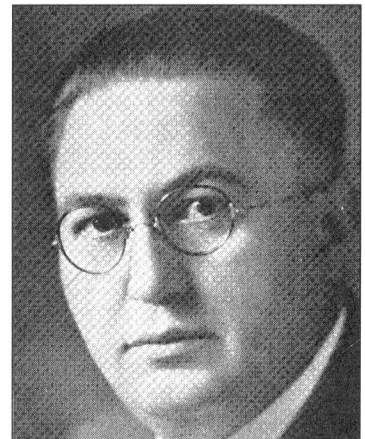

Figure 18-2: Frank W. Elliott

Post-doctoral training in chiropractic during the post-war years was limited. The "Ph.C." (Philosopher of Chiropractic) degree, first awarded to B.J. Palmer in 1908, continued to be issued at several chiropractic institutions, but its requirements varied from school to school and within any given school at different times, and sometimes was an honorary award, rather than an earned certificate (Stout, 1988). Not until 1968 did the ACA's Council on Education rule that the Ph.C. degree was "spurious" (Minutes, 1968). Most education beyond the doctorate was offered for the sake of continuing education requirements of the various state boards. However, several noteworthy examples of more intensive education should be noted. The hospital-based internship training provided by Spears Hospital in Denver has already been noted. The LACC created a "graduate school" in 1948, and the Chiropractic Institute of New York proposed a similar program in 1954 (Announcing, 1954). The LACC's graduate school was launched with the intention of providing coursework in topics not covered or covered to only a minor extent in the school's doctoral program (Laing, 1951, Lupica, 1947; Norcross, 1948, 1949, 1951). The program offered such degrees as "Master of Chiropractic Science" (Chiro.Sc.M.) and Doctor of Chiropractic Science (Chiro.Sc.D.), and required applicants to complete coursework in chemistry and bacteriology as well as clinical subjects (General, 1950; The Graduate, 1951). The LACC may never have awarded the "Chiro.Sc.D.," but several master's degrees were conferred (The Graduate, 1952).

Lee H. Norcross, D.C., N.D. served as the first dean of the LACC graduate school, and organized programs in roentgenology, psychiatry, gynecology and proctology, pediatrics, and ear, nose and throat. Special societies of chiropractors who concentrated their practices in the areas of instruction provided through the graduate school were also established; part of the intent of these societies and educational programs was to preserve broad-scope practice privileges in California and elsewhere (Wentz & Green, 1995). The existence of the graduate program prompted various field practitioners to organize additional societies and course offerings, such as in orthopedics (Hancock, 1963; Wentz & Green, 1995). An "archives center" for chiropractic historical materials was added to the graduate school in 1969 by F. Maynard Lipe, D.C., then dean of the graduate school (Chirogram, 1969a). The "graduate school" eventually became LACC's post-graduate division.

Several efforts were made to integrate chiropractic education into mainstream higher education, although such ventures were at first viewed with great suspicion. John Nugent's early efforts, as NCA Director of Education, to encourage formation of a chiropractic college at the University of Denver met with considerable resistance from the college presidents serving in the Council on Education (Minutes, 1948; see Appendix B). The educators feared that the creation of a university-based chiropractic school might force higher standards on all the colleges, and could result in medical control of chiropractic education. Nonetheless, the Texas Chiropractic College "arranged for its basic science courses to be taught at San Antonio College in 1953" (Wardwell, 1992, p. 146) so as to meet the state's "legal requirement of 60 semester hours in the arts and sciences, and 4200 hours of chiropractic education" (Our, 1972-73). The Northwestern College of Chiropractic (NWCC) developed an affiliation with a local liberal arts college (see below). The Lincoln Chiropractic College attempted to evolve into a liberal arts institution (Exclusive, 1968), but was unsuccessful. The Logan Basic College proposed the creation of a junior college division, and received the permsision of Missouri's Department of Education (Appendix B: Minutes of the Council on Education, June, 1952). The Canadian Memorial Chiropractic College continued its decades long pursuit of university affiliation with schools such as the University of Alberta, Brandon University, Notre Dame University, the University of Guelph, the University of Waterloo, and Waterloo Lutheran University and York University (Brown, 1992, 1994). However, these efforts were not fruitful until the 1990s (Ontario, 1995).

A commendable but apparently limited program of underwriting advanced academic training for college faculty was in evidence toward the end of chiropractic's third quarter. This took the form of a "Faculty Assistance Program" sponsored by the ACA and the FCER (Faculty, 1970). The emphasis at this time was to better prepare instructors to meet the standards expected by HEW's education department; the program provided funds for "tuition, fees, and books" for faculty members while working towards master's and higher degrees. Later on, this program shifted its emphasis to preparing chiropractors for careers in research (Keating, 1992a)

Chapter 19

ON THE THRESHOLD
OF RECOGNITION

As the third quarter of the first chiropractic century drew to a close, the movement to upgrade the chiropractic colleges accelerated its efforts to establish an accrediting agency that the federal government, specifically the Department of Health, Education and Welfare's (HEW's) Office of Education, would recognize. The earliest contacts with the federal education officials had been initiated by John J. Nugent in the early 1950s, and by the end of the decade Nugent reported to the NCA Council on Education:

> Pursuant to the decision we made at our last meeting I have again reopened negotiations with the Federal Department of Education at Washington. I had a long afternoon conference with Mr. Goldthorp, who, as you will remember, is the Specialist for Accreditation, Division of Higher Education...
>
> Our previous decisions to postpone pressing our application were wise from many viewpoints. As we decided, there were many things which the NCA and the schools had to do, and much that had to happen to expose the farcical attempts at accreditation of the ICA...
>
> As Goldthorp said several years ago, "You do not have a disciplined profession. Here are three groups asking for recognition. Get yourselves straightened out, and then come back. We can only accept one agency for each profession" ...we could have persisted at that time...but I was fearful of an investigation of our own schools and an outright rejection that would have been fatal at that stage of our evolution. In a word, our application at that time was premature...
>
> You will be interested in the facts which were influential with Mr. Goldthorp:
> 1. The collapse of the Norcross agency.
> 2. The fact that the ICA was a creature or captive agency of the Palmer School; that all the schools on its list were rejected by our Council; some of these already defunct or about to close and its obvious attempt at deception.
> 3. The fact that the Council on Education was organized after the pattern of accrediting agencies in other professions.
> 4. The close parallel of the pattern which we used in building our schools to that followed by Dr. Abraham Flexner in building the medical schools.
> 5. The concurrent program in the states to raise educational requirements for license, especially the two years of pre-professional college. Our accomplishments here brought praise.
> 6. The affiliation of the Texas School with the San Antonio College with the approval of the University of Texas.
> 7. The recognition by Lewis & Clark and other Oregon universities of credits earned at Western States College.
> 8. The prechiropractic courses in Oregon and Southern California junior colleges inspired by our schools.
> 9. The ownership by our schools of their own plants. The new $300,000 plant at the Lincoln, and the $500,000 building program of the National. The raising of $212,000 in California for the Los Angeles school and other donations for schools elsewhere.
> 10. The scholarships available to students.
> 11. A fact considered most important - The support of our schools by a large segment of the profession as evidenced by the fact that the NCA had accepted the recommendations of the Council on Education and had provided for (1) graduate instruction for faculty members to upgrade instruction, (2) had appropriated $50,000 for operating expenses in 1959 and $50,000 for research and (3) had allocated $100,000 or more annually to be available for our schools beginning in 1960.

...the fact that the Council had been able to win approval for its recommendations of financial support of its schools by the practitioners, as represented by the Directors and House of Delegates of the NCA, was important. I was able to point to a growing list of state licensing boards that are adopting the criteria of the Council, and also to the fact that every chiropractic school in the U.S., with the exception of the Palmer, had applied to the Council for inspection and approval and thus had accepted the authority of the Council...

I left Washington with a gratified feeling of accomplishment and with reasonable hope for our success. I shall keep you advised on developments (Nugent, 1959).

In 1961 the NCA Director of Education reported an initial rejection by the HEW (Minutes, 1961: see Appendix B). The rejection included a bill of particulars specifying the deficiencies in the NCA's Council on Education; Nugent opined that with sufficient financial support and intra-professional cooperation, federal recognition could be achieved. The Council on Education, comprised of the chief executive officers of the various NCA-allied schools plus representatives of the independent (non-NCA-affiliated) Council of State Chiropractic Examining Boards (CSCEB), was greatly distressed in 1961 when Nugent was retired (Gibbons, 1985), this despite the strong endorsement offered by Council representatives to the NCA Executive Board (Minutes, 1961: see Appendix B):

TO THE EXECUTIVE BOARD OF THE N.C.A.

To the full membership of the National Council on Education it is evident that significant progress has been made toward federal accreditation through the efforts of Dr. John J. Nugent as Director of Education of the National Chiropractic Association.

Recent conferences and events in Washington support these facts. We are all, therefor, charged with the responsibility of continuing this program to completion.

It is apparent that a break-through has been accomplished. It is the responsibility of all of us to exploit this break-through.

The members of the Council who over many years have sought with concern and diligence to gain this accreditation, are apprehensive about any change which may weaken our efforts to accomplish this end.

It is evident that the entire N.C.A. membership is vitally concerned about this matter. Expressions by general members, as well as members of the House of Delegates give indication that they demand the maximum of effort which will insure success.

Thus the Council members unanimously and urgently recommend that the services of Dr. Nugent as Director of Education be continued.

The CSCEB (which became the Federation of Chiropractic Licensing Boards/FCLB in 1968; Goldschmidt, 1992) continued to press the NCA/ACA and its Council on Education to increase efforts to achieve federal recognition of chiropractic education. The CSCEB strongly encouraged the NCA's Council to seek accommodation with the International Chiropractors' Association (ICA) (Minutes, 1961: see Appendix B), and endorsed the activities of the "Committee of the Profession on Chiropractic Education," an ad hoc group comprised of association leaders and school administrators (Minutes, 1962: see Appendix B). Little came of this effort, but at approximately the same time the third (and current) National Board of Chiropractic Examiners (NBCE) was established (Holman, 1970, 1971a&b; Saunders, 1965). Edward M. Saunders, D.C., first president of the NBCE reported that:

It was pointed out that we were the only profession without such a board and that soon we would be the only profession left to take the Basic Science Boards in many states, as the other professions would by-pass them through their National Boards. In fact, in some states chiropractors were already having to take the National Medical Board, Part I, instead of the regular Basic Science examination.

In Detroit, at the meeting of The Council of Examining Boards, in 1962, the first National Board of Examiners were formed from members of the Council. Each member was elected from one of five districts of the United States, and each member, with many years of experience, as a member of state examining boards.

The National Board was financed jointly by the NCA/ACA and the ICA organizations, and was charged to make all haste, but to follow the exact procedure of the other National Boards. The National Podiatry and Dental Boards gave their first examination ten years from the date of their inception.

Fortunately, we were able to obtain great help from the Secretaries of the National Dental and Podiatry Boards...In only three years, with their help, we were ready for our first examination. The chiropractic colleges did a tremendous job in forming a pool of some 10,000 to 12,000 questions in thirteen categories... (Saunders, 1965).

Gevitz (1988) has suggested that the eventual repeal of basic science laws in the United States came about because of the dissatisfaction among the medical community. Nonetheless, the acceptance of national board examinations of the several health care professions, including those of the NBCE, by a number of state boards probably helped to encourage the gradual revocation of basic science boards. The NBCE's testing program was several years old when the first state, Florida, repealed its basic science provisions (see Table 19-1). Meanwhile, chiropractic colleges found imaginative ways to improve basic science instruction for their students, thereby deflating the threat of the basic science boards. The Northwestern College of Chiropractic (NWCC), for example, established "an academic relationship with the College of St. Thomas," a private, liberal arts institution (Wolfe, 1970). The arrangement permitted NWCC students to take their pre-clinical, basic science coursework at the College of St. Thomas, from instructors holding advanced academic degrees in the requisite subjects, and earn transferable credits from a regionally accredited institution. The arrangement persisted for only a few years, but helped to raise the credibility of NWCC and chiropractic education generally.

The cooperation between ACA and ICA in supporting the NBCE may have encouraged a continued search for common ground in the college accreditation arena. However, fundamental differences in views of the proper scope of chiropractic practice continued to divide the two camps. The points of contention are seen in a letter from Leonard W. Rutherford, D.C., president of the ICA, to Ted McCarrel, president of a liberal arts school (Cottey College in Missouri) and consultant to chiropractic educators:

Table 19-1: Enactment and revocation of basic science legislation in the United States; states listed in chronological order of revocation (based on Gevitz [1988] and Sauer [1932]); see also Table 7-1

Dates of Enactment & Revocation

1939-1967	Florida
1936-1968	Arizona
1941-1968	New Mexico
1957-1969	Kansas
1946-1970	Alaska
1940-1971	Rhode Island
1937-1972	Michigan
1935-1973	Iowa
1937-1973	Oklahoma
1933-1973	Oregon
1927-1974	Minnesota
1959-1975	Alabama
1925-1975	Connecticut
1927-1975	Nebraska
1951-1975	Nevada
1939-1975	South Dakota
1925-1975	Wisconsin
1937-1976	Colorado
1943-1976	Tennessee
1929-1977	Arkansas
1929-1978	District of Columbia
1949-1979	Texas
1959-1979	Utah
1927-1979	Washington

Dear Ted:

In talking with Dr. Carl Cleveland the other day, he expressed the fear that subjects such as physio-therapy, physical therapy and minor surgery, etc., might be and undoubtedly would be strongly suggested by Janse as proper for a curriculum or electives on standards for the colleges, when you have the next meeting.

Enclosed copy for your information as an example of this little mixing college in Oregon. These underlined are of course medical subjects and would defeat the purpose of chiropractic accreditation as they are already recognized by the proper agency in the Office of Education.

With proper accreditation we can straighten out this Oregon law and others similar. For your information also, Ted, only seven states allow by statue language the practice of physio-physical therapy by chiropractors: Florida, Oregon, Nevada, Alaska, North Dakota, Kansas, and Maryland.

Physical therapy, physio-therapy, electrotherapy, hydrotherapy, minor surgery, dietetics, eye, ear, nose and throat practice, diagnosis, etc., are practices other than chiropractic and must not be included in either standard courses or electives for accreditation... (Rutherford, 1968).

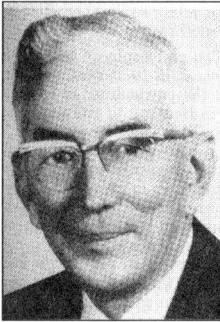

Figure 19-1: William D. Harper, D.C.

Increasing contacts between chiropractic educators and the U.S. Office of Education (USOE) made it clear that one important barrier to federal recognition of any chiropractic college accrediting agency was the divisiveness within the profession, and the lack of independence of proposed accrediting agencies from their respective sponsors (ACA and ICA). The ACA Council on Education, for example, was subordinate to the ACA Board of Directors; in principle, the Board of Directors had the authority to overrule any decision by the Council. Additionally, the government made it clear that a viable accrediting agency had to be well established and national in scope. With Palmer College of Chiropractic as an affiliate, the ICA's Chiropractic Education Commission could claim to represent the largest number of chiropractic students; the ACA's Council could claim the support of a majority of state boards of chiropractic examiners and a history dating to the mid-1930s. Adding to the dilemma was the federal agency's insistence that a chiropractic accrediting agency must show significant financial stability; how to do this without involving the professional associations seemed an impossible dilemma. It is noteworthy that by the late 1960s, the issues of non-profit status of the colleges and the need for a four year curriculum were no longer contested.

Nevertheless, the college presidents sought a forum for united action, one that could exercise some degree of independence from the professional associations (Harper, 1972). An "Association of American Chiropractic Colleges," which would have included both ICA and ACA-affiliated schools, was proposed in 1968 (Articles, 1968; Evaluative, 1968), but apparently was never chartered. At a meeting of college presidents called by William D. Harper, D.C. (Figure 19-1), president of the Texas Chiropractic College, on October 21-22, 1969, in Houston, George Haynes, president of the ACA Council on Education and chief administrator of the LACC, recommended "in principle"

...the following reorganization plan with the statement that the name, number of respective representatives, and even the addition of groups to be represented was open for modification.

1. Name - "The Council on Chiropractic Education."

2. Composition - Institutional members composed of one official representative on the administration level of each member College.

Accrediting Commission composed of representatives from the Chiropractic Colleges, Council of State Chiropractic Examining Boards, International Chiropractic Association and American Chiropractic Association.

3. Purpose - The Council on Chiropractic Education is an autonomous national organization advocating high standards of quality in chiropractic education, establishing criteria of institutional excellence, evaluating and accrediting colleges through its Accrediting Commission, and publishing lists of those institutions which conform to its standards and policies.

The Council on Chiropractic Education is sponsored and supported but not governed by the American Chiropractic Association, the International Chiropractic Association and the Council of State Chiropractic Examining Boards.

Vote on Accreditation - The Accrediting Commission would decide by vote accreditation status. Decisions of the Accrediting Commission on accreditation status may be appealed to The Council on Chiropractic Education (Haynes, 1969).

This proposal, which eventually became the basic plan of organization for today's CCE, was rejected by majority vote of the 11 U.S. chiropractic college presidents in attendance. Several of the ICA schools construed Haynes' proposal as a plan to "absorb" the ICA-affiliated schools into the existing structure of the ACA's Council. Several presidents also objected to the inclusion of non-college representatives on the Accrediting Commission. They feared that "members of the practicing profession and representatives from non-chiropractic academic world were not knowledgeable of the problems of chiropractic education and would tend to demand or impose educational demands that our colleges could not accept" (Haynes, 1969). The ACA college leader noted, however, that based upon his many contacts with the USOE:

Joint professional and school representation appears to be prevalent in the composition of those HEW approved and recognized agencies to grant specialized accreditation to professional schools such as, medicine, dentistry, optometry, etc. (Haynes, 1969).

An alternative proposition was offered by Harper and seconded by David Palmer, D.C. (see Figure 19-2). Articles of incorporation and by-laws for an agency comprised exclusively of college leaders were distributed to the group:

1. Name - "The Association of Chiropractic Colleges."

2. Composition - "The association is and shall be comprised of the presidents, or their chief executive officer or their designated representatives of each of the member Chiropractic Colleges in the United States." (To be called Trustees.)

3. Purpose - "...Specifically and without limitation of the generality of the foregoing, to inspect from time to time all duly recognized chiropractic educational institutes, to set standards, rules and regulations for the administration and conduct thereof, to issue certificates of recognition to withhold or withdraw such certificates and to do all things and have such other powers necessary in order to carry out a complete program of accreditation of chiropractic educational colleges and..."

4. Vote on Accreditation - "A majority vote of all Trustees either in person or by proxy shall be required to accredit a college or, to remove a college from the accredited list" (Haynes, 1969).

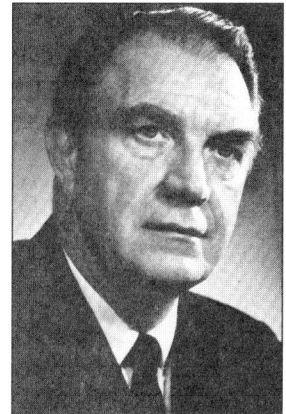

Figure 19-2: David D. Palmer, D.C.

Despite the skepticism expressed by Rex A. Wright, D.C., president of the Council of State Chiropractic Examining Boards, that the government might accredit an agency whose accreditation mechanism was comprised exclusively of executives of member institutions (Haynes, 1969), six college presidents (see Table 19-2) signed the articles of incorporation for the Association of Chiropractic Colleges (ACC) (Federal, 1970). These were filed with the State of Iowa in Scott County on November 3, 1969 (Articles, 1969). Two weeks later ACC's first inspection, of the Texas Chiropractic College, was conducted by Drs. Carl Cleveland, Jr., H. Ronald Frogley, William Kalas, Joseph Mazzarelli and Ted McCarrel (chairman). Palmer College was inspected in mid-December, and received initial approval, with stipulation that it be re-inspected annually. The Texas College was not approved (Association, 1971), and by 1972 had withdrawn from the ACC.

The ACA Council on Education's regulations stipulated that member institutions could not concurrently hold status with another chiropractic accrediting agency. Accordingly, the formation of the ACC in 1969 by the Columbia, Logan and Texas schools greatly reduced the number of ACA-affiliated schools. By the decade's end, only three chiropractic colleges could claim to be "fully accredited" by the ACA's Council (see Table 19-3). The Council's claim to be nationally representative of chiropractic education, considered essential for a favorable rating by the USOE (Haynes, 1970), was therefore further weakened.

Table 19-2: Founders of the Association of Chiropractic Colleges, 1969 (Articles, 1969)

Signatories
Carl S. Cleveland, Jr., D.C., President, Cleveland Chiropractic College of Kansas City
Carl S. Cleveland, Sr., D.C., President, Cleveland Chiropractic College of Los Angeles
William N. Coggins, D.C., President, Logan College of Chiropractic
William D. Harper, D.C., President, Texas Chiropractic College
Ernest G. Napolitano, D.C., President, Columbia Institute of Chiropractic
David D. Palmer, D.C., President, Palmer College of Chiropractic

Canadian Memorial Chiropractic College, Toronto, Ont.	*Los Angeles College of Chiropractic, Glendale, Calif.
Cleveland Chiropractic College, Kansas City, Mo.	*National College of Chiropractic, Lombard, Ill.
Cleveland Chiropractic College, Los Angeles, Calif.	Northwestern College of Chiropractic, St. Paul, Minn.
Columbia Institute of Chiropractic, New York, N.Y.	Palmer College of Chiropractic, Davenport, Ia.
*Lincoln Chiropractic College, Indianapolis, Ind.	Texas Chiropractic College, Pasadena, Tex.
Logan College of Chiropractic, St. Louis, Mo.	Western States Chiropractic College, Portland, Ore.

Table 19-3: Schools of chiropractic in 1970 (Hariman, 1970, pp. 40-1). *"Fully Accredited" by the ACA Council on Eduction.

Chapter 20

FEDERAL RECOGNITION
AND THE ACCREDITATION WARS

The fourth quarter of the first chiropractic century began with multiple achievements in the educational realm. The first of these was the National College's success in obtaining regional accreditation through registration with the state education department in New York:

SED REGISTERS FIRST CHIROPRACTIC SCHOOL

The New York Education Department has approved the professional education program of the National College of Chiropractic, Lombard, Illinois. This is the first chiropractic education program in the country to be approved by the Department under the requirements of the law which became effective January 1, 1968. As a result, persons completing the approved program will be eligible for admission to the New York professional licensing examination in chiropractic.

The registration of this program is the culmination of three years of collaborative effort between the school and the Department, according to Elliott E. Leuallen, assistant commissioner for professional education. During this time, the faculty has been augmented and curriculum revised and the program now meets New York State requirements. In announcing the registration, Leuallen said, "It reflects the dedication of the administration and faculty in their pursuit of excellence in the field" (Beideman, 1995, p. 263).

The New York victory was the result of three years of strenuous effort on the National College's part. The State Education Department's report on the National College in 1969, based upon its first site visit, had noted weaknesses in a variety of areas: an inadequate library budget, the educational credentials of the faculty (e.g., too few Ph.D. instructors in the basic sciences), academic "in-breeding" and lack of faculty development programs, the superficial depth with which some course topics were covered, a lack of "gross pathological material," and inadequate enforcement of pre-professional admissions criteria (Division, 1969). On this basis the Education Department denied National even provisional accreditation, because in the visitation team's opinion, the school could not rectify its deficiencies within two years. The College worked diligently to prove the team wrong, and succeeded on the occasion of its sixty-fifth anniversary (Beideman, 1971). Buoyed by this success, National proceeded to seek additional regional accreditation through the North Central Association of Colleges and Schools, a task that required an additional decade of work to accomplish (Beideman, 1995, pp. 264-5).

The American Medical Association (AMA) was stunned at the capacity of a chiropractic institution to meet the criteria for federally recognized accreditation. Indeed, the organization had believed that it was well along in its plans to "contain and eliminate" the chiropractic profession, as evidenced by an internal memorandum from the allopathic society's Committee on Quackery to the AMA trustees, dated January 4, 1971:

Since the American Medical Association Board of Trustees' decision at its meeting on November 2-3, 1963, to establish a Committee on Quackery, your Committee has considered its prime mission to be, first, the containment of chiropractic, and ultimately, the elimination of chiropractic.

Your Committee believes it is well along with its first mission and is, at the same time, moving toward the ultimate goal. This, then, might be considered a progress report on developments in the past seven years (Trever, 1972).

The AMA did what it could to reverse New York's decision. Ernest B. Howard, M.D., executive vice-president of the AMA, wrote to Ewald Nyquist, Commissioner of Education for New York. In a letter that betrayed his tautological reasoning, Howard objected to National's accreditation on the grounds that 37 of 76 faculty members held the "unrecognized D.C. degree," and that chiropractic was unscientific. Howard continued:

> ...the American Medical Association sincerely requests that the New York Board of Regents reconsider its approval of the professional education program of the National College of Chiropractic, Lombard, Illinois. We believe such approval is a disservice to the public in general, the healthcare consumers in particular and, above all, to the integrity of the accreditation system in the United States (Howard, 1972).

Registration with New York State was not withdrawn. This accreditation created not only a milestone for the college, but for the profession and its accreditation movement, particularly the American Chiropractic Association's (ACA's) Council on Education. National College students, at least those who were residents of New York, could now qualify for federally guaranteed loans and grants, because the New York education department was recognized by the U.S. Office of Education (USOE; a division of the DHEW/Department of Health, Education and Welfare) as a regional accrediting agency (Beideman, 1995, p. 264). National graduates were eligible to take the New York exam for licensure, the only new chiropractors permitted to do so under the terms of the state's 1963 licensing law (a number of D.C.s had received "grandfather" licenses when the law was first enacted). Most importantly, since National College was recognized by the ACA Council on Education, the school's regional accreditation by New York raised the Council's credibility in its quest for USOE status as a professional accrediting agency for chiropractic education.

The second major advance in the accreditation process was the separation of the ACA Council on Education from the parent organization (ACA), and its independent incorporation as the Council on Chiropractic Education (CCE). Prompted by the USOE's concerns about the independence from political influence of a chiropractic accrediting agency (e.g., Haynes, 1970), and perhaps also by the example set by the Association of Chiropractic Colleges (ACC), the CCE was chartered in 1971 as "an autonomous body and the American Chiropractic Association and the Federation of Chiropractic Examiners approved sponsorship of the Council. The International Chiropractors' Association (ICA) gracefully declined to sponsor the CCE, though a place for them has been kept open" (Chirogram, 1974).

With the formation of the CCE, the struggle between the two agencies (ACC and CCE) heated up. In March 1971, William Harper withdrew the Texas Chiropractic College from the ACC, ostensibly because it had been offered "full accreditation by the Education Commission of the A.C.A. and $19,000 provided that Texas College withdrew its application from the Association of Chiropractic Colleges by March 15" (A brief, undated). The CCE's application to USOE was rejected in May 1971 (Ottina, 1971); the following month George Haynes, D.C., M.S. was appointed to chair the Council's "HEW Application Committee" (Haynes, 1972a). Haynes was joined in his effort by John Fisher, Ed.D., CCE Director of Education, and Orval L. Hidde, D.C., J.D. (see Figure 20-1), CCE legal counsel and the new president of the Council (see Table 20-1). Although the CCE's independence from the ACA and the Council's solicitation of support from the International Chiropractors' Association (ICA) satisfied part of USOE's continuing criticism, the federal agency was not willing to recognize two chiropractic agencies, and neither could claim to represent the entire profession nationally, a stipulation for any professional accrediting body.

Pressure for the two agencies to amalgamate came from many quarters, including various state boards of chiropractic examiners (e.g., Fischer, 1972), the Federation of Chiropractic Licensing Boards (FCLB; formerly the Council of State Chiropractic Examining Boards), the National Board of Chiropractic Examiners (NBCE) (Holman, 1974) and, indirectly, the AMA (Frogley, 1973c; Napolitano, 1973b; Roden, 1972; Wright, 1972a). Representatives of the two agencies met outside Chicago in May 1972 to discuss their differences and attempt a merger (Frogley, 1972a; Minutes, 1972), but disagreed over whether the ACC should merge with CCE

Table 20-1: Officers of the Council on Chiropractic Education, 1972 (CCE, 1984; see Appendix A)

Orval L. Hidde, D.C., J.D., President
Leonard J. Fay, D.C., N.D., Vice-President
A. Earl Homewood, D.C., N.D., LL.B., Secretary-Treasurer
Herbert E. Hinton, D.C., Chairman, Commission on Accreditation

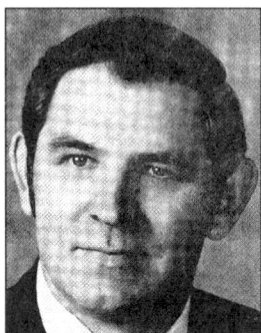

Figure 20-1: Orval L. Hidde, D.C., J.D.

versus the creation of a new, combined organization. Representatives of the ACC were invited to be guest participants at the CCE's regularly scheduled session in June (Hidde, 1972a), but declined the invitation in favor of "joint meetings that are set for the specific purpose of discussing methods, procedures and criteria to achieve a one-voice representation for our chiropractic colleges" (Napolitano, 1972). In August the FCLB issued the following resolution:

> Recognizing the importance and urgency in regard to time, the importance of presenting one plan to the proper agencies, the importance in regard to the future of Chiropractic in solving other controversies;
>
> Be it resolved that all accreditation criteria material from ACC and CCE be submitted to a binding arbitration committee for the purpose of establishing one accreditating [sic] agency, for final presentation to the proper agencies: the committee to consist of one specialist in accreditation from each agency, the third to be selected by the Federation of Licensing Boards and be agreeable to ACC and CCE. Expense of the third arbitrator will be shared by ACC and CCE.
>
> Furthermore, a written acceptance or rejection must be reported to the secretary of the Federation within sixty days.
>
> Resolution passed unanimously by roll call vote. (Hastings, 1972)

The ACC (see Table 20-2) agreed to binding arbitration, and appointed its educational consultant, Ted McCarrel, Ph.D., a former administrator at the University of Iowa and former president of Cottey College, to represent it (Coggins, 1972). The CCE apparently did not officially agree to arbitration as proposed by the FCLB (Marty, 1973), but agreed to several joint meetings with the ACC. Considerable animosity continued between the two agencies. In June 1972, the Florida State Board of Chiropractic Examiners revised its regulations so as to accept applications for licensure only from graduates of schools accredited by the CCE (Vogel, 1972); Utah followed suit in July (McGinn, 1972). In August 1972, the ACC voted to bring suit against the licensing authorities in New Jersey, Utah, and other jurisdictions which required applicants for licensure to have graduated from a CCE-accredited college (Frogley, 1972b). In February of the following year Michael P. Casey of the law firm of Evans, Hoemeke and Casey advised the ACC that the licensing authorities in the states of Connecticut, Minnesota and Vermont were the most vulnerable to an ACC challenge (Casey, 1973). However, the attorney cautioned that the strongest point in any law suit was the CCE's policy which prohibited its member institutions from being accredited by more than one chiropractic agency, a policy that CCE could easily rescind. The possibility of a "multi-state action" charging conspiracy between the CCE, ACA and the FCLB was also considered.

Table 20-2: Officers and Accrediting Commission of the Association of Chiropractic Colleges, 1972 (CCE Archives)

Officers:
President: Dr. William N. Coggins, President, Logan College of Chiropractic, St. Louis MO
Vice-President: Dr. Carl S. Cleveland, Jr., President, Cleveland Chiropractic College, Kansas City MO
Secretary-Treasurer: Dr. Ernest G. Napolitano, President, Columbia Institute of Chiropractic, New York

Accrediting Commission:
Chairman: Dr. H. Ronald Frogley, Executive Vice-President, Palmer College of Chiropractic (College member)
Dr. Ernest G. Napolitano, President, Columbia Institute of Chiropractic (College member)
Dr. William N. Coggins, President, Logan College of Chiropractic (College member)
Secretary: Dr. Carl S. Cleveland, Jr., President, Cleveland Chiropractic College, Kansas City MO (College member)
Dr. William Kalas, Glendale, Arizona (State Board representative)
Dr. Joseph P. Mazzarelli, Pennsaaken, New Jersey (Field practitioner)
Ted McCarrel, Ph.D., Sun City, Arizona (Public representative)

In August 1972, the *ACA Journal of Chiropractic* published an article which claimed that the CCE's standards "are superior to the ACC standards in a number of major areas critical to quality chiropractic education" (Wright, 1972a), a judgment shared by the Kansas State Board of Healing Arts (Coggins et al., 1972; Kansas, undated). At an FCLB meeting in August 1972, attended by representatives of ACC and CCE, Wright asserted that the ACC's publicly released articles of incorporation had been altered so as "to mask the actual focus of power in the college presidents to accredit themselves, giving the impression that the [ACC's] Accrediting Commission does the accrediting, when in fact, its function is only advisory" (Wright, 1972b). This charge was later denied by the ACC (Frogley, 1972c). William N. Coggins, president of ACC, countered by pointing out several apparent conflicts of interest, in that Wright was "a Member of the Examining Boards and also of CCE," while Steve Owens, D.C. was "a member of the Examining Boards, President of the ACA House of Delegates and on the School Board of National College" (Frogley, 1972b).

Despite this friction, plans proceeded for binding arbitration and/or amalgamation of the ACC and CCE. At an "unofficial meeting" in Houston in November 1972, representatives from both agencies met to outline the structure of a single, unified accrediting commission with representation from the ACA, ICA, FCLB and public members (Hidde, 1972b; Memo, 1972). The group (see Table 20-3) met again in Chicago in December, and agreed that the governing body of the combined Council would consist of members of the accrediting commission plus the presidents or representatives of all member schools (Frogley, 1972d). Frogley's (1972d) minutes of this meeting indicate a number of other points of agreement:

> (1) Voting. It was proposed that a three-fourths vote in the Council on all matters requiring a roll call vote which was requested by a member of the Council. Approved.

> (2) The Council will formulate criteria requiring a three-fourths vote for approval. Approved.

> (3) Acceptance of representatives from ICA, ACA, or Federation [FCLB] will be by approval of the Council and a three-fourths vote. Each will be asked for a list of five names, one of which must be approved. NOT APPROVED.

> (4) ICA, ACA and Federation will select their own representatives. Schools will select the school representatives. The new Council will select the lay members. If any group does not appoint a representative, the new Council will appoint a member to fill that slot on a one-year term basis until that post is filled by the group not being represented. Approved.

> (5) Terms for the Commission will be staggered on a one, two, three year basis to begin with. Terms to be selected by "lot". Subsequent terms will be of three years each. Approved.

> (6) Name. Agreed for a new name to be selected. Approved. Suggested name - Chiropractic Education Association or Association of Chiropractic Education. No decision.

> (7) CCE declined to withdraw their present application and it was decided that the ACC will submit their application as a protection. A committee composed of both ACC and CCE groups will go to the U.S. Office [USOE] for assistance in determining acceptable material for combining the two organizations without losing the integrity of their performance record. This will be after a meeting with Mr. Dickey and Mr. Proffitt [of USOE] on December 18 and 19.

Both sides sought a meeting with the USOE to determine the most effective means of amalgamation or the creation of a new agency, such that the progress made by each group was not wasted. A binding arbitration session, scheduled for late in January, 1973 was canceled by the CCE president with FCLB approval until after the CCE's most recent application to the USOE had been acted upon, much to the distress of the ACC (Frogley, 1973a&b). The ACC filed its application with the USOE in December 1972 (Marty, 1973), but was turned down in March 1973, as was the CCE's petition (Ottina, 1973a). The applications both the ACC and the CCE were reviewed by the AMA (Accreditation, 1973a), who requested and received "the opportunity of appearing as an opponent" (Fay, 1973a&b) and was granted 30 minutes of testimony before the USOE against each chiropractic agency.

In rejecting the CCE's application for recognition as a professional accrediting agency, the USOE provided a detailed set of criticisms (Proffitt, 1973a). These concerns included the fact that CCE's claim to be "national in the scope of its operation" was mitigated by the reality that it accredited only half of the chiropractic schools in the nation, and that these schools accounted for "less than 25 per cent" of the total students then enrolled in chiropractic colleges. Here in particular the ACC's rivalry was a distinct barrier to the CCE. The USOE also noted that the CCE could not yet truly claim to be accepted by "the chiropractic profession, its State associations, the chiropractic colleges," and that the profession had not yet decided to accept one accrediting agency over the other. Additionally, CCE's recognition by only a few of the nation's state licensing boards suggested to the federal agency that most jurisdictions did not view CCE schools to be superior to non-CCE accredited institutions. Accordingly, the USOE questioned the validity of CCE's assertion that it served a particular need, specifically the improvement of chiropractic education.

The USOE also challenged the Council's claim to impartiality on the grounds that the president of a CCE college had described the CCE as "a deck stacked against the colleges for political control of not only their actions but now their thinking" (Proffitt, 1973a). The CCE's exclusionary policies, wherein member colleges were prohibited from seeking concurrent accreditation by another chiropractic agency, were seen to reflect the historic "gulf" between ACA and ICA, and were consistent with the notion of an ongoing political agenda. The Council's sole reliance upon the ACA for funding (by route of the Foundation for Chiropractic Education and Research) was also viewed with suspicion. The USOE encouraged the CCE to

ACC Representatives	CCE Representatives
William N. Coggins, D.C. (ACC President), Logan College of Chiropractic	Orval L. Hidde, D.C., J.D. (CCE President), private practice
D.P. Casey, D.C., Logan College of Chiropractic	Leonard Fay, D.C., N.D., National College of Chiropractic
Ernest G. Napolitano, D.C., Columbia Institute of Chiropractic	George H. Haynes, D.C., N.D., M.S., Los Angeles College of Chiropractic
David D. Palmer, B.S., D.C., Palmer College of Chiropractic	John B. Wolfe, B.S., D.C., Northwestern College of Chiropractic
Elmer L. Crowder, D.C., Palmer College of Chiropractic	
H. Ronald Frogley, M.A., D.C., Palmer College of Chiropractic	

Table 20-3: Participants at the combined meeting of the Association of Chiropractic Colleges (ACC) and the Council on Chiropractic Education (CCE), December 2-3, 1972, Chicago (CCE Archives)

"take every necessary measure to assure that its actions and functions are consistent with the formation of an independent judgment regarding the quality of chiropractic education" (Proffitt, 1973a).

The federal agency further faulted the CCE in that the agency's self-studies and those submitted to it by member colleges, although replete with data, were not truly evaluative nor self-critical, particularly reports bearing on the "depth or quality" of basic science instruction. The USOE asked that future reports be more "probing," and that they specifically list the strengths and weakness of the educational area under study. The federal office also questioned the Council's adherence to its own standards, in that several schools had been continued in their "provisionally accredited" status beyond the one year limit set by the CCE (Proffitt, 1973a). Lastly, the USOE recommended that the CCE require its accredited schools to list in their college catalogs not only

> Table 20-4: Participants in the binding arbitration meeting of the Association of Chiropractic Colleges (ACC) and the Council on Chiropractic Education (CCE), Rosemont, Illinois, November 10-11, 1973
>
> *Representatives of ACC*:
>   William Coggins, D.C. (ACC President); Ernest G. Napolitano, D.C.; David D. Palmer, D.C.
> *Representatives of CCE*:
>   Leonard E. Fay, D.C., N.D.; George H. Haynes, D.C., N.D.; Orval L. Hidde, D.C., J.D. (CCE President)
> *Observers*:
>   D.P. Casey, D.C. (Logan College); Elmer R. Crowder, D.C. (Palmer College); John A. Fisher, Ed.D. (CCE); H. Ronald Frogley, D.C. (Palmer College); Harold Kieffer, D.C. (ACA); W. Heath Quigley, D.C., (Palmer College); Richard Vincent, D.C. (FCLB)

the degrees held by the faculty, but also the year and institution which had awarded each degree.

The ACC's application for recognition by the USOE met with similar criticisms (Proffitt, 1973b). The government questioned the scope of coverage (national or something less), need for and impartiality of the ACC, all of which spoke directly to the competition between the two chiropractic accrediting bodies. As it had in the case of the CCE, USOE found the ACC's self-studies to lack critical self-evaluation (see Appendix C). The federal body also felt that ACC did too little to inform the public of its policies and accredited schools. ACC was challenged to better meet the information requests from the USOE, particularly those related to financial matters, and to reconsider its willingness to accredit schools that had failed the standards of the CCE (Proffitt, 1973b). Most damaging, the USOE noted that ACC did not enforce its own standards for pre-professional training among member schools, and did not include basic scientists on its college visitation teams, thereby limiting the expertise available for evaluating basic science instruction. Indeed, Napolitano of the Columbia Institute of Chiropractic in New York was of the opinion that "all too often the D.C. degree has been subordinated to the baccalaureate, Masters and Ph.D. I am not of the opinion that only baccalaureate, Masters or Ph.D.'s are qualified to teach in the Basic Sciences" (Napolitano, 1973a). To add to the agency's shortcomings, its "Candidate for Accreditation," Cleveland Chiropractic College of Los Angeles, had still not acquired non-profit status (Napolitano, 1974).

The failures of the ACC and the CCE to be recognized by the government prompted yet further "unofficial" meetings to discuss amalgamation of the accrediting agencies (Hidde, 1973). A second binding arbitration meeting (see Table 20-4) was held on 10-11 November 1973 outside Chicago (Accreditation, 1973b). The explicit purpose of the meeting was either "to establish a single accrediting agency for chiropractic education acceptable" to the USOE, or to "continue the accrediting program of the ACC and CCE under one authority" (Contract, 1973). Guidelines for a single accrediting agency were signed by Hidde and Coggins, but the following day (November 12) George Haynes wrote, in his capacity as Chairman of CCE's HEW Application Committee, to the U.S. Commissioner of Education to request a review of "recent changes in the structure and accrediting procedures of the Accrediting Commission of the Council on Chiropractic Education" (Ottina, 1973b). The Commissioner was impressed with the CCE's progress and requested that observers from the USOE accompany the CCE's site visitation teams in March 1974. The ACC, meanwhile, reaffirmed its commitment to seek a single college accrediting agency independent of either national professional association (ACC, 1974), and noted that the student bodies in its schools accounted for "more than 71%" of chiropractic students in the United States (see Table 20-5).

The ACC continued to hope for further meetings to amalgamate the accrediting bodies (Coggins, 1974), but aware that CCE might be within striking distance of federal recognition, the Association's consultant, Ted McCarrel, advised the ACC to consider all possibilities (McCarrel, 1974):

  a. Should arbitration develop, just how far are the [ACC] members willing to go?

  b. Should CCE get approval, where do the ACC colleges go from that point? Perish the thought.

  c. How far are the members prepared to go in enlarging the Accrediting Commission of ACC?

  d. Any changes to be made in the officer and accrediting commission setup?

  e. What can be done to make the gamble ACC took in waiting for binding arbitration fully communicated to the profession and the Office of Education?

  f. What effect on ACC does all the attempts of the colleges to go the regional and/or state routes have in the future?

  g. Others too numerous to mention.

Schools accredited by ACC	Students	Schools accredited by CCE	Students
Cleveland Chiropractic College/LA*	485	Los Angeles College of Chiropractic	337
Cleveland Chiropractic College/KC	340	National College of Chiropractic	600
Columbia Institute of Chiropractic	260	Northwestern College of Chiropractic	130
Logan College of Chiropractic	410	Texas Chiropractic College	145
Palmer College of Chiropractic	<u>1965</u>	Western States Chiropractic College	<u>140</u>
Total students in ACC schools	3460	Total students in CCE schools	1352
% of total U.S. chiropractic students	71.9	% of total U.S. chiropractic students	28.1

Table 20-5: Numbers of students enrolled in U.S. chiropractic colleges circa 1974, according to the Association of Chiropractic Colleges (ACC, 1974) *Candidate for Accreditation by the Association of Chiropractic Colleges

The ACC attempted to reactivate its application to USOE, but was ignored; only the CCE's petition for recognition was considered at the federal agency's May 1974 hearings. The struggle, at least between ACC and CCE, was over. Although the ACC's charter continued in force until August 1980, the organization soon faded from the scene (Armstrong et al., 1979, p. 13; Gelardi, unpublished). Sensing the imminence of CCE's triumph, the FCLB resolved to recommend that its members (state boards of chiropractic examiners) revise statutes and administrative codes to require the future license applicants to show evidence of having graduated from a college recognized by the CCE (Vincent, 1974). On 26 August 1974 the CCE was informed by T.H. Bell, U.S. Commissioner of Education, that the CCE's accrediting commission would be added to the Commissioner's "list of Nationally Recognized Accrediting Agencies and Associations" (Chirogram, 1975). Bell's letter to Hidde, chairman of the CCE's Commission on Accreditation, indicated:

> The Advisory Committee on Accreditation and Institutional Eligibility, at its meeting on May 22-24, examined the petition of the Accrediting Commission of The Council on Chiropractic Education for inclusion on the Commissioner of Education's list of Nationally Recognized accrediting Agencies and Associations within the meaning of Chapter 33, Title 38, U.S. Code and subsequent legislation. On the basis of evidence submitted in conformity with the Criteria published in

the Federal Register of January 16, 1969, the Committee has recommended that the Accrediting Commission of The Council on Chiropractic Education be recognized for a period of one year.

In making its recommendation, the Committee determined that the instructions for self-study provided by the Accrediting Commission could be improved by requiring more faculty-student participation in the self-study process and by providing for a more substantive institutional self-analysis, using the information required by the self-study questionnaire. In addition, the Educational Standards for Chiropractic Colleges of the CCE Accrediting Commission appears to the Committee to be too permissive for the rather considerable accreditation job now faced by the chiropractic profession. It was the Committee's judgment that the liberal use of the word "should," rather than the word "shall," in the various statements of standards does not provide the outside observer with a reliable guide to actual Commission enforcement of policy. Similarly, the criteria utilized for "Recognized Candidate for Accreditation" were judged by the Committee to lack clarity regarding the level of compliance with standards which would indicate reasonable assurance that the institution could achieve accredited status within the prescribed three year period.

I concur with the recommendation of the Committee and am pleased to inform you that the Accrediting Commission of The Council on Chiropractic Education hereby is added to the Commissioner's list of Nationally Recognized Accrediting Agencies and Associations for a period of one year.

Please accept my warm congratulations to the Accrediting Commission for its achievements to date and its promise for the future.

Sincerely, T.H. Bell, U.S. Commissioner of Education (Bell, 1974)

Hidde, who had just been succeeded as CCE president by Leonard Fay (see Figure 20-2), had reason to rejoice. Moreover, the following year, on December 11, Bell informed Hidde that the CCE's initial one year recognition by USOE would be extended for a further three years (Bell, 1975). The long path to federal recognition, extending over 40 years (e.g., Watkins, 1934), had at long last been traversed, and the outsiders had become a part of the establishment. It was a time for reflection and self-congratulations (Martin, 1974), and at the top of many lists of those most deserving of recognition was George H. Haynes, who had served as president of CCE from 1961 to 1972 (see Table 20-6), and then for several years as chair of the Council's liaison committee to USOE (Bromley, 1975). In 1976 Haynes retired from his leadership of the Los Angeles College of Chiropractic (LACC) with the rank of President Emeritus (Rehm, 1980, p. 329). By the time he stepped down from LACC's presidency, California had amended its regulations to require graduation from a CCE-accredited college as a condition for licensure (Musick, 1979).

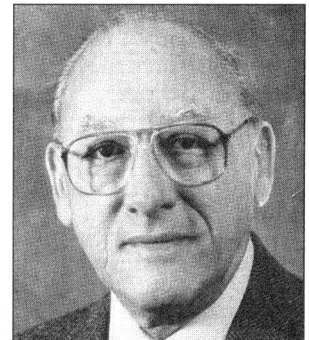

Figure 20-2: Leonard E. Fay, D.C., N.D.

The CCE's success in winning federal recognition produced quick action in many regulatory bodies. Thirty-three days after the CCE's achievement, the FCLB issued the following statement:

Be it resolved that the Federation of Chiropractic Licensing Boards recommends to the various state licensing boards that a rule of law be adopted, either by statute or by administrative regulation wherein it be provided that all applicants for licensure who matriculate in a chiropractic college after October 1, 1975 must present evidence of having graduated from a chiropractic college accredited by the Accrediting Commission of the Council on Chiropractic Education, Inc. (Hidde, 1975a).

In the next few years the Council achieved a number of additional milestones. The CCE was recognized by the Council on Specialized Accrediting Agencies (CSAA) during the Fay administration (1975), by the New York State Education Department (which accepted CCE accreditation in 1976 in lieu of its own evaluations of individual chiropractic colleges), and by the Council on Postsecondary Accreditation in 1976 (Council, 1984; see Appendix A). In January, 1980 the ICA joined the ACA and FCLB as financial sponsors of the CCE and took its seat on the governing board (Council, 1984), thereby adding intra-professional credibility to the Council. Although the two national professional associations continued to feud over many issues, they were at long last united in their support of a single, national accrediting agency for chiropractic education. The ACA "renewed its efforts to get state legislatures to amend practice acts and insert the requirement that to apply to practice within the state, a chiropractor must be a graduate of a college approved by the CCE" or to produce regulatory changes with the same effect (Armstrong et al., 1979, pp. 14, 18, 25-6, 42, 92-104). Also in 1980, the federal government authorized guaranteed student loans of up to $50,000 in its Health Education Assistance Loan (HEAL) program (McAndrews & McAndrews, 1995). Within a short period the majority of U.S. chiropractic colleges were persuaded of the necessity of CCE accreditation (see Table 20-7).

The credibility of the CCE, its policies and procedures prompted the formation of similar agencies in other countries. Communications with the newly forming CCE/Canada commenced during the Fay administration (1974-76), and during James Mertz's presidency (1978-80) the American council recognized the judgments of CCE (Canada) and the Australasian Council on Chiropractic Education (Council, 1984). Full reciprocity between CCE (Canada) and CCE (USA) was established in 1982, and during Ernest Napolitano's presidency (1982-84) the CCE considered the formation of an "International Committee on Accrediting Agencies for Chiropractic Colleges" (Council, 1984).

Napolitano's presidency of the CCE represented the successful integration of the leadership of the previously ICA-accredited and ACA-accredited schools. The president of the Columbia Institute of Chiropractic (renamed the New York Chiropractic College in 1977) had served as an officer of the ACC, and now Napolitano made the transition to leadership of the CCE. Yet, still the accreditation wars went on. New battle lines were formed, this time between the CCE and several newly formed chiropractic colleges, most notably the Sherman College of Chiropractic (SCC) in Spartanburg, South Carolina.

The CCE's continuing adventures involved new leadership (see Table 20-8). Fisher was succeeded as Director of Education by Richard Timmins, Ed.D., whose brief service was ended when he took over as president of Western States Chiropractic College in 1976. Ralph G. Miller, Ed.D. became executive secretary of the CCE, a post he held for nearly 20 years.

Table 20-7: Chiropractic colleges' status with the Council on Chiropractic Education in June 1975 (Current, 1975). RCA: Recognized Candidate for Accreditation.

College	Status with CCE
Los Angeles College of Chiropractic	Accredited
National College of Chiropractic	Accredited
Northwestern College of Chiropractic	Accredited
Texas Chiropractic College	Accredited
Western States Chiropractic College	Recognized Candidate for Accreditation
Canadian Memorial Chiropractic College	Affiliate
Anglo-European College of Chiropractic	Affiliate
Palmer College of Chiropractic	Has applied for RCA Status
Columbia Institute of Chiropractic	Has applied for RCA Status
Sherman College of Chiropractic	Has applied for Correspondent Status
Logan College of Chiropractic	Letter of Intent
Life College of Chiropractic	Letter of Intent
Cleveland Chiropractic College - KC	Letter of Intent
Cleveland Chiropractic College - LA	Letter of Intent

Table 20-8: Educational administrators of the NCA and ACA Councils on Education, the Foundation for Chiropractic Education and Research, and the Council on Chiropractic Education (Schierholz, 1986)

Term	Administrator	Title(s)
1941-1961	John J. Nugent, D.C.	Director of Education, National Chiropractic Association
1961-1964	Dewey Anderson, Ph.D.	Educational Consultant, National Chiropractic Association, Director of Education, National Chiropractic Association, Director of Education, American Chiropractic Association
1964-1974	John Fisher, Ed.D.	Director of Education, American Chiropractic Association, Research Administrator, Foundation for Chiropractic Education & Research
1974-1976	Richard Timmins, Ed.D.	Director of Education, Foundation for Chiropractic Education & Research
1976-1995	Ralph Miller, Ed.D.	Director of Education, Foundation for Chiropractic Education & Research, Executive Secretary (later, Executive Vice-President), Council on Chiropractic Education
1995-present	Paul Walker, Ph.D.	Executive Vice-President, Council on Chiropractic Education

Sherman College of Straight Chiropractic

Sherman College of Chiropractic (renamed Sherman College of Straight Chiropractic in December 1976) was the inspiration of Thom A. Gelardi, D.C. (see Figure 20-3), a 1957 graduate of the Palmer School of Chiropractic. Gelardi's commitment to establish a "college dedicated to locating, analyzing, and correcting vertebral subluxations" and to a vitalistic belief system was made in August 1972 (Gelardi, unpublished). On September 18 of that year he wrote to Ernest Napolitano in the latter's capacity as secretary-treasurer of the ACC, to inquire about membership and accreditation criteria (Gelardi, 1972). President Gelardi's intention to seek ACC accreditation was short-circuited by the CCE's 1974 recognition by USOE. The school (see Figure 20-4) was incorporated on 11 January 1973 (Thompson, 1991), and its formation was announced in *Today's Chiropractic* in April (Gelardi, 1973).

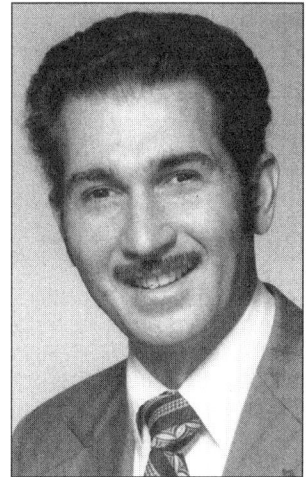

Figure 20-3: Thomas A. Gelardi, D.C.

The first or "pioneer" class (see Figure 20-5), comprised of 63 (Thompson, 1991) or 67 students (Strauss, 1994, p. 220) including Gelardi's wife Betty, matriculated on 27 September 1973 at the first of several temporary campuses in Spartanburg. They graduated in September 1976. By midyear of 1976 Gelardi was also contemplating the formation of a "branch or satellite college" in Northern California (Musick, 1979, pp. 12, 93).

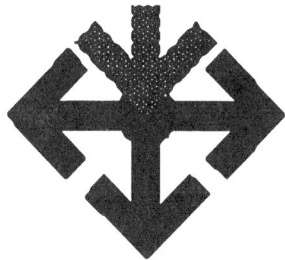

Figure 20-4: Symbol of the Sherman College of Straight Chiropractic

Although SCC did not follow through on its California plans, the idea may have led to the formation of the Pacific States College of Chiropractic on 9 November 1976, and the new school's first president, Thomas Vonder Haar, was first suggested by Gelardi (Musick, 1979, p. 13).

The SCC was named after Lyle W. Sherman, D.C., Ph.C. (see Figure 20-6), longtime Director of the B.J. Palmer Chiropractic Clinic in Davenport (Strauss, 1994, p. 219), member of the ICA Board of Control (1954-1966), director of the ICA's research department (Sherman, 1952) and mentor to Gelardi during the latter's student days at Palmer. Dr. Sherman became a sponsor of the college and a member of its first Advisory Board (see Table 20-9). Sherman's upper cervical adjustive methods (actually, B.J. Palmer's "Hole-in-One") became a strong feature of the institution's technique instruction (Strauss, 1994, p. 220). Palmer graduate Reggie Gold, (see Figure 20-7), who had previously served as dean of the Columbia Institute of Chiropractic, was recruited as dean and later served as vice-president of SCC (Gelardi, unpublished; Strauss, 1994, p. 230).

Sherman College encountered opposition even before it opened. David Palmer, president of the Palmer College of Chiropractic, objected to the SCC on the grounds that it competed for students with other ACC member institutions (Cleveland, personal communication). Gelardi (unpublished) notes that members of SCC's board of trustees were encour-

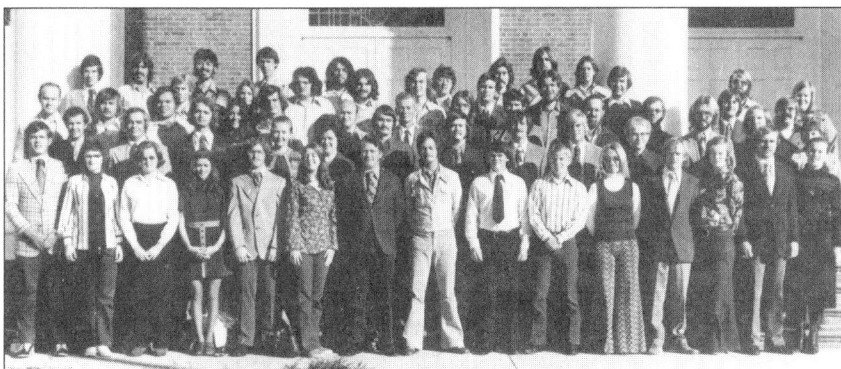

Figure 20-5: First class at the Sherman College of Straight Chiropractic in Spartanburg, South Carolina (courtesy of the Sherman College of Straight Chiropractic)

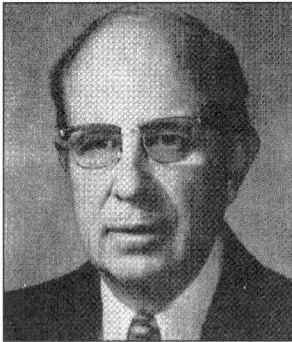

Figure 20-6: Lyle W. Sherman, D.C., Ph.C.

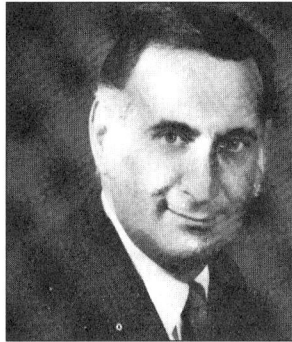

Figure 20-7: Reginald R. Gold, D.C., Ph.C.

aged to resign. Although several did resign, Earl Powel, Ph.D., editor and publisher of *Voice for Health*, resisted this pressure.

The imminent likelihood of CCE recognition by USOE prompted SCC to seek accreditation from the Council, and in February 1974, Gelardi and Marvin Buncher, D.C. met with the CCE and its Commission on Accreditation (COA) for the first of several discussions of the accreditation process (see Appendix D). The College's first application for recognition to COA was submitted in August 1974, when the Council and its COA were first recognized by USOE. Following an extensive process involving a revised application, a site visit by representatives of COA and numerous meetings, SCC's petition for provisional status with CCE was denied in July 1975. An appeal for reconsideration of its application was filed by SCC in October, but the CCE Appeal Panel "sustained the decision of the COA to deny the application of the SCC for Correspondent status (see Apprendix D). Gelardi (unpublished) suggests that the CCE/COA's decision was "political," in support of which contention he notes that SCC was cited for not teaching dissection, although other schools recognized by the Council (Texas College and Columbia Institute) also did not teach dissection at that time. Sherman's president also notes that the Council's standards held that chiropractors diagnose and treat human disease (see Table 20-10), a concept which SCC's board of trustees adamantly rejected as medical in character. The SCC found support for this view from the medical community (Kindig, 1976; Lehman, 1977, 1978). The college did not reapply for CCE recognition for nearly 20 years (Appendix D; Gelardi, unpublished).

Despite its lack of accreditation and the consequent inability of its graduates to sit for licensing exams in most American states, enrollment at the Sherman College of Straight Chiropractic (SCSC) grew to 300 by 1977. At this time the SCSC first occupied its present campus (see Figure 20-8) in Spartanburg, which grew to 81 acres (Gelardi, unpublished). The same year, the college was challenged by the state's legislature to acquire CCE accreditation or fold. The new law was overturned in 1978 after a tremendous political battle between SCSC and the South Carolina Chiropractic Association (Gelardi, unpublished).

Table 20-9: Members of the first Advisory Board of the Sherman College of Chiropractic (Gelardi, 1973)

George Banitch, D.C., Montclair NJ
W.G. Blair, D.C., Lubbock TX
William E. Cameron, D.C., Denver CO
R. Tyrrell Denniston, D.C., Baltimore
Harvey W. Dice, D.C., Memphis TN
Stephen Duff, D.C., San Rafael CA
Ben Evans, D.C., Council Bluffs IA
Robert E. Fitzgerald, D.C., Minneapolis
Charles G. Haynes, D.C., Everett WA
Peter Huggler, D.C., Switzerland
Warren Nolan, D.C., New Zealand
Ray McPike, D.C., Louisville KY
Clair O'Dell, D.C., Wyandotte MI
Earl Powell, Ph.D., Atlanta GA
Lyle W. Sherman, D.C., Spartanburg SC
S.C. Syverud, D.C., Mt. Horeb WI
E.S. Tooma, D.C., Lathrup Village MI
W.E. VanderStolp, D.C., Grand Rapids MI
George Wentland, D.C., Fresno CA

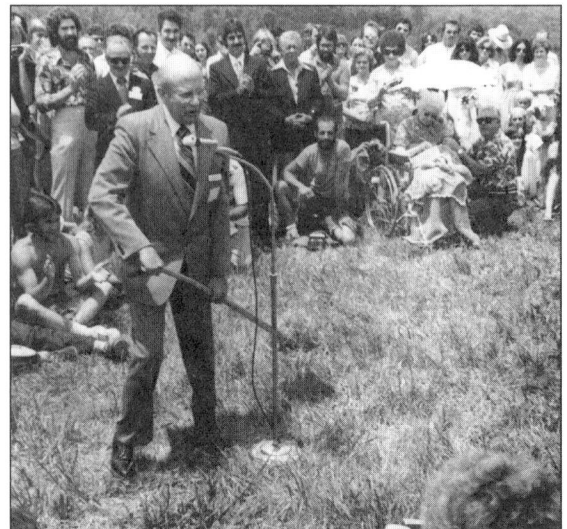

Figure 20-8: Groundbreaking ceremonies for SCSC's Spartanburg campus are conducted by Lyle Sherman.

Sherman's campaign in South Carolina was just the beginning of many legislative and judicial battles, the full breadth and depth of which are beyond the scope of this work. Strauss (1994) devotes a section of his Chapter 13 in *Refined by Fire: the Evolution of Straight Chiropractic* to the legal struggles between adherents to CCE and those who formed the Straight Chiropractic Academic Standards Association (SCASA) as an alternative accrediting agency for chiropractors. Sherman College was joined in this campaign by its sister school, the ADIO (Above-Down, Inside-Out) Institute of Straight Chiropractic, which was founded in 1977 by former SCC vice-president, Reggie Gold. The new Pennsylvania school commenced operations on 4 January 1978 in Levittown (Strauss, 1994, pp. 237-8), and produced chiropractors for more than 15 years.

Sherman College and the ADIO Institute sought to prevent CCE from obtaining further recognition by the federal agency, and brought an unsuccessful suit against the U.S. Commissioner of Education when the CCE was given a three-year renewal of its status in 1979 (Gelardi, unpublished; Strauss, 1994, p. 268). In a report prepared by the Chiropractic Foundation of America (Armstrong et al., 1979), a case was made that CCE had conspired with the ACA and the FCLB to control the profession and eliminate straight chiropractic through control of the educational system for chiropractors. This argument was undermined by CCE's recognition of several "traditional straight" and previously ACC-accredited institutions, such as the Cleveland, Columbia, and Palmer colleges.

However, SCSC's and ADIO's ideas of what "straight chiropractic" meant differed considerably from those of other straight chiropractors. In the case of ADIO founder Reggie Gold, these distinctions became so extreme that he "left the [straight chiropractic] movement in 1979 for almost four years to start Spinology" (Strauss, 1994, p. 259). Gold's spinology was a non-diagnostic, non-therapeutic ideology and practice offered through his "Church of the Triune of Life," which operated "Spinal Tutoriums" or schools in Philadelphia and San Francisco. Gold was adamant that his spinology was not chiropractic, and promotional brochures for his schools declared that the intent of his spinology practitioners was "to restore human beings to harmonious unity of mind, body and spirit for the fulfillment of their life potential." However, the content of his instructional program seemed to harken back to the early days of chiropractic education. Gold's Tutoriums offered a 12-month, 900-hour curriculum (see Table 20-11) in morning or evening classes for $3,000 tuition. Presumably taking his lead from D.D. Palmer's (1914) writings, Gold anticipated that practitioners of his new profession would be protected from prosecution for unlicensed practice under the religious freedom exemptions of many state medical practice acts.

Sherman College and the ADIO Institute persevered in their efforts to train chiropractors without diagnostic skills. Many legal actions followed, including a 1981 suit charging the CCE and the NBCE with restraint of trade (a violation of the Sherman-Clayton Anti-Trust Act) and an investigation of these charges by the U.S. Department of Justice (Strauss, 1994, pp. 269-70). Gelardi (unpublished) notes that the basis of the complaint to the Department of Justice involved a CCE policy which prevented faculty from CCE-accredited schools from lecturing at non-CCE colleges. The Council records that "The CCE participated as intervenor defendant in the U.S. District Court, Washington, D.C., in the case of Sherman College of Straight Chiropractic et al. (vs. U.S. Commissioner of Education). The result was a summary dismissal of the plaintiff's

---

Table 20-10: Excerpt from the foreword to the Council on Chiropractic Education's March 1978 *Educational Standards for Chiropractic Colleges*

> A **Doctor of Chiropractic** is a physician concerned with the health needs of the public as a member of the healing arts. He gives particular attention to the relationship of the structural and neurological aspects of the body in health and disease. He is educated in the basic and clinical sciences as well as in related health subjects.
>
> The purpose of his professional education is to prepare the doctor of chiropractic as a primary health care provider. As a portal of entry to the health delivery system the chiropractic physician must be well educated to diagnose, including, but not limited to, spinal analysis, to care for the human body in health and disease and to consult with, or refer to, other health care providers. It is this concept of the chiropractic physician which serves as the basis for interpretation of the Educational Standards for Chiropractic Colleges...
>
> The Council on Chiropractic Education has validated the "Educational Standards for Chiropractic Colleges." In doing so, it is aware of the importance of these professional colleges to the profession and to the public which it serves. These standards indicate the minimum education received in the approved colleges by doctors of chiropractic as primary physicians...

Table 20-11: Curricular content of the Philadelphia Spinal Tutorium, from a brochure circa 1980

Subject	Hours
Spinology Technic	240
Philosophy and Doctrine	120
Communications	60
Personal Development	60
Ethics & Jurisprudence	60
Innate Matter (Anatomy & Physiology)	60
Spinal Studies	60
Business Procedures & Management	60
Practical Experience	180
Total	900

charges on the part of Judge Hart; the decision reaffirmed the status of CCE as a reliable chiropractic accrediting agency" and that "U.S. Department of Justice satisfactorily closes civil investigation against CCE in that alleged antitrust violations were unfounded" (see Appendix A). Gelardi (unpublished), however, insists that the Justice Department action was dropped only after the CCE changed its policy, thereby no longer forbidding CCE college faculty from lecturing at non-CCE schools. Similar courtroom battles erupted over the years as graduates of the two new "straight" schools were alternately approved for and denied eligibility for licensure in various states. The financial costs to SCSC in pursuing these legal actions were enormous. Student enrollment had peaked in the mid-1980s at around 300-400 students (Gelardi, 1986), further stressing the institution and limiting its revenues.

SCASA Challenges the Establishment

The possibility that the USOE might consider recognition of a second chiropractic educational accrediting agency came to light in a 1978 letter from Ronald S. Pugsley of the USOE to Melvin J. Rosenthal, D.C. The viability of two agencies was ironic, in that the earlier struggle between CCE and ACC had been based, in part, on the premise that USOE would recognize one or the other, but not both. Pugsley wrote:

> We are sensitive to the "straight-mixer" controversy in the field of chiropractic. This particular issue seems to have regenerated itself in recent years with the initiation of some new schools of the "straight" persuasion. In our initial reviews of the Council on Chiropractic Education, which resulted in its recognition in 1974, our staff and the Commissioner's Advisory Committee on Accreditation and Institutional Eligibility attempted to ascertain if CCE accreditation was applicable to both "straight" and "mixer" schools. Our findings were that the CCE's standards, policies, and procedures were relevant to schools of both philosophies. As evidence that CCE continues to perform satisfactorily in this regard, we note that it has granted status to schools which we understand are schools of the "straight" persuasion, including Palmer College of Chiropractic and Life Chiropractic College.

> In response to your specific requests, however, we note the following:

> (1) It is possible for two accrediting agencies which function in the same field of program specialization to be recognized by the U.S. Commissioner of Education. Such is presently the case in four fields - physical therapy, practical nursing, medical assisting, and medical laboratory technician education.

> (2) Each accrediting agency recognized by the Commissioner is reviewed on its own merits, in accordance with the criteria and procedures set forth in the enclosed brochure. The burden of proof regarding establishing compliance with the criteria concerning "need" and "acceptance" is upon the applicant agency, and responses may differ from agency-to-agency. Needless to say, the two concepts are interrelated. Specifically, regarding need, an accrediting agency should show documentation that a need for accreditation exists in a particular field and that the need is being served by the agency... (Pugsley, 1978).

Buoyed by this option, Sherman and ADIO (which was given degree-granting status by the state of Pennsylvania in 1984, and the school was renamed Pennsylvania College of Straight Chiropractic; Strauss, 1994, p. 274), with the assistance of the Federation of Straight Chiropractic Organizations (FSCO), set to work to create the accrediting agency known as SCASA. The new agency was chartered in June, 1978 (Gelardi, unpublished). This project required years of work, but in December 1988, despite recommendations to the contrary from within the federal Department of Education (USDE, successor to USOE), the U.S. Secretary of Education, William Bennett, granted recognition to SCASA. SCASA's credibility had been increased in 1981, when Sherman College was granted "candidate status" by its regional accrediting body, the Southern

Association of Colleges and Schools (SACS). Full accreditation of SCSC by SACS was achieved in 1984, and on this basis (accreditation by an agency recognized by the USDE) Sherman graduates became license-eligible in Minnesota and Delaware the following year (Gelardi, unpublished). Florida followed suit in 1986.

Recognition of SCASA by USDE was continued in 1990. However, SCASA's scope of authority as an accrediting agency for chiropractic education was challenged by the CCE. In California the executives of the national membership associations and of many CCE-accredited schools testified against SCASA at a public hearing in 1989. These leaders charged that SCASA's limited federal recognition as an accrediting body for straight chiropractic education only did not meet the requirements of "equivalency" to CCE as a guarantor of quality chiropractic training in California (Cuneo, 1990). The Council on Post-secondary Accreditation (COPA), which had recognized the CCE, also lent its weight to the CCE's objections to SCASA (Cuneo, 1990).

Sherman College was placed on "probation" by SACS, and USDE notified SCASA in 1992 that, by action of Bennett's successor, Secretary Lamar Alexander (Strauss, 1994, p. 279), the agency's status with USDE would be terminated, effective 4 June 1993 (Gelardi, unpublished). The short life of SCASA was at an end, and graduates of its schools were increasingly barred from licensure in various jurisdictions. With enrollments dipping to as low as 122 students, Sherman College's financial troubles further jeopardized its regional accreditation. Recognition by SACS was lost in 1994. In the meantime, SCSC had re-applied to CCE's accrediting commission for recognition on 14 April 1993. Inspection of SCSC by CCE's COA was conducted in March 1994, and Gelardi and company appeared before the Commission in June. Further reports from the college to the CCE were submitted in December, and on 26 January 1995, CCE recognized SCSC as an accredited institution.

The Pennsylvania College of Chiropractic (formerly ADIO Institute) also applied in 1994, albeit unsuccessfully, for CCE accreditation. In October 1995, the East Coast school announced plans to close its doors and send its records to Sherman College (Pennsylvania, 1995). Joseph B. Strauss, D.C., who succeeded Reggie Gold as president of ADIO Institute in 1979 (Joseph, 1979), views the decisions of the SCASA schools to seek CCE accreditation as capitulation, "just as Palmer, Life and the Clevelands had done in 1973" (Strauss, 1994, p. 283). "In the minds of many," he suggests, "the straight chiropractic movement was finished in the formal education arena." Time will tell.

Not all straight chiropractors have thrown in the towel. Leonard W. Rutherford, former president of the ICA, now heads an organization called the Association for Chiropractic Educational Standards (Rutherford, 1995). Founded circa 1991, the Association for Chiropractic Educational Standards (ACES) believes that:

> ...Chiropractic education and accreditation must be kept within the confines of the legally sound, legally defensible definition and scope of practice of chiropractic principles and practice if our profession is to remain separate and distinct. For education is the molder of the profession (Rutherford et al., 1996).

To accomplish its purpose of maintaining chiropractic as a "separate and distinct" profession by eliminating "mixerism" in chiropractic education and practice, the organization seeks to raise $100,000, and has lodged a protest with the U.S. Department of Education over the legitimacy of the CCE as an accreditor of professional training in chiropractic. The organization also notes that "Legal counsel has been retained for litigation directed against the U.S. Department of Education and the C.C.E." (Rutherford et al., 1996). The profession's internal legal struggles over chiropractic education, it seems, will not end quietly.

Chapter 21

NEW SCHOOLS IN THE MODERN ERA

Sherman College and the ADIO Institute were but two of seven new schools of chiropractic formed in North America during 1973-93 (see Table 21-1). This expansion in chiropractic educational institutions was not predictable; historically, the formation of numerous new schools had been encouraged by the prospect of federal funding for veterans following each world war. We may speculate, however, that the creation of many new schools in the final quarter of the chiropractic century was a result of the CCE's success, and the prospect of federally guaranteed student loans for enrollees at these new institutions. However, several of the emerging colleges, including SCSC, ADIO and Pacific States Chiropractic College in San Lorenzo, California, held strong anti-CCE sentiments. Their births, and that of Life Chiropractic College in Georgia, seemingly had more to do with the revival of strong, straight chiropractic sentiments.

Life Chiropractic College

Sherman College's organization in 1973 was followed in 1975 by the formation of the Life Chiropractic College in Marietta, Georgia. Life College was the creation of Sid E. Williams (see Figure 21-1), a 1956 Palmer graduate who had come to the attention of the straight chiropractic community while still a student, when he was elected vice-president of the Chiropractic Polio Clinic Foundation in Davenport (Chiropractic, 1954). Williams and his wife, Nell, graduated from the PSC in 1956, and returned to rural Austell, Georgia, to establish a chain of 18 chiropractic clinics based on chiropractor George Shears's "G-P-C" principles ("God-Patient-Chiropractor," wherein patients paid the chiropractor only what they could afford). Shears was a founding member of the ICA, and served on its first Board of Control in 1926 (A Tribute, 1951).

By 1960 Williams was teaching his practice-building methods at Parker Seminars (Digest, 1960), and during 1964-70 he collaborated with his wife, former classmate D.D. Humber, D.C. and several other chiropractors in the formation of the non-profit

Table 21-1: Chronology of the formation and renaming of new chiropractic colleges in the North America, 1973-1993 (based on Musick, 1979; Strauss, 1994; Wiese & Peterson, 1995)

1973 (Jan 11): Sherman College of Chiropractic chartred in South Carolina

1973 (Jan 31): International College of Chiropractic Neurovertebrology chartered in California (renamed (1) University of Pasadena, College of Chiropractic, (2) Pasadena College of Chiropractic, (3) Southern California College of Chiropractic, (4) Quantum University)

1974 (Sept 12): Life Chiropractic College formed in Georgia

1976 (Nov 9): Pacific States Chiropractic College chartered in California

1977 (July): ADIO Institute of Straight Chiropractic chartered in Pennsylvania

1978 (Aug 3): Northern California College of Chiropractic chartered in California

1978 (Mar 8): Parker College of Chiropractic chartered in Texas

1980 (Sept 18): Northern California College of Chiropractic became Palmer College of Chiropractic/West

1981: Pacific States College of Chiropractic became Life Chiropractic College-West

1984: ADIO Institute of Straight Chiropractic renamed Pennsylvania College of Straight Chiropractic

1991 (May): Palmer/West and Palmer/Davenport combine as Palmer Chiropractic University

1991: University of Bridgeport, College of Chiropractic is formed

1993: Quebec Ministry of Education forms a chiropractic program at the University of Quebec, Trois Rivieres campus (UQTR)

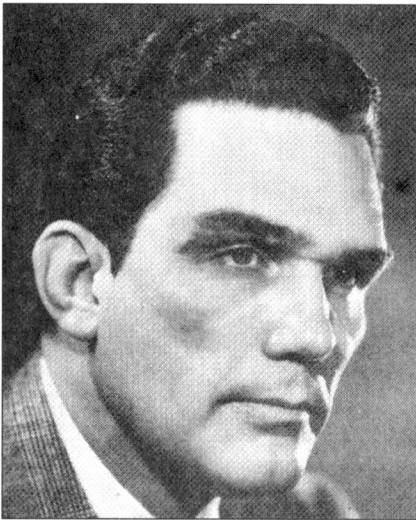

Figure 21-1: Sidney E. Williams, B.S., D.C.

Life Foundation, Inc. and its "Dynamic Essentials" seminars (Dr. Sid, 1995; Lyceum, 1974; Thomas, unpublished). The Dynamic Essentials (DE) seminars became a regular offering for chiropractors who wished to learn: "How to practice with definiteness of purpose...How to enjoy as large a practice as you desire...How to be both happy and prosperous" (Everyone, 1968; It's, 1968). William's intent was to revive the straight chiropractic teachings of B.J. Palmer. In his Life Plan for Chiropractic he described "The Dynamic Essential" as "the 'New Spirit' born into the consciousness after a man becomes aware, humble, and obedient to the will of God within himself" (Thomas, unpublished, p. 98). In 1972 Williams commenced publication of *Today's Chiropractic*, a magazine which eventually became the property and the voice of Life Chiropractic College (LCC); the magazine claims a readership of 65,000 world-wide (Smith, 1996).

By July 1974, the Life Foundation was considering the formation of a chiropractic college, and inquired into the procedures involved in accreditation (Ambrose, 1974; McAndrews, 1974). By September of that year more the $850,000 in pledges for the the new school had been made (Lyceum, 1974), and Sid and Nell Williams incorporated LCC. The first trustees were drawn from leadership of the DE seminars (see Table 21-2). D.D. Humber served as chairman of this first board and as a faculty member. The school opened its doors to 22 students on 20 January 1975 in Marietta, a town just north of Atlanta (Dr. Sid, 1995). Among the original faculty members was Gerard Clum, D.C., who became president of Life Chiropractic College West in 1981. By 1981 the Georgia school had grown to an enrollment of 1,540 students (Life, 1981).

Williams envisioned that his institution would be more than just a school:

> The long-range plan of the Life Foundation is to accomplish a Renaissance - to awake humanity to a dramatically new concept of existence. At the core of the new way of life will be the ancient philosophy that all things are interrelated, that no man is an island, that the slayer and the slain are one...
>
> In the new life, men will flourish together in a spirit of cooperation and harmony. They will regain their faith in nature, and once again experience her as a benevolent, nurturing, healing mother. Each man will be free of the chains of ego, the need for fame and self-aggrandizement. He will experience his own holiness, the holiness of his neighbor, and the holiness of the entire created universe.

Table 21-2: Original members of the board of trustees of Life Chiropractic College, January 1975 (Smith, 1996; Thomas, unpublished, pp. 105-6)

D.D. Humber, D.C., Chairman	Ed S. Ambrose, M.Ed., D.C.
Don Armstrong, D.C.	Richard Baird, D.C.
John Boutwell, D.C.	Ian Grassman, D.C.
Phil Johnson	Tom Morgan, D.C.
Don Parkerson, D.C.	Burl Pettibon, D.C.
Charles Ribley, D.C.	James M. Sigafoose, D.C.
Robert Sottile, D.C.	Joseph Stuckey, D.C.
Nell K. Williams, D.C.	Sid E. Williams, B.S., D.C.

Original administration and faculty of Life Chiropractic College, Marietta, Georgia, January 1975 (Life, 1975a,b,c)

Administration
Sid E. Williams, B.S., D.C., President
Ed S. Ambrose, M.Ed., D.C., Assistant to the President
Ronald J. Watkins, D.C., C.C.R., Dean of Academic Affairs
Marvin Buncher, M.Ed., D.C., Dean of Student Affairs
Robert J. Chadwick, B.B.A., M.A., D.D., Business Manager
Monsignor Richard F. Fitzgerald, M.A., Director of Development
Faculty
W.B. Bean, D.C.
Gerard Clum, D.C.
*D.D. Humber, D.C.
Charles Kalb, D.C.
Nancy Still, M.L.S., Librarian

> We will, in the near future, establish a self-contained community, The City of Life, which will have as its focal point, Life University. This city shall consist of homes, condominiums, retirement cottages, nursing homes, orphan homes, student housing, convention sites, a complete agricultural complex, and shopping facilities. The City of Life shall be founded upon and dedicated to the lofty principles outlined above (Lyceum, 1974).

The school gained professional accreditation of its doctorate through the CCE in 1985, and regional accreditation from SACS in 1986 (Life, 1995a). Among the best known graduates of the institution is Robert A. Leach whose text, *The Chiropractic Theories* (Leach, 1994), has become required reading at many chiropractic colleges. In 1989 Life Chiropractic College was renamed Life College, and broadened its academic offerings. Today, the school boasts bachelor's (business administration, nutrition) and master's degree (sports health science) programs as well as its chiropractic curriculum, and a total student body of nearly 4,200 (Dr. Sid, 1995; Life, 1995a; Smith, 1996). It is the world's largest chiropractic educational institution. Williams' plans include the introduction of a Ph.D. program, attainment of university status, and the formation of additional schools in Europe and the Far East.

Like all CCE-college presidents, Williams serves on the governing board of the Council. His influence extends beyond the educational realm, since, like his role model, B.J. Palmer, he has also served as president of the ICA (1982-85), and during 1985-1995 as chairman of the ICA Board of Control (Smith, 1996). Life College portrays Williams as the "Defender of Chiropractic," and he prides himself for having helped to defeat the proposed merger of ACA and ICA in the late 1980s (Dr. Sid, 1995).

Pacific States/Life Chiropractic College West

Pacific States Chiropractic College (PSCC) was incorporated on 9 November 1976 by George Emmet Anderson, D.C., George F. Wentland, D.C. and James E. Musick, D.C. The trio may have been inspired to create a straight chiropractic school in Northern California by Thomas Gelardi of Sherman College of Straight Chiropractic (Musick, 1979, pp. 12-3, 93), although this has been disputed. Dr. Wentland served on SCSC's first board of advisors (see Table 20-7). When Gelardi's struggles in South Carolina prevented him from establishing a branch campus, Anderson, Wentland and Musick proceeded with the project themselves. Campuses in Santa Cruz and Los Gatos were scouted before settling on a site in San Lorenzo near Anderson's office (see Figure 21-2). Upon Gelardi's recommendation, the Board of

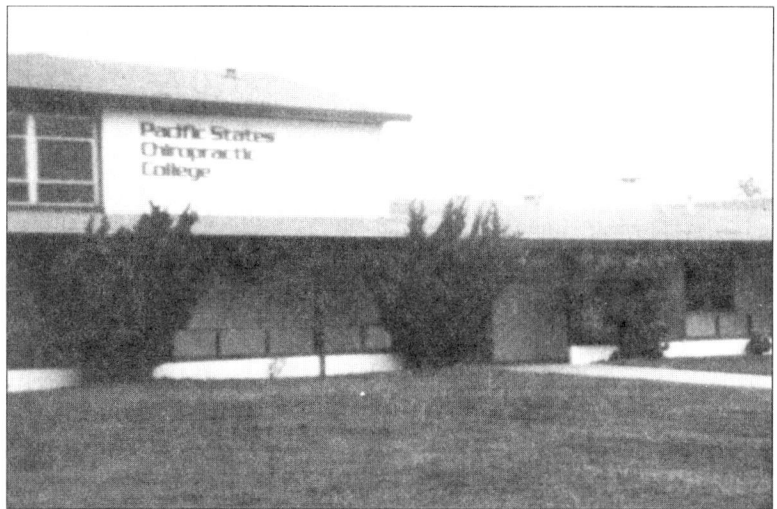

Figure 21-2: Campus of the Pacific States Chiropratic College at 879 Grant Avenue, San Lorenzo, California, circa 1980

Regents of PSCC (see Table 21-3) employed Thomas A. Vonder Haar as an educational consultant. Vonder Haar was an administrator at the University of Missouri in St. Louis (Cleveland, 1975), a speaker at DE seminars (DE, 1976) and a member of the Palmer College "extension faculty" (Palmer College, 1975). He left the University of Missouri and took office as PSCC's first president on 1 September 1977; classes began on 1 March 1978 (Musick, 1979, p. 22). It was later reported that 1953 Palmer graduate Anderson, rather than Vonder Haar, was PSCC's first president (Founder, 1998), but this may refer to presidency of the board rather than the school.

This first college board's original intention was to seek accreditation from the CCE. This goal was imperative, since California voters had approved Proposition 15 in 1976, which seemingly required "that all colleges be approved by the

Council on Chiropractic Education" (Musick, 1979, p. 23). However, several board members, including Anderson and Wentland, had second thoughts about meeting CCE standards, perhaps as a consequence of Sherman College's unsuccessful bid for CCE accreditation in July 1975 and the subsequently revealed possibility of a second, federally recognized chiropractic accrediting agency (Musick, 1979, pp. 92-3). The CCE's standards were viewed as violating straight chiropractic concepts of chiropractic practice. The College's brochure in 1980 offered lofty goals, and seemed to deny concern for intra-professional political disputes:

> ...at PSCC, there is a group of dedicated people - the faculty, the students, and the staff, who are determined to be the first scientific college of chiropractic...A recent controversy in the field has attempted to define the difference between straight chiropractors and mixers (chiropractors who use additional methods of treatment). These terms just don't apply at Pacific States. Labels are not what chiropractic is all about. Making people well is the fundamental basis of chiropractic...

> We teach service to patients and a scientific approach to correcting subluxations. allowing the body to rid itself of dis-ease. If you believe this is what chiropractic is all about, you belong at PSCC (A Brief, undated).

Conflicts developed between some PSCC regents and Vonder Haar, who saw CCE accreditation as essential to the future license eligibility of PSCC graduates. Further disagreements arose over administrative (such as the choice of clinical techniques to be taught) and financial control of the institution (when the board treasurer, Wentland, removed the financial ledgers from the institution). The accounting records, which were ostensibly the responsibility of the chief executive officer, brought the college's operations into violation of CCE standards, and brought members of the board into conflict with one another. The infighting continued, and various board members resigned, only to be re-appointed later on.

Table 21-3: Members of the first Board of Regents of the Pacific States Chiropractic College (Musick, 1979, p. 28). * denotes incorporators of Pacific States; # denotes members of the first Advisory Board of Sherman College of Chiropractic.

*George E. Anderson, D.C., Chairman
Ronald Brennan, D.C., Vice-Chairman
Nan Forrest, Secretary
*#George F. Wentland, D.C., Treasurer
#Stephen Duff, Sr., D.C.
Douglas Dever, D.C.
Don Everingham
Richard Heun, D.C.
*James E. Musick, D.C.
Walter Miller, C.L.U., C.F.P.
Ernest Schulzke, Esq.

The dispute between the president and elements of the board led to Vonder Haar's dismissal on 3 July 1978 (Musick, 1979, p. 69), and a "successful lawsuit" was brought against him (Schultz, 1996a). An exodus of many students and administrators from the PSCC campus took place on July 27; this group later became the founders and organizers of Northern California College of Chiropractic (today's Palmer College of Chiropractic West; see below). The PSCC was reorganized with George Anderson's continuing leadership as chairman of the board and Leon Coelho, D.C., former chairman of Palmer College's radiology department as the new president (Anderson, 1995; Dr. Leon, 1978; Schultz, 1996a). Leonard Rudnick, M.A., D.C., who had participated while still a student in preparing Palmer College's first self-study in 1975, served briefly as academic dean of PSCC (Pacific, 1978). The new administration and a new class of 19 students commenced operations on 25 September 1978 (Pacific, 1978; Schultz, 1996a). Bruce Presnick, D.C. was appointed acting president of the institution in the summer of 1979, and served in that capacity through most of 1980 (Schultz, 1996b). The school moved to its present campus on Via Barrett in January 1980. By 1981, Rita Schroeder, D.C. had been appointed president of the institution, and the PSCC re-applied to CCE for accreditation (PSCC, 1981).

The college's stormy early years and a "rapidly changing economic situation" placed the institution on shaky economic ground. The college established Bingo games as a revenue generator, and considered an alliance with an established chiropractic school. Anderson turned first to Palmer College, and then to Life Chiropractic College. Sid Williams was not initially enthusiastic about adopting the California school, but Gerard W. Clum, D.C. (see Figure 21-3), a 1973 Palmer graduate and member of the Marietta school's first faculty, accepted the presidency of PSCC. Clum subsequently withdrew this acceptance and encouraged George Anderson to re-contact Williams (Schultz, 1996a). On 12 March 1981, a new board of regents was authorized (see Table 21-4); the name of the institution was soon changed to Life Chiropractic College West (LCCW). Although not a member of LCCW's board of trustees, Williams, considered the "founder" of LCCW, selected

Clum as the school's new president (Schultz, 1996c), a position he continues in after 15 years. The Georgia institution granted $500,000 to LCCW, which allowed the California school to successfully reorganize its financial status and meet the standards of the CCE's Commission on Accreditation (Schultz, 1996c). On 4 February 1983 LCCW was granted Recognized Candidate for Accreditation (RCA) status by CCE; full professional accreditation was achieved on 24 July 1987 (Schultz, 1996a).

Shortly after Coelho's 1978 appointment as president of PSCC, he was approached by Robert T. Anderson, Ph.D., professor of anthropology at Mills College in Oakland (Anderson, 1995). Anderson was initiating a medical anthropological study of chiropractic, and had visited the private offices of several Bay area chiropractors. Confused by the diversity of methods and practices he encountered, he came to the school to

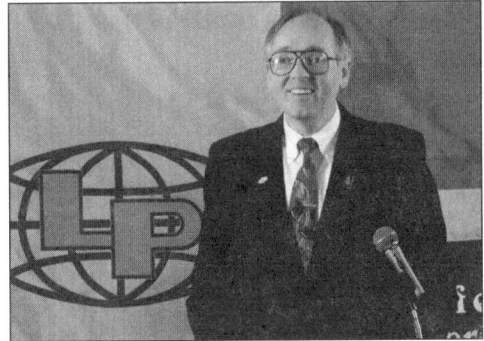

Figure 21-3: Gerard W. Clum, D.C.

learn more about the profession. Anderson's discussions with Coelho led to an arrangement wherein Anderson served as director of research for the young school in exchange for the opportunity to conduct the research. The anthropologist emphasized to Coelho that the college's accreditation efforts could be strengthened by the development of a research program; Coelho and the board agreed (Anderson, 1995).

Anderson was among the members of the first graduating class at LCCW in 1983. The award of the D.C. was delayed until RCA status with CCE was achieved, thereby making LCCW graduates license eligible. During his term as director of research Anderson also served as editor of the *Archives of the California Chiropractic Association*, a short-lived but respectable effort to establish a scholarly periodical. His post as director of research at LCCW has since been held by Daniel Quincy, Ph.D., Robert Jansen, Ph.D. and Charles (Skip) Lantz, Ph.D., D.C.

Especially noteworthy among the several individuals who have served as dean of LCCW has been Marie B. Smith, Ed.D., who earned her doctorate while serving the college, and now holds the position of president of the American River College in Sacramento, California. Smith came to LCCW with a strong background in community college administration. She served as dean of LCCW from 1985 through 1990. Smith coordinated the college's preparations for CCE accreditation in 1986, guided a revision of the college's curriculum which emphasized clinical relevance in basic science instruction, and restructured the academic administration and faculty. She now serves on the boards of directors of LCCW and Life College in Georgia (Schultz, 1996d).

From a student body of 140 at the time PSCC became LCCW (Schultz, 1996c), the college has grown in recent years to more than 800 students (Life, 1995b) and 1,600 alumni (Schultz, 1996c). It boasts a large public clinic in Hayward which provides services to some 1,600 patients per week. Since January, 1995 LCCW has also operated a satellite campus (Schultz, 1996a). The college emphasizes its commitment "subluxation-based education" (Schultz, 1996c) and to Sid Williams' "Lasting Purpose," defined as:

> ...loving for the sake of loving, giving for the sake of giving, serving for the sake of serving and doing for the sake of doing (Life, 1995b).

Table 21-4: Members of the first Board of Regents of Life Chiropractic College West in 1981 (Schultz, 1996c)

John Boutwell, D.C.
Cameron Cassan, D.C.
Ian Grassam, D.C.
Robert Hatch, D.C.
James McGinnis, D.C.
William Remling, D.C.
Charles Ribley, D.C.
James M. Sigafoose, D.C.
Robert Sottile, D.C.
Reverend Carl Standard
Louis Tiscareno, D.C.
Ralph Ungerank, D.C.

Clum's contributions to LCCW and the profession have included service as president during 1990-95 of the Association of Chiropractic Colleges (no relation to the accrediting body which vied with the CCE in the early 1970s for USOE recognition) and creation of the ACC's privately-funded ChiroLoan program for chiropractic students (ChiroLoan, 1996), an alternative to federally funded educational loans. He subsequently held the position of secretary-treasurer of the CCE. He has been a member of the ICA board of control since 1982, and served as the organization's vice-president from July 1988 to March 1991. In 1992 Clum was named ICA's "Chiropractor of the Year" and *Dynamic Chiropractic* magazine's "Man of the Year" (Schultz, 1996c). He has also served as a member of the National Chiropractic Health Care Advisory Committee, and was a participant in the consensus conference which produced the profession's first clinical practice guidelines (Haldeman et al., 1993).

Northern California/Palmer College of Chiropractic-West

On July 28, 1978, 62 students and nine staff personnel of Pacific States Chiropractic College met in Kennedy Park in San Lorenzo, California, to decide whether it was possible to form a new chiropractic college which would not only provide them with the atmosphere and laboratories to obtain a worthy education but would also be an academic anchor for the practicing members of the Profession in Northern California... (Northern, 1980, p. 2).

The walkout of students at the PSCC resulted in the formation of the Northern California College of Chiropractic (NCCC) on 3 August 1978 by six former PSCC students (see Table 21-5). The events were recorded by James E. Musick, D.C., former trustee of PSCC:

> ...Dr. James E. Musick and Robert Hinde delivered the document to the Secretary of State's office in Sacramento. The articles were endorsed and filed August 3, 1978.
>
> With the filing of the Articles of Incorporation with the Secretary of State's office, Northern California College of Chiropractic came into legal existence. It was organized by the former students of Pacific States Chiropractic College. They completed and acted upon the bylaws, established the first Board of Trustees for the college, and actively pursued with Thomas Vonder Haar as President, hired other administrators, and faculty and began the process of looking for a new campus (Musick, 1979, pp. 82-3).

The first classes were held in Kennedy Park in Hayward, California, pending the location of a campus. On the same day that the new school was incorporated, NCCC's first president (see Table 21-6) made a presentation to the California Board of Chiropractic Examiners, and earned the board's preliminary endorsement:

> Mr. Thomas A. Vonder Haar, President of Northern California College of Chiropractic, asked to address the Board.
>
> He indicated the school is currently in operation and incorporated as Northern California College of Chiropractic. Classes are currently being held at Chabot Junior College, but the staff is in the process of negotiating for facilities which provide adequate laboratory equipment. He stated it is the intention of the college to pursue academic excellence and to comply with the regulations of the Board, including gaining status with the Council on Chiropractic Education.
>
> It was moved by Dr. Willard Smith, seconded by Dr. Auerbach, and carried that a vote of confidence be issued to Northern California College of Chiropractic, as to what it was attempting to accomplish (Musick, 1979, p. 82).

In September 1978, Bernard Coyle (see Figure 21-4), a physical chemist and faculty member at San Francisco State University, joined the board of trustees. Over the next 14 years Coyle held most major administrative positions in the college, including Director of Research, Dean of Academic Affairs and acting president, and was responsible for the development of a strong intellectual environment. In the short term, however, the pressing demands of the new school had more to do with meeting payroll, recruiting students, and filling the instructional needs of the institution.

On 18 September 1980 the NCCC was renamed Palmer College of Chiropractic-West (PCCW) when the Palmer/Davenport board of trustees assumed NCCC's half million dollar debt and replaced several of the board members (Mellot & Coyle, 1992). Joseph P. Mazzarelli, D.C., chairman of the board of trustees of the Palmer College in Davenport, assumed the same role on the PCCW board of trustees. John L. Miller, D.C. (see Figure 21-5), vice-president of Palmer/Davenport, was appointed president of PCCW. The school then had 332 full-time equivalent students and 23 full-time equivalent faculty members (Status, 1980, pp. 3-4). Miller, who had led Palmer College in its application process for accreditation by the CCE in the mid-1970s, would now do the same for PCCW, with the assistance of Henry Shull, D.C., another faculty member and administrator from Davenport.

The young institution attained status as a "Recognized Candidate for Accreditation" from the CCE's Committee on Accreditation in September 1981, and full accreditation in June 1985 (Miller, 1995). The first graduating class, comprised of students who had begun their instruction at NCCC, earned their chiropractic degrees in 1982. Among

Table 21-5: Incorporators of the Northern California College of Chiropractic, 3 August 1978 (Musick, 1979)

John Pattison
Stephen Perlstein
Neil Fisher
Don Kelly
Kip Leishman
Robert Hinde

these first PCCW graduates were William C. Meeker, D.C. and Sandy Dutro, D.C., who with Coyle formed the nucleus of the college's research division.

As the 1980s wore on the PCCW developed a reputation as a scholarly environment and leading producer of research. Several 1989 bibliographic surveys (see Table 21-7) of papers published in the profession's leading scientific periodical, the *Journal of Manipulative and Physiological Therapeutics*, revealed that the college faculty, despite its youth, was among the more frequent of authors in the budding scientific literature of chiropractic (Keating, Booher et al., 1989; Keating, Larson et al., 1989). There was irony here, in that the boards of trustees of the two Palmer schools (see Figure 21-6) had anticipated that the acquisition of PCCW would enable the parent school in Iowa to greatly increase its research productivity (Jensen,1980). However, in May 1984 the PCCW board adopted a mission statement which emphasized the role of scholarship in the institution:

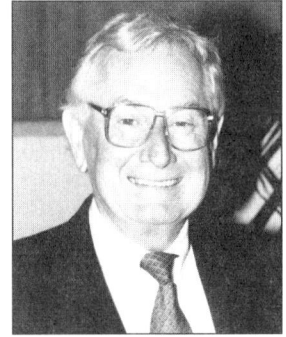

Figure 21-4: Bernard A. Coyle, Ph.D.

> Resolved, that the mission of Palmer College of Chiropractic West is to contribute to the well-being of humankind by advancing the knowledge of chiropractic health science and by developing the skills and nurturing the intellect of students and practitioner.

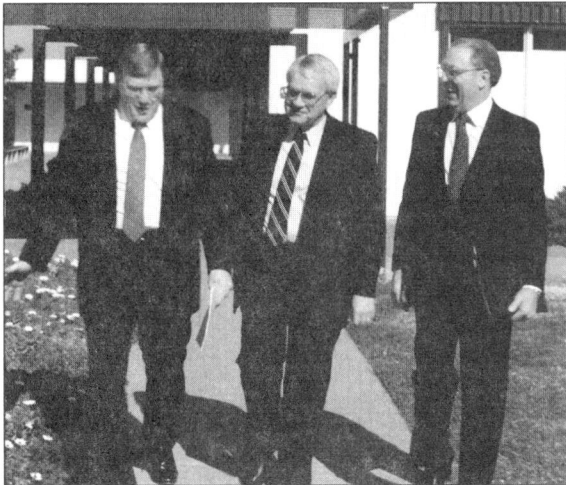

Figure 21-5: L-R: Michael Pedigo, president of ICA, John L. Miller, president of Palmer College of Chiropractic/West and Kenneth Luedtke, president of ACA, stroll on Palmer/West's campus in Sunnyvale, California, during a 1988 visit by the association leaders for a "Chiropractic Unity Day" event

By decade's end it was clear that the new school, with only a fourth of the number of faculty members, had significantly outpaced the Davenport institution in scholarly productivity (see Table 21-8). Credit for the development of a strong academic environment and scholarly productivity belongs primarily to Coyle. During his many years as director of research and later as vice-president for academic affairs Coyle sought to recruit "live wires" to the faculty whenever an opportunity presented itself. As a consequence, in the early 1990s PCCW had on its payroll a great many current and former chiropractic college research directors (Coyle - PCCW; Robert Jansen, Ph.D., - Life Chiropractic College-West; Joseph C. Keating, Jr., Ph.D., - Northwestern College of Chiropractic; William Meeker, D.C., M.P.H. - PCCW and the Palmer Center for Chiropractic Research; Mohan Menon, M.D., Ph.D. - Cleveland Chiropractic College of Los Angeles; and Shawn Moroney, Ph.D., D.C. - Northern California College of Chiropractic) and a number of other active investigators and scholars. Under Coyle's direction PCCW also played a leading role in the formation of the Pacific Consortium for Chiropractic Research (known today as the Consortium for Chiropractic Research), which was established in Autumn 1985 as a collaboration among the West Coast chiropractic colleges (Tolar et al., 1986).

Additional noteworthy members of the PCCW research team were Robert D. Mootz, D.C., D.A.B.C.O., D. Dale Nansel, Ph.D. and Gregory Plaugher, D.C. Mootz, an alumnus of Palmer (Davenport), served on faculty from April 1985 to September 1993, when he was appointed to serve as Associate Medical Director of the State of Washington's Department of Labor and Industry. Nansel, a physiologist, is noteworthy for his development of program of research involving laboratory based studies of spinal adjusting (e.g., Nansel et al., 1989a&b, 1990, 1992), and for his critical assessment of the literature bearing on somatic simulation of visceral disorders (Nansel & Szlazak, 1995). Plaugher, a graduate of LACC, has sought to investigate the clinical methods of Clarence Gonstead, D.C. The PCCW faculty member serves as director of research for the Gonstead Clinical Studies Society, and has edited a volume on these clinical methods (Plaugher & Lopes, 1993). Palmer College West also pioneered in the creation of the "Mentor Model" of clinical training. Designed by Ronald Henninger, D.C., D.A.B.C.O., a Palmer graduate who joined the PCCW faculty in 1980 (Mellott & Coyle, 1992), this program re-arranged the operations within the college's training clinics. No longer would interns operate as free agents to establish their

Table 21-7: Number of articles in the *Journal of Manipulative and Physiological Therapeutics* during 3-year and 9-year periods per chiropractic college (reprinted by permission of the *Journal of Manipulative and Physiological Therapeutics* from Keating, Larson et al., 1989)

Chiropractic College	1978-80	1981-83	1984-86	Total
National	47 (38%)a	33 (36%)	26 (22%)	106 (32%)
Canadian	10 (8%)	13(14%	15 (12%)	38 (11%)
New York	6 (5%)	4	0	10
Palmer	0	4	3	7
Palmer/West	0	1	6 (5%)	7b
Los Angeles	1	1	4	6
Northwestern	2	1	3	6b
Life	0	4	0	4
Western States	1	0	3	4
Cleveland/KC	2	0	1	3
Logan	0	3	0	3
Phillips	0	0	3	3
Texas	0	0	2	2
Anglo-European	0	0	1	1
Life West	0	1	0	1
College totals	69 (56%)	65 (71%)	66 (55%)	200 (60%)
No. of Articles (per period)	122	92	120	334

aPercentage of contribution per period is given in parentheses if 5% or more

bOne article was co-authored by faculty from Palmer/West and Northwestern College

Table 21-8: Scholarly productivity among Palmer and Palmer/West faculty during 1989 and 1990 according to: 1) number of articles published and (mean annual rate of articles per faculty member per College), and 2) according to percent of each College faculty who published papers.

Palmer	Palmer/West	
120	32	Total number of faculty members
36 (0.15)	81 (1.27)	Total number of published articles during 1989-1990 and (annual rate per faculty member per college
24 (0.10)	71 (1.11)	Number of articles published in scholarly journals during 1989-1990 and (annual rate per faculty member per college)
12 (0.05)	10 (0.16)	Number of articles published in trade journals during 1989-1990 and (annual rate per faculty member per college)
18%	59%	Percentage of faculty who authored or co-authored at least one paper during 1989-1990
12%	47%	Percentage of faculty who authored or co-authored at least one paper in a scholarly journal during 1989-1990
7%	19%	Percentage of faculty who authored or co-authored at least one paper in a trade journal during 1989-1990

own "mini-practices" within the school clinic. Instead, patients were assigned to licensed faculty clinicians, who delegated increasing responsibility to individual student doctors based on the faculty clinician's estimate of the interns' progress in developing clinical acumen. It is a more labor intensive system, and sometimes suffers when inadequate clinical staff are available, but promises to produce a more skilled chiropractor.

Southern California College of Chiropractic

The International Chiropractic College of Neurovertebrology was incorporated in California on 31 January 1973 by Arthur J. Garrow, D.C. (see Figure 21-7), Mary E. Stewart and Sharron A. Powell (Articles, 1973). Garrow, a graduate of and former faculty member of the Cleveland Chiropractic College of Los Angeles (Follick, 1996; University, 1976-77), served as the new school's first president, and located the institution in Pasadena. By January 1974, the school had undergone the first of several name changes (see Table 21-9), becoming the University of Pasadena, College of Chiropractic, and reflecting

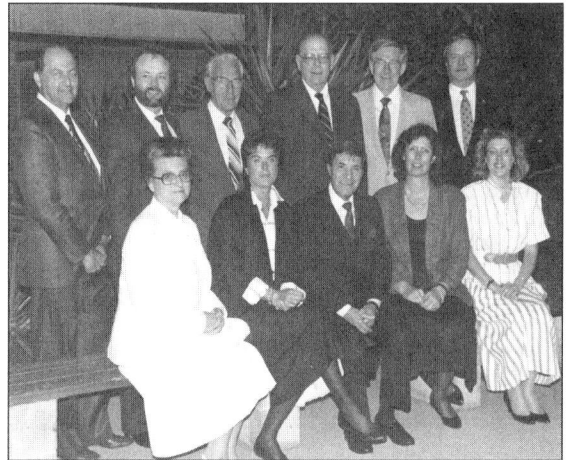

Figure 21-6: Gathering of the Board of Trustees of Palmer College of Chiropractic West in October 1987; L-R (front row): Lelia Schlabach, D.C.; Jenny Sutton, past chairman; Joseph Mazzarelli, D.C.; Marilyn P. Smith, D.C., chairman; Vickie Palmer; L-R (back row): Ron Danis; Paul Peterson, D.C.; Alexander Politis, D.C.; Kent Forney; Harley Gilthvedt, D.C.; Myrvin Christopherson, Ph.D.

Garrow's belief that "the needs of the profession, public and the student would best be served through the development of a university which offered degrees in related fields" (University, 1976-77). Classes for the chiropractic curriculum began in February 1974 and in September the chiropractic school was recognized by the state's Board of Chiropractic Examiners (BCE) for the purpose of licensure. In 1978 the state of California's Department of Education granted approval for the award of the doctorate in chiropractic (Wiese & Peterson, 1995).

The institution's leadership envisioned the creation of a number of health care schools within the university system, and Garrow explored the accreditation process with both the CCE and the ACC (Garrow, 1974). The first commencement exercises were held on June 29, 1975 (California, 1975). By 1976 the student body had grown to 176, and the school planned to phase out its evening division in accordance with accrediting agency requirements (University, 1976). The following year the name of the school changed once more, to Pasadena College of Chiropractic (Wiese & Peterson, 1995).

Pasadena College benefited considerably from a distinguished faculty which drew from the ranks of other chiropractic schools. At various times Wolf Adler, D.O., N.D., D.C. and J. Gordon Anderson, D.C., N.D., both former faculty members and administrators of LACC, served in the same capacity at the young school (Anderson, 1995). Jay D. Kirby, D.C.,

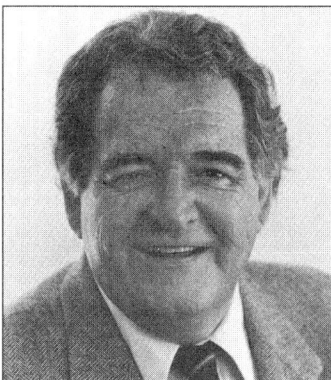

Figure 21-7: Arthur J. Garrow, D.C.

Table 21-9: Various names of the Southern California College of Chiropractic, 1973-1995 (Wiese & Peterson, 1995; Sikorski, unpublished)

Name of Institution	Dates
International Chiropractic College of Neurovertebrology	1973 - c1974
University of Pasadena, College of Chiropractic	c1974 - 1977
Pasadena College of Chiropractic	1977 - 1989
Southern California College of Chiropractic	1989 - 1995
Quantum University	1995 -

F.I.C.C., former professor at LACC (Kirby, 1964) and former editor of its journal (Kirby, 1974; Nilsson, 1972), *The Chirogram*, served as director of clinics in the late 1970s, and George Haynes, long-time president of LACC, served on the Pasadena College's board of trustees (Kirby, 1979).

In the 1980s the campus was relocated to Pico Rivera, California. On 17 October 1987 the school's chairman of the board of trustees, Gene F. Schumann, D.C., announced that Garrow had resigned, and that Carroll T. Lowery had been appointed "Chief Administrative Officer" (Dr. Garrow, 1987). Further institutional changes occurred in 1989, when a new board of trustees was impaneled, with Daniel Kuhn, D.C. as chairman (Wiese & Peterson, 1995). At this time also the school was renamed the Southern California College of Chiropractic, and sought accreditation from SCASA. Full accreditation was granted in May 1992 during the presidency of W. Ralph Boone, Ph.D., D.C., former director of research for the Sherman College of Straight Chiropractic (Wiese & Peterson, 1995). However, with the loss of SCASA's recognition by the federal government the college's status with the California BCE was also rescinded, as of 30 June 1995 (Sikorski, unpublished). In 1995 another change in the composition of the board of trustees and another name change, to that of Quantum University, signaled an end to chiropractic instruction at the 22 year old school.

Parker College of Chiropractic

Named for its founder, James W. Parker, D.C. (see Figure 21-8), a 1946 graduate of the Palmer School who came to be known as the "Dean of Practice Builders" (Baer, 1996), the Parker College of Chiropractic may be seen as an outgrowth of the Parker Chiropractic Research Foundation and the Parker School for Professional Success (Parker, undated), which had been vending products and seminars to the profession since the 1950s. Parker initially considered the purchase of a short-lived institution in Cisco, Texas, the Southwest College of Chiropractic (Dr. James, 1981), but ultimately sought a new charter for his school. The new institution was incorporated on March 8, 1978, and a first campus of 63 acres was purchased in Dallas in 1981 (Parker, undated). In March of that year Parker announced that "it is now in the best interest of chiropractic that a new chiropractic college be opened by September 1981, in the Dallas/Ft. Worth area" (Dr. James, 1981). The stated intention of the Parker College was that "each student will be able to provide during their first year of practice $100,000 of service to chiropractic patients" (Dr. James, 1981).

Fundraising for the new school began at the Parker seminars, and the seminars themselves eventually became a part of the college's curriculum (Parker, undated). On 12 September 1982 the first class of 27 students began their studies at a second campus, located in nearby Irving, Texas, comprising some 22,000 square feet. The first graduation was held in August 1985 (see Figure 21-9), and the student body has since grown to 1,300 (Parker,undated), the third largest student enrollment of any chiropractic institution. Parker initially served as chairman of the board of trustees, and appointed several individuals to serve as president, among them G. Edward Lessard, Ph.D. (September date, 1982) and Harvey Morter, D.C., M.S. In March 1984, Parker took the reins as president of Parker College, which he held until September 1996, when his son, W. Karl Parker, succeeded him. The school achieved regional

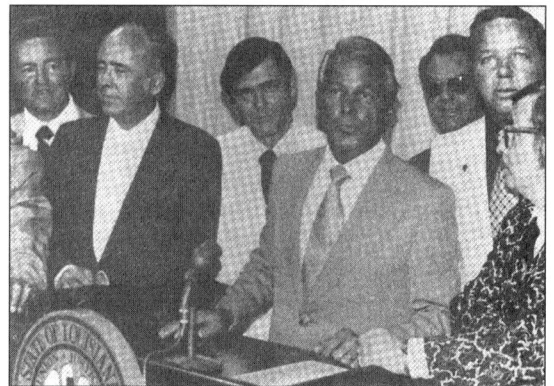

Figure 21-8: James W. Parker, D.C. (far right) is seen here with Louisiana governor Edwin Edwards at the 1974 signing of the first chiropractic law in that state. The Parker Foundation for Chiropractic Research contributed more than $23,000 to the licensing campaign (Cleveland & Keating, 1995)

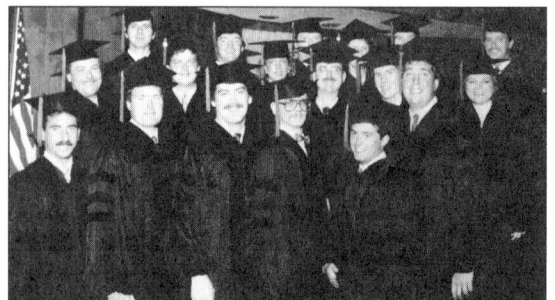

Figure 21-9: First graduating class of the Parker College of Chiropractic, August 1985

accreditation by the Southern Association of Colleges and Schools in January 1987, and was professionally accredited by the CCE in June 1988 (Parker, undated). A bachelor's degree program was approved by SACS and the Texas Higher Education Coordinating Board in 1991, and the school has recently announced that it will give preference to applicants who have a bachelor's degree or who elect to earn their B.S. in anatomy at the College (Preferred, 1996). The school is now located at its "Beta campus" in Dallas.

University of Bridgeport, College of Chiropractic

The University of Bridgeport, College of Chiropractic (UBCC) is unique today as the first university-based chiropractic college in the North America (Graduate, 1994-1995, pp. 49-56), and the only university-based chiropractic school in the United States. The motivation for its creation is credited to Janet Greenwood, Arnold Ciancuilli, Mark Peyser and Robert Matrisciano, who began planning for the college in the summer of 1989 (University, 1995a). This group recruited Frank Zolli, D.C., formerly a faculty member at the New York Chiropractic College (NYCC), to "put together all the necessary information to comply with licensure and accreditation requirements" (Zolli, unpublished), including admissions, recruitment, curriculum, research, continuing education and public relations.

The University administration was already familiar with the chiropractic profession, owing to its pre-chiropractic undergraduate program in the basic sciences, and to its master's level program in nutrition, which had attracted many practicing chiropractors, and had been offered by extension on chiropractic college campuses (e.g., Cleveland, 1981). With the consent of the University's board of trustees, an application for licensure of the chiropractic college was submitted to Connecticut's Department of Higher Education (DHE) in February 1990. The DHE conducted an inspection of the program in August, and authorized the new chiropractic school in December 1990:

> Resolved, that the Board of Governors license a program leading to the Doctor of Chiropractic (D.C.) Degree to be offered by the University of Bridgeport, until December 1992, with the provision that the University submit a library plan to the Department of Higher Education by April 1991, that the University submit in December 1991 a progress report on the implementation of the program, and that there be a full report and site evaluation prior to accreditation (quoted in Zolli, unpublished).

In Spring 1991, Zolli, who had chaired the University's Chiropractic College Committee, was appointed dean of the UBCC (University, 1995a; Zolli, unpublished). Faculty were recruited, an experienced chiropractic librarian was hired, and extensive renovation of an existing structure on the University's campus commenced. Sixteen students entered the program in September 1991, and a second class of 12 students began their studies in Spring 1992.

Accreditation of the chiropractic program by the state DHE was established on 21 April 1993. With this accomplished, UBCC applied for professional accreditation to the CCE. Neil Stern, D.C., former acting president of the NYCC and subsequently executive vice-president of Parker College of Chiropractic, served as CCE consultant to the UBCC. On 17 June 1994 the program was accredited by the CCE (University, 1995a), and in December of that year the school graduated its first class of ten chiropractors (Zolli, unpublished).

University of Quebec at Trois Rivieres, Chiropractic Program

Formation of the doctoral program in chiropractic at Université du Quebec à Trois Rivières (UQTR), the first and still the only state-university-based chiropractic educational program in North America, began in September 1988 with formal discussions between the University and members of the Ordre des Chiropracticiens du Quebec (OCQ), the professional association of the province (Gonthier, 1995). This initiative provoked strong opposition from organized medicine in the province of Quebec, which sought to discredit the university and the provincial ministry of higher education (Université, 1995b).

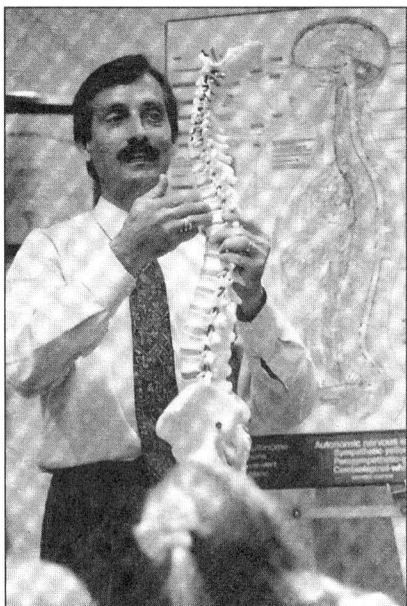

Figure 21-10: Chiropractic education at the Universite du Quebec at Trois-Rivieres

First formal contact between the UQTR's planning committee and the CCE occurred in December 1989 during the Council's meeting in Toronto. Official authorization to commence the doctoral program in chiropractic was granted by Quebec's Minister of Higher Education and Science, Lucienne Robillard, on 16 November 1992 (Gonthier, 1995). The plan included erection of a six million dollar facility to house classrooms, laboratories, administrative offices and an outpatient clinic; construction began in November 1993. The provincial government invested $8.6 million, and Quebec's chiropractors another $1.5 million, to establish the program and facilities. Instruction (see Figure 21-10) began in September 1993, when the UQTR admitted its first class of 45 chiropractic students. André-Marie Gonthier, D.C. was appointed the program's first dean (i.e., Head, Chiropractic Section). Formal application for accreditation commenced in winter 1995 with a letter to CCE (Canada) indicating the University's intent to seek accreditation (Gonthier, 1995). The program, involving 4,800 hours of instruction, will graduate its first class in 1998 (Université, 1995b).

Chapter 22

ACCREDITED EDUCATION SPREADS AND EVOLVES

The CCE's success in achieving federal recognition as an accrediting agency for chiropractic education marked a turning point not only in the academic realm, but in the internal politics of the profession. In 1974 the authority conferred by the USOE meant that the CCE was the proverbial only game in town, and most schools eventually applied and achieved accredited status (see Table 22-1). Competition for students would now be influenced by the eligibility of students at CCE-accredited schools to receive federal grants and guaranteed loans. The former ACC schools soon began to make application to the CCE for recognition; first among these was Palmer College in Davenport.

College	Correspondent*	Recognized Candidate*	Initial Accreditation
Cleveland Chiropractic College, Kansas City		June 1978	June 1982
Cleveland Chiropractic College, Los Angeles		January 1980	January 1985
Life Chiropractic College, Marietta	October 1977*	June 1979	June 1985
Life Chiropractic College-West		February 1983	July 1987
Logan College of Chiropractic		February 1976	June 1978
Los Angeles College of Chiropractic			June 1971
National College of Chiropractic			January 1971
New York Chiropractic College		February 1976	January 1979
Northwestern College of Chiropractic			June 1971
Palmer College of Chiropractic		October 1975	July 1979
Palmer College of Chiropractic-West		July 1981	June 1985
Parker College of Chiropractic		June 1985	June 1988
Sherman College of Straight Chiropractic			January 1995
Texas Chiropractic College			January 1971
University of Bridgeport, College of Chiropractic			June 1994
Western States Chiropractic College	January 1971	May 1975	January 1981

Table 22-1: Dates of initial status with the Council on Chiropractic Education (Miller, 1995)

*Pre Accreditation Status

Palmer College of Chiropractic

David D. Palmer, B.S., D.C., Ph.C. (see Figure 22-1) assumed the presidency of the Palmer College of Chiropractic (PCC) upon the death of his father in 1961 (Rogers, 1961b). Then the largest chiropractic college with an enrollment of more than a thousand students (Hayes, 1963), Palmer opposed the educational policies of the NCA and ACA Council on Education for more than a decade, most especially the introduction of coursework in "physiotherapy, modalities and adjuncts" (Palmer, 1963). Yet, he found accommodation with the idea of chiropractic "diagnosis" (Palmer, 1969), and was also committed to fostering unity within the profession (Dr. Dave, 1968; Palmer, 1969) and with improving the education of

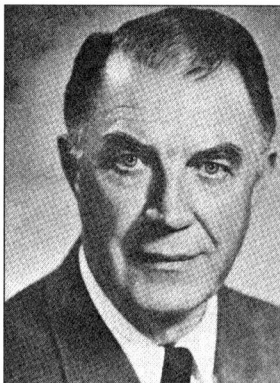

Figure 22-1: David D. Palmer, D.C., grandson of D.D. Palmer and third president of the Palmer College of Chiropractic

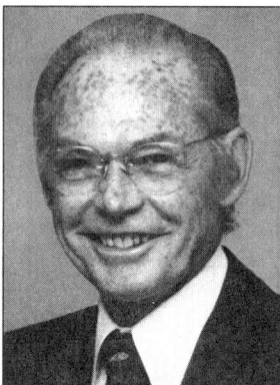

Figure 22-2: W. Heath Quigley, D.C., M.A.

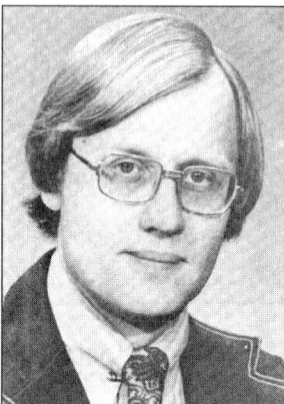

Figure 22-3: Peter Martin, D.O., N.D., D.C., circa 1975

students at his school (Elliott,1963). Dave, sometimes referred to as the "Educator," was responsible for the creation of Palmer Junior College in 1965 and the re-chartering the Palmer College as a non-profit institution in 1966 (Rehm, 1980, pp. 325-6). Active in his community in civic, charitable and business affairs, he fostered a considerable degree of respectability among non-chiropractors for Palmer College .

In October 1969, Dave Palmer joined with the presidents of most U.S. chiropractic schools in a meeting to seek means of unifying their efforts to achieve federal recognition. However, instead of unity, the meeting produced a rival accrediting agency to the ACA Council on Education, the Association of Chiropractic Colleges (ACC), when Palmer "moved the adoption of the Articles of Incorporation and By-Laws presented by Dr. Harper" of the Texas Chiropractic College (Haynes, 1969). The founders of the ACC sought to establish an agency independent of either national professional association, rather than one which would receive the support and sustaining membership of both the ACA and the ICA.

In December 1973, the Educator suffered a stroke which severely reduced his activities as president of the PCC. He continued nominally as president, and assumed the presidency of the college's board of trustees in 1975. In May 1974, Palmer appointed William Heath Quigley, D.C., (see Figure 22-2), nephew of Mabel Palmer, former director of the Clear View Sanitarium (a mental hospital operated by the Palmer School), and a member of the ACA, to serve as the Administrator of the PCC (Palmer homecoming, 1975; Quigley, 1996; Rehm, 1980, pp. 325-6). During his administration the college achieved a number of milestones, including eligibility for federally guaranteed student loans, expansion of the training clinics and the creation of satellite clinical facilities, development of a new curriculum including physiotherapy instruction (offered as an elective through the PCC Division of Continuing Education), the formation of a Faculty Senate, and a fund drive for the erection of a new building on the Davenport campus (Palmer homecoming, 1975). Quigley (1995) is also proud of the weekly Philosophy Committee meetings he established, which came to focus on the need for serious scientific investigation at the PCC, and led to the formation of the college's research division.

In 1975 Peter A. Martin (see Figure 22-3), future president of Palmer College of Chiropractic-West and a 1968 Palmer graduate, was appointed by Quigley to head the PCC Post Graduate School of Chiropractic Studies (Palmer Homecoming, 1975). Martin later served in a similar capacity at the LACC during Quigley's term as president of the West Coast institution.

Quigley was also responsible for the 1974 promotion of John L. Miller, D.C., a 1954 Palmer graduate then serving as dean of his alma mater, to the position of vice-president for academic affairs (Quigley, 1995). Quigley had been serving as chair of a college task force which explored the accreditation issue, and following CCE's recognition by the USOE in August 1974, he initiated discussions with the CCE about an application from PCC for accreditation. The job of preparing an institutional self-study, a requisite component of the application to CCE, was assigned to Miller, who appointed himself, students Leonard Rudnick, M.A., Dave Williamson, M.B.A. and Galen Politis, B.S., and secretary Carol Wright to prepare the document (Rudnick, 1996). Cloistering themselves for several weeks, the group sought to find a delicate balance between the CCE standards and the attitudes of traditionalists within the Palmer community, including those of its invalid president, Dave Palmer (Rudnick, 1995). The PCC achieved candidate status with the CCE in 1975, and full accreditation in 1979. However, by August 1976, Quigley had fallen from favor with Palmer and the board of trustees, perhaps as a result of his accreditation efforts (Rudnick, 1996), and was asked to resign. An "Administrative Executive Committee" headed by Galen R. Price, D.C. and composed of Miller (see Figure 22-4), vice-president of development E.L. Crowder, D.C., and the vice-president of business affairs W.B. Gehlsen, was appointed to "conduct the affairs of

Palmer College of Chiropractic until such time as another chief administrator is appointed" (Palmer homecoming, 1976).

Dave Palmer died in 1978 (Rehm, 1980, pp. 325-6). He was succeeded as president by Galen Price, D.C., a long time faculty member at the PCC. Joseph Mazzarelli, D.C. (see Figure 22-5), who served as president of the ICA during 1974-1979 (Gibbons, 1986), became the chairman of the PCC Board of Trustees. Price was succeeded as president of the college in 1979 by Jerome F. McAndrews, D.C. (see Figure 22-6), a 1956 Palmer graduate who had served under Mazzarelli at ICA as executive vice-president of the straight chiropractic society (Gibbons, 1986). When Mazzarelli and the PCC board elected to acquire Northern California College of Chiropractic in 1980 and transform it into Palmer College of Chiropractic-West, McAndrews was also appointed to head the short-lived Palmer College Federation (Jensen, 1980). The concept of the Federation was revisited in 1991 with the formation of Palmer Chiropractic University System (PCUS).

McAndrews' eight and a half years (1979-1987) as president of the oldest chiropractic school saw a number of changes. The institution committed itself to achieving regional accreditation through the North Central Association of Colleges and Schools for both its bachelor's and D.C. programs, and to this end major renovations to campus facilities for instruction in the basic and clinical sciences were made (McAndrews, 1996). A greatly expanded and more stable faculty was recruited, and computer equipment was introduced for instructional and research work. To further the effort for regional accreditation, McAndrews initiated the first long-range planning process in the college's history.

McAndrews' administration was also noteworthy for the commitment made to scholarly development. The Davenport institution created the Palmer Research Institute (PRI), which was located at the former ICA headquarters at 741 Brady Street. Seed money for the institute and other research activities reached as much as $650,000 annually in internal budgeting, which allowed the PRI to hire a number of investigators and provided release time for research for other faculty members. A policy requiring scholarly productivity from the PCC faculty members was implemented, with the intent that "never again would faculty enter the classroom without the discipline of science" (McAndrews, 1996). While this mandate for research may have done more to intimidate faculty than it did to raise scholarly output, it bespeaks a growing awareness of the importance of scientific investigations within the Palmer community.

In addition to the formation of the PRI, McAndrews was also responsible for the establishment of an internal grants program for faculty research, for the development of a master's degree program, and for investigation of possible affiliation between the PCC and a state university. The latter plans were set aside by school's board of trustees following the McAndrews' replacement as president by Donald Kern, D.C. Palmer Chiropractic University was established 17 May 1991 (Crawford, 1996), through the combination of PCC and Palmer College-West in California; at that time Michael Crawford, M.A. (see Figure 22-7) was appointed chancellor of the expanded, dual campus institution.

On 28 October 1994, Virgil V. Strang, D.C., Dean of Philosophy with 44 years of teaching experience was appointed the seventh president of the Fountainhead. He guided the first chiropractic college through two centennial celebrations: one in 1995 honoring the profession, and one in 1997, recognizing 100 years of Palmer chiropractic education.

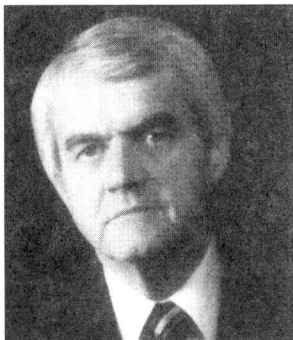

Figure 22-4: John L. Miller, D.C.

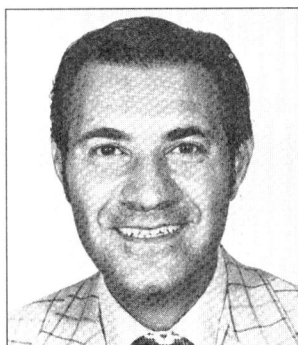

Figure 22-5: Joseph Mazzarelli, D.C.

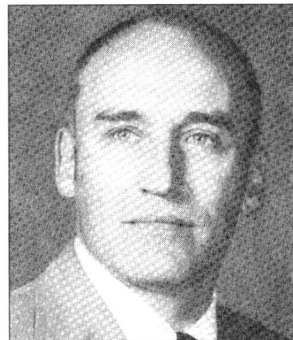

Figure 22-6: Jerome F. McAndrews, D.C.

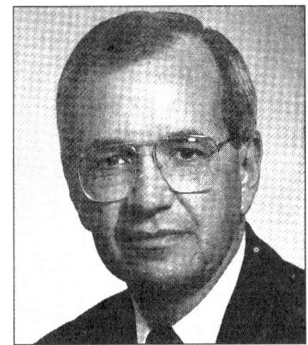

Figure 22-7: Michael Crawford, M.A.

Cleveland Chiropractic Colleges

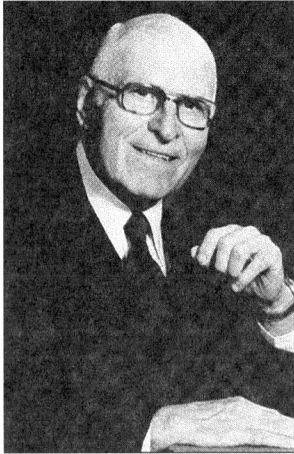

Figure 22-8: Carl S. Cleveland, Sr., D.C.

Headed by Carl S. Cleveland, Jr., D.C. as president since 1967 (Report, 1971; Appendix C), the Cleveland Chiropractic College of Kansas City (CCCKC) resisted the CCE until the latter's recognition by the USOE in 1974. With the decision to achieve CCE recognition came many changes. Late in December 1976, after 46 years at its Troost Avenue site, the institution began a relocation to its present Rockhill Road campus, the former First Church of the Nazarene (Cleveland, 1977). Library facilities were substantially improved, and the school's evening division, which had operated since the CCCKC's founding in 1922, was discontinued. The college made its first application to CCE in 1976, and received "Recognized Candidate for Accreditation" (RCA) status in June 1978. Full accreditation by CCE was achieved in June 1982 (Miller, 1995). By this time CCCKC had also been granted "Candidate for Accreditation" status with the North Central Association of College and Schools (NCACS), the regional accrediting agency for schools in the Midwest. Full accreditation was received from NCACS in 1984 and in September 1995, CCCKC commenced its baccalaureate program, which allows students to earn the B.S. in Human Biology while studying for the doctorate in chiropractic.

The Cleveland Chiropractic College of Los Angeles (CCCLA), successor to the Ratledge Chiropractic College, acquired its present campus at 590 North Vermont Avenue in central Los Angeles in 1976. Carl Cleveland, Sr. (see Figure 22-8), founder of the Kansas City institution in 1922 and purchaser of the Ratledge school in 1951, lived to see both institutions attain federally recognized accreditation. The California school received RCA status with CCE in January 1980 (Miller, 1995), and was granted full accreditation by the agency in January 1985. The CCCLA interns serve a diverse patient population in Los Angeles and have available interdisciplinary rotations at the Coast Plaza Doctors Hospital and Whittier Hospital Medical Center.

Leadership of the Cleveland schools is now vested in Carl S. Cleveland, III (see Figure 22-9), who serves as president of both colleges. A graduate of the University of Missouri at Kansas City who earned the D.C. from CCCKC in 1975, this third generation of Cleveland family chiropractors served in

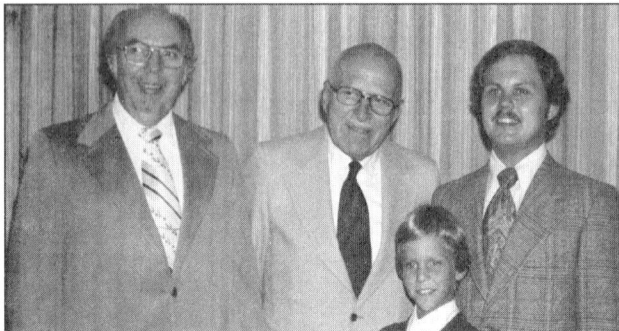

Figure 22-9: Four generations of the Cleveland family pose for this photograph in the late 1970s. Left to right are Carl Jr., Carl Sr., Carl IV and Carl S. Cleveland III.

various administrative and faculty positions at the Kansas City school his grandfather founded, and became president of the institution in 1981. He assumed the presidency of the Los Angeles school in 1992. Current plans call for reorganizing the two Cleveland colleges under one board of trustees; each school will operate as a branch of a multi-campus system.

Among the most noteworthy of Cleveland alumni is 1982 CCCLA graduate Rand Baird, M.P.H., D.C. (see Figure 22-10), who was the prime mover in the 1983 campaign to reverse the American Public Health Association's anti-chiropractic position (Vear, 1987). The former hospital administrator commenced his chiropractic teaching career as an instructor in public health while still a student at the Los Angeles school (Vear, 1987); Baird now serves as professor at LACC and as a member of the board of trustees of his alma mater.

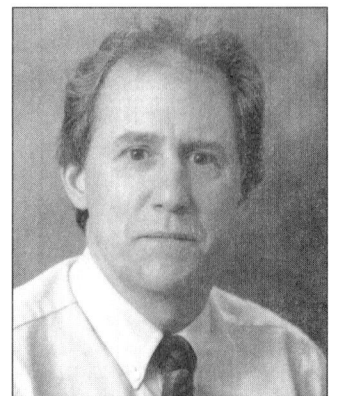

Figure 22-10: Rand Baird, M.P.H., D.C.

Los Angeles College of Chiropractic

Twenty years after taking possession of its Glendale campus, the LACC had once again outgrown its facilities, and commenced a search for larger quarters. The college flirted for a while with the purchase of a convent school nestled in the hills of Los Gatos, California, in the mid-1970s (Los Gatos, 1975a-c; Smallie & Smallie, 1975), but was unable to obtain the finances and local zoning changes necessary for the operation of a busy campus. Not until 1980 and the inauguration of Maylon Drake, Ed.D. as LACC president was the school's present campus in Whittier acquired (LACC, 1986).

The leadership of the institution changed significantly during the 1970s. The changes troubled Ralph J. Martin, D.C., N.D., who had brought about the 1947 merger of the LACC with its non-profit ancestor, the Southern California College of Chiropractic (SCCC), and who had served for many years in the governance of the ACA, the FCER and the NCA/ACA Council on Education. Martin, whose clinical orientation was very broad-scope, reflected upon the evolution of the LACC's board during his term as chairman:

> As I completed my services with the American Chiropractic Association in 1972, I was invited to return to LACC as chairman of the Board of Regents of the California Chiropractic Educational Foundation, where I served until February 1977, when the Board was taken over by a combination of 'straights' and 'orthopedists' with restrictive concepts of chiropractic, including 'straight' philosophy and orthopedics. I could not feel at home in that environment, especially since it had permeated across the country and in the ACA (Martin, 1986).

A number of changes in the senior administration of the college also occurred (Los, 1995, p. 5). In 1976 George Haynes had retired after two decades as chief executive officer of the LACC (Rehm, 1980, p. 329), and A. Earl Homewood, who had twice previously presided at the Canadian Memorial Chiropractic College (CMCC), succeeded Haynes to the LACC presidency. His term was short, however, and before the year ended Heath Quigley, former chief administrator at Palmer College, was appointed president of the LACC. J. Gordon Anderson, D.C., N.D., a 1946 SCCC alumnus who had served on the LACC faculty since his graduation (Anderson & Dishman, 1992), was appointed dean and vice-president, and served in this capacity until 1978 (Anderson, 1992). Maynard Lipe, D.C., who had served as dean of the LACC graduate school (postgraduate division), retired in 1976 (LACC, 1986), and Quigley appointed Peter Martin to the post of vice-president of development and dean of continuing education (Martin, 1992).

With a student body of about 700 students crammed into its two-acre Glendale campus, disharmony within the board, administration and student body, and with mounting economic problems, the LACC was placed on confidential probation by the CCE's Commission on Accreditation in the late 1970s (Anderson & Dishman, 1992; Drake, unpublished). The college board of trustees (see Table 22-2) decided to appoint E. Maylon Drake, Ed.D., a professor and administrator at the University of Southern California, to head the institution.

The Drake administration commenced on February 1, 1980, and purchased the present 38 acre campus in Whittier, California, in the summer of 1981 from the Fullerton Union High School District (Drake, unpublished; LACC, 1986; Los, 1995). Acquisition of the new facility was made possible in part by the college's receipt of the assets of the Seabury Foundation, in excess of $750,000 (LACC, 1986). A down payment of $2,000,000 was made, and the college was also successful in obtaining California Educational Facilities Act (CEFA) bond issues in 1983 and 1985 which helped to finance the

Table 22-2: Trustees and senior administrators of the Los Angeles College of Chiropractic in 1979 (Drake, unpublished)

Trustees
Anthony Bazzano, D.C., Chairman
Leonard Savage, D.C., Vice-Chairman
Franklin Schoenholtz, D.C., Secretary-Treasurer
Howard Essegian, D.C.
Robert Moore, D.C.
Carl Nixon, Jr., D.C.
Ordean Syverson, D.C.
Dr. C.C. Trillingham
Vierling Kersey, Pe.D.
Charles Crecelius
Wanda Lindsey
Administrators
W. Heath Quigley, D.C., M.A., President
Matthew M. Givrad, Ph.D., Executive Vice-President
Tuan Tran, Ph.D., Vice-President of Academic Affairs
Robert B. Jackson, D.C., N.D., Vice-President and Clinic Director
Robert Heinbaugh, Vice-President of Development

Table 22-3: Professional educators recruited in the 1980s to assist in the academic and fiscal development of the Los Angeles College of Chiropractic (Drake, unpublished)

John Beckman, Ed.D.
Truman Case, Ed.D.
E. Maylon Drake, Ed.D.
Frank Kittinger, Ed.D.
Joseph Laurin, Ph.D.
Gary Miller, Ph.D.

remodeling of the new campus and lower the mortgage interest. Classes began on the new campus on 9 September 1981.

With these successes in expanding facilities, reorganizing the college's financial picture and re-establishing the school's status with the CCE, the Drake administration turned its attention to regional accreditation. By the mid-1980s a number of chiropractic colleges in other regions of the nation had been successful in achieving dual accreditation status, that is, recognition of their chiropractic professional programs by the CCE and institutional accreditation by the respective regional accrediting body. However, the regional agency for institutions of higher education in California and Hawaii, the Western Association of Colleges and Schools (WASC), had a reputation for being among the most demanding in the nation. The LACC applied to WASC in 1984 and received candidacy status in 1986 (Los, 1995). However, WASC was wary of the standards in chiropractic colleges, and special efforts were required to convince the agency that indeed, LACC functioned as an institution of higher education.

To meet this challenge a number of professional educators were added to the LACC family (see Table 22-3), and the college's research programs were expanded. Reed B. Phillips, D.C., Ph.D., D.A.C.B.R. (see Figure 22-11), formerly the director of research for the FCER and a medical sociologist as well as a chiropractic radiologist, was recruited to head the college's research division. Phillips was joined in his research efforts by Alan H. Adams, D.C. (see Figure 22-12), formerly the academic dean of the CMCC, and like Phillips, a National College graduate. With Adams as stimulus, the administration explored various innovative training programs for health care providers, such as those pioneered at the medical schools of Harvard and McMaster universities. In September 1990 the LACC commenced operation of its "Advantage Curriculum," which seeks to organize the training of doctors around specific competencies rather than subjects, and encourages the student to function as an active self-learner in a problem-based instructional program (Los, 1995). The Advantage program produced a major shift in the distribution of student time in lecture vs. laboratory and practice-relevant experiences (see Figures 22-13a&b).

Impressed with these developments, the WASC's Accrediting Commission for Senior Colleges and Universities granted LACC initial accreditation status in June 1993. By this time, however, Drake had retired as president (he now serves on the college's board of trustees), and was succeeded for a short period by Matthew

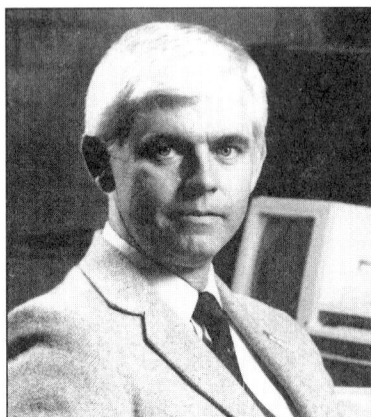

Figure 22-11: Reed B. Phillips, D.C., Ph.D., D.A.C.B.R.

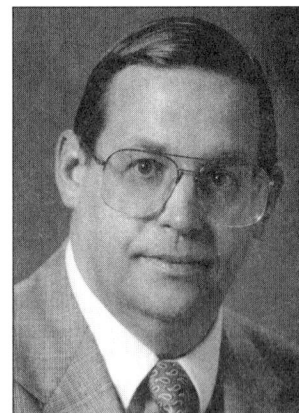

Figure 22-12: Alan H. Adams, M.S., D.C.

Givrad, the former executive vice-president. The board of trustees appointed Phillips, the LACC director of research, to serve as acting president on 19 November 1990 (Drake, unpublished). Phillips' appointment to the presidency on 1 September 1991 diminished his active participation in the research agenda, and exemplifies a problem that has come to plague chiropractic institutions world-wide: the loss of scientists to administrative positions (Ebrall, 1995b).

Despite the personnel changes at LACC, the institution continued to expand its scientific capacities under the stewardship of its Acting Director of Research, Alan Adams. A measure of recognition of this research sophistication was attained on 29 September 1994, when the federal government's Health Research and Services Administration awarded the College $889,671 for a controlled clinical trial of chiropractic treatment for myofascial pain syndromes.

Figure 22-13a: Contrast in hours per week spent in lecture before vs. after implementation of the Advantage Curriculum at the Los Angeles College of Chiropractic (courtesy of Gary Miller, Ph.D.)

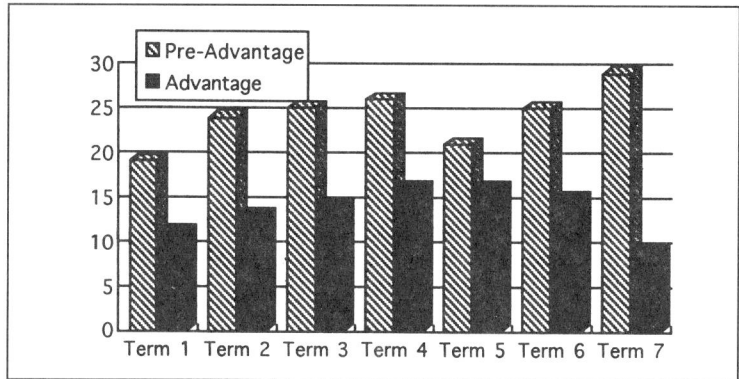

Figure 22-13b: Contrast in hours per week spent in laboratory before vs. after implementation of the Advantage Curriculum at the Los Angeles College of Chiropractic (courtesy of Gary Miller, Ph.D.)

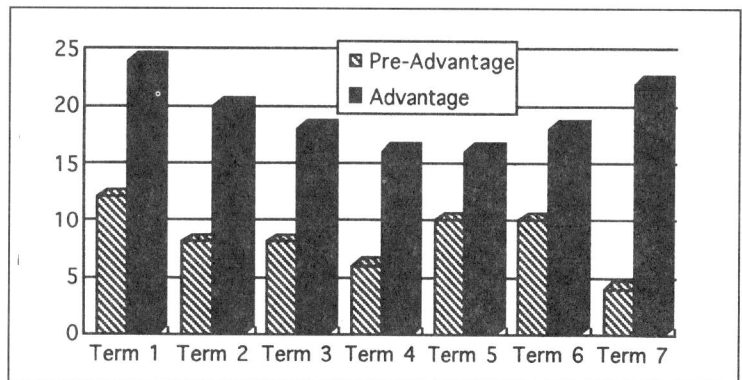

Northwestern College of Chiropractic

The leadership at the Northwestern College of Chiropractic (NWCC) changed in 1984, when Donald M. Cassata, Ph.D. (see Figure 22-14) succeeded founder John B. Wolfe to become the second president of the school. The change in leadership followed soon after the acquisition of a new 25 acre campus for the school in Bloomington, Minnesota (New, 1983). Under Cassata's supervision the college's division of research was expanded, and plans for the development of a research center, the Wolfe-Harris Center for Clinical Studies, took shape. Cassata was succeeded in 1991 by John Allenburg, D.C., the former dean of NWCC during the last years of Wolfe's presidency.

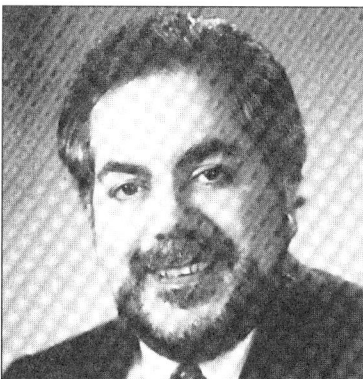

Figure 22-14: Donald M. Cassata, Ph.D.

Western States Chiropractic College

Prompted by the NCA Director of Education, John J. Nugent, Western States College split off its naturopathic division following W.A. Budden's death in 1954, and became the Western States Chiropractic College in 1967 (WSCC) (see Figure 1-6). Robert E. Elliot, D.C. (see Figure 22-15) assumed the presidency of the college in 1956, succeeding Ralph M. Failor, D.C. (see Table 22-4). For the next two decades the institution continued to operate at its limited facilities at 4525 S.E. 63rd Avenue in Portland, which it had purchased in 1946. In 1973 the school relocated to its present 22-acre campus, the former Marycrest Catholic school, in northeastern Portland. Elliot resigned in 1974, and was succeeded by Samuel G. Warren, a retired educator who had served on the college's board of trustees (Western, 1975).

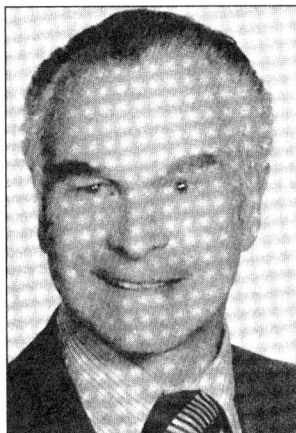

Figure 22-15: Robert E. Elliot, D.C., president of WSCC (1956-74)

The WSCC repeatedly gained and lost accreditation from the NCA and ACA Council on Education, usually owing to its poor finances and under-qualified instructors (Stonebrink, 1974), which in turn were attributable to its small student body. Wardwell (1992, p. 93) notes that:

> ...During the 1956-1970 period WSCC's total enrollment never exceeded 38; it survived only because of personal and financial sacrifices of dedicated board member Milton I. Higgins and Presidents Ralph M. Failor (1954-1956) and Robert E. Elliott...

The school was not among those listed by Hariman (1970, pp. 40-1) as "fully accredited" by the ACA the year before CCE's independent incorporation. However, WSCC claimed "correspondent" status with CCE in 1974 (H.E.W., 1974), which provided eligibility for its students to receive federally guaranteed loans. "Recognized candidate for accreditation" (RCA) status with CCE was achieved in May 1975 (Hidde, 1975b), and expansion of the faculty, library and laboratory facilities was also noted (Western, 1976). On July 1, 1976, Richard H. Timmins, Ed.D., a former executive secretary of the CCE, former administrator with the FCER and former president of Huron College in South Dakota, was appointed president of WSCC (Western, 1976). The college anticipated an enrollment of 430 students for its Fall 1976 term (Western, 1976).

Western States' status with CCE was again jeopardized in the late 1970s, during Timmins' presidency. The college's RCA status with CCE was lost in 1979, this time for reasons having more to do with the structure and activities of the board of trustees and administration (Vear, 1979, 1995). At this time Herbert J. Vear, D.C. (see Figure 22-16), then serving as academic dean of WSCC, was appointed to succeed Timmins, and the chairman of the board of trustees was prevailed upon to resign. Availing themselves of the CCE's appeal process, Vear, with the assistance of John B. Wolfe, president of Northwestern College of Chiropractic, made a strenuous effort to recover RCA status. This was granted in January 1980, and full accreditation was approved during the Council's mid-year board meeting (Vear, 1995) and granted on January 23, 1981 (Catalog 1992-94). In September 1986, the college achieved regional accreditation from the Northwest Association of Schools and Colleges (Catalog 1992-94), and now offers a bachelor's degree in addition to the chiropractic doctorate.

The WSCC has long had a reputation for teaching one of the broadest scopes of practice in the profession, including minor surgery and obstetrics. Although there has been a significant decline in chiropractic involvement in these practices (perhaps owing both to state attorney general's rulings and to the difficulty of purchasing malpractice insurance for these practices), Wardwell (1992, p. 141) noted that as many as 194 deliveries were attended by chiropractic physicians in Oregon

---

Table 22-4: Presidents/Directors of the Western States Chiropractic College and its ancestor institutions, 1904 to present

Institution	Owner/President/Director
Chiropractic School and Cure	John Marsh, D.C. (1904-1909)
D.D. Palmer College of Chiropractic	D.D. Palmer (1908-1910)
Pacific College of Chiropractic	William O. Powell, D.C. (1909-1913)
Oregon Peerless College of Chiropractic & Neuropathy	John E. LaValley, D.C. (1911-1913)
Pacific Chiropractic College	William O. Powell, D.C. (1913-1916)
	Oscar W. Elliott, D.C. (1916-1926)
	Lenore B. Elliot (1926-1929)
	William A. Budden, D.C., N.D. (1929-1932)
Western States College, School of Chiropractic & School of Naturopathy (non-profit)	William A. Budden, D.C., N.D. (1932-1954)
Western States College (non-profit)	Ralph M. Failor, D.C. (1954-1956)
Western States Chiropractic College (non-profit)	Robert E. Elliot, D.C. (1956-1974)
	Samuel G. Warren (1974-1976)
	Richard H. Timmins, Ed.D. (1976-1979)
	Herbert J. Vear, D.C., F.C.C.S.[C] (1979-1986)
	William H. Dallas, D.C. (1986 to present)

Figure 22-17: Western States College's flow chart for the evaluation of chiropractic methods, better known as the "Kaminski model"; reprinted by permission of the *Journal of Manipulative and Physiological Therapeutics* (from Kaminski et al., 1987)

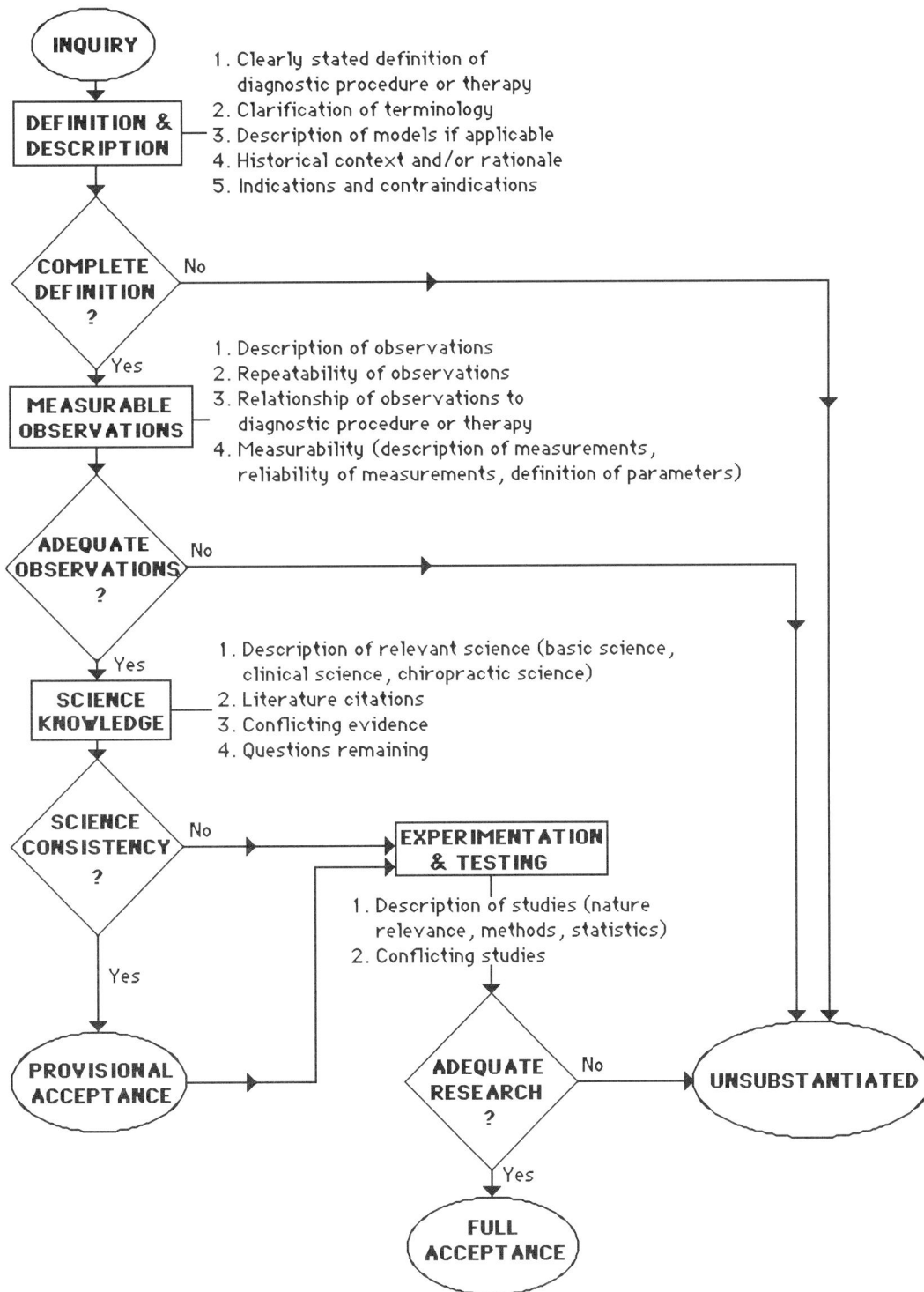

during 1981. The College has continued its broad-scope tradition, and plans have been underway since 1993 to develop a "Doctor of Chiropractic Medicine" degree program. The proposed curriculum seeks to train chiropractors to make use of pre-scription pharmaceuticals. Great consternation has been voiced in the profession in reaction to this proposal.

The Vear administration saw WSCC return to the academic leadership role it had played during Budden's years as president. Exemplary was the formation in the early 1980s of the Chiropractic Library Consortium and its *Index to the Chiropractic Literature* (Whitehead, 1990). Kay Irvine, M.L.S., library director at WSCC, served as editor of the index from its inception until 1997. At about the same time, the college established its residency program in radiology under the supervision of Appa Anderson, D.C., N.D. In the early 1980s the school co-spon-sored several research conferences organized by Scott Haldeman, D.C., Ph.D., M.D. Earlier, while serving as academic dean, Vear had proposed the creation of a Committee on Chiropractic Technique to "oversee the teaching of all undergraduate technique programs at WSCC" and to "identify and recommend additional tech-nique programs" at the college (Vear, 1977). By the mid-1980s this faculty com-mittee had developed an algorithm for the scientific evaluation of chiropractic assessment and treatment procedures (see Figure 22-17). The algorithm (Kaminski et al., 1987), which has come to be called the "Kaminiski model" after its first author, has been well received within the scientific community in the profession.

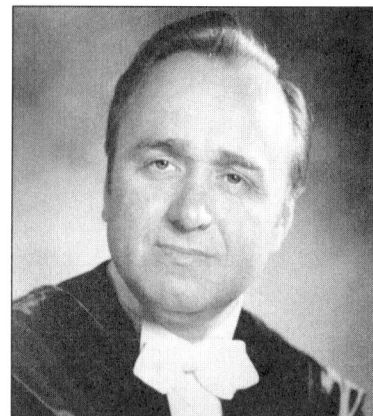

Figure 22-16: Herbert J. Vear, D.C. F.C.C.S.(C)

Despite its small size (fewer than 400 students), the college has evolved into one of the strongest sources of research data in the profession. Credit for this is attributable in part to the Vear legacy, and to the outstanding faculty which has been assembled. Noteworthy for their various contributions to the scholarly litera-ture are Joanne Nyiendo, Ph.D., director of research, Robert Boal, Ph.D., Richard Gillette, Ph.D., Mitch Haas, D.C. (see Figure 22-18) and Mark Kaminski, M.S.

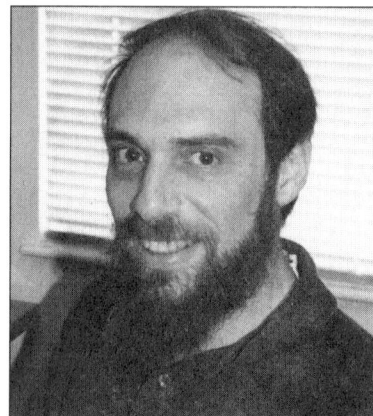

Figure 22-18: Mitchell Haas, M.S., D.C.

Other Forms of Accreditation

When the National College of Chiropractic achieved status with the New York State (NYS) Department of Education in 1971, it marked the first step into federal recognition for chiropractic education. However, the nature of National College's accomplishment was not the professional accreditation today offered to chiropractic schools via the CCE. Accreditation by NYS was a form of regional accreditation. Regional accreditation in the United States provides certification of the overall academic quality of an institution, rather than approval for any particular curriculum or program offered by the institution. Elsewhere, comparable recognition typically depends upon college affiliation or integration with universities (e.g., Australia, Canada, Denmark). The distinction between regional vs. professional accreditation became salient among American chiro-practors when Sherman College of Straight Chiropractic, although not recognized by the CCE, achieved accreditation status with the Southern Association of Colleges and Schools, a federally recognized regional accreditor. In some jurisdictions, licensing regulations which required applicants to have graduated from institutions accredited by an agency recognized by the U.S. government were revised to mandate graduation from CCE-accredited schools.

Regional accreditation of chiropractic colleges also opened the door to a broader range of degree programs. Principal among these has been the baccalaureate degree, which is still not a requirement for admission to most chiropractic colleges. However, responding to demand, a number of chiropractic schools have implemented programs whereby coursework within the chiropractic curriculum (e.g., biology and the physical sciences) is also recognized as liberal arts credit. Several schools have developed programs wherein pre-chiropractic, liberal arts study plus chiropractic study are combined, and students are offered the opportunity to earn a B.S. in human biology with the doctorate in chiropractic. The details of such dual-degree programs vary among regional accreditors and among chiropractic colleges. These programs, in combination with the growth of university-based chiropractic education, have resulted in a variety of non-chiropractic degrees awarded by or through chiropractic institutions (see Table 22-5).

College or University	Accrediting or Awarding Body	Academic Degrees Awarded
Anglo-European College of Chiropractic, Bournemouth, England	University of Portsmouth	B.Sc.
Cleveland Chiropractic College, Missouri	North Central Association of College & Schools (North Central)	B.S.
Life College, Georgia	Southern Association of Colleges & Schools (Southern)	B.S., B.B.A., M.S.
Logan College of Chiropractic, Missouri	North Central	B.S.
Los Angeles College of Chiropractic, California	Western Association of Colleges & Schools	none
Macquarie University, Sidney, Australia	Australian government-funded institution	various
National College of Chiropractic, Illinois	North Central; New York State Department of Education	B.Sc.
New York Chiropractic College	Middle States Association of Colleges & Schools	B.A., B.S.
Northwestern College of Chiropractic, Minnesota	North Central	B.S.
Palmer College of Chiropractic, Iowa	North Central	B.Sc., M.S.
Parker College of Chiropractic, Texas	Southern	B.S.
Royal Melbourne Institute of Technology, Australia	Australian government-funded institution	various
Sherman College of Straight Chiropractic, South Carolina	Southern	none
Technikon Natal, South Africa	Certification Council for Technikon Education	various
University of Bridgeport, Connecticut	New England Association of Schools & Colleges	A.A., A.S., B.A., B.E.S., B.F.A., B.M., B.S., M.S., M.B.A., Ed.D.
Western States Chiropractic College, Oregon	Northwest Association of Schools & Colleges; Oregon Office of Educational Policy & Planning	B.S.

Table 22-5: Regional accreditation and non-chiropractic degrees offered through several schools providing chiropractic curricula, 1995 (College, 1995; Graduate, 1994; McNamee, 1994-95; Western, 1992).

The CCE has also considered the possibility of establishing accreditation procedures for post-doctoral (license renewal and specialty) education, paraprofessional training and for seminars in practice-building (e.g., CCE, 1976; Cleveland, 1996). However, no definite programs in these areas have been established.

International Accreditation

While developments in the accreditation of chiropractic colleges outside the North America are beyond the scope of this work, the development of reciprocal agreements between the CCE and similar agencies in Canada, Europe and the Pacific deserve mention, and suggest the influence that the CCE has had internationally. In most jurisdictions which grant chiropractic licensure, a chiropractic diploma granted by a school accredited by any of the international chiropractic educational councils (see Table 22-6) will be recognized as meeting the requirements for practice. Parenthetically, O'Neill (1994) provides a detailed account of the development of chiropractic education and accreditation in Australia.

The Chiropractic Curriculum

Training programs for chiropractors are typically divided between the basic sciences, clinical sciences and an internship (McNamee, 1994, p. 11). Owing to the profession's continuing conflict with organized medicine, the chiropractic curriculum

Table 22-6: Dates of formation and reciprocity between foreign accrediting agencies for chiropractic education and the Council on Chiropractic Education (USA) (McNamee, 1994, pp. 20-3; Walker, 1995)

Agency	Date of formation	Date of reciprocity with CCE/USA
Australasian Council on Chiropractic Education	1976	February 2, 1986
Council on Chiropractic Education-Canada	May 26, 1978	March 27, 1982
European Council on Chiropractic Education	early 1980s	January 23, 1993

Table 22-7: Comparison of allopathic and chiropractic curricula in California (Haynes, 1975); reprinted by permission of the American Chiropractic Association. NL = Not listed (Catalog lists no description of this particular area of study).

General Factors	LACC	Stanford	Loma Linda	UCLA	UCSF	USC
Entrance requirements semester units	60	90	85	90	90	90
Length of course (yrs.)	4	4	4	4	4	4
Quarter or semester system	S	Q	Q	Q	Q	S
Tuition per quarter (semester to quarter equivalent)	400	1500	910	227	500	1013
Offer Bachelor's degree	Yes	Yes	Yes	?	?	?
National Board Examination required for graduation	Yes	Yes	Yes	?	Yes	Yes
Curriculum						
Anatomy	810	264	450	564	252	Yes
Biochemistry	162	120	170	288	120	Yes
Physiology	324	300	180	264	120	Yes
Microbiology	180	108	190	99	120	Yes
Pathology	288	156	315	348	120	Yes
Pharmacology	36	96	115	138	96	Yes
Public Health	144	Yes	82	NL	Yes	?
Obstetrics & Gynecology	144	Yes	328	Yes	Yes	Yes
Pediatrics	36	Yes	440	Yes	Yes	Yes
Psychiatry	108	Yes	500	Yes	Yes	Yes
Radiology	126	Yes	47	Yes	NL	NL
Physical Therapy	120	NL	0	NL	NL	NL
Diagnosis & Treatment	1884	Yes	1279	Yes	Yes	Yes
Miscellaneous	162	Yes	162	Yes	Yes	Yes
Surgery	72	Yes	690	Yes	Yes	Yes
Nutrition	108	NL	0	NL	NL	NL

Table 22-8: "Representative Curricula in Medical and Chiropractic Schools" (Corporate, 1991, pp. 76-7); reprinted by permission of the Foundation for Chiropractic Education and Research.

Medical School[1]: First Academic Year (40 weeks)

	Lecture	Lab**	Total
Gross Anatomy & Embryology	60	111	171
Histology	44	57	101
Biochemical Molecular & Cell Biology	86	9	95
Preventive Medicine	10	0	10
Nutrition	10	0	10
Physiology	52	32	84
Pathology	40	40	80
Human Behavior	27	0	27
Microbiology	74	44	118
Neuroscience	44	38	82
Human Sexuality	12	15	27
Human Genetics	16	0	16
Clinical Medicine I	19	44	63
Clinical Correlation	10	0	10
Total	504	390	894

Chiropractic School[2]: First Year (3 Trimesters or Quarters)

	Lecture	Lab**	Total
Gross Anatomy & Embryology	163	120	285
Histology	90	45	135
Biochemistry	90	30	120
Physiology	120	30	150
Pathology	45	0	45
Neuroscience	105	0	105
Chiro. Principles & Therapy	165	105	270
Diagnostic Imaging	37.5	45	82.5
Neuromusculoskeletal	45	15	60
Physical Diagnosis	45	30	75
Professional Literature	15	0	15
Human Sexuality	0	10**	10
Health Science Terminology	15	0	15
Total	937.5	430.0	1367.5

Second Academic Year (33 weeks)

	Lecture	Lab**	Total
Pathology	48	44	92
Pharmacology	78	18	96
Pathophysiology I (e.g., resp., cardiovasc.)	75	32	107
Pathophysiology II (e.g., renal, endocrinology)	52	26	78
Pathophysiology III (e.g., gut, lab. diag.)	61	40	101
Pathophysiology IV (e.g., inf. dis., skin, eye)	47	7	54
Clinical Medicine II	0	44	44
Clinical Medicine III (tutorials: med., peds., fam.med., neuro.)	192	0	192
Total	553	211	764

Second Year (3 Trimesters or Quarters

	Lecture	Lab**	Total
Microbiology	60	60	120
Pathology/Clinical Pathology	127.5	60	187.5
Cardiology/Respiratory	60	45	95
Gastrointestinal/Genitourinary	75	15	90
Infectious Disease	30	0	30
Chiropractic Principles & Therapy	150	195	345
Diagnostic Imaging	120	37.5	157.5
Clinical Chiropractic	45	60**	105
Public Health	30	0	30
Nutrition	60	0	60
Physical Diagnosis	60	30	90
Neuromusculoskeletal	120	60	180
Total	937.5	562.5	1500

Third and Fourth Academic Years (72 weeks)

Six Weeks Each in Required Externships in:
Medicine I (basic)
Medicine II (advanced)
Obstetrics-Gynecology
Pediatrics
Psychiatry
Surgery
Outpatient Medicine-Clinical Medicine IV
Neurology or Surgical Specialties
Electives - 24 Weeks

Third and Fourth Years (Four Trimesters)

	Lecture	Lab**	Total
Diagnostic Imaging	30	45	75
Obstetrics-Gynecology	60	7.5	67.5
Endocrinology	30	0	30
Geriatrics	30	0	30
Pharmacology	30	0	30
Dermatology	15	0	15
Mental Health	90	0	90
Pediatrics	30	0	30
Clinical Chiropractic	45	60**	105
Chiro. Principles & Therapy	0	30	0
Clinical Nutrition	45	0	45
Clinical Case Studies	0	34**	34
Emergency Proc./Minor Surgery	22.5	30	52.5
Practice Management	75	0	75
Legal Aspects of Chiropractic	30	0	30
Internship	0	832**	832
Total	532.5	1038.5	1571.0

has often been compared with that for medical students in terms of the topics covered and number of hours of time devoted to each topic. One such comparison was provided by LACC president George Haynes during his final year (1975-76) as school leader and member of the CCE's governing body (see Table 22-7).

On the surface, comparisons such as those found in Table 22-7 seem to suggest that chiropractic students receive more extensive training in the basic sciences, and less extensive clinical training than medical students. However, this comparison may be misleading in several respects. Given the greater selectivity in medical school admissions, the typical allopathic student commences her/his medical school experience with a stronger background in the biological and medically-relevant physical sciences than does the chiropractic counterpart. The contrast between M.D. vs. D.C. students in terms of hours spent in the study of obstetrics and gynecology, pediatrics, psychiatry, and minor surgery also merits further explanation. Such topics are taught primarily via classroom lectures at chiropractic colleges, whereas medical students' education in these subjects relies heavily upon third and fourth year practica (externships or clinical rotations) in addition to didactic instruction and readings. Such differences are more readily apparent in a 1991 report prepared for the FCER by the Corporate Health Policies Group (see Table 22-8).

Perhaps the most important difference between the training of D.C.s and M.D.s occurs at the internship level. Whereas the medical internship is a post-doctoral, supervised, hospital-based experience, the chiropractic internship takes place prior to the award of the doctorate during the final year of the 3.4 year (10 trimesters or 12-13 quarters) chiropractic curriculum. Therefore, any comparison between chiropractic and medical education (such as seen in Table 22-7 and Table 22-8) ought to recognize that the most intensive part of the allopathic physician's supervised clinical training, the internship, is in addition to the four-year medical school experience. Moreover, too often the pre-doctoral interns at chiropractic schools have been:

> ...left to assimilate locally-determined professional and clinical concepts largely on their own; they have no standardized preceptor or clear clinical role model to follow around and learn from.
>
> Typically, a new student in a chiropractic college clinic (be he as talented, well educated and prepared as a student of medicine) is often turned loose to develop and practice his own brand of diagnostic, therapeutic and patient management procedures with minimal contact or detailed clinical instruction from qualified chiropractic clinicians. He essentially sets up and largely operates independently within the college's training clinical version of a private practice. By and large chiropractic clinical students recruit, examine and treat their own patients, without routine availability of clinical faculty to preceptor them in the step-by-step aspects of patient care and chiropractic professionalism (DeBoer, 1983).

DeBoer's (1983) criticisms may have been part of the impetus for the development of the "Mentor Model" of clinical training designed by Ronald Henninger, D.C., D.A.B.C.O., then serving as chief of clinics at Palmer College of Chiropractic-West. Consistent with DeBoer's recommendations, the Mentor Model established a corps of "Clinical Professors" (licensed chiropractic clinicians) within the training facility who assume all responsibility for the management of individual patients. Interns' participation in the care of patients then becomes a delegated responsibility of the attending doctor/mentor, who assigns progressively greater duties to an intern as the latter progresses through the training experience and demonstrates her/his capacity for greater independence. Henninger subsequently implemented a version of the Mentor Model at the training clinic of the Western States Chiropractic College, where a favorable supervisor/intern ratio of 1:7.5 was eventually achieved.

Other initiatives for improving the clinical training of chiropractors are noteworthy. "Externship" programs for clinical students, which permit the advanced intern to practice under the supervision of field chiropractors, date at least to 1981 when John Allenburg, then dean of the Northwestern College of Chiropractic, introduced the "Preceptor Associate" program (Walker, 1981). The program was modeled after the Rural Physicians Associate Program at the University of Minnesota's medical school, and was not unlike the practice-based training that has been available within osteopathic education (American, 1979; Design, 1980). A number of chiropractic colleges have since implemented similar programs, which are generally well-received by chiropractic students, owing to their practical nature and to the diversity and volume of patients and patient-problems encountered. Multiple "satellite" training clinics, often serving the indigent and co-sponsored with social welfare agencies, have become quite common within chiropractic schools. It should also be noted that, although the volume and diversity of patient populations has been problematic for many chiropractic colleges, this is not universally the case. The Cleveland Chiropractic College of Los Angeles training clinic, which is situated in a low-income district, has been able to function as a source of primary care to local residents, thereby providing a broad range of supervised experience for its students.

A number of chiropractic colleges have been active in seeking hospital-based clinical practica for their pre-doctoral students. Such articulation arrangements are still exceptional, however, perhaps owing to the lingering animosity between chiropractors and organized medicine. Their importance rests in the broader exposure to types of health problems, and to the increased opportunity for inter-disciplinary dialogue and exchange. In even fewer cases, such as the collaboration between CMCC and the University of Saskatchewan and between LACC and the University of Colorado (University, 1996), post-doctoral training in tertiary care teaching hospitals has become available to chiropractic residents.

The curriculum of any educational institution is subject to continual revision and improvement. In recent years, however, several chiropractic schools have sought to produce even more fundamental improvements in the manner in which chiropractors are trained. The LACC's "Advantage" curriculum has already been mentioned; similar programs to provide small group, problem-based learning experiences have also been implemented at the National College of Chiropractic (Swenson, 1996; Winterstein, 1996) and the CMCC (CMCC, 1996; Moss, 1996). Under consideration at this time are innovations involving extensive use of the internet, or what has come to be known as "telemedicine" (Distance, 1996); it is anticipated that such strategies will serve to increase inter-disciplinary dialogue.

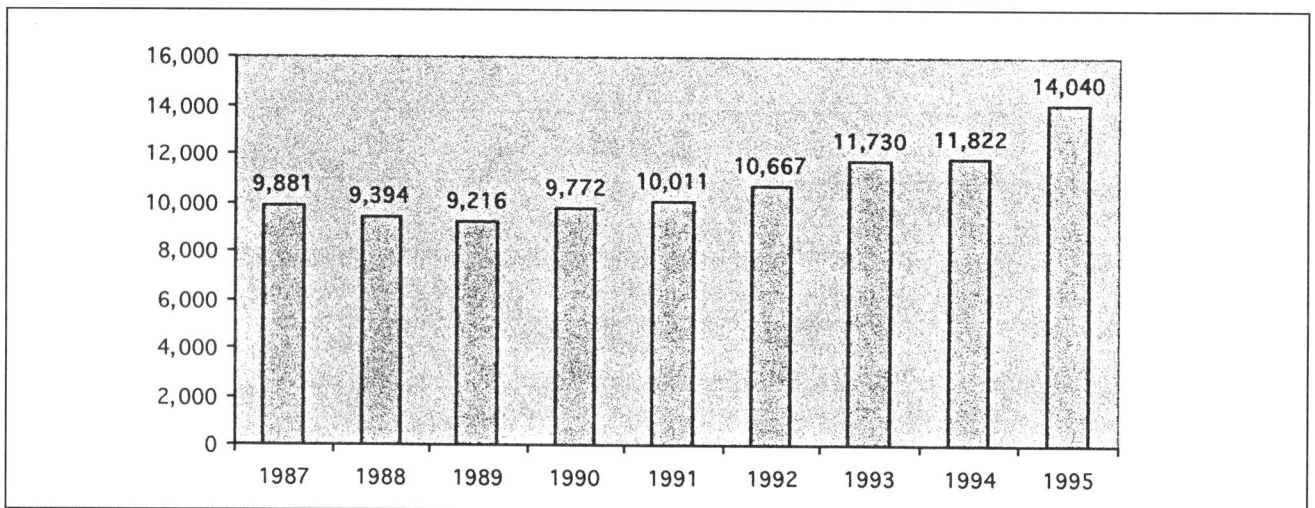

Figure 22-19: Number of students enrolled in chiropractic college in the United States during 1987-1995 (based on Cleveland, 1996)

Each chiropractic college's curriculum is significantly influenced by the institution's finances, which in most cases are dependent most heavily upon tuition. A 1978 survey of 11 schools indicated that the average tuition-dependency was 75%, and that 40% of program costs went to instructional activities (Miller, 1978, pp. 44, 53). The typical chiropractic college, it was noted, involves three years and three months of training in academic terms (usually trimesters) of approximately 16 weeks duration, for a total of approximately 4,777 student contact hours. The number of faculty members required to implement any particular school's training program was importantly related to the number of hours allocated to the curriculum of the clinic and to the instructional methods employed in the clinic (Miller, 1978, p. 52). The sizes of incoming classes of students varied considerably among those schools sampled (from 30 to 160 students), and student attrition was considered "high" (Miller, 1978, pp. 52-3). The colleges were varied in the number of new classes admitted per year.

Chiropractic colleges have been exceptional in their success at developing professional educational programs with practically none of the public funding which has characterized most other health care professions. Gibbons (1980b) has noted:

> Few, if any of the other professions can match this unique experience. Alone among health professions, it has presided over its own destiny, despite intense ideological debate and dissension, and brought forth a professional school system acceptable to the accrediting agencies of the federal government and leading university regents. And in a time when virtually every other aspect of public health training is subsidized by government, the profession has achieved this without any federal or taxpayer assistance.

Figure 22-20: Numbers of U.S. chiropractors 1900-1990 (based on
Wardwell, 1992, pp. 102-3)

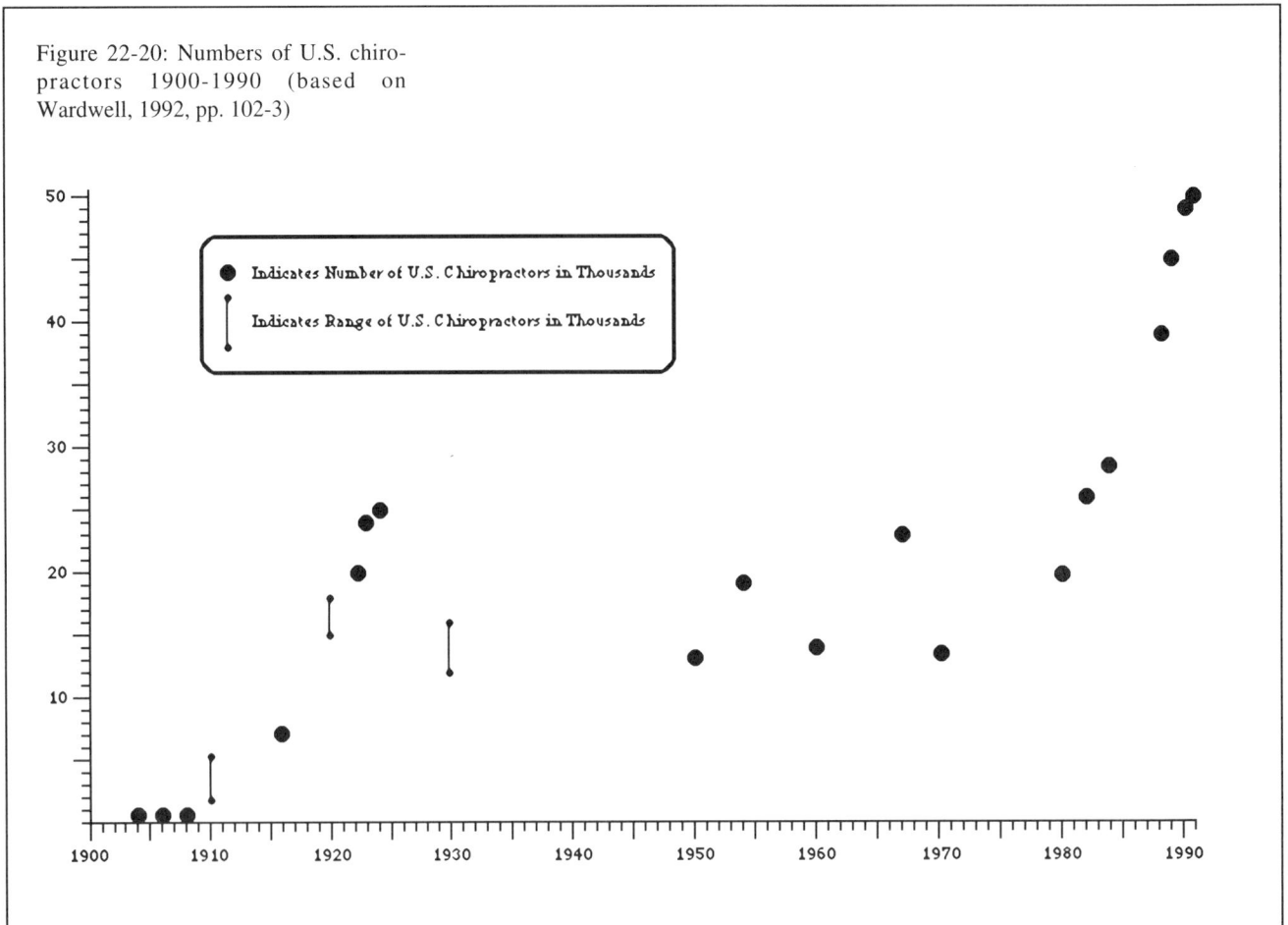

● Indicates Number of U.S. Chiropractors in Thousands

| Indicates Range of U.S. Chiropractors in Thousands

Moreover, the educational enterprise in the profession has been decidedly successful in increasing the number of chiro-practors (see Figures 22-19 and 22-20), based overwhelmingly upon student tuition. As the profession proceeds to its second century, however, a continuing curricular challenge will involve the search for additional sources of income for further cur-ricular improvements. Among these will be greater funding from state and federal government sources, private philanthropy, and expanded services to patients. Finances have been, and for the foreseeable future will continue to be, an important limit-ing factor in the training of chiropractors.

Collegiality and the Formation of the Second ACC

The history of the Association of Chiropractic Colleges (ACC) can be traced to the Clinical Competency meetings pulled together by the National Boards (NBCE), when clinic directors and deans of chiropractic sciences met in Colorado (Clum, 1998). This first intercollegial group was followed by meetings of the Deans and then the Presidents of the colleges. Today's Association of Chiropractic Colleges annual meetings include administrators and academicians of various stripes, from librarians to public relations people. Faculty present papers on teaching methods and educational research. Admissions professionals plan joint recruiting events in arenas such as the American Public Health Association and National Association of Allied Health Professionals' annual conventions. At these venues, chiropractic education presents a unified front to the rest of the education world.

This very civilized state of affairs is not one that would have been easily predicted, considering the bitter climate between colleges in the 1970s and 1980s. The formation of the ACC exemplified the best and worst of chiropractic politics (Cleveland, 1998). The earliest formal action to establish the "Association of Chiropractic College Presidents" (ACCP) came by a motion from Dr. Rick Timmins, former Executive Director of CCE and Former President of Western States Chiropractic College. An association that could potentially challenge the ACA's dominance met with substantial resistance from Joseph Janse, the President of the CCE, and in addition, certain members of the incumbent CCE Executive Committee members (Cleveland, 1998).

In January 1984, the ACCP met and unanimouly supported a definition of "Chiropractic science." Other definitions that were also agreed upon were "applicant, qualified applicant, accepted applicant and matriculant." It was felt that this would assist college admissions officers in the gathering of pertinent information in regard to the prospect pool and multiple applications. Carl Cleveland III, D.C. was charged to draft bylaws for the function of an "organization of Chiropractic Colleges," a non-incorporated organization (Association, 1984).

In 1985, the group changed their name to the Association of Chiropractic Colleges, the same name that had been used by the rival accrediting agency in the previous decade (see Chapters 19 and 20). Those involved interpret the ACA's resistance to this new organization in slightly different ways. It may have been a confusion with the earlier ACC and a concern this new group would be a dividing mechanism of accreditation (Miller, 1998; Fay, 1998), or a more pervasive fear of loss of control (McAndrews 1998, Clum 1998). But everyone agrees there was resistance.

Just as the ACA's FCER had withheld Grant-in-Aid funds in 1969 to ensure the colleges comply with the two-year preprofessional education requirement (Schierholz, 1986), once again money was used as leverage to ensure the colleges toe the ACA line. As the ACC moved toward incorporation, colleges whose votes would be necessary were forgiven loans in exchange for their opposition to the incorporation. As a 501(c)6 trade association, the Association would be a political organization which could proselytize and hire a legislative representative. In 1986, the ACC established an office in Washington and engaged Howard Holcomb as a lobbyist. In 1988, the ACC report to the CCE stated:

"We are also working on the modification of bylaws and articles of incorporation...The corporation itself, and its major project, coordination of the burgeoning tendency for groups within the colleges to network with each other, including the colleges, will be major objectives of concern."(Association, 1988)

Jerome McAndrews, D.C. became President of the ACC shortly after he joined the group in his role as president of Palmer College. He "ran the meetings under the assumption that everyone in the room had full veto power"(McAndrews, 1998). The ACC has focused on those matters that are germane to chiropractic education. An entrance examination for chiropractic students has been on the agenda for a number of years, but a fear of dictated national definition of chiropractic practice guidelines make some schools reluctant to support the exam.

One of the great successes of the group was the establishment of the ChiroLoan program. Chiropractic's participation in the HEAL (Health Education Act Loan) program was in jeopardy after President George Bush declared that chiropractic and podiatric students were "unworthy of public trust." The establishment of the ChiroLoan allowed students to finance their education independently of the U.S. Government. The program also allowed the ACC to become financially independent of any one of the colleges or professional organizations (Clum, 1998).

The first ever coordinated and expanded meeting of the ACC was held March 17-20, 1994. The convocation in Las Vegas brought together many of the institutional subgroups that had met on a random or regular basis including academic officers, the directors of financial aid, admissions and marketing, registrars and librarians (Association, 1994). A track was included for teaching faculty. Although more limited in scope, these paper sessions supplanted the Congresses of Chiropractic Educators, which had been held in 1989 at Palmer, in 1990 at Palmer West and in 1994 at Life.

In July 1996, the ACC released the ACC Chiropractic Paradigm (Figure 22-21). The schematic shows patient health through quality care built on a foundation of the science, philosophy and art of chiropractic and surrounded by a number of issues facing the profession.

One of the enduring projects sponsored by the ACC is the publication of *The Journal of Chiropractic Education*. The *Journal* was started as a personal project of Grace Jacobs, D.A., in 1987 (Jacobs, 1987) "For some time faculty members at chiropractic colleges have expressed a desire [to] have their counterparts share ideas relevant to the teaching of chiropractic." In 1989, in its third year of publication, the *Journal* was ensured stability through the financial support of the ACC.

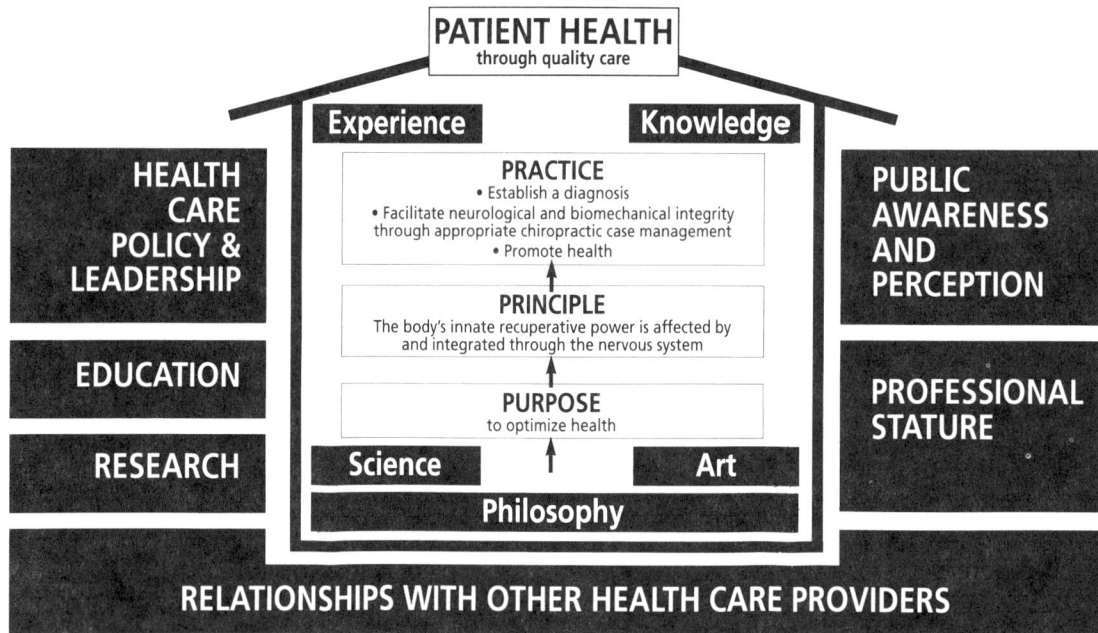

Figure 22-21: The ACC Chiropractic Paradigm

Chapter 23

THE EMERGING SCIENCE OF CHIROPRACTIC

In the final quarter of chiropractic's first century the importance of scientific investigation and its role in chiropractic education finally became apparent to the school leaders (Corporate, 1991; Janse, 1978; Phillips, 1995). Although some awareness of the necessity of documenting chiropractic outcomes had been in evidence earlier on (e.g., Hildebrandt, 1967; Martin, 1969; Muilenburg, 1970; Watkins, 1944), this now grew more rapidly, not only within the academic community (Dr. Goldstein, 1975; Haldeman, 1975), but in the leadership of the professional associations (e.g., Dallas, 1975). Stimulus for this emerging awareness was provided by the history-making conference sponsored by the National Institutes of Health in Bethesda, Maryland, during February 1975, which has been described as "the 'great watershed' in the science of chiropractic" (Gitelman, 1984). The conference brought together leaders from the allopathic, chiropractic and osteopathic professions as well as scientists interested in manipulative methods (see Table 23-1), and resulted in a monograph entitled *The Research Status of Spinal Manipulative Therapy* (Goldstein, 1975). For the first time chiropractic, osteopathic and medical providers and critics of manual methods of health care came together under one roof to discuss what was known (and especially what was not known 20 years ago) about manipulation.

That this conference took place at all must be credited to the persistence and determination of Chung Ha Suh, Ph.D. and the ICA (Cleveland & Keating, 1995). Suh, trained in biomechanical engineering at the University of California at Berkeley, was professor and chairman of the Department of Engineering Design and Economic Evaluation at the University of Colorado at Boulder in the early 1970s. Intrigued by the research questions raised by the interests of several Colorado chiro-

Thomas H. Ballantine, Jr., M.D.	Joseph W. Howe, D.C., D.A.C.B.R.	Harry D. Patton, M.D., Ph.D.
William Bromley, D.C.	Joseph Janse, D.C., N.D.	Edward R. Perl, M.D.
Robert E. Burke, M.D.	Martin Jenness, D.C., Ph.D.	David E. Pleasure, M.D.
Thomas N. Chase, M.D.	William L. Johnston, D.O.	Santo F. Pullella, Ph.D.
Carl S. Cleveland, Jr., D.C.	Christopher B. Kent, D.C.	Richard Remington, Ph.D.
Jerome Cornfield	Igor Klatzo, M.D.	Akio Sato, M.D., Ph.D.
James Cyriax, M.D., M.R.C.P.	Andries M. Kleynhans, D.C.	Herbert H. Schaumburg, M.D.
William S. Day, D.C.	Irvin M. Korr, Ph.D.	Robert Shapiro, M.D.
J.S. Denslow, D.O.	Elizabeth Lomax, M.D., Ph.D.	Seth Sharpless, Ph.D.
Giovanni DiChiro, M.D.	Horace W. Magoun, Ph.D.	Chung Ha Suh, Ph.D.
David Drum, D.C.	Robert Maigne, M.D.	Sir Sydney Sunderland, M.D.
Gustave Dubbs, D.C.	Peter A. Martin, N.D., D.O., D.C.	Peter Tilley, D.O.
Karl Frank, Ph.D.	Joseph P. Mazzarelli, D.C.	Donald B. Tower, M.D., Ph.D.
Lyle A. French, M.D., Ph.D.	Fletcher H. McDowell, M.D.	Walter I. Wardwell, Ph.D.
Ronald Gitelman, D.C., F.C.C.S.(C)	James H. McElhaney, Ph.D.	Edmund B. Weis, Jr., M.D.
Murray Goldstein, D.O., M.P.H.	John McM. Mennell, M.D.	Henry G. West, Jr., D.C.
Philip Greenman, D.O.	William D. Miller, D.O.	Augustus A. White, III, M.D.
E.S. Gurdjian, M.D., Ph.D.	Alf Nachemson, M.D., Ph.D.	Andrew B. Wymore, D.C.
Lloyd Guth, M.D.	George W. Northup, D.O., F.A.A.O.	
Scott Haldeman, D.C., Ph.D.	Sidney Ochs, Ph.D.	

Table 23-1: Participants in the National Institutes of Health workshop on spinal manipulative therapy, Bethesda, Maryland, February 2-4, 1975 (Goldstein, 1975)

practors who were developing instruments for adjusting the upper cervical spine, the Korean-born scientist resolved to explore the effects of spinal nerve root compression upon nerve conduction. He obtained initial support for his pilot investigations from the ICA, and prepared a research grant proposal to submit to the National Institutes of Health (NIH) for funding. In this case, however, his proposal, although scientifically worthy, received a low funding priority rating (Cleveland & Keating, 1995).

Suh, who had an established track record of attracting external funding, including federal money for his scientific studies, was informed confidentially that his proposals would not be funded by NIH so long as the term "chiropractic" was employed (Cleveland & Keating, 1995). Offended by this blatant intrusion of inter-disciplinary politics upon the scientific process, Suh collaborated with William S. Day, D.C., president of the ICA, in appealing directly to the U.S. Congress for support. The pair spoke before the House Appropriations Committee, Subcommittee on Labor, Health, Education and Welfare on May 18, 1973, and at a similar Senate Committee hearing in July. The House Appropriations Subcommittee reported (Cleveland & Keating, 1995):

> The committee believes that in view of the recent inclusion of chiropractic services under Medicare, this would be an opportune time for an independent, unbiased study of the fundamentals of the chiropractic profession. Such studies should be high among the priorities of the NINDS and a budget of as much as $2 million should be earmarked for this study and chiropractic research to be conducted by chiropractors...

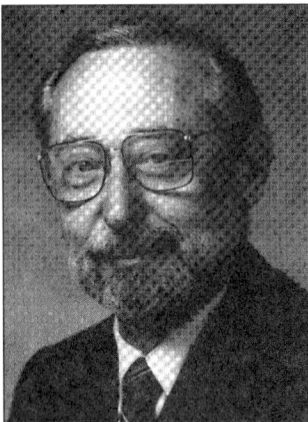

Figure 23-1: Murray Goldstein, D.O., M.P.H.

These funds were appropriated, and the National Institute of Neurological Disorders and Stroke (NINDS), part of the NIH, awarded Suh $238,000 for his studies. Dr. Murray Goldstein (see Figure 23-1), the associate director of the NINDS, decided to use some of the balance of funding to underwrite a conference on chiropractic. In order to encourage the participation of osteopathic and medical doctors, the meeting was promoted as an interdisciplinary conference on spinal manipulation. Goldstein became a featured speaker at chiropractic convocations (e.g., Dr. Goldstein, 1975; Schierholz, 1986, p. 34).

Perhaps the most important outcome of the NIH conference was the recognition among all participants that the scientific validity of manipulation was very far from established. Certainly, the mere fact that practitioners of manipulation from diverse disciplines had laid aside their traditional antagonisms long enough to critically discuss their methods (both the similarities and the differences) was of considerable importance, and many enduring alliances among individual participants have been apparent (see Table 23-2). Another benefit was the creation of the Chiropractic Research Abstracts Collection (CRAC) by the faculty of the Canadian Memorial Chiropractic College (CMCC) (Gitelman, 1984). The CRAC brought together much if not all of the available literature from multiple disciplines concerning manual methods of health care; successive editions were published by the CMCC and later by Williams & Wilkins, Inc., a medical publishing house. Since there was, at the time (1975), no other index to the chiropractic literature, the CRAC provided the first extensive inter-disciplinary index for the literature on manipulative procedures.

But if the 1975 NIH conference on spinal manipulation was a "great watershed," it was also the "great eye-opener" (Gitelman, 1984) for chiropractic and its academic community:

> We were in the ball game, but just barely so. We took a look at our potential research personnel and facilities and realised that we were quite deficient...

> Having reviewed all the previous chiropractic research, we found it wanting, for with a few notable exceptions, such as Illi, Janse, Gillet, Liekens, Johnson and Grice, who had made worthwhile contributions, most of the work of early researchers was questionable. I use the word "questionable" in order to be kind, for I feel that much of it must have been based on a "voice heard in the middle of night"...But strange as it may seem, many have swallowed such a dubious ball of wax, sold with a sugar coating of Innate Intelligence, a smattering of science and such inane phrases as "The power that made the body will heal the body," "Above down and inside out," "Put the bone in motion and Innate will do the rest." These systems were death to thought and undermined our educational institutions, leaving no room for research other than by their chauvinistic [technique] founders, who dared not do legitimate research (Gitelman, 1984).

The NIH conference and the U.S. Office of Education's admonition to CCE in 1976 that its criteria should indicate "There shall be research instead of should be research" (Schierholz, 1986, p. 36), seems to have prompted a spurt of activity among the chiropractic colleges. Richard Timmins, Ed.D., ACA Director of Education and Research Administrator for the FCER, delivered a similar message to the FCER's board of trustees. Goldstein, the NIH organizer of the conference, urged the CCE's leadership to "get research into chiropractic colleges and get your applications in for help on training personnel. You should be able to get 11-12, maybe a few more from each graduating college interested in research In 3-4 years you should have a formidable team to work with" (Schierholz, 1986, p. 34).

Although several more decades would pass before substantive federal funding for chiropractic investigations at the colleges was acquired, the conference had helped to set several of the schools on that pathway. The CMCC developed coursework in research methodology (Gitelman, 1984), expanded the CRAC, approved the formation of the College of Chiropractic Science (Canada) (see Table 23-3) and established a residency program in conjunction with William Kirkaldy-Willis, M.D., an orthopedic surgeon at the University of Saskatchewan (Gitelman, 1984; Keating, 1992, pp. 71-2). The College of Chiropractic Sciences was organized specifically to train future chiropractors as researchers and scholars who could populate the ranks of the chiropractic college faculties in future years (Vear, 1974).

Table 23-2: Members of the editorial board of the National College of Chiropractic's *Journal of Manipulative and Physiological Therapeutics*, September 1980. Asterisks indicate those members who had participated in the 1975 NIH conference on spinal manipulation (see also Table 23-1)

Barry S. Brown, Ph.D.
Robin R. Canterbury, D.C., D.A.C.B.R.
Barry P. Davis, Ph.D.
William C. Davis, Ph.D.
Pierre-Louis Gaucher, D.C.
*Ronald Gitelman, D.C., F.C.C.S.(C)
*Philip E. Greenman, D.O.
Adrian S. Grice, D.C.
*Scott Haldeman, D.C., Ph.D., M.D.
*Andries M. Kleynhans, D.C.
*Irvin M. Korr, Ph.D.
Reed B. Phillips, D.C., D.A.C.B.R.
C.A. Pinkenburg, D.C.
Stanley Plagenhoef, Ph.D.
*Akio Sato, M.D., Ph.D.
Bertram Spector, Ph.D.
Ralph S. Stowe, D.C.
Pat Thomason, Ph.D.
Tuan A. Tran, Ph.D.
*Walter I. Wardwell, Ph.D.
James F. Winterstein, D.C., D.A.C.B.R.

At the Anglo-European College of Chiropractic in Great Britain, research director Alan Breen, D.C. (see Figure 23-2) overcame the traditional ostracism experienced by chiropractic authors when his paper, "Chiropractors and the Treatment of Back Pain," was published in the medical journal, *Rheumatology and Rehabilitation* (Breen, 1977). At Palmer College of Chiropractic, president Jerome McAndrews directed that all faculty members must publish. The National College commenced fund-raising to erect its research center (Gitelman, 1984), and the administration encouraged greater scholarly efforts from the campus community:

TO ALL STAFF MEMBERS TO INCLUDE ADMINISTRATION, FACULTY AND CLINIC STAFF:

There is a marked and ever-increasing need within the chiropractic profession to present subjects of critical study, innovative investigation and research in the form of well-prepared papers that will appear in major publications within the profession, as well as clinical and scientific journals outside the profession.

The entire scientific and clinical community is seeking information from the chiropractic profession relevant to the major concepts, hypothesis and conjectors [sic] that comprise the thinking of our people. We are being challenged at every level, not necessarily in a mitigating or derogatory manner. People are interested in us and they want to know how we think and ideate and what we have done on an investigatory basis.

For these reasons, may I submit to you the most sincere request that if at all possible you commit yourselves to

Table 23-3: Charter members of the College of Chiropractic Science (Canada)

David Churchill, D.C.
David Drum, D.C.
Glen Engel, D.C.
Ronald Gitelman, D.C.
Adrian Grice, D.C.
Scott Haldeman, D.C., Ph.D.
Edgar Houle, D.C.
Robert Johnston, D.C.
Lyman Johnson, D.C.
Thomas Maxwell, D.C.
Herbert J. Vear, D.C.

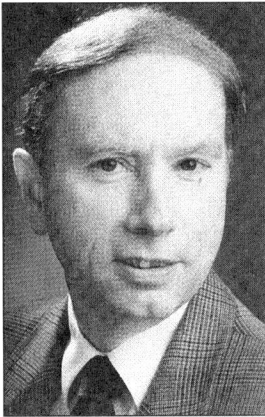

Figure 23-2: Alan Breen, D.C., Ph.D.

the preparation annually of two scientific papers and submit them to the Chairman of the Department of Editorial Review and Publication, namely, Dr. Roy W. Hildebrandt.

As you well know, we here at the College have embarked upon a great adventure that has already become a commanding challenge and has already provoked commendable comments and observations. I refer to the quarterly published by the College, namely, THE JOURNAL OF MANIPULATIVE AND PHYSIOLOGICAL THERAPEUTICS. Then there are the scientific and clinical sections of the JOURNAL OF THE AMERICAN CHIROPRACTIC ASSOCIATION, the JOURNAL OF THE INTERNATIONAL CHIROPRACTORS ASSOCIATION, the SWISS ANNALS OF CHIROPRACTIC and the DIGEST OF CHIROPRACTIC ECONOMICS. On several occasions I have received requests from Journals outside of the profession and of significant stature for articles and papers.

So, indeed, your literary talents are very much needed and it is my hope that you will see fit to respond with a sense of happy involvement (Janse, 1978).

The 1975 NIH conference was followed by a variety of intra-chiropractic and interdisciplinary meetings on spinal manipulative therapy (SMT). Irvin M. Korr, Ph.D., physiologist and long-time researcher within the osteopathic community, moderated a second NIH conference on SMT in October 1977 (Gitelman, 1984), which led to the publication of his edited volume, *The Neurobiologic Mechanisms in Manipulative Therapy* (Korr, 1978). With the assistance of Joseph P. Mazzarelli and Jerome F. McAndrews, chairman of the board and executive vice-president respectively of the ICA, Scott Haldeman (see Figure 23-3), a 1964 Palmer graduate serving as an associate clinical professor in neurology at the University of California at Irvine, School of Medicine, organized an interdisciplinary meeting which produced the first chiropractic text (see Table 23-4) to be published by a medical publishing house (Haldeman, 1980). In his capacity as chairman of the board of trustees of the PCC, Mazzarelli also organized the World Chiropractic Conference held in April and May 1982 in Venice, Italy; the conference produced an edited volume of papers concerning SMT (Mazzarelli, 1982), including the earliest known experimental effort to differentiate between the effects of segment-specific adjusting and more generalized manipulative methods (Cleveland, 1982). On the West Coast several chiropractic colleges sponsored an interdisciplinary conference which featured Haldeman's perceptions of the research status of SMT (see Figure 23-4). In the middle 1980s, Palmer College of

Table 23-4: Contributors to *Modern Developments in the Principles and Practice of Chiropractic* (Haldeman, 1980)

Leon R. Coelho, D.C.
John H. Coote, Ph.D.
H.F. Farfan, M.D., C.M., F.R.C.S.(C)
Richard A. Gerren, Ph.D.
Russell W. Gibbons, B.A.
Ronald Gitelman, D.C., F.C.C.S.(C)
Adrian S. Grice, D.C., F.C.C.S.(C)
Scott Haldeman, D.C., Ph.D., M.D.
Andries M. Kleynhans, D.C.
Marvin W. Luttges, Ph.D.
Reed B. Phillips, D.C., D.A.C.B.R.
Akio Sato, M.D., Ph.D.
Chung Ha Suh, Ph.D.
Sydney Sunderland, M.D., D.Sc., F.R.A.C.P., F.A.A.
John J. Triano, D.C., M.A.
Walter I. Wardwell, Ph.D.
Henry G. West, Jr., D.C., F.I.C.C.

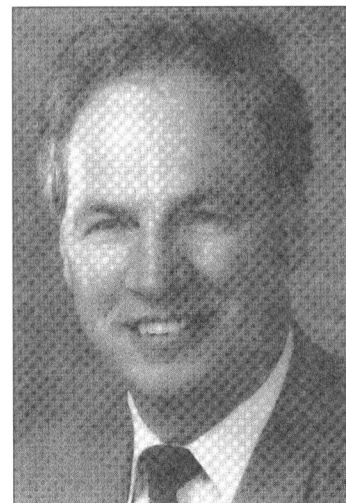

Figure 23-3: Scott Haldeman, D.C., Ph.D., M.D., F.C.C.S.(c)

Chiropractic West co-sponsored research conferences with the American Back Society, an interdisciplinary group composed of orthopedic surgeons, neurologists, chiropractors, physiotherapists and others concerned with back disorders.

The NIH conferences also inspired investigative activity, albeit on a small scale, at several schools. Ronald L. Rupert, D.C., future developer of CHIROLARS (Rupert, 1990), first became involved in research at his alma mater, the Cleveland Chiropractic College of Kansas City, in 1978 during Alex Warner's term as Director of Research. The following year Rupert collaborated with Marvin Luttges, Ph.D., in sensory studies at the University of Colorado. During Rupert's term as Director of Research at CCCKC, various collaborative projects with the Kansas City College of Osteopathic Medicine and the University of Missouri dental school were established. In the early 1980s Rupert and basic science instructor Robert J. Wagnon, Ph.D. (future director of research for Palmer College in Davenport and later at the Sherman College of Straight Chiropractic), obtained funding for a small-animal laboratory from the FCER (Rupert, 1996). In 1981, a "research fellowship" was established at the Kansas City college.

Sometimes the growing concerns for scientific and scholarly development produced amusing tactics. Exemplary were the directives issued by a few college administrators requiring all faculty to engage in research and to publish. Similarly, the CCE's adoption of a formal definition of "chiropractic science" at its January 1984 annual meeting (Appendix A), although well intentioned and perhaps of some political value within the profession, had little if any influence on those scholars and scientists who were actually engaged in exploring the boundaries of chiropractic knowledge. The definition suggested that:

> Chiropractic is the science which concerns itself with the relationship between structure, primarily the spine, and function, primarily the nervous system, of the human body as that relationship may affect the restoration and preservation of health.

Predictably, chiropractic investigators ignored such official pronouncements and pursued their own agendas. Only in the last decade, as significant sums of money became available for substantive research grants (National, 1994) and as the number of qualified researchers has grown, has a focus for chiropractic research begun to take shape.

National College of Chiropractic and the Scholarly Literature

Joseph Janse's commitment to scholarly development was exceptional, and included concern for the epistemologies employed by chiropractors, the meager resources available within the profession for substantive scientific development, and the paucity of legitimate scientific periodicals. His own writings, spanning four decades, evidence his personal growth toward a critical, skeptical attitude regarding clinical phenomena and his gradually increasing recognition of the need to conduct clinical experiments in order to determine cause and effect relationships between what chiropractors do and how their patients respond.

Owing to its relatively strong economic status and the absorption of several intellectually more advanced chiropractic institutions, such as the Chiropractic Institute of New York and the Lincoln

You are cordially invited...
to attend

THE FIRST INTERCOLLEGIATE RESEARCH SYMPOSIUM

Cleveland Chiropractic College
Los Angeles Chiropractic College
Pasadena University Chiropractic School

presented on

MARCH 19, 1978

- at -

Cleveland College Campus (Host)
590 North Vermont, Los Angeles

- by -

The International Society For The Advancement of
CLINICAL CHIROPRACTIC
and
SPINAL RESEARCH

featuring:

COLLEGE DEANS

CARL CLEVELAND, JR..............................of C.C.C.
W. HEATH QUIGLEY................................of L.A.C.C.
ARTHUR GARROW..................................of P.U.C.S.

RESEARCHERS

MARY DITTO, D.D.S., Ph.D........................of C.C.C.
TUAN TRAN, Ph.D..................................of L.A.C.C.
RICHARD STUART, Ph.D.........................of P.U.C.S.

SPECIAL ADDRESS
"WHY RESEARCH?"
Scott Haldeman, D.C., Ph.D., M.D.

Figure 23-4: Announcement for research symposium appearing in the March 1978 issue of the *World-Wide Report*

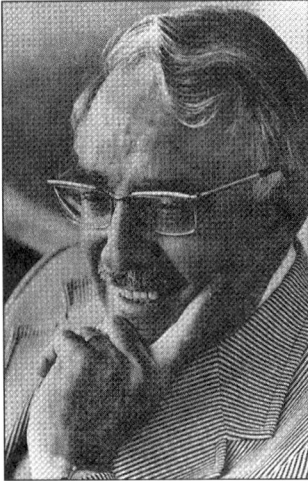

Figure 23-5: Joseph Janse, D.C., N.D.

Chiropractic College, the National College was better prepared than most chiropractic schools to meet the new challenges of research that loomed larger after the 1975 NIH conference on spinal manipulation. Janse (see Figure 23-5) also recognized that the profession and the colleges had done relatively little work to create the infrastructure necessary for scientific investigation in the profession (Keating, 1992). In particular, he was concerned that no credible outlet for scientific publishing had been established, and to this end he repeatedly petitioned the ACA to establish a science journal. Unfortunately, his concerns, like those of C.O. Watkins in the 1940s, 1950s and 1960s, went unheeded by the nation's largest professional association. The society continued to identify its trade magazine, the *Journal of the American Chiropractic Association*, as a "scientific publication" as recently as September 1995 (Guidelines, 1995).

Frustrated at the trade association's unwillingness to fill this professional need, Janse resolved that the National College would establish its own science journal. For this he turned to Roy W. Hildebrandt, D.C., a Palmer graduate and former chairman of his alma mater's department of roentgenology who had joined the National College faculty. Hildebrandt believed that the creation of such a periodical required a significant financial commitment from the institution, perhaps as much as $100,000, in order to sustain the magazine in its first few years irrespective of the initial interest (or lack thereof) in the field. He also determined that a credible science journal must adhere to several critical standards, such as the autonomy of its editor and the establishment of a blind-peer-review process for manuscripts (Keating, 1992, pp. 67-70, 299-311). Janse consented to these terms, and appointed Hildebrandt to serve as the new periodical's first editor. In March 1978, the first issue of the *Journal of Manipulative and Physiological Therapeutics* (JMPT) was released (Hildebrandt, 1978).

Table 23-5: Several scholarly journals established during the 1980s

Founded	Name of Journal	Affiliation of Journal or Editor
1981	Chiropractic History	Association for the History of Chiropractic
1984	Research Forum*	Palmer College of Chiropractic
1987	Chiropractic Sports Medicine	None
1987	Journal of Chiropractic Education	Northwestern College of Chiropractic
1988	American Journal of Chiropractic Medicine**	None
1989	Chiropractic Technique	Northwestern College of Chiropractic

*Merged with several other periodicals
**Discontinued in 1991

The rate of scholarly contributions (Keating, Larson et al., 1989; Keating, Booher & Door, 1989) and of subscriptions to JMPT grew slowly. Interest in a science journal was limited at first, owing to a lack of scholarly tradition as well as to inter-college rivalry. However, as the JMPT's durability and the quality of its contents became apparent, a flurry of new periodicals was seen, and many of these were affiliated (or their editors were affiliated) with chiropractic colleges (see Table 23-5). The annual rate of published contributions to the JMPT tripled during its first 11 years, from about 40 papers per year during 1978-80 to an average of 124 papers per year during 1987-88 (see Table 23-6). Although the average annual percent of original data reports grew very little during 1978-1988 (from 24% to 27%), a clear increase in some categories of original data reports were apparent, such as measurement evaluations; normative, survey and actuarial studies; and case reports. The JMPT also became a communication forum for a small group within the profession, some of whom were located at chiropractic colleges (Keating & Young, 1987), who sought to create a substantive, scholarly literature and to raise intellectual standards within the profession (e.g., DeBoer, 1983, 1988).

The JMPT's eventual success was also attributable to achieving international and interdisciplinary indexing (see Table 23-7). When first published in 1978, neither the JMPT nor any other periodical in the profession was recognized by the U.S. National Library of Medicine (NLM), publishers of the *Index Medicus*. This was a significant limitation for the chiropractic literature (Hildebrandt, 1981a&b; Keating, 1992, pp. 307-310) in that *Index Medicus* provides access to citations from several thousands of bio-medical journals world-wide, and exclusion renders a journal somewhat invisible to the scientific community. The JMPT's founding editor, Roy W. Hildebrandt, repeatedly petitioned the NLM for inclusion of JMPT, but was rebuffed on the grounds that there was little interest in chiropractic subjects within the health science community. In response, Hildebrandt conducted a comprehensive survey of all mentions of chiropractic within journals included in *Index Medicus*. His survey revealed several hundred such mentions, all of them derogatory and most of which were anecdotal reports

Table 23-6: Number of data reports and non-data reports appearing in the *Journal of Manipulative and Physiological Therapeutics* during 3-, 2-, and 11-year periods (1978-1988); from Keating, Booher & Door, 1989; reprinted by permission of *Chiropractic Technique*

Type of Article	1978-1980	1981-1983	1984-1986	1987-1988	Total 1978-88
Data Reports					
Controlled Trials	1	1	1	1	4
Measurement Evaluations	4	11	8	12	35
Clinical Analog	6	4	5	5	20
Clinical Series	7	8	7	6	28
Normative, Survey & Actuarial Studies	4	8	12	14	38
Case Reports	7	13	19	28	67
Basic Science	1	1	2	1	5
Subtotal	30	46	54	67	197
Non-data Reports					
Reviews	23	14	21	23	81
Technical Reports	9	5	7	3	24
Editorials	11	10	8	15	44
Letters to the Editor	33	15	29	139	214
Special Reports & Reprints	16	2	1	1	20
Subtotal	92	46	66	181	385
Total	122	92	120	248	582

of injury supposedly incurred by chiropractic care. Armed with these data, Hildebrandt argued that the NLM's policy toward chiropractic literature helped to create the situation with which it sought to justify excluding the JMPT. In other words, suggested Hildebrandt, the scant apparent interest in the chiropractic literature was perpetuated by *Index Medicus'* biased and exclusionary attitude, which had previously allowed only medical physicians to comment on chiropractic. On this basis the NLM relented (Hildebrandt, 1981a&b); JMPT was first included in *Index Medicus* in 1982, and has since achieved inclusion in a number of other scholarly, interdisciplinary indexes, such as BIOSIS and *Excerpta Medica*.

Table 23-7: Indexing and topics covered in several scholarly journals of chiropractic. All are indexed in the Chiropractic Library Consortium's *Index to the Chiropractic Literature* and CHIROLARS, an electronic data base which includes citations from "every issue of scientific journals" (Rupert, 1990).

Journal Title	Other Indexes	Journal Topics
Chiropractic History	Bibliography of the History of Medicine of the National Library of Medicine (USA)	History
Chiropractic Journal of Australia	Australasian Medical Index, British Library Complementary Medicine Index	Science, history, professional issues, education
Chiropractic Sports Medicine	Biosciences Info Services, Excerpta Medica, Physical Education Index	Science, professional issues
European Journal of Chiropractic	Current Awareness Topics Service (British Library)	Science, history, professional issues, education
Journal of the Canadian Chiropractic Association		Science, history, professional issues, education
Journal of Chiropractic Education		Education, science and history
Journal of Chiropractic Technique		Science, history, professional issues, education
Journal of Manipulative and Physiological Therapeutics	BIOSIS, Current Contents, Excerpta Medica, Index Medicus, USSR Academy of Sciences	Science, history, professional issues, education

The development of scholarly periodicals within chiropractic was significant not only because of its important function as part of the infrastructure of the science of chiropractic, but also because of the long-standing discrimination experienced by chiropractors (e.g., Gaucher-Peslherbe, 1996) in their attempts to publish in the wider health science literature. As recently as 1987, for instance, the editor emeritus of the *Journal of Bone and Joint Surgery* expressed his sentiment that "The Journal offices would be firebombed if a chiropractor were to appear as a co-author. Old feuds die hard, and I doubt if the Journal's readers are ready for that yet" (Curtiss 1987).

The JMPT became a model for other scholarly publications in the profession. In addition to the new journals introduced in the 1980s, substantive improvements in a number of periodicals published by national professional associations outside the U.S. were seen. Among the association magazines now recognized as scholarly publications are the *European Journal of Chiropractic*, the *Journal of the Canadian Chiropractic Association*, and the *Chiropractic Journal of Australia* (formerly the *Journal of the Australian Chiropractic Association*).

Developing Research Skills and Awareness

In the aftermath of the 1975 NIH conference, the leaders of the FCER and the CCE paid greater attention to research skills development within the profession. A few individuals, such as Logan College graduate John J. Triano, D.C. (see Figure 23-6), had already availed themselves of the training options provided within Suh's engineering department at the University of Colorado. Taking heed of the recommendations from Goldstein of NIH and FCER Director of Education Richard Timmins, the Foundation committed itself to developing research sophistication among a few more chiropractors. Triano became the first recipient of the FCER's Schierholz Fellowship Award in support of his doctoral studies in engineering/biomechanics at the University of Chicago (Schierholz, 1986, p. 39).

Although Scott Haldeman's 1977 call (Haldeman, unpublished) for the creation of a "Chiropractic Research and Postgraduate Educational Institution" (see Table 23-8) and regional "Spinal Research Rounds" went unheeded, the FCER did establish a fellowship

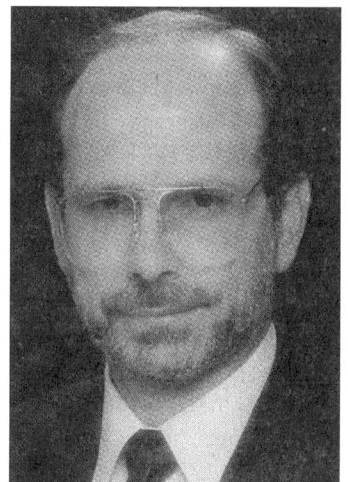

Figure 23-6: John Triano, D.C., Ph.D.

program (circa 1977) which provided funds for graduate training (Schierholz, 1986, p. 37). Among the early recipients of these fellowships were National College graduate Reed Phillips (for work towards his master's in community medicine at the University of Utah School of Medicine) and Northwestern College of Chiropractic alumnus and faculty member Thomas Will (for his M.S. in epidemiology at the University of Minnesota School of Public Health). Haldeman received a small grant for support during completion of his medical internship (Schierholz, 1986, p. 37).

The FCER also took the advice of Paul Silverman, Ph.D., a consultant to the National College, who encouraged the formation of a Chiropractic Research Commission (CRC) to promote greater interaction and collaboration in research matters among the colleges. A task force consisting of one representative each from the

---

Table 23-8: Goals of Scott Haldeman's 1977 proposal for the establishment of an institution for chiropractic research and post-graduate education (Haldeman, unpublished)

1. To attract the finest chiropractic researchers, clinicians and educators into an environment which would permit them the greatest degree of freedom of inquiry.
2. To conduct clinical research into the efficiency of chiropractic and the testing of chiropractic therapeutic procedures and diagnostic instrumentation.
3. To conduct experimental research into the principles of research.
4. To train chiropractic educators to the highest level possible in order to upgrade the undergraduate programs of the chiropractic colleges.
5. To provide courses and internship programs from one week to one year in length for practicing chiropractors wishing to upgrade their clinical skills or academic knowledge.
6. To organize continuing education seminars of the highest possible standards to the field practitioners of chiropractic.
7. To publish textbooks of the highest possible standard for the profession.
8. To upgrade the standard of articles in chiropractic journals.

ACA, the CCE, the FCER and the various schools convened in Chicago in August 1977 to create the CRC. At the group's third meeting, in March 1978, the Commission resolved to sponsor a "Chiropractic Research Symposium" (Schierholz, 1986, p. 37), which became an annual event held at a different chiropractic college each year (e.g., Davis, 1982). By 1989 this conference was transformed into today's International Conference on Spinal Manipulation (ICSM) (Proceedings, 1989). Reed Phillips became the FCER's director of research in Autumn 1979 (Phillips, 1996), the first person to hold this position since Clarence Weiant in the late 1940s. Phillips established several priorities for research proposals (Schierholz, 1986, p. 40):

1. research development grants

2. basic science research grants

3. clinical science research grants

4. education and training grants

The Dawn of Experimental Chiropractic

Martin (1994) has noted that chiropractors since D.D. Palmer have construed chiropractic as a science. However, the epistemology of science accepted by chiropractors more closely resembled the "nineteenth century, natural history approach to science" rather than the "experimental control of variables in a carefully regulated laboratory environment" which characterized biomedical research in the twentieth century (Martin, 1994). While the medical community built laboratories and developed a technology for controlled clinical trials (Bull, 1959; Doll, 1991; Lasagna, 1955; Lillienfeld, 1982), chiropractic colleges built museums for their collections of anatomical specimens. By mid-century B.J. Palmer (see Figure 23-7) wrote of *Chiropractic Controlled Clinical Trials* (Palmer,1951), but apparently none of the studies conducted at his research clinic in Davenport employed rigorous experimental methodology (Keating et al., 1995; Mannello et al., 1996). And although occasional papers in the chiropractic literature acknowledged the need for controlled research (e.g., Hildebrandt, 1967; Watkins, 1948), not until the eye-opening 1975 NIH conference was recognition of the paucity of experimental studies of manual methods widely appreciated.

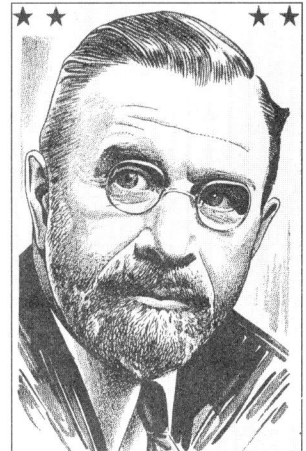

Figure 23-7: B.J. Palmer, D.C., Ph.C., circa 1949

In the aftermath of the Bethesda meeting a small but meaningful scientific literature began to emerge in the pages of the JMPT and several other scholarly periodicals. Clinical experimentation came slowly, however. In its first nine years of publication, only three randomized, controlled clinical trials (RCTs) were published by the JMPT, and none of these dealt with spinal manipulation. An experimental literature bearing on SMT developed in non-chiropractic journals (Keating, 1992, pp. 413-7; Shekelle et al., 1991a). The first RCT of spinal adjusting for any health problem (in this case, low back pain), which was conducted by Gerald N. Waagen (see Figure 23-8) at Palmer College in Davenport, did not appear until the mid-1980s (Waagen et al., 1986). Although a few in the profession question the existence of a science of chiropractic (Dunn et al., 1990), faculty investigators at the chiropractic colleges have contributed RCTs of adjusting and related therapeutics for a small number of clinical conditions, such as low back pain (Bronfort, 1989; Hsieh et al., 1992; Triano et al., 1995), childhood nocturnal enuresis (Leboeuf et al., 1991; Reed et al., 1994), headache (Boline et al., 1995), and high blood pressure (Yates, 1988). Additional such trials are now in progress at CMCC, LACC, National College of Chiropractic, Northwestern College of Chiropractic and both Palmer schools.

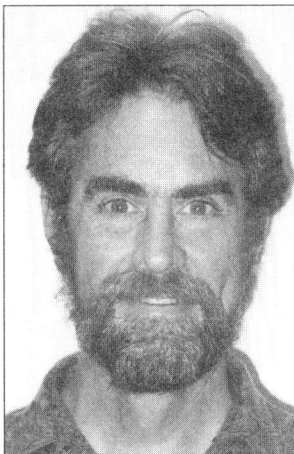

Figure 23-8: Gerald N. Waagen, Ph.D., D.C.

In addition to RCTs, other forms of controlled clinical studies have been recommended, such as time-series experimental methodology (Center & Leach, 1984; Keating, Giljum

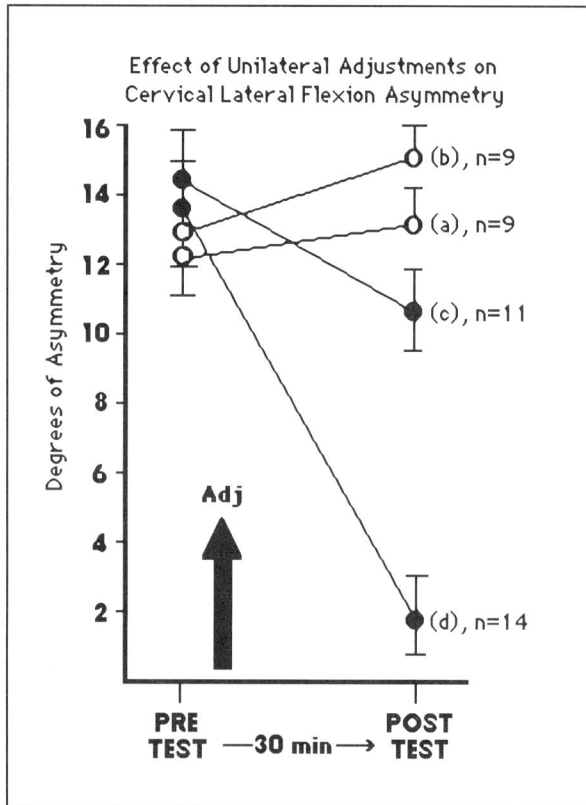

Figure 23-9: On pretest, all groups exhibited mean cervical lateral-flexion end-range asymmetries of about 14°. Strong and statistically significant post-adjustive change was evident among those subjects adjusted on the most restricted side, as predicted. No significant change was seen among those subjects (Groups b and c) who received no adjustments. Some change was seen among subjects who received thrusts on the hypothesized "wrong" side (i.e., side with less restriction in cervical lateral flexion end-range of motion). These data suggest that the measurement system was sensitive to change produced by adjusting. (Adapted from Nansel et al., JMPT 1989; 12(6): 419-27; reprinted by permission of the *Journal of Manipulative & Physiological Therapeutics*)

et al., 1985). These procedures have enabled a few faculty investigators to explore cause-effect relationships in the clinical situation with very small sample sizes by means of within-subject comparisons. A few examples of this sort of clinical investigation have appeared in the scholarly literature in chiropractic (e.g., Giesen et al., 1989; Levine et al., 1990; Meyer et al., 1990). The potential for these sorts of investigation to empower practitioner-researchers in the college clinics and in the field has yet to be explored to any significant extent.

Experimental designs have also been employed in several "measurement evaluations" and "clinical analogue" studies (Keating, 1992a). Haas and co-workers at Western States Chiropractic College have employed experimental methods to demonstrate the sensitivity of motion palpation methods to changes produced by adjustive procedures directed to the thoracic spine (Haas et al., 1995). Another good example is the work of Nansel et al. (1989b, 1990) at Palmer College of Chiropractic West, who explored the trial validity and temporal distribution of inclinometric (pendulum goniometric) measurement of cervical lateral flexion asymmetry in end-ranges of motion. In the first of these studies this research team tested the notion that the optimal side for unilateral adjustment in the cervical spine is the side demonstrating the greater restriction in cervical lateral flexion (see Figure 23-9). Nansel et al.'s (1989b) work is also noteworthy as the only known example of a triple-blinded clinical experiment in the chiropractic literature. Nansel's "experimental adjustory" established at PCCW is also important an example of programmatic research and a sustained opportunity for chiropractic students to observe (as subjects) and participate in (as research assistants) the conduct of critical scientific investigations.

Experimental methodology has also been employed in studies of the effects of adjusting and manipulation on physiological parameters. Cleveland (1982) sought to demonstrate that segment-specific thrusts produced greater changes in sensory functions than other manual methods. A collaborative project between investigators at CMCC and the Royal Melbourne Institute of Technology (Terrett & Vernon, 1984) showed that osseous adjusting had a profound effect on the threshold for perception of paraspinal cutaneous pain. Harris and Wagnon (1987) at Cleveland College in Kansas City explored the effects of adjusting on skin temperature. The effects of manual methods on immune function have been experimentally studied at the National College (Brennan et al., 1991, 1994) and at CMCC (Vernon et al., 1986). National College investigators have also explored several electromyographic parameters which distinguish low back pain patients from normal subjects (Humphreys et al., 1989; Triano & Schultz, 1987). Nansel et al. (1993) have studied the effects of cervical adjusting on lumbar muscle tone.

Other Areas of Scholarship

The growth in scholarship in chiropractic since 1975 involves a variety of activities in addition to the conduct and report of RCTs (see Table 23-6). Evaluations of the measurement methods involved in assessing and monitoring aspects of bodily dysfunction, and particularly the clinical lesions or targets of chiropractic intervention, have become numerous. Demographic studies of chiropractic patient populations have appeared, and large-scale descriptive studies comparing chiropractic and medical outcomes are underway at the Western States Chiropractic College (WSCC).

In the past decade WSCC has become a leader in the chiropractic research community. The college played a central role in the formation of the Pacific Consortium for Chiropractic Research in 1985 (Tolar et al., 1986) when Robert L. Tolar, Ph.D. (see Figure 23-10), appointed Vice President/Dean of the College by Herbert Vear in 1981 (Western, 1981) collaborated with Bernard Coyle, then vice president for academic affairs at PCCW. Tolar, whose doctoral dissertation dealt with the problems of consortiums (Coyle, 1992), joined with Coyle to present a plan for the organization to the California Chiropractic Association, which became a sustaining member of the agency. The Consortium (the term "Pacific" has been dropped), a fund-seeking and research-conducting organization, has brought

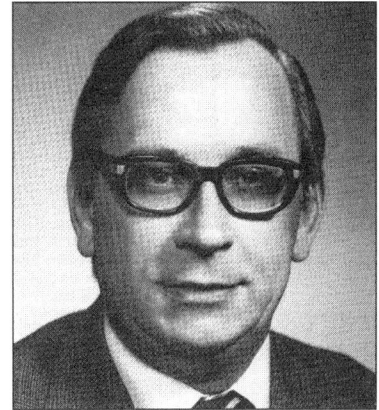

Figure 23-10: Robert L. Tolar, Ph.D., co-founder of the Pacific Consortium for Chiropractic Research

together the talents of research directors and faculty members at a number of chiropractic colleges throughout the United States. Although initially perceived as a rival to the ACA's grant-making body (Coyle, 1992), the FCER, the difference between grant-seeking (Consortium) and grant-making (FCER) functions has lessened such tensions.

The research efforts of several faculty members at WSCC provide good examples of important investigations other than RCTs. The college's research director, Joanne Nyiendo, Ph.D., is primarily responsible for the previously mentioned large-scale, prospective, longitudinal, descriptive comparison of chiropractic vs. medical outcomes and practice activities with patients suffering low back pain. This is a collaborative project with the Oregon Health Sciences University, and involves the first large research grant from the federal government, specifically, the Health Resources and Services Administration. Nyiendo has also reported a number of other demographic surveys of patient populations at chiropractic college clinics (Nyiendo & Haldeman, 1987; Nyiendo & Olsen, 1988; Nyiendo et al., 1989). The work of Mitchell Haas, M.A., D.C. is also noteworthy; Haas has explored the reliability and validity of a variety of traditional chiropractic techniques (e.g., Haas et al., 1993a-c, 1995). Several of WSCC's basic science faculty have also been active contributors to the scholarly literature, including Robert Boal, Ph.D. (e.g., Kaminski & Boal, 1992), Richard Gillette, Ph.D. (e.g., Fine et al., 1994; Gillette et al., 1993a&b) and Mark Kaminski, M.S. (e.g., Kaminski et al., 1987).

Health care policy issues have in very recent years become a topic of concern for some chiropractic scholars, as evidenced by efforts to encourage the creation of clinical, educational and reimbursement guidelines for the practice of chiropractic (e.g., Haldeman et al., 1993; Mootz, 1996; Mootz et al., 1996; Savage et al., 1987; Shekelle et al., 1991; Vear, 1992). College faculty have also contributed to the literature on cost-effectiveness and relative outcomes of chiropractic services vs. medical care for musculoskeletal disorders (Ebrall, 1992; Jarvis et al., 1991; Johnson et al., 1985, 1989; Nyiendo, 1991a&b). However, as Mootz et al. (1995) have noted, chiropractic colleges have done very little to encourage or prepare future D.C.s for careers in health care policy. An optimistic sign in this area is the recent recommendation by the Ontario government (Ontario, 1995) that chiropractic education be brought into the mainstream of postsecondary education:

> The Chiropractic Services Review report released by the Ontario Ministry of Health examines "Health Human Resources Planning and Education" in its second chapter. "Appropriate location and funding for chiropractic education" is examined, with two resulting recommendations:
>
> R2.1 That chiropractic education be placed in the multidisciplinary atmosphere of a university, and be funded in a manner similar to other health professions.
>
> R2.2 That the government develop a health human resources (HHR) plan with respect to chiropractic services.

Specifically, the report called for "placing chiropractic education in an Ontario University," and listed the benefits, including:

*Expose chiropractic students to a multidisciplinary atmosphere.

*Develop a more constructive relationship between chiropractors and (medical) physicians and other health professionals.

*More cooperation in practice between chiropractors and other health professionals, especially (medical) physicians and physiotherapists.

*More effective patient care.

*Facilitate necessary basic science and clinical research.

*More equitable access to chiropractic as a career.

*A chiropractic profession more representative of the Ontario population (Ontario, 1995).

Table 23-9: Founders (and their academic affiliations) of the Association for the History of Chiropractic, 1980

Founder	Academic Affiliation
Cheri D. Alexander, D.C.	-
Eleanore B. Busch	-
Fern L. Dzaman	-
Leonard E. Fay, D.C.	National
Russell W. Gibbons	-
Vern Gielow	Palmer
A.E. Homewood, D.C., N.D.	Western States
Herbert K. Lee, D.C.	Canadian Memorial
Joseph E. Maynard, D.C.	-
Ernest G. Napolitano, D.C.	New York
Arthur L. Nickson, D.C.	Logan
Viola M. Nickson, D.C.	Logan
James E. Ransom, D.C.	-
William S. Rehm, D.C.	-
James M. Russell, D.C	-
Richard C. Schafer, D.C.	-

In May 1995, CMCC signed a "Letter of Intent" to affiliate with York University (Moss, 1996). Plans call for the CMCC's relocation to the campus of the University and the award of the chiropractic doctorate by the University. The affiliation bodes well for all areas of chiropractic scholarship.

Chiropractic history as an area of scholarship has become somewhat more common among college faculty in the past decade. The formation of the Association for the History of Chiropractic (AHC) in 1980 (see Table 23-9), and their publication of a scholarly journal, *Chiropractic History*, helped to raise consciousness about the importance of preserving the profession's story. However, despite an annual Conference on Chiropractic History held on a rotating basis at various chiropractic college campuses, the early contributions of historical research from college faculty was minimal, amounting to less than a third of all papers published in the journal during its first eight years of publication, and less than the number of papers contributed by private practitioners and professional associations (see Table 23-10). This trend has not changed significantly in the past decade (Green, 1995), although with the National College's 1991 introduction of the periodical *Philosophical Constructs for the Chiropractic Profession* (since renamed the *Journal of Chiropractic Humanities*) and the profession's centennial, some greater interest in the profession's past has become apparent at the colleges. Other scholarly journals have also shown a strong interest in publishing historical research; among these are the *Chiropractic Journal of Australia*, the *European Journal of Chiropractic*, the *Journal of the Canadian Chiropractic Association* and the *JMPT*.

Critical discussions of philosophical issues in scholarly journals has also grown in recent years (e.g., Coulter, 1990, 1993; Jamison, 1991; O'Malley, 1995; Phillips, 1995b). These discussions have called into question some of the traditional tenets and root metaphors which have guided the profession heretofore. In comparison with the philosophical literature in allopathic medicine, recent works in the philosophy of chiropractic have been far more concerned with epistemological than with ethical issues, although several papers in the latter category are noteworthy (e.g., Brennan, 1995; Ebrall, 1995c; Keating & Hansen, 1992). The methods by which chiropractors acquire new knowledge seem likely to dominate philosophical discourse for the foreseeable future, owing to the traditional diversity of epistemologies (Keating, 1992a) offered by chiropractors and the pressing need to amplify research and other scholarly activities.

Epilogue

Further significant growth in the science of chiropractic will necessarily involve the continuing evolution of the colleges. Scientific research has not yet become "a major part of the fabric of any [chiropractic] institution" (DeBoer, 1983) in part because of the paucity of qualified investigators at the colleges and in part because:

> ...research has traditionally been separated from teaching; it is something that is done in a separate department, by separate research faculty. It has been said that education without research is like confession without sin. The culture within chiropractic schools of separating teaching, service and research into distinct tasks for different individuals may prevent scholarship and critical appraisal skills from developing within the faculty, within the student body, and among practitioners (Mootz et al., 1995).

Indeed, the recently convened, federally-sponsored workshop organized by William C. Meeker, D.C., M.P.H., Director of the Palmer Center for Chiropractic Research in Davenport, revealed a number of distressing facts. Meeker notes that fewer than 9% of the 960 chiropractic college faculty members in the United States "have any involvement whatsoever in conducting chiropractic research" (Meeker, 1996). He notes a vicious cycle (not unlike that seen in Figure 23-11), wherein "Lack of research capacity leads to lack of research which leads to lack of funding which leads to lack of research, etc.," and offers several proposals for breaking out of the loop:

1. development of a culture which reinforces research activities
2. development of the recognition of the need for hard data for decision-making
3. collaboration with researchers in non-chiropractic institutions
4. development of financial resources for scholarly work

Employment of much greater numbers of D.C./Ph.D. faculty scholars is a challenge which is necessarily embedded within the economic limitations of the colleges' traditionally heavy tuition dependence. And although scarce resources may continue to justify the existence of distinct research departments at many chiropractic colleges, the promotion of greater scholarship among non-research-department faculty is a challenge to administrators, who are responsible for recruitment and faculty development. More scholarly faculties will presumably be better equipped not only for the research imperatives confronting the profession, but also better prepared to meet the new challenge of preparing doctors for an uncertain health care market and to deal with the seemingly perpetual controversy within the profession: what is a chiropractor?

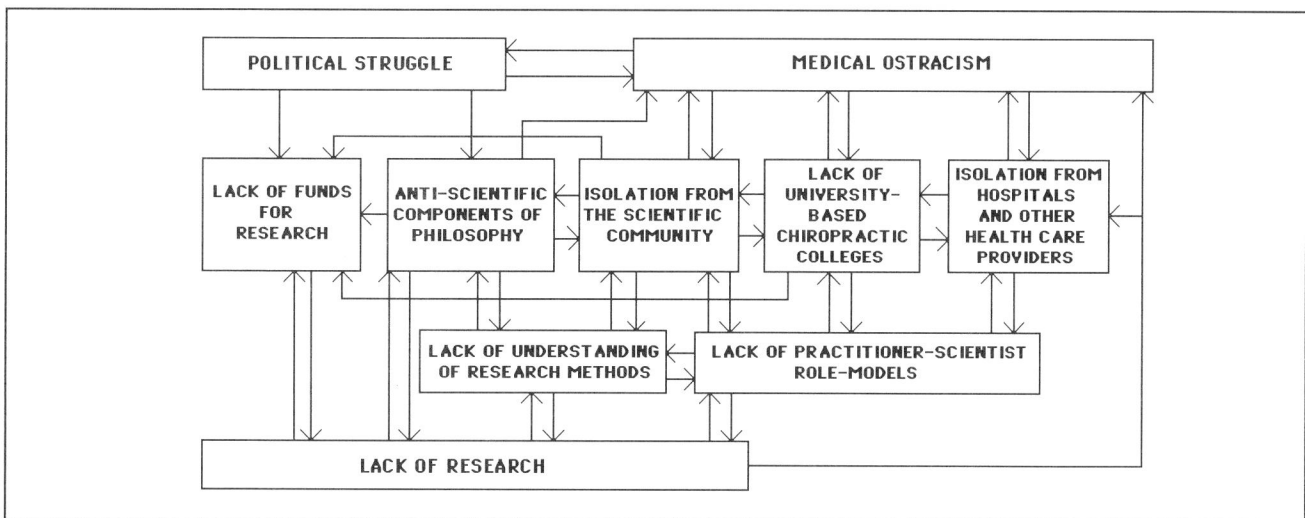

Figure 23-11: Pattern of inter-locking impediments to the development of chiropractic science (redrawn from Keating, Mootz & Nelson, 1986)

Chapter 24

EXPECTATIONS: PREDICTIONS FROM THE COUNCIL ON CHIROPRACTIC EDUCATION

In 1995, members of the Council on Chiropractic Education were invited to give their predictions for the future of chiropractic education. These are their responses.

**Council on Chiropractic Education,
1995 Board of Directors**

John F. Allenburg, D.C.
Merydith H. Bakke, D.C.
Carl S. Cleveland, III, D.C.
Gerard W. Clum, D.C.
William H. Dallas, D.C.
Shelby M. Elliott, D.C.
Thomas A. Gelardi, D.C.
Meredith A. Gonyea, Ph.D.
George A. Goodman, D.C.
Bruce Gundersen, D.C., D.A.B.C.O.
Randolph C. Harding, D.C.
John D. Hemauer, D.C.
Thurston E. Manning, Ph.D.
Peter A. Martin, D.O., N.D., D.C.
Kenneth W. Padgett, D.C.
James W. Parker, D.C.
John P. Pecchia, C.P.A.
Reed B. Phillips, D.C., Ph.D., D.A.C.B.R.
William C. Remling, D.C.
Charles E. Sawyer, D.C.
Virgil Strang, D.C.
Sid E. Williams, D.C.
James F. Winterstein, D.C., D.A.C.B.R.
Frank A. Zolli, D.C.

John F. Allenburg, D.C., President,
Northwestern College of Chiropractic, Bloomington, Minnesota
Colleges, Associations, Practitioners Can Secure Profession's Future

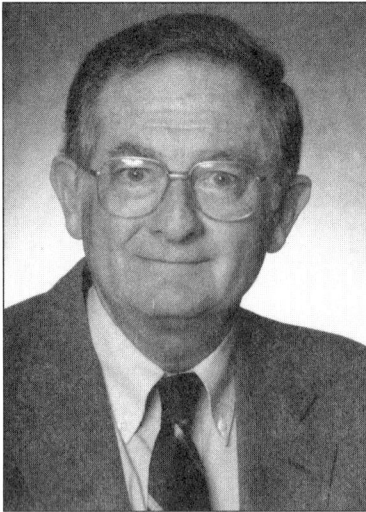

The future of the chiropractic profession is my most important non-family concern. At Northwestern College, 600 of the best young men and women anywhere have chosen our profession and career to serve people's heath and to earn a living. For their commitment, they are entitled to all of the satisfaction that I have had.

In the more than 40 years that I have gratefully been a member of the chiropractic profession, during which time significant challenges have never been absent, there hasn't been a time like the present with so many problems and so much opportunity.

We Know What the Problems Are.

> Exclusions by Managed Care, gatekeeper systems, and limited networks have deprived patients of freedom of choice and access to chiropractic care and have taken away a substantial segment of the market share that our profession has earned during the past 100 years.

> Health policy decision-makers, public and private, do not yet understand or accept that Doctors of Chiropractic are qualified to be first contact gatekeeper practitioners, able to diagnose, refer appropriately and manage the health of patients.

> Managed care organizations are determining health care needs, not the patients' doctors. Often, this necessitates either patients paying for necessary care without reimbursement or doctors providing care without appropriate compensation.

There are Answers

To firmly establish a rightful position for our profession, the following are a few of the "key" things that we need to do as colleges, as professional organizations and as practitioners.

Our Chiropractic Colleges Must

> Graduate doctors with clinical experience, personal and professional integrity, dependence on science and research, convictions about the benefit of chiropractic health service, human relationship attributes and commitment to share the responsibilities of the profession and be participators in its affairs.

> Carry out research to advance chiropractic science and build the credibility of the profession. Eventually, every door that is closed because of questions about effectiveness can be opened by evidence derived from clinical outcomes research. The most important factor shaping health care policy will be reliable evidence of effectiveness of diagnostic and treatment procedures.

Our Professional Organizations Must

> Continue to develop and implement state and national agendas and action plans directed toward legislators, health policy makers, and health care purchasing organizations with an overwhelming focus on enabling direct access to doctors of chiropractic for the diagnosis, prevention and care of health problems appropriate to chiropractic practice. These minimally must include neuromusculoskeletal disorders, primarily the spine; physiologic system disorders which relate to the spine and nervous system; and problems associated with unhealthful living practices.

> Carry out an effective public information program to bring about high levels of understanding, appreciation and utilization of chiropractic health care services.

> Inspire and lead members of the profession and their patients to persistent communication with legislators and health purchasers in demands of equal access to doctors of chiropractic for appropriate care.

Chiropractic Practitioners Must

> Continue our clinical education in order to consistently deliver the highest quality care. In the "Era of Assessment and Accountability," care will need to be more evidence-based which will necessitate on-going attention to current literature.

> Support the educational and research infrastructure of the profession which resides in the colleges.

> Be active members of the communities in which we practice. It builds our personal and professional stature and positions us for input to and influence on public policy.

> Support our state and national associations through membership and with additional contributions for political action and public information. Only our associations can lead concerned efforts to gain access equity for the public to chiropractic practitioners.

And, We Must Work Together

If we will work in cooperation, with mutual respect as a character attribute, each fulfilling our expected responsibilities, I have the most profound confidence that we can gain for our profession and for our patients everything that is right and deserved.

Merydith H. Bakke, D.C., DeForest, Wisconsin

The future of chiropractic education rests with the educational institutions, the Council on Chiropractic Education (CCE) and its Commission on Accreditation (COA). Our education focus and process must be responsive to the needs of our patient public. Chiropractic education must prepare our doctors to responsibly provide competent evaluative and diagnostic procedures, as well as to deliver chiropractic treatment reflective of the standards within the profession. It is also imperative that our doctors can maximize the public's exposure to chiropractic with an attitude of cooperative, cost-effective care within the total range of safe and effective health care opportunities for our patient public.

I believe the key to the future of chiropractic education lies in a successful blending of our chiropractic philosophy of natural health care, scientific research that contributes to our informational base, and the development of consenses regarding responsible and effective treatment protocols.

As always, the future of chiropractic is in our hands!

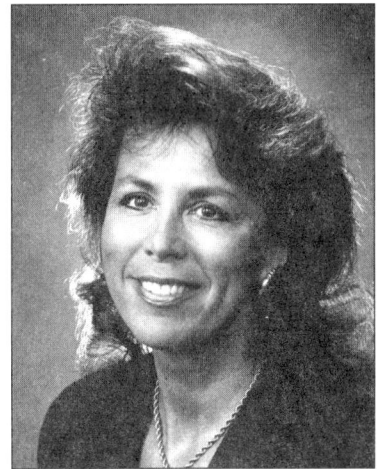

Carl S. Cleveland, III, D.C., President, Cleveland Chiropractic Colleges, Kansas City, Missouri and Los Angeles, California

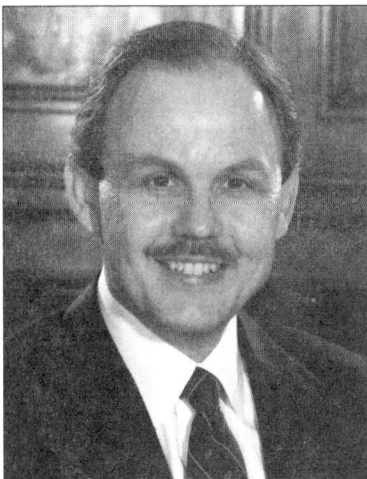

The future: a fourth generation chiropractor's prediction.

Multiple factors will impact the chiropractic profession and its role in the changing health care delivery system. It is projected that three major dynamics will drive chiropractic's acceptance and utilization. These include research, the future healthcare structure and reimbursement system, and consumer attitudes regarding health and wellness.

Research: The chiropractic research agenda will move beyond the initial success of the low back pain studies of the 1990's to undertake studies on spinal adjustment/manipulation and the management of headache. The resultant guidelines will substantially impact public awareness and enhance opportunities for interdisciplinary referral between doctors of medicine and chiropractic. In addition, isolated symptomatic care studies will demonstrate a role for chiropractic in specific forms of allergies, digestive diseases and certain neurological disorders. The greatest impact for the profession, however, will result from an understanding of spinal function and its interface with joint nociception, mechanoreception and related neurobiologically mediated activity. Further, studies demonstrating the relationship between the maintenance of proper spinal mechanics and nervous system activity and its effect on patient function and well being, as may be assessed on generic non disease-specific surveys (RAND 36-item Health Survey or MOS SF-36) will contribute to chiropractic's role as a "wellness" practitioner. The profession will then gradually exchange its public image from that of "back pain" practitioner to doctor of "spinal hygiene" and structural health. Patients will then routinely seek regular spinal exams as today's health conscious consumer seeks regular dental examination.

Healthcare systems and reimbursement: Substantial changes will occur in the corporate healthcare structure and reimbursement systems. Reimbursement will become guidelines driven and focus on those procedures demonstrated to be outcomes effective. Patients will become more empowered with information and take an aggressive role in healthcare choices. In addition, reimbursement entities will expand inclusion of chiropractic to cut costs and to remain competitive in response to patient demand. In the urban setting, the corporate health care conglomerates will define primary care as a collective function served through group multi-disciplinary provider centers rather than a single provider's office. This will be driven through the need to share overhead expenses, accommodate guidelines directed interdisciplinary referral and provide quality patient care. It is projected that a substantial portion of referrals to doctors of chiropractic will be from doctors of medicine, in part because of reimbursement guidelines and because the medical practitioners will not have the skill to effectively manage those conditions related to spinal function. While limited numbers of medical practitioners including osteopaths will express interest in manipulation, few will take time to adequately gain competency in this procedure. Substitution of manipulative procedures via physical therapists will continue to be a competitive element for chiropractic. Debate over terminology such as mobilization, manual therapy and spinal manipulation will be battled in state legislatures. The chiropractic profession will triumph in these confrontations due to the practitioner's neuro-musculoskeletal diagnostic competencies and adjustive technique. The technical understanding of the components of vertebral subluxation complex and its relationship to health, plus the distinction to be made between mobilization and manipulation as compared to the specific vertebral adjustment will become key points in defining the profession's role in this debate.

Consumer Attitude: Patients will continue to become more informed and empowered regarding healthcare choice and treatment. Patient interest in physical fitness, diet, nutrition, naturally grown foods, self-care, prevention and wellness will continue to expand. The chiropractic profession will benefit from the growing public interest in "alternative health care" coupled with an increased dissatisfaction with chemical and invasive medicine. Greater public understanding of chiropractic's role in spinal hygiene and wellness will increase patient willingness to pay out of pocket for services. Colleges must prepare graduates to function in a cash based as well as managed care based practice environment. The profession must be cautious of peddlers of eclectic or "all things natural" remedies that will attempt to ride by association on the respect and advancement of chiropractic. The profession will risk embarrassment from adverse media exposure resulting from practitioners attempting to profit from consumer interest in alternative procedures through prescription of nutritional, homeopathic or botanical therapies for treatment of specific diseases.

Trends in Education: The chiropractic educational institutions will continue to take a dominant lead on behalf of the profession. The Council on Chiropractic Education will serve to bring the colleges to the discussion table for issues regarding accreditation. However it will be the Association of Chiropractic Colleges that will take the predeminent position as the leader of the educational and research community and provide consortial services to its members and related constituencies. Many of the educational institutions will pool resources to fund regionally positioned research centers associated with interdisciplinary centers or universities. Specific institutions will form multi-campus partnerships both nationally and internationally sharing specific administrative and educational components between geographic locations. Distance learning technology will revolutionized health care education and will foster sharing of faculty and inter-institutional faculty appointments. Certain colleges will broaden their institutional mission and develop programs in addition to the chiropractic degree program. While the colleges will cooperate collectively on multiple issues, scope of practice and philosophical differences will continue between institutions.

Within the historically broad-scope chiropractic institutions, certain colleges will attempt to present a chiropractic program with the inclusion of limited pharmaceuticals as an adjunctive procedure to chiropractic practice. Others within the broad-scope camp will remain "drugless" but attempt to capture the consumer's interest in alternative healing and offer programs such as homeopathy, naturopathy and related forms of "holistic" healing. Yet other colleges will remain broad-scope, but reject the eclectic holistic programs based on lack of scientific basis. On the other side of the spectrum, certain institutions will continue the passion for "by hand only" chiropractic, and will qualify the value of the diagnostic methodology solely as part of the instructional process, and propose limited application as part of the clinical experience.

The majority of institutions, however, will represent a balance of the philosophy, science and art of chiropractic and present a "hands on" emphasis to specific adjustment of the spinal column, with intense neuroscience and biomechanical curricular emphasis associated with a focus on the vertebral subluxation complex and its clinical manifestations. Within these institutions the diagnostic process and its related parameters will serve as manifestations of "physiology gone wrong" and become a component of research or an indicator to monitor progress of spinal function correction, or in certain instances serve as indicator for patient referral. Patients may be co-treated between doctors of chiropractic and medicine. Vertebral subluxation complex will serve as a diagnostic entity and in itself may be the only indication for care thus becoming the basis for chiropractic spinal maintenance care. At these institutions the utilization of adjunctive procedures will be selective and limited to the preparation or support for the adjustive process, or for management of extremity or non-spinal injuries. The most effective educational experience will come from the institutions providing a balanced approach to the philosophy, science and art of chiropractic blending the traditions of the past with the demands of contemporary healthcare, and yet instilling in the graduate a passion and commitment to the unique perspective and principles of this profession. The future has never looked better. Our best days are yet to come.

Gerard W. Clum, D.C., President,
Life Chiropractic College West, San Lorenzo, California

In our first century of chiropractic as a profession and discipline, we focused on the uniqueness of our views and perspectives. The second century of our existence will be marked by a recognition of the value, utility, and practicality of our views and perspectives.

Throughout our history we have identified the chiropractic profession as being based on the trilogy of philosophy, science and art. At this moment in time, our philosophical perspectives on life, health and healing are being embraced by all segments of our society. From consumers to providers we have awakened to the ability of the body to heal itself, and we have explored and adopted those strategies that will support this new realization.

Our society is running headlong into a changing paradigm of health and into changing models of health care delivery. According to the former U.S. Surgeon General C. Everett Koop, the medical paradigm is crumbling. When intervention was more profitable than prevention, intervention was the order of the day. When prevention assumed the status of economic wisdom, it began to occupy a new place in people's lives. Regardless of the motivation behind the shift in emphasis, the reality is clear: we have far more dominion over our health and wellness than we ever knew or chose to exercise.

The non-invasive, minimally iatrogenic nature of chiropractic care, with its cost-effective attributes, has blended with the movement of the public consciousness from an acceptance of the status quo of health care to a new vision of all matters related to health.

This union has caused a redefinition of health, wellness, sickness and disease. It has allowed new thought to enter what was once a stifled realm of activity. In his text, Healing Word, Larry Dossey, M.D., noted, "I came to realize the truth of what many historians of science have described: A body of knowledge that does not fit with prevailing ideas can be ignored as if it does not exist, no matter how scientifically valid it may be." The changes of the society relative to matters of health, well-being, vitality and wellness have created a climate open to new ideas as well as the reconsideration of old ideas. These changes have also heralded a movement from a quantity-of-life view to a quality-of-life discussion. This has allowed the public mind to entertain the logic and reason (or lack thereof) of everything from heroic measures to the motives of their providers.

As much as the philosophy of health care has changed, so too has the role and significance of science of our culture. The public has become remarkably pragmatic relative to science. The move to outcomes-based research in health care is a prime example.

Aside from becoming more pragmatic, the other colossal change relative to science in health care has been the availability of science to the individual. The emergence of the Internet has placed great stores of scientific information and a vast

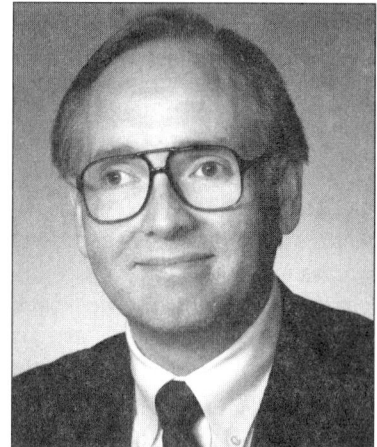

array of opinions in the hands of non-scientists.

In recent years new avenues of information have been sought. These have reflected what doesn't work and at what cost in monetarily and human terms. We have seen the rage of one day become the reject of another. We have seen the days of the "miracles of antibiotics" followed by the "end of the antibiotic era."

Specific to chiropractic, the emergence of a reality perspective in health care-related research has been linked with tremendous advances in neurologically oriented research to yield a union that has opened vistas once only dreamt of in the chiropractic world.

The culture has removed the deity status once provided the medical arts and its practitioners and it has allowed itself to question concepts and practices once followed with blind faith and loyalty. This change has resulted in a shift from who's right to what's right.

The chiropractic profession is poised to move to a new level of understanding and appreciation, in the public mind, through an honest and open application of science. The musculoskeletal aspects of chiropractic science have been acknowledged, and a wider appreciation of the neuromusculoskeletal role of the profession is emerging. We will soon see the realization of a greater application of our views in matters related to visceral function and ultimately to neuroimmune-related aspects of healing and wellness.

The art of chiropractic will continue to unfold in an erratic and uncoordinated way as is the nature of any art form. The realization of the public's appreciation of the body's ability to heal, combined with the understanding of the mechanisms of healing identified by the scientist, will lead to a refinement of the art of chiropractic.

To the practitioner it is abundantly clear that the chiropractic adjustment yields wonderful and near miraculous results. What we have failed to do is develop our art to the level that the near miraculous is an hour-by-hour event rather than the sporadic pattern of profound outcomes we now enjoy.

The power of the adjustment will be understood and appreciated at a new level and we in turn will experience a renaissance in the efforts to enhance the application of our clinical skills. We will demand greater clinical accountability and expertise of each other as the public demands more of the profession at large.

The challenge of the immediate future will be to recognize the monumental shifts that are underway in our world as to health and healing. We must understand that the present tumult involving all matters related to health is a transitional process and not an end in itself. We must realize and take great strength from the movement of thought toward our time-honored views. Finally, we must be good and noble stewards of the philosophy, science, and art of this phenomenon called chiropractic. Its principles and practices will exist for all time but its banner must be held high and protected, so that the public may soon come to realize the value of our contribution to their health and wellness.

Countless men and women sacrificed greatly to bring the chiropractic profession to its present position. They stood tall and advocated a new approach to health care when all they had was a poorly developed theoretical model and superb outcomes of care. Fullness of time has revealed to us how right our forebears were. Whether by chance, coincidence, inspiration, or divine intervention, a vision was realized and advanced against all odds. As challenging as those introductory years were, we must be diligent and conduct ourselves wisely to ensure that the years of our acceptance are not more dangerous and treacherous than anything we've ever known.

Shelby M. Elliott, D.C., President,
Texas Chiropractic College, Pasadena, Texas

> Positive thinking is the belief in our own self-worth and in the value of everyone else. That belief leads to self confidence, respect for others and a lifestyle based on strong values.

While reading the above statement by Mrs. Ruth Stafford-Peale, widow of Reverend Norman Vincent Peale, it occurred to me how that statement sums up the talents represented by the Board of Regents, Alumni Board, faculty, staff and brilliant students of Texas Chiropractic College. As a family unit, we are exuberant and have a strong confidence, respect and appreciation for one another, our college and the chiropractic profession. TCC has a great heritage and can be proud that we have graduated some of the most outstanding doctors since 1908.

As a veteran chiropractor, it has been my privilege over the years to see and live many changes in chiropractic and health care. When I was a student, the greatest challenge was getting chiropractic licensed in the state of Texas. Basic Science Examining Boards designed to eliminate chiropractic were springing up in many states. Accreditation was a taboo. Hospital privileges and insurance coverage were simply unheard of. There was constant abuse from medical doctors — political forces — afraid of compromise. Yes, there has been much change!

Why? One might ask. Due to the unrelenting work of dedicated chiropractors, we stand here today in the midst of a revolution won. In the U.S. government's research published in December, 1994, chiropractic was proven to be twice as effective at half the cost of standard medical care over the last decade. Recent polls indicate that the percentage of chiropractic patients from all sectors of the population is rising. One can only imagine that the percentage of patients from the sports and entertainment arenas are probably twice that of the general population.

Today, chiropractic remains to be the third most popular method of health care used to rid the world of disease. As we are continuing to scratch the surface, the sophistication of chiropractic education has advanced to even greater heights. Reaching untapped resources, Texas Chiropractic College draws tremendously bright and aggressive students from more than forty U.S. states and ten foreign countries. Chiropractic educational institutions across the nation are all experiencing growth.

Realizing the strength of partnership in our profession, D.C.s and students are teaming up across the nation in support of legislation to: a) continue research efforts for chiropractic within the allopathic world, and b) further enhance the inclusion of chiropractic care in managed care programs, mainly PPOs and HMOs. At the American Chiropractic Association's National Legislative Conference held in Washington, D.C., March 7-8, 1996, it was a pleasure to see so many people, especially students, lobbying for chiropractic. Senator Harkin summarized it best when he said, "...now is the greatest time in history for students to be in chiropractic college. They do have a bright and wonderful future." In fact, TCC students were well organized and had the most appointments with the numerous legislators.

Now, we have more bipartisan legislators working hard for chiropractic. Robert E. Mills, lobbyist for the American Chiropractic Association, feels certain that he is going to get government research for chiropractic. Senator Edward Kennedy and a majority of Democrats are already committed and many Republicans are working in the same way. Overall, Mills believes there is minimal resistance and the future looks bright for research and federal funding as programs continue to be the driving force manipulating reform in government attitudes.

TCC is definitely doing its share to continue research efforts. In fact, we are participating in a collaborative study with the Texas Back Institute/Institute for Spine and Biomedical Research on the "Influence of Neonatal Exposure to Estrogen and Skeletal Tissue." To reflect the profession's remarkable milestones through research, TCC's Susan Grigsby, Ph.D., director of research, remains an integral part of the emergence of research being done at the college. Her efforts have been phenomenal in that she has built an outstanding program for student research and various research projects for the college. Last year, 1994 TCC graduate, Sarah Combs, D.C. was named TCC's first postdoctoral fellow. Currently, she is conducting chiropractic research and gaining expertise in chiropractic research methodology at the Texas Back Institute.

Slowly, doors are being opened to us from the University of Texas Medical Branch. Representatives from St. Joseph's Hospital have invited us to meet with them to teach them more about our college and chiropractic. A group of individuals from the college have met with the City of Houston's Health and Human Services Department executives, the University of Houston's College of Optometry, the University of Texas Medical and Dental Branches, and various civic, social and media organizations regarding our efforts to launch the "Well Child Project." This project will be a vehicle (literally) that will bring diagnostic health care services and resources to the doorstep of many underprivileged children in the Houston Metropolitan area. Still in its formative stages, this customized motor home will be transformed into a mobile clinic, learning and distribution center with interns working together from TCC, UT's Medical and Dental Schools, and U of H's College of Optometry.

As TCC's president, my goal to see chiropractic education in the public university system will soon be a reality. Our efforts so far have met little or no resistance. Once this has been accomplished, I'm certain that this will set the tone for others to follow. When this happens, we will not have to worry about the level of prechiropractic education or grade point aver-

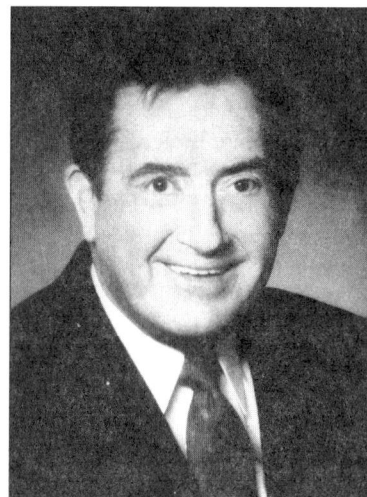

ages. With the increased amount of applicants, top colleges will have the opportunity to pick quality students. Naturally, our top priority is always making sure our students receive the best chiropractic education. Our finished product is measured by the success of our graduates.

In the future, there will be a much greater degree of cooperation, an interchange of ideas and research among the various health care professions. The true strength of this great profession lies within our ability to perform this healing art. As one individual committed to the profession, I am truly thankful for the discovery of chiropractic one hundred years ago by one individual who believed. With the start of the second century, many transformations will be witnessed in the philosophy and practice of chiropractic. Somehow I doubt they will equal the profound change that was witnessed when D.D. Palmer made his consequential leap of reason on September 18, 1895.

George A. Goodman, D.C., F.I.C.C., President,
Logan College of Chiropractic, Chesterfield, Missouri

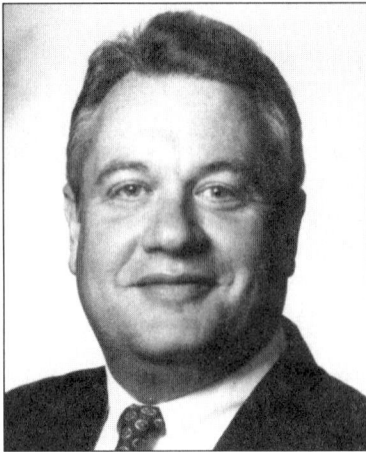

The expectation of chiropractic education is that it will not be a static knowledge base. We, as a profession, have not reached our potential. The profession of chiropractic will only be as strong and significant as the educational environment of our colleges. If our educational institutions and faculty provide static sources of the same information year after year without growth and development, society will pick up on this immediately. It is incumbent on the institutions of chiropractic education to provide faculty who can generate effective teaching that motivates learning and growing as a profession. Therefore, one of the most important missions that chiropractic education can provide for the future is the attraction, development and retention of quality faculty.

I can only speak for Logan College of Chiropractic and state that the core of our commitment to the future students, alumni, and the profession, is our dedication to teaching and learning. We see our mission to provide quality practicing and clinically competent clinicians as a standard to the future of the profession. It is our firm belief that our future will be collectively significant if our practitioners have the resolve to be responsible for standard-setting for the anticipated changes in health care.

Technology that surrounds health care should be incorporated into our institutions, such as interactive simulations, teaching clinical skills that could be shared among all chiropractic colleges electronically. Imagine chiropractic students in a class being presented a case history with different aspects of the case being continually changed and brought to a virtual reality depending on the student's response on diagnostic and treatment algorithm. It is this kind of education which will allow a more clinically based curriculum to be established in chiropractic colleges in a practical and a more affordable manner.

Through the use of computer simulation models, which would include the integration of distance and interactive learning concepts and virtual reality simulation technologies, our students would be able to deal with case scenarios and continually improve their skills prior to graduation. As managed health care increases to put pressures upon practitioners to maximum efficiency, we must provide the most efficient doctors within our resources. The academic setting is very important to provide a scientific, well rounded, knowledgeable doctor of chiropractic. We must carry this educational opportunity to its natural conclusion of a clinically based curriculum.

Chiropractic education must set standards for the profession and be a strong advocate to society concerning both the chiropractic profession, including education, and the patients served by doctors of chiropractic. We visualize the establishment of standards in the area of ethics, clinical practice, science, wellness and prevention concepts, and of course, greater admission and educational requirements.

Chiropractic education must take a leadership role in the establishment of educational partnerships with other institutions of higher learning and state agencies. An example would be the role of chiropractic health care in the correctional institutions of America. Educational partnerships with other institutions of higher learning would provide scientific technology and supplementation to our tuition-driven, single focused institutions. The educational component will certainly be challenged to provide performance and outcomes-related research. We will be forced to take an active role to speak out and critically perform clinical research.

It is my expressed opinion that in order to provide significant meaning to the concepts of wellness and prevention, it must be a curricular practice and a clinical outcome. Treatment guidelines in this arena of constant transition in health care must again have a significant awareness in the educational component. It is clear that prevention and wellness, along with strong research programming, directed at the development of specialized "niche" provide studies that will assist in the lowering of such areas as Workers' Compensation costs. The future will also demand treatment principles that will deliver "state-of-the-art" scientific information that blends well with conservative health care, based on a safe and sound understanding from research documentation.

In conclusion, we at Logan College of Chiropractic see a strong and significant need for chiropractic physicians well into the next century. It is incumbent and absolutely necessary that chiropractic education be strengthened institutionally and professionally. Chiropractic educational colleges and their association in the future must communicate and promote public policy and chiropractic issues. This will increase the options for doctors of chiropractic and our patients.

Finally, we can count on change, always change — change seen as a beginning for something better or a catalyst for opportunity and achievement, never as an enemy to be feared.

To those of us within the chiropractic profession, spinal adjusting and structural integrity for the treatment of low back pain has been a mainstay of this profession, but only addresses a part of what chiropractic has to offer. Therefore, it is encouraging that the future will finally catch up with the chiropractic past and "discover" the other many benefits of chiropractic care.

Bruce Gundersen, D.C., D.A.B.C.O., Salt Lake City, Utah

In order to provide a reasonable projection on chiropractic education of the future, it is necessary to understand the current relationship between the actual market for chiropractic services from a pure supply and demand point of view.

Currently, a local government related insurance carrier provides benefits for chiropractic services under a managed panel. This appears to be the destiny for the next five years, although it will certainly evolve. There are no deterrents to seeing a chiropractic physician. It is managed on an equal basis with other providers; same co-payments, premiums, etc. There is, perhaps, a better listing in the directory of services for the chiropractic group. The utilization rate in a population of 100,000 lives for 1995 was 9,227 people who sought the services of a chiropractic physician at least once. This represents a 9.2% demand. A private carrier with traditional disincentives has a demand rate of 3.4%, which seems to be more typical. The number of providers who saw at least one of those was 321. Some saw only one and some saw many more than one. The steering mechanisms of the panel, location, individual provider appeal and individual provider marketing have not been measured here. Perhaps it is these immeasurable items that conflict with the expected laws of supply and demand. For this discussion, we will assume that all chiropractic providers are equal at least in some ways.

If all things were doled out on an equal basis, this would equate to not quite 29 patients per provider per year or 2.3 patients per month. The fees paid per patient per year were $231.00 averaged for the panel and the non-panel visits. Using $100,000 gross annual income as the minimum necessary for a provider to survive equates to 433 patients per year which determines the actual demand for providers at 21 providers per 100,000 lives in a system where unlimited access will exist.

The current supply of providers with active licenses and whose addresses are within the same geographic boundaries as the population of about 1,900,000 is 464. If the utilization rate of this entire pool were 9.2%, 174,000 would use the service allowing 403 providers to survive at 100,000 per year each. The HMO market which affords no access to chiropractic at this

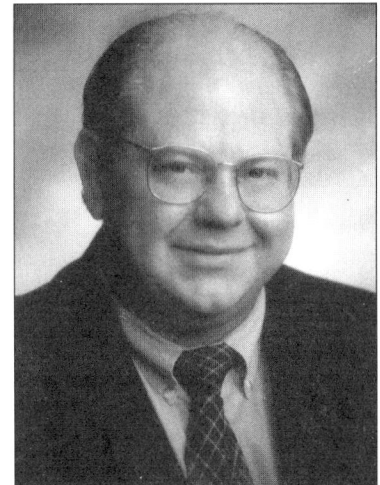

time represents about 480,000 and the uninsured about 350,000 leaving an available market of 1,070,000 lives; who do not actually utilize at 9.2% but more like 4-6% on the average. Taken at 6%, or 64,200 lives using the service would allow only 148 providers to survive.

During the past 12 months, there have been 86 new licenses granted. This represents a 23% increase in one year. Twelve months ago, the HMO market share was 380,000 and the uninsured was estimated at 330,000. Thus the market diminished by about 6% while the provider pool expanded.

This trend defines this inherent need for chiropractic education to deal with both aspects of supply and demand in the next ten years. The supply of new chiropractic providers must be measured precisely to fit the projected need based on the trend discussed above. This may be accomplished by a number of mechanisms which include a student cap, different entrance screening and requirements. Should the educational institutions take a proactive measure and employ these steps on a graduated basis, chiropractic medicine is likely to become the paramount portal of health care access which it is positioned to inherit.

In order to accomplish this task, the demand side of the equation can be affected by the chiropractic institutions. Setting a standard of making primary access providers will gradually accomplish this. Putting out graduates who are most qualified as initial entry managers will force government, private insurance and public opinion policy makers to steer people to this portal.

This will require a better integration into the health care education system. Becoming part of the state education and university systems may be a step in that direction. Creating departments of chiropractic medicine in the teaching hospitals will not only demonstrate the benefits of chiropractic medicine employed in serious musculoskeletal cases and allow for intra-professional referrals, it will also open the door for employment on internal disorders of eventually all kinds.

Both of these steps will be taken by the prudent directors of chiropractic education and the public stands as the penulti-mate beneficiary. The steps must be taken carefully and simultaneously in order for chiropractic to fulfill its possible destiny as a primary entry science and application method. As this occurs, both government and private industry will recruit support for the chiropractic educational process which will ease the dependence on tuition survival.

Randolph C. Harding, D.C., Holiday, Florida

Our chiropractic colleges will be preparing students to be doctors of Chiropractic who will be serving as a portals of entry into the health care delivery system. The students the colleges select will be of the higher caliber of not only academic intelligence but also one that has concern and compassion for people and the society in which we live. The student will be in tune or in agreement with the philosophy of the chiropractic approach to health care.

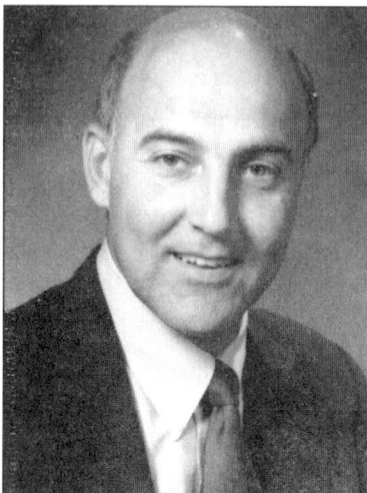

Chiropractic colleges will prepare students with an educational system that will use a modern high tech educational approach. This approach will allow for a lower instructor/student ratio with more emphasis on self study and small group studies with the instructor serving as a mentor/resource person. Through world wide electronic communication with other educational centers and colleges, the students will be capable of hearing and seeing "famous" professors. They will be able to directly communicate their own questions, thoughts and ideas with world renown educators. Through increased student dialogue, the instructors themselves will be probed and intellectually stimulated. There will be less traditional classroom lecture and more self study small group interdisciplinary dialogue. All this will allow the instructor to be a mentor and source of information for the student, thus allowing the student/instructor to develop a closer rapport.

The computer will be a valuable educational tool to be used not only in the basic sciences such as anatomy and dissection, but also in the clinical sciences. Students' notes will be maintained on computers and the traditional text book will give way to CD disc. The college libraries will have less hard copy resource material and will be predominantly electronic libraries where resource information is stored on computer tape and disc. The resources of Internet and the World Wide

Web will be routinely used. The learning process will also include training using "Virtual Reality" experiences. Every conceivable experience can be created, demonstrated and taught. Conditions and clinical situations that are routine can be varied to deal with the "not so routine." Various conditions and clinical situations will be taught and experienced so students can be exposed to these situations and gain confidence in the knowledge of knowing how to properly handle and manage a given problem. In the clinical setting, the students will maintain patient records electronically and will communicate via various telecommunication technologies in delivering and meeting the health care needs of patients. Clinical laboratory and imaging techniques, as well as other medical data, will be processed electronically. Overall, the thrust of the chiropractic education will be to allow the student to have and gain more hands on experience early in their training. The chiropractic training will prepare students to do and perform highly complex diagnostic testing in an office setting that by today's standards might only be done in large sophisticated institutions. The teaching clinics will expose the student to a wide variety of clinical experiences that will prepare them as portal of entry practitioners.

Our students will be trained to render a service that will be based on sound proven methods as being the most appropriate form of care for a given condition. The students will be trained to perform a diagnostic work-up that will be state of the art, one that follows a logical sequence and not a random unorganized testing system. Chiropractic will be the treatment of choice for a number of conditions that have been proven to respond to spinal manipulation and other natural health care means as the most appropriate and cost effective approach.

When our students graduate, they will be thoroughly prepared to enter into a health care delivery system that considers the chiropractor as part of the health care team. They will be prepared to work in an environment that will include the traditional office setting or larger interdisciplinary clinical setting. Our graduates will be concerned with patient education for the prevention of disease and maintenance of good health as well as provide expert knowledge to industry for ergonomics and prevention of on the job injuries. In addition, a certain number of DCs will be trained to work in an administrative role as state and federal government workers and/or in the private sector as administrators and overseers of various health care systems. The resources of the colleges will be available to the field practitioner through telecommunication linkups.

As new and inventive ways are developed to educate and train students, the colleges will explore and determine if these are the best ways to educate and train our students. The schools will adopt new methods of teaching for the sake of quality education in order to prepare the students for the awesome responsibilities they will be assuming.

John D. Hemauer, D.C., Whittier, California

The chiropractic profession and its educational institutions have undergone an unbelievable metamorphosis during the past four decades. The negative perceptions of the 1950s have been replaced by very positive ones in nearly every aspect of the chiropractic profession's societal and scientific roles. The impetus for this change, in my opinion, has been the coordinated effort of the chiropractic educational community to develop uniform educational standards and the acceptance of those standards by regional and specialty accreditors.

The challenges for the twenty-first century are enormous. With a high community wide regard for the value of chiropractic procedures, there are those in sister professions who would like to adopt and monopolize them. The only way to prevent this from occurring is for chiropractic educators to continue to refine their educational processes, with emphasis in those areas that are uniquely chiropractic, especially chiropractic adjusting/manipulation. Excellence in this area can only be achieved by continued general educational progress, particularly in more comprehensive clinical training and research. That means the very best qualified technique programs must be developed and expanded. Additionally, there must be a very high priority placed on clinical research related to manipulative procedures.

Assuming these educational goals can be achieved, it will be mandatory that chiropractic health care become fully integrated into mainstream health care delivery, with full and co-equal participation with all other primary health care providers in third party reimbursement programs, including the widely projected expansion of managed care.

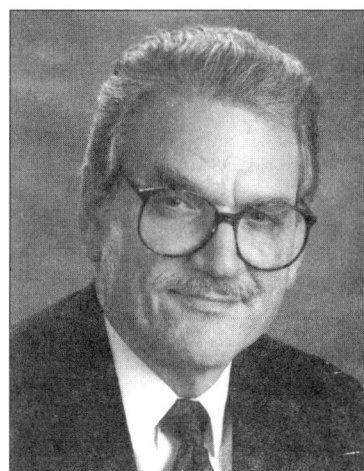

Peter A. Martin, D.O., N.D., D.C.,
President, Palmer College of
Chiropractic-West, San Jose, California

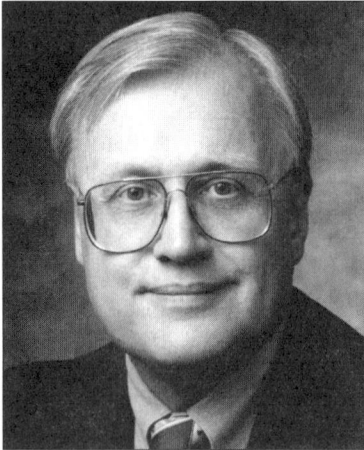

Virgil Strang, D.C., President,
Palmer College of Chiropractic,
Davenport, Iowa

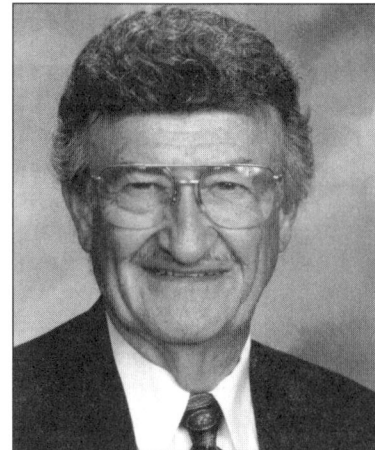

The administration of the Palmer Chiropractic University System, including its two presidents, sees a bright future for chiropractic and chiropractic education.

We're optimistic because the chiropractic paradigm is increasingly well received in the marketplace, the shift to managed care holds opportunities for our graduates, and evolving educational standards will mean better faculty, better chiropractors and, we would hope, a better health care system.

We aren't optimistic out of naiveté or indifference to the sometimes destructive forces roiling society and its health care delivery. Nor do we expect changes favorable to chiropractic to come without hard work and persistence. Our confidence lies in the conviction that chiropractic, tempered in the furnace of its historic struggles, today can exhibit the philosophical strength and muster the pragmatic flexibility to carve out its own future.

Clearly there is a massive shift to managed care, but it is not so clear who will end up doing the managing. The transfer of financial control to insurance companies is not automatically improving health care. In profound ways people's health is still not being managed. Health care is a consumer-driven enterprise, and consumers will continue to demand more efficacious and cost-effective health management. That presents an opportunity for chiropractic.

Who is better equipped to become primary care gatekeepers and help people manage their health than doctors of chiropractic, who understand and teach that health management begins with prevention and wellness? When people's health is managed from the point where they begin to depart from good health (if not before), costs will automatically go down because there will be less need for heroic care. While there will be plenty of room in the new environment for a chiropractor to be a "super specialist," we still see chiropractors ideally positioned for the generalist role. However, the demands upon tomorrow's chiropractic graduate will be greater than those on today's.

We see four major implications for chiropractic education if the profession is to fulfill its potential in the emerging health care system.

First, chiropractic students need firmer grounding in the holistic philosophy that is the essence of chiropractic's unique successes. That stronger foundation includes improved communication and teaching skills so that as doctors they can help patients take responsibility for their own health. Chiropractic philosophy must be presented and applied so as to broaden chiropractic's scope of thinking. For too long, philosophy has been used to develop apologetics for personal beliefs and practices, contributing to fragmentation within the profession and isolation from other health care providers. Instead, philosophy ought to emphasize a balanced understanding of the various factors relating to health so that the practitioner can function most effectively in his or her preventative care role.

This broader philosophical perspective must be coupled with more sophisticated examination, diagnostic and documentation skills appropriate to a portal-of-entry role. We're not talking about only diagnosing disease but about analyzing the person's entire health lifestyle. We're talking about a sophisticated patient education program being a significant part of every chiropractor's services and every chiropractic patient's experience. We're also talking about an outreach mentality that prompts everyone in the profession to be conscious of building public and policy-maker awareness of what chiropractic has to offer.

Second, chiropractic education must become more clinic-driven, with greater attention to outcomes. Quality care, not just low-cost care, will separate the winners from the losers in health care delivery. Quality care requires improved utilization of practice guidelines, outcome measurements, documentation and quality assurance in college clinics. It also directs that the basic sciences, much of which will have to be learned in pre-professional education, will need to be further integrated with the chiropractic clinical sciences. This will go hand in hand with a sharper chirocentric focus throughout the entire curriculum. Everything must relate directly to the actual delivery of chiropractic care. Of course, this clearer focus of chiropractic education ought to be reflected in refined testing measurements for state and national board examinations.

Third, because scientific validation is mandated in the new, structured health care environment, chiropractic education must become more research-oriented. Chiropractic colleges will have to devote financial and human resources to gathering a critical mass of scientific evidence through rigorously designed research projects. Because the demands for research are too great for the chiropractic profession on its own, chiropractic colleges will need to mount every effort to share in projects with universities and other non-chiropractic research forums. And while this research is being done, priorities must be maintained so that results are delivered to the profession expeditiously. For that matter, chiropractic research results ought to be delivered to the public in down-to-earth terminology that helps ordinary people appreciate chiropractic's scientific foundation.

Fourth, chiropractic education must broaden its influence through far-reaching and well-marketed continuing education. The health care system will continue to change, and those who will succeed in this environment must be adaptable to change. They will need to be life-long learners, and chiropractic colleges (which will be held accountable more than ever for what their graduates do) must supply, at times and locations convenient to busy practitioners, post-graduate education that keeps pace with new developments. College faculty and other conducting continuing education programs themselves must become more adaptable to change. They absolutely must stay up to date with the oncoming explosion of scientific knowledge and with the changing complexities of the health care system in the real world. That all means colleges will need to implement vigorous, broad-based faculty development programs. Again, involvement with other institutions and perspectives is critical to this increased enlightenment.

It is evident that chiropractic education faces enormous challenges. Yet the prospects are also very exciting. If we can react insightfully when the givens suddenly become question marks and if we can maintain our focus on the condition of patients rather than the condition of pocketbooks, we will survive the shakeout and find ourselves in an enviable professional position.

A deeper philosophical understanding and increased public awareness of it, true outcomes-based, efficacious and cost-effective clinical management, more scientific validation translated into appropriate professional behavior, and readily available, progressive post-graduate education will all promote greater unity within the chiropractic profession itself, with other academic institutions and with the health care system. That means chiropractic can find its rightful place in the mainstream without compromising its integrity. The ultimate beneficiaries will be consumers, who at long last will have a more rational system to help them manage their health.

Kenneth W. Padgett, D.C., President, New York Chiropractic College, Seneca Falls, New York

I believe that the primary battle within the profession today is no longer "straight" vs. "mixer," it is "primary care physician" vs. "neuromusculo-skeletal specialist." The heat being generated by this controversy is significant in the field, and consequently has been reflected in the schools. This has always been the pattern in chiropractic. The schools have tended to play a "Johnny come lately" role, latching on to whatever ideas are generated or techniques promulgated by charismatic chiropractic personalities, be they forward-thinking or reactionary.

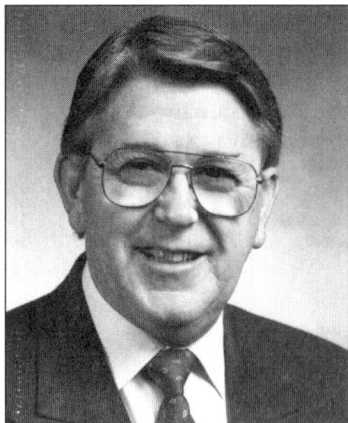

As a point of reference, look at the medical profession, and at where all of the major advances in allopathy have come from over the past 50 years. They have come from the medical schools and teaching hospitals. In contrast, chiropractic colleges have done little to "advance" the chiropractic profession. "Advances," such as they have occurred, have typically been generated from the field, and usually from entrepreneurs.

The time has come for that to change. The colleges must be on the front line in establishing the profession as a viable force in the health care field. We must offer programs which are innovative and progressive. We must take technique away from the technique entrepreneurs. In the controversy of "primary care" vs. "NMS specialist," I think we must be ready, willing and able to provide programs which produce both types of chiropractors. Additionally, we must acknowledge that the way we deliver our curriculum must be more reflective of the needs of our stakeholders - students, faculty, and the public. Our "easy in - quick out," 36-to-40 month programs must cease. We need to upgrade our admissions requirements, and stop contributing to the "burnout" of our students and faculty in our nearsighted devotion to outmoded trimester or quarter programs that leave little or not time for research or reflection.

I believe we are now moving as a profession in this direction. The question is, are chiropractic educators willing to do what it takes to make this happen? We often say we are, but resist change when confronted with it. The future is in our hands as educators. Either we meet this challenge head-on or go about business as usual. This will mean establishing higher educational standards and maintaining a level of quality with other similar professions.

Here are some examples of admissions standards we're currently reviewing at NYCC: 1) Require 90 college credits. This incrementally grants more opportunities for academic and personal growth, and elevates the baseline for chiropractic program admission to that which exists for virtually all the recognized primary health-care professions. It also provides additional flexibility to strengthen any chiropractic prerequisite, undergraduate course requirements which might be deemed necessary in the future. 2) Place emphasis on the caliber of the undergraduate preparation (e.g., the institution where the credits were earned, an assessment of course content and difficulty, etc.) rather than solely on GPA. 3) Initiate a national pre-screening/qualifying examination that measures a student's academic preparation for and potential of success in chiropractic studies. Strengthen the admission interview process.

As a profession we must be continual watchdogs of our educational standards, keeping them at a level of quality equal to our sister professions. The eyes of the world are upon chiropractic, which has become one of the world's fastest growing professions. This is the dawning of a new era for health care. This new era could well become the age of chiropractic, putting the burden of our success squarely on the shoulders of chiropractic education. Let us draw from our rich beginnings and build toward the rewards of a promising future. The chiropractic foundation is solid as we have just attested to during our centennial celebrations. We must sustain the momentum.

We must also remember that to establish chiropractic as a primary form of health care in the future will take LEADERSHIP! Who will lead chiropractic into this new era of health care? The heirs apparent are currently in our chiropractic colleges. Bright, enthusiastic future doctors of chiropractic can be found within the parietal walls of each of our chiropractic colleges. I constantly tell students to get involved in the profession, both educationally and politically, if they are to carry our profession into its second century. Our students truly are the doctors of tomorrow who will be thoroughly equipped to assume leadership positions. This is the essence of the paradigm shift, as I perceive it. And it will be reached through the profession's sincere desire to maintain its total commitment to academic excellence. At this juncture, some will opine that we need to fill the seats to keep our colleges alive. But this thinking is deceptive. Our focus must always be on the quality of education our students receive. If we have to sacrifice numbers to keep our standards high, so be it. The stakes are high. Our educational standards must be just as high. This cannot be over-emphasized.

James W. Parker, D.C., President,
Parker College of Chiropractic, Dallas, Texas

The Chiropractic profession and the C.C.E. have come a long way in their relatively short histories, and this profession has learned well from the histories of other professions. Chiropractic did not need a "Flexner" report to upgrade its educational programs; it did so after due consideration, including lessons learned from the trials and tribulations of the medical profession.

Medicine has sacrificed itself to a rigid, mechanistic model, virtually devoid of humanizing principles. As a result, it has lost public confidence, compiled a research literature that even it describes as "of appalling poor average quality," and foundered in the face of the chronic ills that continue to plague us. Chiropractic should also learn from the history of our first cousin in the healing arts, osteopathy, which succumbed to the temptation to embrace that same model and now struggles on a daily basis in search of its own identity.

The future, therefore, is clear, from the history of both of these mechanistic healing arts, as it relates to chiropractic. We must strive for professional excellence within our own healing paradigms. The profession has prospered now for over 100 years because of its results and patient satisfaction, the latter of which is about the only common denominator in all the official reports for chiropractic generated in the last 15 years. The *Journal of Alternative and Complementary Medicine* (January 1996) stated "Chiropractic has much to offer patients beyond the mechanical effects of manipulation." It further stated, to support that statement, "When the chiropractic profession was examined in order to isolate a paradigm for chiropractic education and research, the pattern emerged was of a profession that incorporates the principles of vitalism, holism, humanism, conservatism and rationalism." We must maintain our "separate but equal" posture, and not be blended into the exclusively mechanistic healing paradigm. Therefore, our education system in the future must:

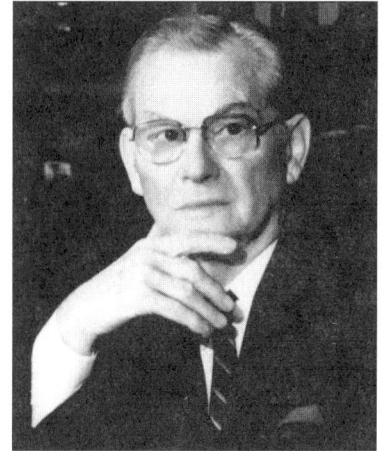

1. Seek Those Who Are Best Qualified To Be Doctors of Chiropractic

The future Doctor of Chiropractic must possess those social skills and the prerequisite broad-based science training that will afford a firm foundation for the education that he or she seeks at a chiropractic college and the social skills to communicate properly with colleagues and patients. To that end, a serious study should be made with respect to the present prerequisites required by chiropractic colleges. To merely elevate the length of time one spends in Liberal Arts programs prior to entering a chiropractic college serves little to no purpose. The study should not only evaluate predictors of academic success, but also those disciplines that embrace more practical education, so that the graduate can communicate in oral and written formats and in socio-economics; we need fewer "scientific eggheads" and "social outcasts" and more "well-balanced" students.

2. Streamline Curricula So That College Offerings Address the Needs of the Profession and the Missions of Each Institution

Curricula are driven today by "the lowest common denominator" of several State Boards. Institutions need the freedom and authority to construct curricula which address the needs of the profession, the Missions of the institution, and training for its graduates to fit our paradigm to serve in a constantly changing health-care environment. This must be done without undue political interference, and college Boards of Trustees must also be safeguarded from those intrusions.

3. Produce Research Which Is Ongoing and Continue to Search for Truth

Research must embrace not only "bench research," but also the occurrences that materialize daily in the practice of vitalistic, holistic, patient-centered healing, especially with energy as its base. Are these occurrences not valid because they cannot (at this time, with our present base of mechanistic scientific knowledge) be understood, predicated or replicated? We as a profession must begin to accept simple truths to problems, and blend them with science. To have the pendulum of Research go to the far left will not do, nor will it serve any purpose to go to the far right. The pendulum must fall within a median range, where science serves to enrich practice, and practice serves to inform and confirm science. All too often has humanity blindly reacted to "scientific" research, only to find out later that the truth was something quite different.

4. Serve Humankind

The colleges must develop a network of public service vehicles to bring a chiropractic awareness to sick and suffering humanity. The overall "drugless, knifeless, natural form of health care" should become the symbol of chiropractic by the public. Efforts must also be made to establish a "chiropractic base" in under-served or unserved countries.

Therefore, latitudes in the admissions process must be made to accommodate those from foreign countries, who wish to study Chiropractic in the States, an opportunity that can only enhance the health of people worldwide, including their precise scientific requirements and even their grade level based on the chiropractic population, if any, especially in third world countries.

Reed B. Phillips, D.C., Ph.D., D.A.C.B.R.,
President, Los Angeles College of Chiropractic, Whitter, California

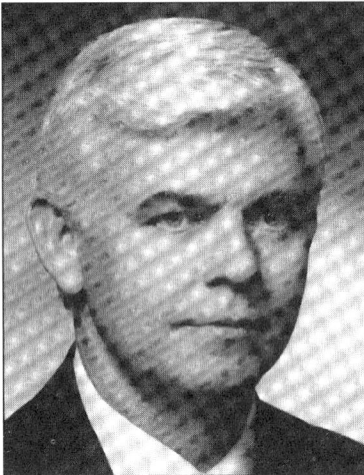

"Education is what survives when what has been learned has been forgotten."
— B.F. Skinner

To discuss the future of something, we must first define what that something is. Education is the focus but what do we mean by this term? Traditionally, education in chiropractic has included the formal process of obtaining a doctor of chiropractic degree (DC) and some form of continuing education to meet requirements for relicensure or to seek some specialty designation in the profession. Throughout our hundred-year history, wide variation in quality and content has existed in both components of the educational process. Only in the last twenty years have standards for the pre- DC degree program been established by the Council on Chiropractic Education (CCE) thus reducing (but not eliminating) the variation among the institutions providing such programs. At the conclusion of our centennial anniversary, the post-DC training continues to function devoid of standards and replete with variation in quality and content.

During this past centennial, chiropractic education has made significant strides toward offering a professional education. That is to say, the trend toward a foundation based on science and increased emphasis on research, expansion of the duration of the educational experience to encompass a greater sphere of knowledge and the increasing requirements for access have lifted the social acceptance of chiropractic education to a level similar to other doctoral degree granting programs. Full acceptance by other professionals continues to wane however, due to the persistent lower requirements for access to chiropractic education as compared to other professional programs.

The traditional educational model chiropractic follows is consistent with the typical model of education developed as a product of the Industrial Age. It is a seat-bound, time-framed program that in today's Information Age, limits access. In the typical model, the knowledge network is controlled by the teacher who practices his/her religious ritual in the cathedral of the university, much like the physician in the hospital. The teacher determines what is to be taught and how learning is to be evaluated. The university determines when and where the teacher will teach. The learner is an obedient subject who gains great stores of knowledge by rote memorization and faithful acceptance of the gospel as espoused by the professor. If the words of Skinner quoted above are true, what is left after what is learned in school is forgotten.

Today the Information Age demands a new model. No longer is education limited to courses taught during certain semesters in certain rooms with limited seating, limited visual aids and limited faculty. The knowledge network continues to be the domain of the teacher but a network of learners has emerged that drives a new model. To learn, one only needs to turn on the television or computer and an abundance of information is readily available. The enhanced access to information coupled with the expanded knowledge base that now revises itself every five-to-seven years, has literally brought the world into the living-rooms of the learner. "Distance-free" education with immediate access presents opportunities for learning never before conceived. The concept of continuing education is being transformed into the concept of "perpetual learning." To stop learning is to become obsolete.

So where is chiropractic education headed? It could remain within the limits of the traditional model it has evolved into and run the risk of obsolescence and potential extinction. It could transition itself by incorporating new technology into the current model and add a new level of excitement to the learning process. Or, it could transform itself into a process that meets the needs and expectations of the rapidly developing learning network. Such a transformation is not abrupt but evolutionary, and is being impelled into the next century at a rate far beyond any Darwinian expectation.

Chiropractic education needs to re-think its mission and take a serious look at how well it is fulfilling that mission. We are indeed training students to be doctors of chiropractic. But, we are training them to function in a twentieth-century model of health care. Exposure to technology is minimal. Challenges from the rigors of critical thinking and problem solving are not encouraged. Research is preached but rarely practiced. Our industrial model of education has produced able technicians claiming to be professionals. The informational model will provide an opportunity for a self-selection process between those who wish to become life-long learners and those who do not.

Chiropractic education should be a front-line participant in the life-long, distance-free learning process. We need to develop opportunities for faculty training to manage the knowledge network that will be accessed by the learning network. Chiropractic education must take the lead in the preparation and dissemination of educational material and programs, or some other entity will fill the void, a void that is yet to be clearly defined.

Chiropractic education must free itself from the fetters of the past. While traditional buildings with traditional faculty and traditional programs will persist, we must make room for new concepts in learning methodology, new avenues to accessing knowledge, new formats for evaluation of competence and new forms of recognition for achievement. The DC degree must remain, but how one achieves and maintains this status must be scrutinized to assure the most effective and efficient transfer of knowledge and competence. We are like the pioneers of the past, blazing new trails in a world envisioned by only a few. Chiropractic will remain as long as it serves the needs of the patients. Chiropractic education will remain as long as it meets the ever changing needs of the perpetual learner.

William C. Remling, D.C., F.I.C.A., Glendale, New York

During our first hundred years, the profession has seen tremendous growth in the presence of formidable opposition. As the strongest trees are those that grow and exist in the severest winds and conditions, so too with our profession. We have seen our institutions grow from unaccredited to accredited, from small rented facilities to full college campuses, some with dorms. We have seen the extent of education and the quality of applicants for admission increase dramatically.

Are we any better today than even 40 years ago? Are our graduates any better anchored in their understanding of chiropractic, its purpose, design and contribution to health care of the patient? Is chiropractic any more secure because of the development of the educational process? Are we developing new and better methods of testing and evaluating patients, chiropractically? Are we researching the basic premise of chiropractic? Or are we producing more educated, less committed, direct access technicians attempting to function allopathically?

We are in turbulent times, chaotic times, as the entire health care reimbursement industry is in the process of reform. Managed care is growing in popularity with the promise of "complete medical care" and little or no expenditure for the patient. Chiropractors and students are reacting with panic and the fear of exclusion that is prevalent among all health professionals. Will we ever appreciate our raison d'etre as established by our founding fathers? Will we ever lead the patients to responsible health care? Will we ever simply remove the interference to the body's innate ability to heal and respect and honor the creating intelligence?

The future is bright for those who understand and appreciate the context that is uniquely chiropractic. The vitalistic approach to chiropractic is anchored and provides a real alternate approach to the present day medical, treatment paradigm. This is the message that resonates with the public. We are seeing them "rise up" like the phoenix to take responsibility for themselves and their "world." We have the education, knowledge and philosophical perspective that makes us a logical, conservative, cost effective choice of the growing number of those who wish to avoid the medical model at all costs. Science supports our tenets. Other health professions are beginning to appreciate them. All we need is for Doctors of Chiropractic to appreciate them, develop them and practice them, with the pride and confidence they are contributing a safe, cost effective, valuable service that can improve the quality of life without compromising it.

We will more fully appreciate our fundamentals and forefathers. The education process will return to rest on a firm foundation of chiropractic principles and practice. Research will be focused on testing for aberrant nerve function as a result of altered biomechanics, its effect on the body's physiology and its correction by the chiropractic adjustment. We, in practice, will educate patients on physiology, prevention and chiropractic.

As managed care continues on its road to socialized medicine, we will see the fall from predominance of the pharmaceutical industry and the medical establishment as many patients waiting to receive their "free medical services" realize they didn't need them in the first place. The alternate approach, chiropractic, is an oasis of teaching and coaching available to people to help them avoid health crises and take responsibility for themselves by removing the interference to their normal physiology and unrealized potential.

Sid E. Williams, D.C., President, Life University, Marietta, Georgia

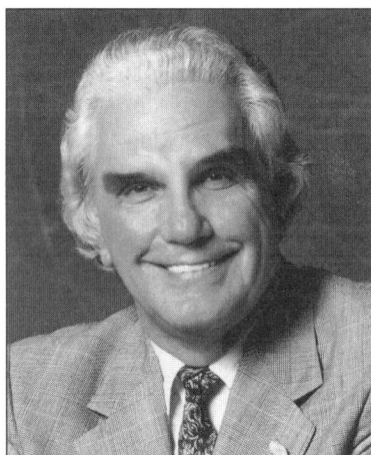

The future of chiropractic is as unlimited as the horizon. With each brave step that we take in our noble journey around the globe, a challenging new horizon appears before us. Beginning in 1895 and for many decades thereafter, simply providing chiropractic care for patients without suffering the indignity of imprisonment was a worthy goal. Next we sought and achieved legal recognition in every state as well as in many other countries. We battled to bring an end to the illegal discrimination practiced against our profession by the AMA and won an historic but tenuous victory there. And now, as we come even closer to the top of the mountain, we should not be surprised as we find the opposition even stronger and more determined than ever to stop us.

Why is there so much resistance to chiropractic? Because ours is the first profession in the history of mankind to solve the very mystery of life which has been puzzling the scientific world for thousands of years. We have demonstrated beyond a shadow of a doubt that the critical difference between healthy, happy, vigorous, productive, long-living human beings and those who, in an identical environment, remain sickly, diseased and depressed is their spinal hygiene.

The truly inspiring news, of course, is that, as chiropractors, we can provide the primary component of spinal hygiene by correcting neural interferences and allowing the wonderfully-made human body to begin the phenomenal natural process of healing itself. Medical men since Hippocrates have searched for that great, mysterious life-giving principle for these thousands of years. However, because a rigid mechanistic model for human functioning was established and enforced, especially in the western world, conflicting ideas have been either ignored or ridiculed. So, while medical researchers were trying to come up with another drug or procedure to support their entrenched theories, D.D. Palmer reached out with his skilled hands and demonstrated the life-giving thrust that has been felt throughout the world ever since. His zeal and tenacious defense of the bigness of his discovery has made our profession possible and is the primary reason we have been able to attract a parade of millions of champions of chiropractic care. And we, as modern chiropractors, are the privileged heirs of that astounding discovery and the great historical tradition which surrounds it.

Already, as major magazines declare that the end of the drug era is here, chiropractic's march continues to pick up momentum and enthusiasm. I anticipate that long before another 100 years have passed, our view of spinal hygiene will be universally accepted. To reach our full potential, however, we must never forget that chiropractic is a unique specialty field limited to certain procedures that we are trained to perform. That is the only reason we have been able to gain licensure in all 50 states in the U.S., all the provinces of Canada, and in many foreign countries — which is miraculous in itself.

Chiropractors who mimic our medical foes by denying the validity of this scientific process are denying the very principles that set our profession apart and makes it a unique and very marketable science. As patients and third-party payers alike are reaching out to health care vendors who stress wellness, disease prevention and the least invasive intervention techniques, chiropractic stands out like a morning star! The professionally trained and licensed chiropractor who understands and appreciates the scientific validity of the spinal subluxation, as proved scientifically more than 20 years ago by Dr. C.H. Suh, is now fully equipped to do the job. And no other health care profession can make that claim.

I envision the day when we will have at least a million fully trained chiropractors to serve the needs of the world's billions of suffering people. Yet, chiropractic care is not something that should be left entirely to the professionally trained person. Just as informed parents know how to apply basic first aid, they should also be trained to provide family members with basic spinal hygiene, which includes both preventive and corrective techniques. As we continue to embrace new tools and technologies in our curriculum at Life College, it is my intention to include Spinal Hygiene as a separate course to provide a means for teachers, parents or anyone else who is interested in learning the basics of maintaining and enjoying the health benefits of a healthy spine. Spinal Hygiene also should be introduced in public education from elementary through high school to give every person a firm grounding in this vital subject. Over a period of time, then, this appreciation of chiropractic will spill over into business, industry and government as well as higher education. And, as the world is exposed to both spinal hygiene and "innate philosophy," the end result will be that more people will seek chiropractic care and achieve better health at a lower overall cost.

As one way to carry the chiropractic message to the world, I am no building a radio and television network (Healthy Living Network), scheduled to begin broadcasting this year before the 1996 Olympics begin in Atlanta. I envision that HLN will reach 50 million households before the year 2000, and before the end of this century, spinal hygiene will be a household term and regular viewers will know how to provide chiropractic first aid for their families. We must do everything possible to reach out even more creatively and with even more compassion to fulfill the crying needs of the suffering billions in the world.

Understandably, our old foes in organized medicine will continue to fight to preserve their historic domain, but that alone cannot stop us. We can, however, defeat ourselves. It is age-old wisdom that tells us that a house divided against itself cannot stand. It is for that reason that I call upon every man and woman of whatever age and whatever alma mater who now enjoys the precious privileges won through the blood and sweat and tears of pioneer chiropractors to stand with us under a common banner. We are chiropractors all. Let us think as one, act as one, and love as one. And we will have no need ever to regret our past or be fearful of our future.

James F. Winterstein, D.C., D.A.C.B.R., F.I.C.C., President, National College of Chiropractic, Lombard, Illinois

I received an excellent article the other day, authored by Stephen L. Carter and titled "The Insufficiency of Honesty." The following is a quote from this article. "The first point to understand about the difference between honesty and integrity is that a person may be entirely honest without ever engaging in the hard work of discernment that integrity requires: she may tell us quite truthfully what she believes without ever taking the time to figure out whether what she believes is good and right and true."

I could write about the rosy picture of chiropractic education as the profession "expands beyond everyone's wildest dreams as people finally become aware that the chiropractic paradigm of health is better and greater than any other. While I might passionately believe that statement to be true, and stating it would be honest on my part, if I am to have integrity I must "engage in the hard work of discernment that integrity requires."

Some might say, "don't be so pessimistic," however, as educators in the profession of chiropractic, our first responsibility must be to fulfill a mandate to those whom we serve that all of our words and actions send a clear and an unassailable signal, that their confidence in our integrity is well placed. We have been a distrusted profession, and in many ways that has not been our fault, however inasmuch as we are often unable to change others, the responsibility for elevation and progression in chiropractic education falls squarely upon our shoulders. We must, as chi-

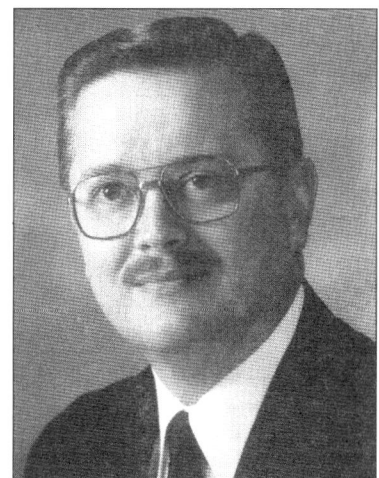

ropractic college presidents, always strive to be above reproach.

Having thus set the stage, I hope that the reader will look upon my words as my best understanding of the signals that guide my thoughts as I attempt to do what no one can truly do - look to the future.

These are not easy times because we have collectively matriculated a student body that is larger than any in our record-ed history. This fact must loom large in the minds of those who look to the future in a country where managed care has established an exceptionally strong foothold as the currently accepted paradigm for health care delivery, for we have a responsibility to provide at least a reasonable expectation for those who enter the profession, that they can successfully prac-tice, and to those who are presently practicing, that we will not overpopulate the profession.

That there are problems with managed care is no secret, and while I do not see the current state of affairs persisting far into the future, I do believe that the time for major improvements will extend over more than just a few years. This suggests a true dilemma regarding chiropractic institutional size, student numbers and resulting financial support of those institutions. In our capitalistic society, competition is the strongest driver and I see that despite the current interest in alternative care methods, there will be a declining student enrollment in chiropractic colleges beginning within the next two to five years. Because many chiropractic colleges are quite tuition dependent, we could see some severely strained budgets. Whether my view is optimistic or pessimistic, I do believe it is quite firmly rooted in the current reality.

Once we get out beyond twenty years, one can only guess. When I engage in that game, I do believe that the profession of chiropractic will be alive and well and I think that it will have expanded in a real sense to include a greater intra-profes-sional awareness of the multiple faces of prevention beyond the effects of disturbed spinal biomechanics. As we mature, we will discover more about our special paradigm of "neurobiomechanical harmony" and the part it plays in total human health and disease, and we will also learn that it is not the total answer.

I believe and hope that chiropractic colleges will shrink in size. There is no other professional model of education that enrolls thousands of students in any one school. The reason for this is simply the improbability of providing a high quality professional education in a setting where students vastly outnumber faculty and massively overtax facilities and legitimate, well developed clinical opportunities.

Chiropractic education will be expanded; first with increased pre-requisite education to the extent that the great majority of our students will hold the baccalaureate when they matriculate in chiropractic college. Within a decade, chiropractic stu-dents will be spending a longer period of time in the clinical setting beyond what is typical at this time. I look for the estab-lishment of residencies as an eventual requirement for regular chiropractic practice. While there will be some integration of chiropractic students into the hospital settings, simple numbers tell me that it will not be widespread. This is based upon cur-rent projections of diminishing hospital beds with resulting closing of hospitals. This means there will be less opportunity for residency openings. That is not bad because it will result in more residencies being conducted in ambulatory care centers where primary care of patients takes place; a setting that is more appropriate for chiropractic residencies than the tertiary care setting of the hospital. Some of these ambulatory care centers will surely be operated in conjunction with hospitals so our future chiropractic residents could get the advantage of exposure to both settings.

Some chiropractic colleges will merge and some will close and there will no doubt be new ones. Some will seek entry into the public university settings and I think some will be successful. Those who pursue such affiliation will discover the pros and the very large "cons" of the circumstance as well. Some chiropractic colleges will remain free standing and in the long run, I believe a mixture is a good thing.

In summary, my hopes are pinned on personal and institutional integrity, strengthening of prechiropractic education, lengthened internships or the establishment of post professional general chiropractic residencies and a marked change in size of chiropractic colleges to institutions of less than 1,000 students. With these changes our prosperity will be markedly strengthened.

Frank A. Zolli, D.C., Dean, University of Bridgeport, College of Chiropractic, Bridgeport, Connecticut

As chiropractic enters its second century, the profession as always, is confronted with challenges. In our first one hundred years, members of the profession fought for survival and legitimacy. In our first one hundred years, ours was a pro-fession deeply divided by philosophical differences. Despite individual interpretations of what chiropractic is and is not, there is an inescapable fact which has surfaced: chiropractic works. While the previous statement may be simplistic, it is also accurate. Whether chiropractic is practiced by a "straight" or "mixer," a philosopher or scientist, it seems to matter little, all chiropractic practitioners get sick people well. Chiropractic, in the hands of practitioners with divergent points of view, has helped millions of people. As a result, chiropractic has become the largest drugless healing profession in the world. Where do we go from here?

An essential element in the expansion of chiropractic is the educational foundation afforded chiropractic students. Chiropractic education has the responsibility of providing every student the opportunity to learn the most contemporary, comprehensive information available to support their understanding and practice of the chiropractic healing art. Chiropractic students should understand the history of the profession and its evolution. For only in our knowledge of the past will we be able to prevent mistakes in the future. Fundamental basic science information should be integrated and correlated with clinical material to provide an interesting and relevant academic experience for students. The clinical component of our training must emphasize the chiropractic approach to health care and wellness. The art of chiropractic: the ability to adjust a patient and stimulate the natural recuperative powers of the body must remain the fundamental component of chiropractic care.

As society enters the twenty-first century, all too often there is the human cry of depersonalization in an ever increasing technical world. It is the responsibility of chiropractic education to continue to develop chiropractors with highly developed humanistic skills. Laboratory tests and diagnostic imaging studies are a common element of all health care professions. The manner in which the information from these tests is both interpreted and communicated to the patient is what separates a technician from a doctor.

Chiropractic is not, nor should it ever be, limited to the treatment of low back pain or musculoskeletal conditions. Chiropractic is a natural approach to health which incorporates manipulation, nutrition and exercise in an effort to help the patients we serve. Unlike other health care therapies, chiropractic, properly applied, does not produce toxic side effects.

It is incumbent upon chiropractic education to build upon the principles and positive attributes established by our chiropractic pioneers. We need to produce practitioners who emphasize the principles and practice of chiropractic in patient care, yet have the ability to cooperatively work with other health care practitioners.

Other areas of education which need to be developed and initiated include courses to help graduates establish their practices on sound business practices, as well as articulation agreements with hospitals. The latter arrangement would serve several functions simultaneously. It would expose chiropractic interns to a wide variety of clinical cases, as well as the prevailing diagnostic technologies in use. It would also provide the opportunity for members of different professions to learn about the strengths and weaknesses of their respective professions. It could also provide the framework for building cooperative relationships which could help bridge the gap between professions, while focusing upon the ultimate aim of all health care professions effective patient care.

Chiropractic's second century is filled with opportunities. While remaining vigilant to protect those rights and privileges which were secured in our first hundred years, we must aggressively promote our distinct, natural approach to health care. Fundamental to our future success as a profession will be the continued evolution of chiropractic education. It is the academic foundation established in chiropractic institutions which will enable future leaders and practitioners to continue chiropractic's growth.

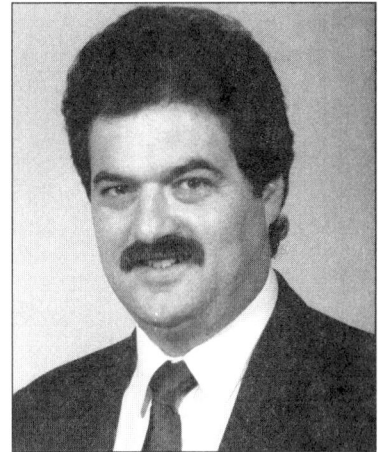

Appendix A

Historical Developments of Important Aspects of Chiropractic Accreditation

The Council on Chiropractic Education

THE HISTORY

The importance of quality education was recognized early in the chiropractic profession. Voluntary efforts to improve chiropractic education were undertaken as early as 1935 when a Committee on Educational Standards (CES) was created by the National Chiropractic Association (NCA) which later became the American Chiropractic Association (ACA). At the conclusion of the annual convention of the NCA, its Board of Directors, acting on instruction from the House of Delegates, appointed the CES.

The Council on State Chiropractic Examining Boards (CSCEB) also undertook to improve chiropractic education at about the same time as the NCA. And in 1938, both groups merged into a new Committee on Educational Standards. Under the direction of this committee, the first college self-study questionnaire was sent to all colleges actively engaged in chiropractic education. At this time, 37 such colleges were in existence.

1940 NCA EDUCATION REPORT

In 1940, a report was submitted to the House of Delegates of the NCA at its annual convention. It included the following observations.

1. All chiropractic colleges were proprietary institutions.
2. Chiropractic colleges differed in their teachings.
3. A broad spread of program length was apparent; they ranged from 18 to 36 months, with some schools seeking to support curricula of two lengths.
4. Some schools possessed two charters, one in chiropractic and another either in drugless therapy, naturopathy or mechanotherapy.
5. A marked variation of course depth was apparent, especially in the basic science and diagnostic subjects.
6. An on-campus atmosphere of individualized concepts was being administered.
7. A general need of laboratory and classroom facilities was evident.
8. A heterogeneity in curriculum composition and emphasis was apparent.
9. A need for coordination among the various colleges was noted.
10. Greater emphasis had to be placed on standardization in entrance requirements, faculty selection and student academic progress.

THE COMMITTEE ON EDUCATIONAL STANDARDS

Work was completed in 1939 on educational criteria that were presented for approval of the chiropractic colleges. Funds were subsequently appropriated by the NCA to employ an inspector to visit the applicant institutions for the purpose of evaluating their progress against their self-studies and educational criteria. In its early years, the Council received applications for membership from the colleges listed:

• Atlantic States College of Chiropractic, Brooklyn, New York. In 1962 it was amalgamated with the Columbia Institute of Chiropractic.
• Canadian Memorial Chiropractic College, Toronto, Canada.
• Carver Chiropractic College, Oklahoma City, Oklahoma. Discontinued functioning both in 1952 and 1964. Its registry and alumni were affiliated with the Logan College of Chiropractic.
• Chiropractic Institute of New York.
• Cleveland Chiropractic College, Kansas City, Missouri.
• Cleveland Chiropractic College, formerly Ratledge Chiropractic College, Los Angeles, California.
• Columbia Institute of Chiropractic. Columbia Institute of Chiropractic became New York Chiropractic College in 1977.
• Detroit College of Chiropractic, Detroit, Michigan. Discontinued functioning in 1948. In 1967 its registry and alumni were affiliated

with the National College of Chiropractic.

• International College of Chiropractic, Dayton, Ohio. Discontinued functioning in 1954.

• Kansas State Chiropractic College, Wichita, Kansas. Discontinued functioning in 1952 and in 1965 its registry and alumni became affiliated with the National College of Chiropractic.

• Lincoln Chiropractic College, Indianapolis, Indiana. Discontinued functioning and in 1971 its registry and alumni became affiliated with the National College of Chiropractic.

• Logan College of Chiropractic, St. Louis, Missouri.

• Metropolitan College of Chiropractic, Cleveland, Ohio, which discontinued functioning in 1948.

• Missouri College of Chiropractic, St. Louis, Missouri. In 1964 it was amalgamated with the Logan College of Chiropractic.

• National College of Chiropractic, Lombard, Illinois.

• Northwestern College of Chiropractic, Minneapolis, Minnesota.

• Oakland College of Chiropractic, Oakland, California. Discontinued functioning in 1950 and its registry and alumni became affiliated with the Los Angeles College of Chiropractic.

• Ross-O'Neil Chiropractic College, Fort Wayne, Indiana. Discontinued functioning in 1948.

• Texas Chiropractic College, Pasadena, Texas.

• University of Natural Healing Arts, Denver, Colorado. Discontinued functioning in 1958 and in 1964 its registry and alumni became affiliated with the National College of Chiropractic.

• Western States College of Chiropractic, Portland, Oregon.

In 1941, the CES issued its first list of institutions with status. The list consisted of 12 provisionally approved colleges.

Throughout the 20 year period from 1941 to 1961, the Committee continued to function to strengthen chiropractic education. Many of the weaker colleges were merged with other institutions to create stronger academic programs. A number of the substandard institutions were simply closed. The number of active colleges had been reduced to ten by 1961.

EDUCATIONAL STAFF MEMBERS

Because the CES functioned on a part-time basis, their efforts received no immediate or direct attention from the administrations of chiropractic colleges.

To solve this problem, the House of Delegates of the old NCA instructed its Board to select and appoint a Director of Education on a salaried, full-time basis. Accordingly, at the annual convention of the NCA in 1941, Dr. John J. Nugent was appointed to this position. A man of vigor, courage and indomitable determination, Dr. Nugent served in this capacity until 1959.

John J. Nugent, D.C. - First NCA Director of Education: 1941-1959

During his tenure, John Nugent spearheaded the initiation, partial or complete fulfillment of the following upgrading accomplishments in chiropractic education:

1. The conversion of a major number of the chiropractic colleges from proprietary status to that of an evolving eleemosynary status.

2. The formation and preparation of criteria for chiropractic colleges. In the beginning, these criteria were submitted simply as guidelines and recommendations. Later they were published as an issue from the Office of the Director of Education. They progressively underwent several revisions with the assistance of the membership of the Council on Chiropractic Education (CCE). Eventually, in 1959, they were adopted by the CCE as the criteria to be fulfilled and conformed to by the participating school members of the Council. Since then they have undergone other revisions.

3. An accrediting committee was established to function in the area of evaluating and classifying chiropractic colleges, which began to assume accreditation supervision. At first this committee was conservative in its efforts, probing and searching for effective means of helping the institutions.

4. Many state boards of chiropractic examiners were aware of the importance of their function and the exactness of their responsibilities and the great need for standardizing examination procedures. State boards' contacts with Dr. Nugent led to a more effective cohesion and liaison between and among the various boards.

5. With unrelenting determination Nugent instituted a program of upgrading entrance requirements and pre-professional college requirements.

6. Dr. Nugent should be credited with the accomplishment of divorcing chiropractic colleges from naturopathic courses. The problem was complex. In some instances, existence of the naturopathic course was justified by the fact that in certain states the practice of chiropractic was so limited (due to the licensure restriction in some states) that in order to maintain diagnostic and practice scope, resort had to be made to naturopathy.

7. Dr. Nugent also spearheaded the effort of establishing contact with state and federal agencies of education, dealing with approval and accreditation. He foresaw the significance of this recognition and sought to emphasize and encourage expansion of all efforts in these areas of responsibility.

8. Dr. Nugent also provided initiative and momentum to the program of subsidies for educational institutions by means of profes-

sional grants. In the beginning, this was not too popular in its impact. Hesitancies were encountered, but eventually the program was successfully instituted. Indeed, the name of Dr. John J. Nugent will always represent in the history of chiropractic, determination, integrity and accomplishment of one of its outstanding members.

Dewey A. Anderson, Ph.D. - Second Director of Education: 1959-1963

Following the retirement of Dr. Nugent, Dr. Dewey A. Anderson, Director of the Public Affairs Institute, Washington, D.C., was appointed as Director of Education. Dr. Anderson had already served the NCA on a consulting basis. He had also written a dissertation on chiropractic which was later published by the Public Affairs Institute.

Dr. Anderson served in the capacity of Director of Education of the NCA from 1959 to 1963, acting in concert with the Council on Chiropractic Education. During his tenure, Dr. Anderson sponsored and significantly emphasized a number of programs:

1. Colleges were encouraged to subsidize continuing education of faculty members who evidenced strong pedagogical capacity, yet needed to fortify their background with additional education. The wherewithal for this purpose was primarily forthcoming through special grants from the NCA.
2. Dr. Anderson, supported by Dr. Emmett J. Murphy, the then NCA Washington representative, alerted the profession to the need of establishing contact with the Office of Education (USOE) of the U.S. Department of Health, Education and Welfare for the purpose of accomplishing two goals:
    (a) Achieving eligibility recognition by the USOE for chiropractic educational institutions
    (b) Establishing minimum qualifications for federal assistance in certain areas of research, education, facilities and
        housing.
3. While Dr. Anderson became Director of Education after the NCA House of Delegates instructed the Board of Directors to establish the Foundation for Accredited Chiropractic Education (later to become known as the Foundation for Chiropractic Education and Research), he may be credited with being a leader in the encouragement of its educational and college programs. Therefore, the already successful program of recurring, reputable grants-in-aid to chiropractic institutions of education gained added momentum through his efforts.

John A. Fisher, Ed.D. - Third Director of Education: 1963-1974

By the time Dr. Fisher was appointed, the NCA changed its name, and merged with other organizations to form the American Chiropractic Association (ACA). Dr. Fisher, having been an educator and college administrator, came to his position with a broad spectrum of knowledge and years of experience which would serve the educational arm of the profession well. In cooperation with CCE and the Administrative personnel of the chiropractic colleges he encouraged and afforded guidance in a number of important areas of concern, among others. He:

1. Assisted the CCE in making the transition from a department of education of the American Chiropractic Association to an autonomous national accrediting agency status in 1971.
2. Established a standard auditing and financial reporting method for all the colleges.
3. Effectively helped the CCE standardize its on-campus inspection and evaluation procedures to make them sophisticated and acceptable to the scrutiny of state and federal agencies in education.
4. Encouraged proper departmentalization of college functions and relating personnel; helped to develop a more academic atmosphere in procedural matters involving the staffs, affairs, on-campus relationships and relationships with the educational work in general.
5. Insisted upon establishing an exact understanding of the requirements that confront any accrediting agency and its sponsoring organization. He then sought to encourage the administrations of the participating colleges to seek means and ways to fulfill these requirements.
6. Counseled the various college administrators on the mechanics of college administration in such important areas as budget planning, auditing, records, admissions, evaluation of credits, faculty governance, curriculum development and campus planning.
7. Assisted the CCE in acquiring reliable accrediting agency status and eligibility in recognition from the United States Office of Education (USOE) in 1974. Eligibility recognition was renewed thereafter.

Rick Timmins, Ed.D., CCE Executive Secretary: 1974-1976

At the time Dr. Timmins was appointed to the position of Executive Secretary of the CCE, it had just achieved eligibility recognition with the USOE. The CCE became, therefore, a nationally recognized accrediting agency for chiropractic education.

Ralph G. Miller, Ed.D., CCE Executive Secretary: 1976-1987, Executive Vice President:1987-1995

When Dr. Timmins accepted the presidency of Western States Chiropractic College in 1976, a search for a replacement resulted in the appointment of Dr. Ralph G. Miller as Executive Secretary. Dr. Miller, experienced as an educator and college administrator, provided assistance to the CCE in a continuing program of growth and service to chiropractic education.

Dr. Miller submitted the following as the more significant achievements during his 19 year tenure.

1. The transition of the CCE accreditation standards to meet the changing requirements of the U.S. Department of Education

(USDE) and the Council on Postsecondary Accreditation (COPA). Beginning in 1987, CCE Standards began to include institutional and programmatic educational outcomes and the related assessment mechanisms. The CCE's COA maintained continuous recognition by first the USOE and later the USDE from 1974 on, and the COPA and its successor organizations from 1976 on.

2. The CCE mission statement was restructured to clarify the CCE's threefold mission of accreditation, educational improvement and public information. The CCE adopted a comprehensive set of operational manuals which were based upon a CCE Model of Institutional Effectiveness which would assess the success of the CCE in achieving its own goals.
3. The membership of the COA was redefined and term limits established.
4. The CCE Board of Directors accepted a White Paper that covered six basic themes and which gave impetus to the development of a strategic plan of operations.
5. A second public member was added to the CCE and its COA.
6. Financial reserves were established to comply with the USDE and COPA requirements ensuring the COA had sufficient budgetary and administrative autonomy from related, affiliated or associated trade associations or membership organizations to carry out its accrediting functions independently.
7. Clinical Competency Delineations became a part of revised standards which assess the institution's success in educating students to practice the science and are of chiropractic.
8. The number of U.S. chiropractic institutions and programs which received the COA award of Accredited Status grew from four to nineteen.
9. CCE USA established reciprocal recognition of CCE Canada, the Australasian CCE, and the European CCE only after intensive review of their accreditation papers and processes, and status reviews of their colleges.
10. CCE and its COA planned and implemented a continuing validity/reliability program of Council standards, and the validation of the COA decision-making process.
11. The Executive office established the chiropractic profession's second largest microfiche collection of historical documents.
12. The Executive office created biennial reports which coincide with and depict the achievements of each new administration.
13. The Council on Chiropractic Education and its Commission on Accreditation Executive Offices were moved from West Des Moines, Iowa, to Scottsdale, Arizona, in 1994.

Paul D. Walker, Ph.D., CCE Executive Vice President: 1995-
    In 1995, the Council on Chiropractic Education Board of Directors conducted a national search for a new Executive Vice President. Dr. Paul D. Walker, an experienced educator and college leader, was selected from a large pool of highly qualified candidates. Dr. Walker assumed the position of Executive Vice President on June 12, 1995. He continues in this leadership role.

Council of Educational Institutions

    Through the encouragement of the original CES, a group of interested administrators of the NCA called a meeting of chiropractic colleges at the annual convention of the National Chiropractic Association in 1942. Its purpose was to form the Council of Educational Institutions (CEI). The colleges originally represented on the CEI were the National College of Chiropractic, the Lincoln Chiropractic College, the Eastern Chiropractic College, the Los Angeles College of Chiropractic, the Western States College of Chiropractic, the Missouri Chiropractic College, and the University of Natural Healing Arts. In the beginning, the meetings were of an exploratory nature. They were held in conjunction with the CES. Topics of significant discussion dealt with:
1. The need to standardize course length and curriculum composition;
2. Common problems of concern about chiropractic education;
3. Standardizing concepts in chiropractic principles and clinical procedures; and,
4. Studies of state licensing laws, state boards of examiners' actions and procedures.
    Minutes were kept, a president and secretary were elected. Those serving originally were Dr. Craig Kightlinger of New York and Homer G. Beatty as president and secretary, respectively. No binding commitments were concluded upon. It was a volitional gathering of school men and members of the CES in an effort to discuss problems and issues in chiropractic education. In 1945 Dr. Kightlinger resigned as president of the Council due to retirement. Soon thereafter, Dr. W.A. Budden, President of the Western States College of Chiropractic, was elected president of the Council and Dr. Clarence W. Weiant appointed as secretary.
    At the 1946 convention of the NCA, the CEI membership and the NCA Committee on Educational Standards formalized their organization and their professional relations. Instructions were assigned to the officers and the director of education to come prepared with definite recommendations at the 1947 annual convention.

THE COUNCIL ON CHIROPRACTIC EDUCATION
    Formal and official establishment of the Council on Chiropractic Education (CCE) was effected at the annual convention of the National Chiropractic Association on August 4, 1947, in conjunction with institutional representatives and members of the Committee on

Educational Standards.

At this time, the CCE received the approval and support of the House of Delegates, and the Board of Directors were instructed to include it as one of the NCA's Councils and provide it with financial support to cover its operating expenses.

EARLY COMPOSITION OF CCE

Essentially, the composition and voting of the authority of the CCE consisted of:

1.   The five member Committee on Accreditation - each member holding one vote.
2.   The director of education - holding one vote.
3.   The Council of Educational Institutions (CEI) with one person representing each institution. The institutions were grouped as follows:
    (a) Those participating in the accrediting program and possessing some classification. The representative of each of these had one vote. The total number of votes carried from time to time depended upon the number of participating institutions.
    (b) Those simply sitting in as observers and not seeking approval or accreditation status.

It may be noted that originally, chief school administrators as well as the director of education had voting authority in relation to accreditation status; the determination of accreditation status was the result of three voting groups: (1) the accrediting Committee, (2) the Council on Educational Institutions and (3) the director of education.

While the CCE has served uninterruptedly since 1947, it was incorporated as an autonomous national organization in 1971; its purposes and functions have been progressively clarified and refined.

In 1963, at the annual convention of the NCA, significant and far-reaching changes were made:

1.   The old NCA and other groups were reorganized as the American Chiropractic Association.
2.   The CCE was reorganized to the following extent:
    (a) While the director of education was assigned to serve both the accrediting agency and the colleges, he was held responsible directly to the ACA Board of Governors and the ACA executive director. His vote on institutional status was rescinded making him a neutral element, functioning only on an advisory, counseling and staff basis.
    (b) The accrediting committee of the CCE became officially known as the Accrediting Agency of the American Chiropractic Association and was provided with full authority to conclude upon the status of accreditation of any of the participating institutions of education. The membership of the Committee consisted of:

    Walter B. Wolf, Chairman - Eureka, South Dakota
    Orval L. Hidde, Secretary - Watertown, Wisconsin
    Herbert E. Hinton - Dania, Florida
    John Richard Quigley - Tacoma, Washington

    (c) The CCE members representing the educational institutions did not have voting authority in relation to the accreditation status of any of the participating colleges; it was considered a conflict of interest for any school person to have a right to vote on the status of any other institution. Their voting authority in relation to all other CCE matters was retained. Actually, the accrediting agency gained full autonomy in the area of accreditation.
    (d) To the membership of the CCE was added three appointees of the Council of Chiropractic Examining Boards (CCEB), namely the president, vice-president and the secretary. They were, however, only auditing members and did not possess voting authority in relation to any CCE affairs.

The CCE was incorporated in 1971 as an autonomous national organization and continues to function in this capacity. During the CCE's early years just after its incorporation, a public member was added to the Commission on Accreditation and the CCE Board of Directors; this person was appointed from the ranks of the educational community at large and served to represent the interests of the many publics served. A second public member was added in 1980.

The five years after 1971 saw the CCE grow from an accreditation agency which established minimum standards for chiropractic colleges in the United States to one which received the approval of the prestigious Council on Postsecondary Accreditation (COPA) and eligibility recognition from the United States Office of Education (which was to become the Department of Education in 1980).

CCE PURPOSE, STRUCTURE, AND FUNCTION: 1980

The CCE received well-deserved praise and recognition since its creation because of the manner in which it met its challenges and achieved its goals. The purposes of the CCE, as a reputable national organization, can be briefly stated as:

(1) advocating high standards of quality in chiropractic education;
(2) establishing criteria of institutional excellence for educating primary health-care chiropractic physicians;
(3) inspecting and accrediting colleges through its Commission on Accreditation; and
(4) publishing lists of those institutions which conform to its standards and policies.

The CCE is composed of two sections. The institutional members section is composed of one official representative of each member college (16 programs and institutions as of January 1996). The second section is the Commission of Accreditation which is composed of nine members: two members from member colleges, two members appointed by the Federation of Chiropractic Licensing Boards (FCLB), three members appointed by the sponsoring national associations (ACA/ICA), and two public members elected by the full council.

The CCE's Commission on Accreditation monitors the quality of education offered by the chiropractic institutions through the accreditation process. Institutions are evaluated against their own objectives and against the Educational Standards for Chiropractic

Colleges by highly specialized teams of education experts. These standards have been developed over many years and represent the minimum requirements an institution must meet to acquire status.

They cover every aspect of an institution's operation and include such topics as objectives, administration, finance, scholastic regulations, faculty, library and physical plant, research and continuing education.

THE LICENSURE RELATIONSHIP

Due to the quality standards exhibited by the CCE, the Federation of Chiropractic Licensing Boards recommended to the various state licensing boards that applicants for licensure should be graduates from chiropractic colleges having status with the CCE's Commission on Accreditation or a college meeting equivalent standards. The licensing jurisdictions of a vast majority of states recognized the wisdom of this recommendation.

As a responsible accrediting body, the CCE standards had to provide for the educational needs of all licensing jurisdictions in the United States. In some states, chiropractors are licensed to utilize treatment procedures that exclude only prescription drugs and major surgery. In other states, however, treatment procedures are more limited by definition. CCE does not interfere with institutional philosophy. If an institution chooses not to prepare students for practice in all states by limiting its teaching of treatment methods, it may do so provided it properly informs the student consumer of the practice limitations of that education as well as the current states in which he or she will not qualify for licensure. If, on the other hand, an institution does in fact undertake to prepare students for practice in the states with liberal statutes by offering courses in the broad range of treatment procedures, it must then also provide adequate clinical experience in those treatment procedures. This assures the student the opportunity for both knowledge and the development of clinical skills necessary for competent application.

THE PROCESS OF STATUS REVIEW

The CCE began its national autonomous position in 1971 with three categories of status recognition for chiropractic colleges:
• Correspondent Status: A pre-accredited status which indicated that an institution had given evidence of sound planning and the resources to implement those plans, and had indicated an intent to work toward accreditation. Correspondent status was not accreditation, nor did it imply or assure eventual accreditation.
Correspondent Status was dropped as a category in 1975.
• Recognized Candidate for Accreditation Status (RCA): A pre-accredited status which indicated that an institution had given evidence of sound planning, the resources to implement those plans, and had an intent to work toward accreditation. Recognized Candidate for Accreditation Status was not accreditation, nor did it imply or assure eventual accreditation. Recognized Candidate for Accreditation was dropped as a category in 1982.
During the changes in statuses, in order to protect students, first, colleges in the correspondent status were given two years to obtain either RCA or fully Accredited status. Then, RCA status holding colleges, and any chiropractic institution having degree granting authority prior to July 1, 1982, could apply for accredited status by January 1, 1987.
• Accredited Status: The Accredited status indicated compliance with all essential standards of the CCE.

Elected CCE Officers and Goals: 1971-1997

With the incorporation of the CCE in 1971, Dr. George H. Haynes was unanimously reelected as president. Haynes had served for many years before the incorporation; his administration was noted for moving the CCE in the direction which eventually resulted in CCE's national status as an independent accrediting agency. Below, each administration and its officers are listed along with some of the more significant achievements of each.

1971-1972: THE HAYNES ADMINISTRATION OFFICERS:
Dr. George H. Haynes, President
Dr. Richard Simon, Vice-President
Dr. John B. Wolfe, Secretary-Treasurer
Dr. Herbert E. Hinton (January, 1971, Acting Chairman; June, 1971, Chairman), Chairman, Commission on Accreditation
Achievements:
1. Articles of Incorporation and By-laws adopted.
2. CCE incorporates as a national autonomous accrediting agency.
3. Officers elected under the newly modified by-laws.
4. Preparation for USOE initial application.
5. First CCE position paper adopted.
6. Standards for continuing education adopted.
7. CCE incorporates research as an educational standard.

1972-1974: THE HIDDE ADMINISTRATION OFFICERS:
Dr. Orval L. Hidde, President
Dr. Leonard E. Fay, Vice-President
Dr. Earl A. Homewood, Secretary-Treasurer
Dr. Herbert E. Hinton, Chairman, Commission on Accreditation
Achievements:
1. The Chiropractic Oath adopted by the CCE.
2. The first public member seated.
3. Intensive effort in preparing the document for initial recognition of CCE by the USOE.
4. Numerous meetings held with USOE officials in Washington, D.C., regarding CCE application.
5. Continued work toward developing more comprehensive standards.
6. CCE central office established.
7. Conferences of college staff groups begin, i.e., academic officers, clinical directors, etc.

1974-1976: THE FAY ADMINISTRATION OFFICERS:
Dr. Leonard E. Fay, President
Dr. John B. Wolfe, Vice-President (1975)
Dr. Earl A. Homewood, Secretary-Treasurer (1974); Vice-President (1975)
Dr. J.R. Quigley, Secretary-Treasurer ((1975)
Dr. Orval Hidde, Chairman, Commission on Accreditation; Past President (1974-76)
Achievements:
1. Initial listing of the CCE by the U.S. Office of Education (Initial listing by USOE: 1974; continued in 1975)
2. Renewal of USOE listing for an additional three years.
3. CCE becomes a member of the Council on Specialized Accrediting Agencies (CSAA).
4. Correspondent status dropped.
5. Expansion of the CCE membership.
6. Communications with the newly forming CCE (Canada), ACCE (Australia).
7. Expansion of CCE's Executive Offices: services, programs.
8. The development of an independent CCE budget.
9. CCE Executive Committee formed, 1974.
10. First Executive Secretary appointed.

1976-1978: THE WOLFE ADMINISTRATION OFFICERS:
Dr. John B. Wolfe, President
Dr. James A. Mertz, Vice-President
Dr. J.R. Quigley, Secretary-Treasurer
Dr. Orval Hidde, Chairman, Commission on Accreditation
Dr. Leonard Fay, Past President
Achievements:
1. CCE status decisions accepted by the New York State Department of Education, 1976.
2. CCE receives initial Council on Postsecondary Accreditation (COPA) recognition; 1976.
3. CCE logo adopted.
4. Adoption of the CCE Position Paper on Ethics.
5. Further major revisions made to the CCE Standards for Chiropractic Colleges.

1978-1980: THE MERTZ ADMINISTRATION OFFICERS:
Dr. James A. Mertz, President
Dr. Patrick H. Sullivan, Jr., Vice-President
Dr. Leonard E. Fay, Secretary-Treasurer
Dr. Orval Hidde, Chairman, Commission on Accreditation
Dr. John B. Wolfe, Past President
Achievements:
1. Acceptance of procedures, policy, rules of CCE (Canada), ACCE (Australia).
2. CCE member appointed to the CCE (Canada) Board.
3. USOE eligibility recognition renewed.
4. Adoption of five year plan by CCE.

5. Evaluation team workshops instituted.
6. CCE consultant workshops instituted.
7. Adoption of chiropractic principles paper.
8. Adoption of the CCE position/policy paper on diagnosis, treatment, and referral.
9. Publication of booklet entitled "The Council on Chiropractic Education and the Accreditation Process for Chiropractic Colleges."

1980-1982: THE SULLIVAN ADMINISTRATION OFFICERS:
Dr. Patrick H. Sullivan, Jr., President
Dr. Ernest G. Napolitano, Vice-President
Dr. John Barfoot, Secretary-Treasurer
Dr. Orval Hidde, Chairman, Commission on Accreditation (1980)
Dr. James A. Mertz, Past President (COA Chairman, 1981)
Achievements:
1. CCE accepts propedeutique program as equivalent to its own pre-professional requirements.
2. The International Chiropractors' Association becomes a CCE sponsor alongside the ACA.
3. Auxiliary fund raising program initiated.
4. CCE status as a reliable accrediting agency for chiropractic colleges is reaffirmed in the Sherman College vs. U.S. Commissioner of Education case.
5. Panel of experts provides evidence to demonstrate acceptable methods, as x-ray alternatives, for the clinical determination of vertebral subluxations.
6. FCER/FACTS representatives review status of chiropractic research before CCE.
7. Second public member seated by CCE.
8. Adoption of the CCE policy statement on instrumentation.
9. CCE accepts the Swiss Federal Matura and First Medical Propedeutical as equivalent to its own pre-professional requirements.
10. Clarification of CCE's position on adjustive therapy.
11. Publication of chiropractic student oriented booklet entitled "The Role of Accreditation in Chiropractic Education."
12. Validity and reliability program of the CCE criteria and standards is encouraged and initiated upon the recommendation of the U.S. Department of Education.
13. Negotiations started to establish interagency agreements regarding the team visit procedure with six regional accrediting agencies.
14. U.S. Department of Justice satisfactorily closes civil investigation against CCE in that alleged antitrust violations were unfounded.

1982-1984: THE NAPOLITANO ADMINISTRATION OFFICERS:
Dr. Ernest G. Napolitano, President
Dr. John B. Barfoot, Vice-President (1982), Secretary-Treasurer
Dr. Marino R. Passero, Secretary-Treasurer (1982); Vice-President (1983)
Dr. Beatrice Hagen, Secretary-Treasurer (1983)
Dr. Neil Stern, Chairman (1982), Commission on Accreditation
Dr. James A. Mertz, Chairman (1983), Commission on Accreditation
Dr. Patrick H. Sullivan, Jr., Past President
Achievements:
1. CCE continued and substantially broadened its workshop program to embrace college self-study personnel and business officers.
2. CCE recognition by the Council on Postsecondary Accreditation continued without impediment through 1986.
3. CCE recognition continued by United States Department of Education through 1986.
4. Full reciprocal agreement initiated and ratified in June 1982 on the chiropractic college accreditation process between the CCE (USA) and the CCE (Canada).
5. A paper entitled "The Community of Interest" was unanimously approved. Its thesis describes the CCE as a broadly representative chiropractic college accrediting body dedicated to upholding the qualitative and quantitative aspects of the CCE criteria.
6. CCE moves to a one level accreditation status by deleting its Recognized Candidate for Accreditation status category.
7. The concept and bylaws for an International Committee on Accrediting Agencies for Chiropractic Colleges (ICAACC) approved; to foster cooperative efforts in international chiropractic education and accreditation.
8. Task Force of the CCE Clinical Quality Evaluation Committee undertakes to determine the status of competency based clinical education as it pertains to the newly graduated doctor of chiropractic.
9. Development of an index of chiropractic literature through 1980.
10. The CCE obtained from the North Central Association of Colleges and Schools a tentative agreement to establish an interagency agreement between the two organizations; consummation of the document depended upon ratification by the executive committee of the North Central organization.
11. The CCE developed a comprehensive career information/public information package consisting of updated and revised additions

of: "The Future Depends on You," "The Role of Accreditation in Chiropractic Education," and "The Council on Chiropractic Education and the Chiropractic Colleges."

12. CCE obtained membership in the American Council on Education.

13. A vastly improved complaint procedure was implemented.

14. A further clarification of definition of multi-campus units was implemented.

15. The Broad Spectrum Group of the Validity/Reliability Program finalized the first phase of the program; its conclusions and recommendations were made to the CCE Executive Committee.

16. Major efforts were undertaken to establish and determine the need for CCE to establish standards for chiropractic assistants, and chiropractic radiologic technology.

17. The matter of confidentiality and disclosure in accreditation was implemented to determine its implication for the CCE and its COA.

18. CCE implements a major effort to identify and clarify the issue of research as it applies to chiropractic, via a presentation by Dr. Cheryl Montefusco, during the 1984 CCE Annual Meeting.

19. CCE institutes and implements The Workbook for Calculation and Interpretation of Indicators of Financial Condition for Chiropractic Colleges.

20. CCE becomes a patron of the National Association of Advisors to the Health Professions, October 1983; CCE to participate in the first such program in June 1984.

21. CCE undertakes, for the first time, a $10,000 matching gift fund program.

22. CCE approves the Richmond College Pre-chiropractic Program, London, England.

23. CCE undertakes a survey of the colleges to determine diagnosis and patient referral, as well as to determine qualifications of instructors for clinical experience.

24. CCE establishes a Committee on Chiropractic History which would create a chiropractic history syllabus and course outline for optional use by chiropractic colleges.

25. The term of office of CCE officers is extended from one to two years.

26. The initiation of long range planning for the CCE was initiated in 1982, and actual feasibility studies submitted in 1983.

27. CCE President invited to address the Canadian Memorial Chiropractic College's commencement convocation on May 8, 1982, in Toronto, Canada. The special significance of this was the fact that the graduates were the first to receive their diplomas from a chiropractic institution which had obtained Recognized Candidate for Accreditation status from both the CCE (Canada) and the CCE (USA), via the reciprocal recognition of the two agencies.

28. CCE approved and endorsed the following definition of CHIROPRACTIC SCIENCE at the 1984 annual meeting: Chiropractic is the science which concerns itself with the relationship between structure, primarily the spine, and function, primarily the nervous system, of the human body as that relationship may affect the restoration and preservation of health.

1984-1985 THE PASSERO ADMINISTRATION OFFICERS:
Dr. Marino Passero, President
Dr. Beatrice Hagen, Vice-President
Dr. Jerome McAndrews, Secretary-Treasurer
Dr. Neil Stern, Chairman (1984), Committee on Accreditation
Dr. Patrick Sullivan, Chairman (1985), Committee on Accreditation
Dr. Ernest Napolitano, Past President
Accomplishments:
* Clinical competencies were delineated to identify the cognitive, affective, and psychomotor skills implicit in the first professional degree awarded by a CCE-accredited chiropractic college.
* The establishment of financial indicators which would assess the financial stability of the colleges.
* A task force on admissions was formed to clarify interpretations of the Standards.
* Continuing cooperation of the Council on Chiropractic Education USA with the Council on Chiropractic Education Canada and the Australasian Council on Chiropractic Education.
* Celebrated fifty years of chiropractic education through accreditation.
* Three colleges were newly accredited.
* The ICA Spinal Roentgenology Program was added to the specialty councils.
* Chiropractic representation was established in the American Public Health Association.
* Development of a data base for state licensing information.
* The first annual report (1985) was distributed to the CCE's constituencies.

1986-1987 THE HAGEN ADMINISTRATION OFFICERS:
Dr. Beatrice Hagen, President
Dr. Jerome McAndrews, Vice-President (1986-1987)
Dr. Maylon Drake, Vice-President (1987)

Dr. Neil Stern, Secretary-Treasurer
Dr. Patrick Sullivan, Chairman, Committee on Accreditation
Dr. Marino Passero, Past President
Accomplishments:
* Draft checklist for site teams to use in evaluating clinical experience was distributed by the Clinical Quality Assurance Panel.
* Task Force on Standards of Care formed to establish a guiding standard for the chiropractic institutions. It produced a document that embraces expectations without prescription.
* Established reciprocal relationships with Australasian Council on Chiropractic Education and Council on Chiropractic Education Canada.
* The process of a major review and revision of the standards for accreditation was begun. The first phase was a validity/reliability study of the purposes of the CCE and the accrediting process.
* Sponsored a presentation to the National Association of Advisors to the Health Profession to provide a greater understanding of chiropractic to those important in guiding potential students to chiropractic programs.
* Continued strategic planning process.
* Applied for and received renewal of status with Council on Postsecondary Accreditation and the U.S. Department of Education.
* Workshops were held in the areas of clinical quality assurance and financial indicators.

1988-1989 THE DRAKE ADMINISTRATION OFFICERS:
Dr. Maylon Drake, President
Dr. John Miller, Vice-President
Dr. James Winterstein, Secretary-Treasurer
Dr. Patrick Sullivan, Chairman, Committee on Accreditation
Dr. Beatrice Hagen, Past President
Accomplishments and Concerns:
* The greatest concern was the U.S. Department of Education approved the Straight Chiropractic Academic Standards Association's petition for recognition.
* Draft revision of Standards presented to the college presidents which included a new Mission Statement and focused on outcomes assessment. The Standards emphasize planning as a major critical component and function of expectation for the institutions, while allowing more freedom for individual differences between institutions.
* CHIPEDS (Chiropractic Education Data System) developed which would allow trend analysis.
* Three ad hoc panels were organized: (1) on Institutional Indicators; (2) on Procedures Implementation; (3) on Strategic Planning.
* The Clinical Competency Delineations became the part of the revised Standards which assess the institutions' success in training students to practice the science and art of chiropractic.
* Four significant changes were made to the CCE Standards: 1) faculty standard, requiring that members of the clinic staff must hold first professional degrees in health sciences or an appropriate terminal degree and have three years full-time practical experience; 2) advanced standing standard, allowing applicable credit to those who have taken professional clinical work in another healing arts program; 3) standard on organization, outlining board criteria, and; 4) a resolution on Specialty Councils.
* The CCE appointed an ad hoc blue ribbon panel to review and make an analysis of the Council and Commission membership to include all individuals from supporting organizations.
* CCE-USA approved a first level agreement with the European Council on Chiropractic Education, which recognized its educational standards and Constitution.
* CCE Panel on Ethics was transferred to the Association of Chiropractic Colleges.

1990-1991 THE JOHN MILLER ADMINISTRATION OFFICERS:
Dr. John Miller, President
Dr. James Winterstein, Vice-President
Dr. Carl Cleveland III, Secretary-Treasurer
Dr. Matthew Givrad, Chairman, Committee on Accreditation
Dr. Maylon Drake, Past President
Accomplishments:
* The accreditation process and the Standards were modified with a transition plan being introduced. The purposes were restated as mission and functions, based upon a Model of Institutional Effectiveness. The accreditation process will include a system of review which will be driven by quantitative (data) assessment, as well as empirical and qualitative assessment through peer review.
* The Manual of Operations was revised and the first use of the Manual in self studies took place in Fall 1990 in three chiropractic institutions.
* The Board adopted a revised set of manuals including: 1) Bylaws, 2) Standards, 3) Manual of Operations, 4) Policy Manual, 5)

Procedure Manual: Commission, 6) Procedure Manual: Executive Office, 7) Procedure Manual: Site Visitation Teams, 8) Procedure Manual: Institutions, and 9) Manual of Manuals.
* The CCE Executive Vice President was made a nonvoting ex officio member of the CCE Executive Committee and the COA Executive Committee.
* The CCE's mission statement was revised, the better to more clearly identify the functions of the CCE.
* Changes were made to the Standards to clarify the governance of a chiropractic program within a university.
* In the clinical portion of the Standards, it was clarified that a student must perform a minimum of 80% chiropractic spinal adjustments during at least 250 separate patient care visits.

1992-1993 THE WINTERSTEIN ADMINISTRATION OFFICERS:
Dr. James Winterstein, President
Dr. Carl Cleveland III, Vice-President
Dr. William Dallas, Secretary-Treasurer
Dr. Marino Passero, Chairman, Committee on Accreditation
Accomplishments:
* The CCE Panel on Planning recommended acceptance of a White Paper that covers six basic themes which give impetus to a strategic plan for the future.
  1) Expand the scope of activities to include accreditation of postgraduate programs in chiropractic offered by any institution with an accredited D.C. program and chiropractic paraprofessional programs offered in any U.S. institution of postsecondary education. 2) Emphasize programmatic accreditation functions. 3) Play a leadership role in improving the quality of chiropractic education, which includes instruction, research, and service. 4) Study ways to improve the balance between the educational community and the chiropractic profession in the governance structure of CCE. 5) Serve on behalf of the profession to raise the critical issues. 6) Assume a focused role in promoting chiropractic education.
* Established a reciprocity agreement with the European Council on Chiropractic Education.
* Eliminated "confidential probation" and made all decisions of the Commission on Accreditation placing a program or institution on probation a matter of public knowledge. Created a procedure for reinstating the accredited status.
* Bylaws changes included clarifications and changes to protect the autonomy of the Commission on Accreditation.
* Five new or revised manuals were adopted.

1994-1995 THE CLEVELAND ADMINISTRATION OFFICERS:
Dr. Carl Cleveland III, President
Dr. William Dallas, Vice-President
Dr. John Allenburg, Secretary-Treasurer
Dr. Marino Passero, Chairman, Committee on Accreditation
Dr. James Winterstein, Past President
Accomplishments:
* The CCE participated in the Chiropractic Centennial Foundation's 1995 Grand Celebration of 100 years of chiropractic.
* The Committee on Ethics reported that it surveyed codes of ethics from all CCE programs and several other professions before recommending selected materials to the Council and its Commission on Accreditation to guide their activities.
* An orientation program was developed for new directors.
* The Board of Directors restructure the mission statement to clarify the Council's threefold mission of accreditation, educational improvement and public information.
* Bylaws changes ensure that the Commission on Accreditation has sufficient budgetary and administrative autonomy from related, associated or affiliated trade associations or membership organizations to carry out its accrediting functions independently. The membership of the Commission was redefined and term limits established.
* Major revisions to the Standards allowed conformity to the 1992 Higher Education Act and the 1994 publication of the USDE Secretary's Procedures and Criteria for Recognition of Accrediting Agencies.
* The Task Force on Admissions studied the Mexican bachellerato degree, but did not approve it as sufficient pre-chiropractic education.

1996-1997 THE DALLAS ADMINISTRATION OFFICERS:
Dr. William Dallas, President
Dr. John Allenburg, Vice-President
Dr. Gerald Clum, Secretary-Treasurer
Dr. Marino Passero, Chairman, Committee on Accreditation
Dr. Carl Cleveland III, Past President
Accomplishments:

There are three components in the mission statement of the CCE that constitute the backbone of higher education. These are instruction, research and service. The CCE has continued to strengthen infrastructure and organizational leadership to meet the needs of the instruction component, and to a lesser degree, the service element. Attention has been concentrated on curricula, clinical experience and operations and facilities.

During this administration, CCE can best be described as having solidified the foundation for assurance that each member college is addressing the criteria for adequacy in the instruction aspect of our mission. Our standards are established and improving and the operational components of our system in place. The CCE Executive Office is stable and under sound professional leadership.

Appendix B

MINUTES OF THE NCA/ACA COUNCIL ON EDUCATION, JULY 1940, 1941, AND 1948 THROUGH 1968.

Inventory of Minutes, Dates and Locations of 36 Meetings:

July 28, 1940, Minneapolis	June 15-18, 1958, Miami Beach
July 22-23, 1941, Baltimore	January 3-6, 1959, Dallas
January 23-25, 1948, Chicago	July 6-9, 1959, Chicago
June 1948, Portland OR	July 3-7, 1960, Minneapolis
January 5-7, 1949, Chicago	June 11-17, 1961, Las Vegas
July 25-29, 1949, Chicago	February 19-22, 1962, Los Angeles
February 1-3, 1950, Chicago	June, 1962, Detroit
July 31-August 4, 1950, Washington	January 19-24, 1963, Los Angeles
July 22-27, 1951, Detroit	June 24-26, 1963, Chicago
January 16-19, 1952, Indianapolis	January 12-16, 1964, Palm Springs CA
June 23-26, 1952, Miami Beach	January 16-21, 1965, Des Moines
July 26-31, 1953, Los Angeles	June 19-25, 1965, Hollywood FL
February 11-13, 1954, San Antonio TX	January 18-22, 1966, Des Moines
February 9-11, 1955, New York	June 22-25, 1966, Los Angeles
July 4-8, 1955, Atlantic City NJ	February 7-10, 1967, Atlanta
February 15-17, 1956, Toronto	June 28-July 1, 1967, St. Louis
July 1-6, 1956, Chicago	February 1-4, 1968, Las Vegas
January 5-8, 1957, Miami Beach	June 30-July 5, 1968, New York

Source

The following pages present the Minutes of the NCA (later ACA) Council on Education and related materials made available by the National College of Chiropractic Library, Special Collections and the Council on Chiropractic Education. They are not complete, and include some illegible data. We are grateful to James F. Winterstein, D.C., D.A.C.B.R., President and Ronald P. Beideman, D.C., N.D., Archivist, of the National College of Chiropractic, and to former CCE Executive Vice-President, Ralph G. Miller, Ed.D., for access to this information. Some minor changes have been made, such as in spelling, and page layout.

Minutes of the semi-annual meeting of the COUNCIL ON EDUCATION held in Chicago, January 23, 24, and 25, 1948, at the Congress Hotel, Dr. Thure C. Peterson presiding.

The following persons were in attendance: The Institute of Chiropractic of New York (accredited) - Dr. Thure C. Peterson; The Lincoln College of Chiropractic (accredited) - Drs. James Firth and Arthur Hendricks; Western States College of Chiropractic (accredited) - Dr. W.A. Budden; The Los Angeles College of Chiropractic (accredited) - Dr. Ralph J. Martin; The Canadian Memorial College of Chiropractic (accredited) - Drs. R.O. Mueller and S.F. Sommacal; National College of Chiropractic (accredited) - Dr. Joseph Janse, Dr. R.C. King and Mr. O.J. Turek attended the Sunday session; Northwestern College of Chiropractic (provisionally accredited) - Dr. John B. Wolfe; Carver College of Chiropractic (provisionally accredited) - Dr. Paul Parr; Denver University of Natural Healing (non-accredited) - Dr. H.C. Beatty; The Missouri College of Chiropractic (solicited provisional accrediting) - Dr. H.C. Harring; The Logan Basic College of

Some of the Players

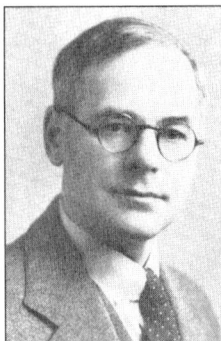
W.A Budden

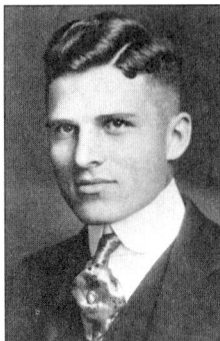
Carl S. Cleveland, Sr.

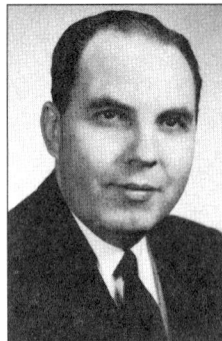
Carl S. Cleveland, Jr.

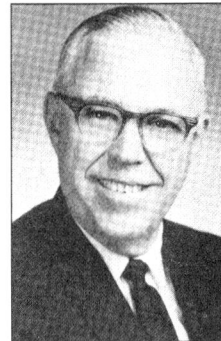
William N. Coggins

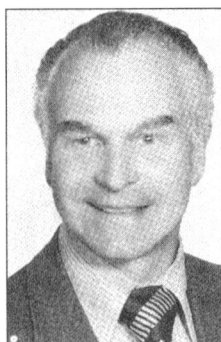
Robert E. Elliot

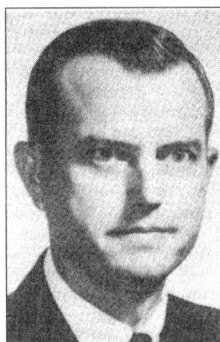
Jerry England

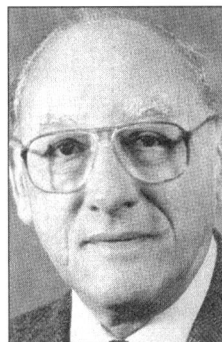
Leonard Fay

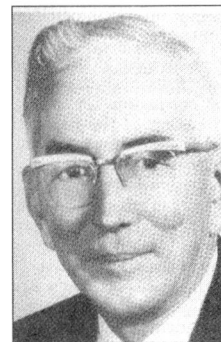
William D. Harper

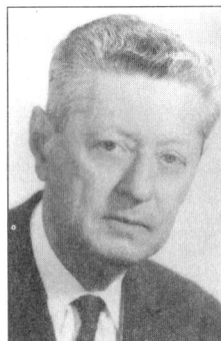
George Haynes

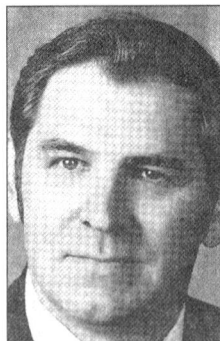
Orval Hidde

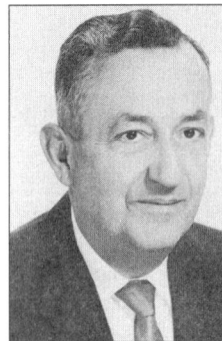
Henry G. Higley

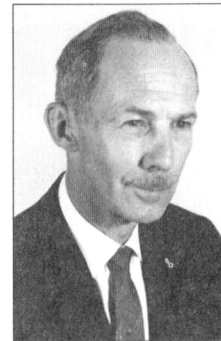
A. Earl Homewood

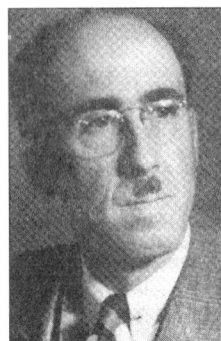
Fred W. Illi

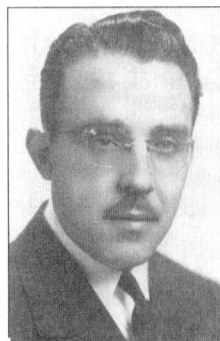
Joseph Janse

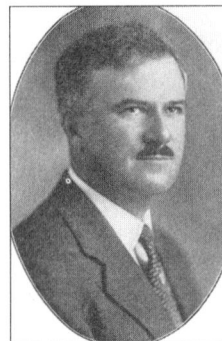
Craig M. Kightlinger

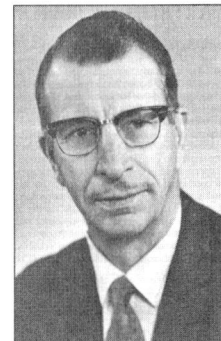
Ralph J. Martin

Chiropractic (solicited full accrediting) - Drs. Fern M. Logan, Wm. M. Coggins, and Hedburg; Dr. John J. Nugent, Director of Education.

The following members of the Committee on the Accrediting of Chiropractic Colleges: Drs. Walter Wolf, E.H. Gardner, T.J. Boner, Dr. Justin Wood having sent in his excuse.

Dr. Herman Schwartz attended the first two days representing the NCA Committee on Psychology.

The meeting was opened by Dr. Thure C. Peterson and he expressed the opinion that inasmuch as a number of people in attendance were there for the purpose of presenting the case of their respective colleges for recognition and accrediting by the Council that a closed meeting be held for a short time, attended only by those who held a voting power in the Council to discuss the status and the qualifications of those seeking membership. This was fully agreed upon by the members of both groups concerned. After the separation Dr. John J. Nugent, Director of Education, was asked to give a detailed report on his inspection of some of the schools that were seeking full recognition.

THE ATLANTIC STATES COLLEGE OF BROOKLYN, NEW YORK. Dr. Nugent advised the group that Dr. Phillips, formerly associated with Drs. Kightlinger, Peterson, and Trubenbach in Eastern College of Chiropractic, as well as the Chiropractic Institute of New York, had organized this new college. He stated that the school is located in the basement of a privately operated commercial high school known as Colby College. According to his report physical plant of this new college was exceedingly poor consisting of only a few drab and ill-equipped rooms. Dr. Phillips and his X-ray assistant represented the primary personnel of the faculty, as well as a few local practicing chiropractors who came in to give a few lectures now and then. At the present time the school has matriculated some 20 students and Dr. Nugent advised that he would recommend no further consideration of the application of this institution, this recommendation being unanimously accepted by the Council.

THE COLUMBIA COLLEGE OF CHIROPRACTIC, BALTIMORE, MARYLAND BRANCH. Dr. Nugent advised the Council that Dr. Dean, the president of the Columbia College of Chiropractic of New York, a little over a year ago had organized a branch college in Baltimore, Maryland. At that time Mr. Earl T. Hawkins of the Maryland Department of Education, asked Dr. Nugent why this school was not recognized by the National Chiropractic Association. Dr. Nugent advised Mr. Hawkins that as yet the college had not made application for a thorough inspection. After some time Mr. Hawkins granted the institution a charter and rendered it temporary recognition on the basis of 12 provisional stipulations. Dr. Nugent received a copy of these 12 provisions and after studying them he advised Mr. Hawkins that if these provisions were fully complied with the National Chiropractic Association would extend the Baltimore Branch of the Columbia College full recognition. It is to be noted that neither the Maryland State Chiropractic Association or the Maryland Board of Chiropractic Examiners favor the institution or the dispositions of Dr. Dean. About this time Mr. Hawkins resigned from his position and his successor was induced by Dr. Dean to give the college full recognition.

Dr. Dean proceeded to buy an old residential building in which this group is at present time housed. At this point Dr. Peterson asked Dr. Nugent whether Dr. Dean had asked for an inspection and NCA approval. Dr. Nugent answered no, but that his investigation of the situation had been solicited by the Maryland State Chiropractic Society and Board. Then Dr. Peterson wanted to know whether Dr. Nugent would, if he deemed it advisable, recognize the branch school in Maryland when the original school in New York had not been approved. Dr. Nugent insisted that if the branch school possessed those qualifications to warrant recognition he would recognize the same, regardless of the status or position of the New York school. At this time the suggestion was made that further investigation and considerations be conducted before any specific decision be reached.

THE LOGAN COLLEGE OF CHIROPRACTIC. Dr. Nugent then proceeded to give a detailed report of his inspection of the Logan Basic College of Chiropractic. He said that he had spent a lot of time at the school proper and that the physical equipment was very good and that Dr. Logan had instituted a very fine and extensive building program, that the procedures of registration and bookkeeping and the handling of finances and students was in good order. The curriculum he said was somewhat off balance, yet the course was a full four-year course. Certain corrections had already been made in the curriculum and he had been asked by Dr. Logan to return and help reorganize the schedule, as well as prepare a catalogue. The faculty, Dr. Nugent asserted, was fairly good, there being at present three very competent men and others less competent but possessing the potential of becoming good instructors.

Dr. Nugent advised the group that Dr. Logan's anti NCA attitudes had changed noticeably and that he was sincerely desirous of receiving NCA approval and becoming a member of the Council. Because of these and other contributing factors Dr. Nugent advised and suggested that the Council give the Logan College full approval.

The following discussions ensued.

Dr. Budden asked the question whether Dr. Logan had agreed to do away with this matter of making his undergraduates as well as postgraduates sign a contract of secrecy with reference to the technic that they had been taught. Dr. Nugent advised that Logan was really conducting two schools; one, an undergraduate school which was on a full non-profit basis and two, a postgraduate and extension school which was his personal and private business, and that he saw no reason why Dr. Logan should be asked to discontinue the latter. At this point Dr. Janse advised the opinion that if Dr. Logan is as frankly desirous of recognition and inclusion by and in this Council he should be more than willing to desist from demanding any contracts of secrecy of any of the people whom he teaches, whether undergraduates or postgraduates. Furthermore that Dr. Logan should stop encouraging cliques and attitudes of separation, which served so viciously in creating dissentions and differences among state groups and our national unity. He further expressed the belief that Dr. Logan's tendency to go about the country putting on special technic courses for which he charges rather exorbitant fees should also be discontinued.

Dr. John B. Wolfe at this time interjected his opinion that the contentions of Drs. Budden and Janse were fully correct, that at one time he had contemplated putting in a chair of basic technic in the Northwestern College and that the stipulations and contract impositions demanded of him by Dr. Logan were such that they represented an abuse of his integrity and consequently he refused any such proposition. Dr. Peterson, at this point, advised the opinion that the Logan College be permitted a period of six to twelve months for purpose of readjustment and during which provisional recognition would be extended them. Dr. Nugent expressed the belief that Dr. Logan would not be satisfied with a provisional recognition but that it would have to be a full recognition or none. At this time Dr. James Firth said that he, like the rest, did not approve of the contract element in basic technic or the secretiveness and separatism that heretofore had been practiced. He mentioned, however, that much of this Dr. Vinton Logan had inherited from his father and consequently it was not entirely his fault or creation. Furthermore, Dr. Firth informed the group that the postgraduate courses as taught by Dr. Logan were not held at the college but in a downtown St. Louis Hotel. He also said Dr. Logan had advised him that he was aware of the fact that some of his conduct of the past had been somewhat untoward and that the element of secretiveness in basic technic was at an end.

Dr. Arthur Hendricks commented that it was his opinion that all of the previous speakers were justified in their attitudes towards the Logan situation. He suggested that Dr. Logan be fully and frankly confronted with the aversions expressed and the suggestions made and that if he were sincerely willing to comply with certain stipulations full recognition should be afforded.

Dr. W.A. Budden made a motion that Drs. Nugent and Gardner and the Committee on Accrediting of Colleges meet with Dr. Fern Logan and her associates who were waiting on the outside and discuss with them the four primary issues that were in question. This motion was seconded by Dr. Firth. Dr. John J. Nugent was then handed the four stipulations that were to be considered by the Logan people before the Council would proceed with the approval of their institution. These stipulations were:

(1) That in both undergraduate and postgraduate instruction no contracts of secretiveness with reference to basic technic be demanded of those who take the work.

(2) That the Logan College or anyone associated with the Logan College refrain from conducting money making classes all over the country in form of special technic courses.

(3) That a conscientious effort be made on the part of Dr. Logan and his associates to avoid the establishment of any technic cliques or the practice of group separatism within state and national organizations.

(4) That the element of commercialism, as well as the teaching of high pressured courses in salesmanship, be discontinued.

Dr. Nugent and the Committee on the Accrediting of Colleges then proceeded to meet with Dr. Fern Logan, an associate of Dr. Vinton Logan in the administration of the college, Dr. Wm. M. Coggins, the dean of the college, and Dr. Hedburg, who is a field representative of the Logan College, and following is the report and a continued discussion by the Council with the Logan representatives about the situation at hand.

Dr. Nugent advised the Council that they had met with the Logan representatives and that Dr. Fern Logan, the spokesman, had informed him that the secretiveness clause had already been discontinued, at least in their undergraduate work, that it never had been their intention to promulgate a principle of separatism, and that because of the augmented enrollment they had been forced to cut down their postgraduate and extension course work to a minimum.

At this time Dr. Nugent advised Dr. Logan that it was the general consensus of opinion that Dr. Vinton Logan's claims and addresses on unity and group amalgamation had been somewhat inconsistent and ill sustained and he advised here that these attitudes must change before full acceptance of their college as an accredited school of the NCA could be realized. Furthermore, that if the other accredited schools be desirous of teaching basic technic that such privileges should be accorded without necessarily any contractual agreement with the Logan school other than contacting the Logan College and obtaining their advice and approval upon the instructor, and who is to have had full and competent instruction in basic technic. At this point Dr. Fern Logan expressed the desire that every decision she held in abeyance until she and her associates have an opportunity of contacting Dr. Vinton Logan directly and explain to him the exact attitude and disposition of the various members of the Council and the Accrediting Committee with reference to the circumstances of the Logan College. Dr. Budden then made the following motion, that none of the accredited schools shall venture to teach basic technic or any other special technic without consulting the colleges directly in which these technics found origin, as to the qualifications of the instructor who is to teach the technic, and this was seconded by Dr. H.E. Gardner.

Dr. Thure C. Peterson was then instructed to contact Dr. Logan in New York and advise him of the dispositions of the Council and also of the four points that were brought to the attention of his representatives at the private meeting held with them and Dr. Nugent and the Accrediting Committee. Dr. Peterson was then to relay to the members of the Council a detailed report on the reactions and opinions of Dr. Logan with reference to the same.

This decision was fully agreeable to the Logan representatives and they left assuring the members of the Council that they felt that every due and kind consideration had been extended them and that a definite understanding would be reached to effect a harmonious solution to the problems that existed.

NOTE BY DR. PETERSON: A meeting was held at the National Republican Club the following Friday from 6 to 11 P.M. attended by Drs. Vinton Logan, John Nugent and Thure C. Peterson. All of the opinions of the members of the Council were presented in substance to Dr. Logan and all avenues of possible conformation by the Logan College to the wishes of the Council were explored. Dr. Logan was reluctant to have the approval hinge upon conditions and it was finally decided to have Dr. Logan take up the matter with his Board of Directors when he returned to St. Louis. Up to the time of publishing these minutes there has been no further word from Dr. Logan.

Dr. Peterson informed the Council in general session that Dr. Wilford Biron of Antioch, Illinois, at the suggestion of several members of the profession, had contacted him requesting an audience of the Council so that he might present them a program that had been elaborated by the College of Audiometry of 894 Main Street, Antioch, Illinois. Dr. Biron was invited into the Council and advised that he would be rendered 30 minutes to explain and present his proposition to the group. Dr. Biron announced himself as a practicing chiropractor in Antioch, Illinois, who had become acutely interested in the field of help for the deaf. He asserted that he had in his private practice found that in many instances chiropractic was of benefit but that at times certain adjunctive measures have to be added and consequently he turned to the field of audiometry, which he defined as that science which dealt with the methods employed in determining the degree of auditory deficiency as well as estimating the proper type and use of various hearing aid devices. Dr. Biron asserted that this investigation lead him to become affiliated with the College of Audiometry of Antioch, Illinois, whose president is Dr. Frank Keefe. He said that they wanted to present their work to the chiropractic profession because it was their opinion that the work was so closely related to that of the chiropractor that probably a cooperative program could be established. He informed the Council that they would like to propose a program consisting of three points: 1. for the purpose of encouraging the members of the profession to take a greater interest in the science of audiometry: 2. to create a regular and substantial course of audiometry in all of our chiropractic colleges; 3. to obtain the privilege to write articles for the NCA Journal and to advertise in the same.

Inquiries were then made of Dr. Biron as to the extent and nature of the college in question, as well as the course they were now conducting. He informed the group that the college was not a resident college but was really an extension college consisting of correspondence work and the conducting of special classes in various sections of the country, these special group instruction courses consisting of eight Sundays and costing $200 each, and were only given to men with professional licenses. After presenting his program Dr. Biron was excused and then the brief following discussion ensued.

It was the consensus of everyone present that no credence or recognition could be given this program or group. First, because it appeared that as yet their efforts were not too substantial and more or less of the correspondence course status. Secondly, it appeared as if it were an effort on this group's part to gain recognition on the strength of our professional reputation, and thirdly, as an entree to advertise themselves without cost with our professional publications. For that reason the entire membership of the Council felt that the proposition and program should not experience any further consideration.

At this time Dr. Peterson proposed that the Council now proceed to consider the various resolutions that had been referred to the Council by the House of Delegates at the Omaha convention. For purpose of dispatch and clarity they shall be considered in their order as they were presented to the Council.

Resolution 1: Be It Resolved that all accredited colleges shall teach a course in X-ray of not less than 240 hours, this to include spinography and general radiology.

This resolution was considered rather extensively by the members of the Council and it was sincerely felt that the spirit of the resolution was quite proper and certainly warranted our consideration. However, it was the general opinion that we could not go on record as specifically designating 240 hours as a must for the X-ray course in all of the accredited colleges, the reason being that if this request were granted other groups representing other favored projects could and would demand the same and this would run into the danger of over loading our college curricula with augmented hours in various specialties. It was the consensus, however, that greater emphasis should be placed upon the teaching of diagnostic roentgenology, the opinion being expressed that the teaching of spinography alone or as a major in X-ray could not be sufficient. Consequently the following resolution was passed. The Council on Education has decided that rather than the specification of a set number of hours the colleges provide basic instruction in the fundamentals of roentgenology, with special emphasis upon the diagnostic values including both osseous and soft tissue consideration as well as spinography. Further studies in this subject should be graduate work leading to specialization.

Resolution 2: Be It Resolved that the National Chiropractic Association require Physical Therapy as a necessary part of the curriculum for the approval of chiropractic colleges by the National Association.

This resolution provoked a rather extensive discussion especially by the delegates from California. They, in defense of the resolution, maintain that if all of the accredited chiropractic colleges were forced to include a substantial course in physio therapy in their curricula it would serve to lend legal percentage and support to such states as California where the practice of chiropractic is broad in its inclusion of physio therapy. Dr. Martin then proceeded to read a letter as prepared by Dr. Duane M. Smith, the California NCA delegate. This letter proceeded to detail the reasons why this resolution should be passed. It made the assertion that the resolution at the Omaha convention had been opposed by the Lincoln College of Chiropractic and the Chiropractic Institute of New York, both colleges not teaching physio therapy. This assertion was, of course, immediately contested by all members of the Council and attention was drawn to the fact that at the Omaha meeting those representing the colleges that teach physio therapy as well as those representing the colleges that do not teach physio therapy vigorously opposed any coercion in this matter, and consequently denied the passage of the resolution and Dr. Martin was instructed to advise Dr. Smith of the same.

In his letter Dr. Smith stated that if the resolution as it was written could not be passed that the Council at least accept an alternate proposal, namely, that Dr. John J. Nugent be instructed to change the wording of his manual, "An Outline of a Standard Course in Chiropractic Education," as it relates to the subject of physio therapy be not considered an elective subject. Dr. Nugent expressed his opinion that this should be done and this suggestion was most agreeable to the entire Council and consequently the proper alterations were made and Dr. Martin was instructed to advise Dr. Smith of the same.

Resolution 3: Be It Resolved that the NCA adopt a policy for the professionally owned schools which are approved by the NCA Council on Education whereby the first year's dues of a graduate will be added to the tuition and scattered over the four years of instruction. These dues would, of course, be the junior membership dues, or one-half of the regular dues and would include membership in the NCA, and also cover the fee of the student membership. If for any reason the student did not complete the course, these monies would be refunded.

The Council was advised that this resolution had also been proposed by the California delegation at the annual meeting in Omaha. It was, however, the very frank and general opinion that it would be rather untoward to expect the colleges to make every student join the National Chiropractic Association by including this charge in his first year's tuition. The majority of the schoolmen maintained that a goodly percentage of the students coming into our colleges were referred to our institutions by non-NCA members and they felt that it would be an abuse of confidence and really an issue of coercion if all students, regardless of their attitude or inclinations, were made to comply with such a stipulation. Attention, however, was drawn to the fact that in all of the recognized colleges and also the provisionally accredited colleges Junior NCA chapters have been organized and the greater percentage of the student body are members of the same. At this time the opinion was expressed by all that the Executive Council of the NCA should have their attention drawn to the fact that very seldom did any member of the official NCA visit any of the colleges and take the opportunity of explaining to the student body the reasons why membership in the NCA is so imperative and to outline to the student groups what the NCA is doing in relation to our professional security and future, and consequently the following answer to the resolution was passed upon.

It was decided against any mandatory policy of inducing student membership in any organization or any dues-collecting arrangement by the colleges. The colleges invite the visits of members of the official family of the NCA with the view to stimulating the interest of the students in the organization and its aims.

Resolution 4: Be It Resolved that the Delaware Chiropractors' Association, Inc. recommends that the National Chiropractic Association, through its Committee on Educational Standards, change or enlarge the curricula of the schools it accredits so as to give the undergraduate student a comprehensive training in dynamic psychology. At least 200 hours of study should be devoted to this subject so that the graduate chiropractor shall have a greater understanding of mental health and mental disease, thus being more fully equipped to aid the sick, and to raise the prestige of our profession.

Be It Further Resolved that copies of this Resolution be sent to the Executive Board, to the Committee on Educational Standards, and to the Secretary of the National Chiropractic Association.

Dr. Herman Schwartz, a member of the Committee on Psychology, personally presented this resolution and in very friendly as well as considerate terms outlined the Committee's reasons why they felt this resolution should be passed. He gave to each member of the Council a prepared brief of these reasons and invited the Council to study the same carefully. In the discussions that followed everyone agreed that the study of abnormal psychology should represent a primary part of the various clinical courses that were presented. Furthermore everyone agreed that a substantial number of class hours be dedicated to the subject of abnormal psychology specifically. However, the Council was disinclined to commit itself to prescribe a definite 200 hour course to this subject fearing that it may represent an overload as far as the rest of the curricula was concerned. Recognition was made of the fact that in all clinical courses, and even in the subject of chiropractic principles, the realization that neurological medications penetrate the psychic field as well as the physical field should be taken cognizance of. In fact everyone agreed that any delineation between the mental and the physical ailments was somewhat of an obsolete and unfounded procedure. As a result of these discussions, and to the complete satisfaction of Dr. Schwartz, the following answer to the resolution was prepared and passed upon.

We heartily approve of the increased interest created by the Committee on Psychology for the study of abnormal psychology. We would encourage all colleges to consider the subject of abnormal psychology and its clinical application to the chiropractic premise as of major importance. It is to be strongly recommended that in all clinical studies the element of the mental and emotional influences, normal or abnormal, upon the health and the diseased states of the patient, be impressed upon the students' thinking. Consequently the necessity of stipulating a specific number of didactic class hours assigned to this subject is not considered advisable. Furthermore, we recognize the fact that further qualifications in this subject should be supported by additional study in the form of a specialty.

Resolution 5: The following proposal is made to the National Council on Educational Institutions. It is a fact that not enough interest has been taken in the new graduate doctor of chiropractic going out into the field to begin the practice of his profession. The first few years, in most instances, are tough years on the young doctor, as he often finds himself up against many obstacles he is not seasoned to cope with. Consequently, some give up the ship and fall by the wayside, and go back to their former vocations or work, and never start back in practice again, and perhaps a would-be chiropractor is lost. The young doctor starting out needs help and seasoned guidance.

The following plan is suggested to remedy such a condition as stated above. The colleges must formulate a follow-up plan for their students after graduation. Often an encouraging letter or a word of kindness and a genuine interest in the new doctor while he is struggling would mean the factor between failure and success. Also the college should try and place each graduate student for a one year time in the office of a successful older graduate practicing chiropractor. The older doctor would welcome the help afforded by the young doctor in the part of relieving him from overwork, and what a blessing for the young doctor. The personal training and correct approach of each personality in patients that the older doctor understands and will be glad to teach the young doctor would mean success in almost every case of the young doctor. After this one year training in the office of the practitioner, the college should issue a certificate of credit to the young doctor. We do hereby implore the colleges to adopt this proposal and plan and give it a trial. Such a plan cannot but bear fruit.

Every member of the Council fully approved of the good intent of this resolution but felt that the heterogeneous circumstances of practice that exist in the chiropractic profession today would not permit the chiropractic colleges to take advantage of the suggestions made by this resolution and in answer to the resolution, the following decision was passed upon. The colleges are in complete accord with the ideals expressed in this resolution but are of the opinion that they are unable to assume responsibility of sponsorship of this plan. It is recommended that the initiative be taken by the committee proposing this resolution in the preparation of master lists of chiropractors willing to cooperate in the plan and that such a list be furnished to each college. The colleges furthermore agree to cooperate wholeheartedly in this proposal.

Resolution 6: The proposal to establish a chair of chiropractic in the University of Denver. Preliminary steps have been taken in conferences by Drs. Nugent and Bishop. The matter is referred to the Council on Education for further action.

This resolution provoked a great deal of discussion and inquiry. Dr. Beatty of Denver, Colorado, was asked to speak upon the subject. He advised the group that probably greater clarification of the issue could be obtained if specific questions were asked of him and he would attempt to answer the same. Dr. James Firth asked the question, Is it true that Denver University is willing to sponsor a chair of chiropractic in one of its colleges? To this question Dr. Beatty answered by stating that the Denver University, within recent years, had established a policy under which it was willing to sponsor any profession or trade regardless of the nature of the same as long as it enjoyed proper recognition. Furthermore that this sponsorship was based upon two stipulations. One, that the college pertaining to this profession or trade be properly financed by the profession representing it. Two, that in the case of a chair of chiropractic the University would have to be assured of specific NCA and C.R.F. support.

Then Dr. Janse asked the question as to whether the subjects pertaining to chiropractic proper would be taught on the campus and within the buildings of Denver University proper. To this question Dr. Beatty answered that it was his opinion that they would not be but that the course would be only under the auspices of the Denver University and that the chiropractic subjects would either be taught in the buildings of the now existing Denver University of Natural Healing Arts or those of the Spears Sanatorium.

Then Dr. Budden asked the question as to whether the Council thought that having a chair of chiropractic in a state university would be of benefit to the chiropractic profession and furthermore whether such a situation would not cause the University of Denver to lose its rating with the North Central Committee on the Accrediting of Colleges and Universities. To this inquiry Dr. Nugent expressed the opinion that neither apprehension had basis. The attitude of Dr. Nugent, however, was rather vigorously opposed by all of the other schoolmen, the general consensus being that in all of this resided quite a severe danger that might result in the eventual subjugation of chiropractic education to the authority and dominance of not only the medical profession but also the hierarchy of academic standards of American education. In fact, following represents a brief resume of the individual opinions expressed.

Dr. Janse felt that the entire issue was somewhat nebulous and certainly indefinite in its aspects. He advised the group that he could not comprehend how Denver University could retain its rating by the North Central Association and still sponsor a chair or a college of chiropractic. Furthermore, it was his contention that if such a college were organized at the Denver University every member of that college faculty, whether they taught pre-clinical or clinical subjects, would have to possess an academic degree besides that of a Doctor of Chiropractic, if Denver University were to expect to retain its rating. This then, he maintained, would give us a chiropractic college all of whose faculty members possessed either Ph.D., M.S. or B.S. degrees. He voiced the apprehension that this was setting a precedence toward which the medical exponents could make reference in their legislative battles against us and which may force upon all of the other accredited colleges the same stipulations. Dr. Janse questioned whether any of the other colleges at the present time would be able to comply with such a regulation or would even want to because he felt that in many of our chiropractic colleges were men who, although they did not possess an academic degree, but as the result of the training that they received at their colleges and as a result of their personal efforts, possessed teaching capacities and an understanding of their subject matter that placed them in the category of being extraordinarily capable and he felt that it would represent an abuse to have to sacrifice men of this caliber. It was his conviction that those graduating from our accredited colleges, were men whose degrees in every respect, were comparable in knowledge and information possessed to any master of science degree that a person could have obtained from a state university. He asserted that we should strive for higher educational standards and better qualification among our faculty members on strength of our own attainments and educational procedures rather than to plagiarize the methods and efforts of others.

Dr. Firth seemed to be of the same opinion as Dr. Janse in many respects. He expressed the opinion that the venture was wrought with a certain amount of hazard and that he felt that great caution should be exercised along these lines. He informed the group that in his numerous contacts with the field he had experienced a rather reluctant attitude on the part of the average practitioner with reference to the idea of affiliating our chiropractic colleges with universities. He said that following were some of the inquiries that he had encountered.

First, if for example by virtue of the C.R.F. and NCA the University of Denver were to be granted a certain amount of money or buildings to maintain and house the proposed chiropractic college, what would happen to the same if for some reason or another Denver University were to decide that the venture was not worthwhile. Second, is it consistent with the maintenance of the individuality as well as autonomous legality of our profession to attempt to incorporate chiropractic education with orthodox professional education of various types? He expressed the opinion that the matter as yet appeared to be quite indefinite and consequently he felt that extensive deliberations should be made before any specific commitments are gone into.

Dr. Hendricks voiced the same opinion and expressed the idea that he was rather fearful that if such amalgamation were realized it would represent the possibility that our professional concepts, theories and methods would suffer and probably be overcome by the orthodoxy surrounding them.

Dr. Budden expressed the definite opinion that such an amalgamation would endanger the life and the integrity of chiropractic as an independent profession. Furthermore he expressed the opinion that we should not seek to emulate standard educational procedure or medical education for the sake of prestige and position alone but that the nature of our concepts and clinical procedures were such that our educational methods and approaches should be conditioned accordingly and that if we were to assume the orthodoxy completely it would be like fitting a round peg in a square hole. He severely criticized the idea that a man must possess an academic degree before he can represent a good educator in our chiropractic colleges. Furthermore he expressed the opinion that it would be grossly unfair and unjust to impose regulations and stipulations upon the faculty of a recognized chiropractic college that would compel them to obtain their academic degrees or discontinue their efforts. (It might be said that his opinion represented the consensus of attitude.)

Dr. Harring definitely supported the contentions of the various schoolmen.

Dr. Mueller drew the Council's attention to the fact that the homeopaths had ventured the same thing and resultantly they had lost their professional identity.

Dr. Martin voiced the opinion that nothing ventured, nothing gained, and consequently he felt that a chance should be taken.

Dr. Parr felt that great danger resided in the eventual outcome of the venture and advised that it should be sidestepped.

Dr. Nugent was then asked to give his frank opinion. He said that it was his conviction that all of the apprehensions and concerns expressed were ill founded. He believed that in no way would it represent a danger of eventual absorption by the medical profession, or orthodox education. Furthermore he expressed the conviction that probably here was an opportunity to set a precedence whereby greater professional recognition could be obtained and other universities be induced to do the same and he asked the question why shouldn't that be our ambition. He said that he felt that in no way would this represent a hazard or a competitive danger to the now existing chiropractic colleges and that he could not see how the fact that a university affiliated chiropractic college possessing a faculty of men with degrees only would inflict the same necessity upon the now existing chiropractic colleges. He also voiced the opinion that he could very readily stock such a college with a faculty of men with degrees exclusively, and yet who possessed chiropractic training. He maintained, however, that it was not his opinion or understanding that those teaching the clinical subjects of chiropractic at the proposed Denver University College of Chiropractic would have to possess an academic degree. He insisted that he would continue careful negotiation with Denver University and that if affiliations were feasible he would vigorously recommend such a move. He then proceeded to detail his conversations with the various representatives of Denver University. He advised the group that in the company of Drs. Ohlson and Bishop he met with Chancellor Gates of Denver University as well as the University Treasurer and legal counselor. He advised the Council that he informed these gentlemen that he would not favor a chair of chiropractic at the University but would definitely approve of a college of chiropractic. He narrated the fact that Chancellor Gates at this time spoke rather abundantly and acutely of his dislike for the monopoly that medicine had established. At this time Dr. Nugent was advised to consult with the Dean of Professional Colleges of the University, as well as to contact the President of the Board of Trustees to obtain their opinions as well as consent. In consulting with the Dean of Professional Colleges this gentleman told Dr. Nugent that all students entering this affiliated chiropractic college would have to have two years of pre-professional college work in the liberal arts, and then four years of chiropractic training. Dean Allen, however, proposed a plan to Nugent that would allow the chiropractic students to obtain these two years of liberal arts training concurrently with their chiropractic education and Dr. Nugent expressed the belief that this would be the desired and most advisable procedure.

Then Nugent advised the group that at this time Chancellor Gates had been replaced by Chancellor Price and he had been advised that the whole matter be dropped until the new Chancellor had been contacted. That represented the amount of work and the extent of contacts established up to the time of the Omaha convention. Since then Dr. Nugent advised not too much work had been done, although he had been advised by Drs. Ohlson and Bishop that Chancellor Price was favorably inclined and that they felt that negotiations could be continued. At this time Nugent advised the group that he felt that the venture should not be dropped, and that every sincere and conscientious effort should be made to investigate the situation further. He told the group that such were his intentions and he had been instructed by the Executive Board of the NCA to do so.

At this time Budden expressed the opinion that Dr. Nugent should be instructed not to continue any negotiations or to make any commitments that would involve the educational program of the NCA especially in relation to the Denver University situation without having fully advised the Educational Council of his intentions. This seemed to represent the general attitude that prevailed and consequently the following answer to the resolution was proposed.

Discussions of this resolution supplemented by reports given by Drs. Nugent and Beatty disclosed that specific action by the Council on Education at this time would be premature. However, the Council is against any commitments being made by the NCA or the Chiropractic Research Foundation in such negotiations relative to professional or pre-professional requirements without the consent of the Council. At this time Dr. Peterson expressed the opinion and suggestion that Dr. Janse be instructed to present the answers to the various resolutions and especially review the discussions with reference to the last one as pertaining to a college of chiropractic at the University of Denver with the Executive Council of the NCA that was meeting at the Stevens Hotel the following week.

NOTE: This is to inform the members of the Council that on Wednesday afternoon, Feb. 3rd, Dr. Janse was invited by the Executive Board to present the answers as well as the general attitudes and discussions of the Council on Education on the resolutions that had been referred to for consideration. Dr. John J. Nugent was present and he informed the Executive Council, as well as the Executive Secretary that Dr. Janse had given a proper and fair presentation of the Council's decisions with reference to the resolutions. It might also be mentioned that some discussion was made as to the Council's suggestions on the nature and type of educational programs that would most likely be most receptive to those attending the NCA convention in Portland this coming summer. This Dr. Janse did and it is gratifying to note that nearly all of the suggestions as elaborated by the Council were received and put into application.

On Sunday afternoon, January 25th, the majority of the members of the Council were the guests of the National College of Chiropractic at a luncheon. At the end of the same Dr. Peterson, in behalf of the Council, expressed his gratification at the fact that constructive work had been accomplished and also gave voice to the fact that all of the schoolmen present and members of the Council were sincerely and deeply appreciative of the fine work that Dr. John J. Nugent, Director of Education, was doing, and assured him of the full and frank support of the Council with reference to his future endeavors. The entire body stood in compliment to Dr. Nugent and in respect for his efforts.

Before the Council was dismissed to make an inspection of and a visit to the National College of Chiropractic several more discussions were gone into. In relation to the matter of audiometry, the following resolution by the Council was prepared. Namely, the Council was thoroughly in favor of the principles of audiometry, yet it feels that no special recognition should be extended to any special group sponsoring it. Furthermore, all articles and advertisements that might appear in the Journal with reference to audiometry be thoroughly screened for scientific exactness; that the issuance of a degree in consequence to having taken either a correspondence course or a course by special class training is disapproved of.

Dr. Peterson then announced that Dr. Weiant had been contacted by the Randon Foundation and requested that he supply them with specific answers to a goodly number of questions pertaining to chiropractic as a profession as well as a clinical procedure. It was the decision of the Council that many of the questions and their answers would require so much detailed work that certainly at the present time complete compliance with the request by the Randon Foundation would be impossible, but Dr. Weiant should be encouraged to maintain his connections with this Foundation and give them all of the data available.

Dr. Nugent then advised the Council that he had rearranged the wording of his manual on educational standards as they pertain to physic therapy. This correction was read for observation and all in attendance agreed that it was very proper and definitely in order. At this time Dr. Gardner asked the representatives of the schools that do not teach physio therapy to express the reasons why they did not include physio therapy in their curriculum. Dr. Peterson said that he, as a representative of the Chiropractic Institute of New York, could simply answer Dr. Gardner by stating that in New York the inclusion of physio therapy would involve them in legal difficulties that might eliminate the favorable circumstances they had built up. Furthermore it was their sincere conviction that the teaching of physio therapy robs from the importance of chiropractic and consequently they did not feel that they would want to sacrifice this importance for the sake of an adjunct.

Dr. Firth, in answer to Dr. Gardner's inquiry, said that they certainly at Lincoln College were not radicals and do not frown upon physio therapy. They have for a number of years, he maintained, sponsored the following definition of chiropractic. Chiropractic is the science of finding and removing nerve disturbances. He voiced the opinion that if, by means of physio therapy, this could be accomplished a little more readily he saw no reason why it shouldn't be used or taught by those who desire to do so. He informed the group that a number of years ago his institution conducted a survey and it was found that approximately 82% of the chiropractors used some form of physio therapy. However, when this 82% was asked whether they would advise that the Lincoln College put in physio therapy, 90% of them voiced the opinion that Lincoln should stay as it is - namely, a college that teaches no physio therapy.

At this time Dr. Nugent was called upon to give a report on the provisionally accredited colleges.

1) The Kansas State College of Chiropractic at Wichita, Kansas. According to Dr. Nugent this college did have a program of expansion. However this program was lagging to some degree because of lack of money and unified interest. He said that if no further progress had been made upon his next inspection of the college we will have to take the same from the provisionally accredited list.

2) The Northwestern College of Chiropractic at Minneapolis, Minnesota. With reference to this institution Dr. Nugent said that of recent date a goodly number of favorable discussions had been conducted with Dr. Wolfe, the president, and he felt that if certain deficiencies could be rectified full recognition could be afforded the institution within a reasonable time. At this point, Dr. J.B. Wolfe, the president of the Northwestern College, asked Dr. Nugent to be more explicit in pointing out to him and his associates just exactly what stipulations would have to be met before he could expect full recognition. He informed Dr. Nugent that the continuance of the Northwestern College was heavily contingent upon full approval and therefore he was very anxious that he be instructed specifically as to what he must do to acquire full approval. He felt that he should be given an opportunity to attain the status within a short time and if his institution could not fully conform with the stipulations he would then resign himself to the necessity of reconstructing his entire program.

3) The Denver University of the Natural Healing Sciences. At this point Dr. Homer C. Beatty asked for inspection and provisional approval and Dr. Nugent advised him that this inspection will be made within the near future.

4) The Missouri College of Chiropractic. Dr. H.C. Harring also advised the Council that he was seeking inspection and full

approval and the Council was advised by Dr. Nugent that a thorough inspection of this college would also be conducted as soon as possible.

5) The Carver College of Chiropractic. Dr. Paul Parr, the president of this institution, emphatically contended that he was in Chicago to obtain full approval for his institution. He maintained that since the last inspection by Dr. Nugent the college had improved to at least 200% and felt that on the basis of these improved conditions, including a new x-ray laboratory, visual education facilities, new school furniture, new clinical and chemical laboratory, added faculty, etc. full approval should be accorded him. At this time Dr. Peterson advised Dr. Parr that until the Council could grant his institution full approval Dr. Nugent, as the Director of Education, and the Committee on Accrediting of Colleges must present to the Council their decisions and suggestions in relation to approval or disapproval. For that reason it was the opinion of the Council that especially in the case of the Northwestern College of Chiropractic and the Carver College of Chiropractic Dr. Nugent should, between now and the Portland convention, make a full and thorough inspection of these colleges, and that he and the Committee on the Accrediting of Colleges should come to a definite decision which was to be relayed to the Council before or at the time of the Portland convention so that these institutions at that time would know just exactly where they stand.

Minutes of the COUNCIL ON EDUCATION
The sessions were held in conjunction with the National Chiropractic Association's Convention held in Portland, Oregon, June 18 to July 3, 1948, Dr. Thure C. Peterson, President of the Council, presiding.

The first session of the Council meetings were held the morning of June 28th. Those present included:

(A) Members of the Committee on Educational Standards
   Dr. John J. Nugent
   Dr. Edward H. Gardner
   Dr. Justin C. Wood
   Dr. Walter B. Wolf
   Dr. T.J. Boner

(B) Members of the Committee on Educational Institutions
   Dr. W.A. Budden, President, Western States College of Chiropractic
   Dr. Arthur Hendricks, Vice President, Lincoln College of Chiropractic
   Dr. Thure C. Peterson, Administrator, Chiropractic Institute of New York
   Dr. Raymond Houser, Dean, Los Angeles College of Chiropractic
   Dr. Ralph J. Martin, President of the Board of Directors of the Los Angeles College of Chiropractic
   Dr. Lee H. Norcross, Dean of the Graduate School of the Los Angeles College of Chiropractic
   Dr. John B. Wolfe, President, Northwestern College of Chiropractic
   Dr. Paul O. Parr, President, Carver College of Chiropractic
   Dr. Homer C. Beatty, President, University of Natural Healing Arts
   Dr. Joseph Janse, President, National College of Chiropractic

(C) As a special guest, Mr. C.P. Von Herzen, special attorney of the California Chiropractic Association, was present at several of the sessions.

Dr. Peterson, as the presiding officer of the Council, drew the attention of those present to the fact that the schools were now confronted with the possible problem of losing students as the result of the draft. A motion was made that special recommendations be made to Dr. Emmett J. Murphy, national legislative representative, to attempt to attain proper consideration in behalf of our chiropractic students, at least to the degree of obtaining deferments until the school year is completed. This motion was seconded, and Dr. Janse, as Secretary of the Council, was instructed to write a formal letter to Dr. Murphy to this effect.

Dr. Peterson then drew attention to his belief that in certain respects the Connecticut Basic Science Board was somewhat inordinate and unfair in the manner in which it conducted its examination, the nature of the questions that were asked, and also the fact that the applicant had to divulge the school of practice he graduated from in order to qualify for the examination. He made the suggestion that an effort be made to have applicants for the Connecticut Basic Science Board gather to form a special preparatory course for several weeks or months before the examination. His ideas were heartily approved of by the remainder of the Council and the suggestion was made that this matter be looked into very carefully, and if such a program could be organized every conscientious cooperation should be made.

Dr. Peterson was then asked to make a report on the conference that he and Dr. Nugent held with Dr. Vinton Logan in New York this past winter in relation to the probability of rendering recognition to the Logan Basic College of Chiropractic.

(1) Dr. Peterson stated that a more complete report of his and Dr. Nugent's conference would be made when the report of the Accrediting Committee was submitted but did make the general statement that Dr. Logan's attitude was rather adamant and

somewhat hypercritical of the National Chiropractic Association and of the National Council on Education.

(2) Dr. Parr said that he felt that if Dr. Logan and his associates desire to fully cooperate with the NCA program and become a part of the Council membership he should make a personal appearance at the Council meetings and thrash the issue out across the Council table. He said that he had had a number of personal conversations with Dr. Logan and that Logan had expressed certain criticisms of the Accrediting Committee, as well as the Council on Education.

(3) Dr. Budden voiced the opinion that Dr. Logan and his associates should not necessarily demand any special considerations or treatment and if they desire to become an integral part of the NCA and the Council they would have to abide by the same formalities of good will and friendly intention as the rest of the members.

(4) Dr. Hendricks said that he disapproved of the attitude of superiority sustained by these people in their relation to the NCA and the Council.

(5) Dr. Beatty voiced his similar opinion.

(6) Dr. Janse expressed the opinion that the Logan people should be expected to make the same concessions and comply with the same stipulations as the rest of the members of the Council.

At this time Dr. Budden drew the Council's attention to the fact that the Executive Board as yet did not fully understand and realize that the Council on Education should and does represent the final voice of decision in all educational affairs of the NCA

(1) Dr. Peterson elaborated further by stating that it was his opinion that Dr. Nugent, although the Director of Education, is subject to the decisions and authority of the Council, and that his investigations, decisions, and commitments should always be subject to the final approval of the Council.

(2) Dr. Parr voiced a similar opinion and stated that he felt that both the NCA Executive Council, as well as Dr. Nugent, should be specifically instructed accordingly.

Next Dr. Budden drew the Council's attention to the situation that had arisen in Nevada. Two graduates of the Western States Chiropractic College and two graduates of the Los Angeles College of Chiropractic had taken the Nevada State Chiropractic Board, at which time these four people were advised by the members of the Board that their Nevada licenses would be withheld because they were considered incompetent technicians, and that it was recommended that they take postgraduate work, preferably at the Palmer School of Chiropractic.

(1) Various members of the Council voiced their frank disapproval of such prejudiced and discriminatory conduct and it was concluded that Dr. Nugent should be instructed to immediately investigate this situation and to establish a correction of this discrepancy.

Dr. Hendricks drew the Council's attention to a rather pertinent problem affecting the chiropractic graduate primarily from a financial standpoint. He said that as the result of the fact that a goodly number of chiropractic boards only held their examination once or twice a year, it happened quite frequently that a young graduate having about a month or so left to go before completing his resident work would make application to take the examination on the stipulation that if he passed his license would be withheld until he had finished his school work and obtained his diploma. In some instances, Dr. Hendricks asserted, this request was complied with. In others it was denied and as a result the graduate would have to wait anywhere from six to ten or more months after the time he graduated until the next meeting of the examining board, and consequently impose on him an inconvenience of loss of time as well as an interim during which he could not proceed to establish himself and develop an income.

(1) It was then made a resolution that the Secretary of the Council be instructed to write the various Chiropractic State Boards and acquaint them with this circumstance, and to obtain their conscientious cooperation in solving this problem.

Dr. Janse stated that an effort would be made on the part of the various college administrations to be more exacting in their initial orientation of the incoming student as to what states he, upon graduation, would qualify for. Dr. Janse gave as an example the state of Pennsylvania, which demands that the chiropractic matriculant possess one year's college training in physics, chemistry, and biology. Yet, he maintained, that it had happened that Pennsylvania students had been accepted for enrollment who did not possess these pre-professional qualifications and who had not been advised of this necessity.

Every schoolman present fully agreed with this suggestion and committed himself to the assumption of this responsibility.

The second session of the Council convened in the afternoon of Monday, June 28th. Dr. Thure C. Peterson, President of the Council presided. At this time he reiterated the purpose and functions of the Council, stating that the intra-mural set-up within the Council between the Committee on Educational Standards on the one hand and the Committee on Educational Institutions on the other, could and should work toward the benefit of all concerned. He expressed the keen desire that members of both committees fully realize their responsibilities to the Council and the profession as a whole. He expressed his appreciation for the cooperation experienced in the past year and voiced the confidence that the Council would progress to the point where it would represent a dynamic agent for good and progress in the profession.

Dr. Peterson then called upon Dr. E.H. Gardner, President of the Committee on Educational Standards to make his report. In substance the following items were the ones emphasized by Dr. Gardner in his report.

(1) Essentially no marked changes in the status of any of the various colleges of chiropractic had taken place.

(2) He acknowledged the fine and thorough work done by Dr. John J. Nugent, the NCA Director of Education, and a member of his Committee.

(3) He stated that he had been authorized by his Committee to report the following in relation to the various colleges that had been

under the surveillance:

(a) Los Angeles College of Chiropractic, Full status of approval

(b) Lincoln College of Chiropractic, Full status of approval

(c) Western States College of Chiropractic, Full status of approval

(d) Chiropractic Institute of New York, Full status of approval

(e) Canadian Memorial College of Chiropractic, Full status of approval.

(f) National College of Chiropractic, Full status of approval

(4) Dr. Nugent at the present time along with the Committee were making a careful survey of the situation in relation to the Oakland College of Chiropractic.

(5) The Kansas State College of Chiropractic was in a rather difficult situation and the opinion in general was that it would take some time before it would even come near to portraying qualifications that would merit approval.

(6) The University of Natural Healing essentially was in the same position that it was a year ago and consequently its rating being status quo.

(7) Missouri College of Chiropractic, very little changes had taken place, and consequently remained in rating status quo.

(8) Carver College of Chiropractic, noticeable improvements had been made yet the committee felt that full approval would have to be withheld until additional progress had been made and resultantly felt that its rating should be as yet status quo.

At this point it was moved and seconded that the report of the Committee on Educational Standards as given by Dr. Gardner be accepted and approved.

Dr. Peterson was then called on to make a complete report of his and Dr. Nugent's meeting with Dr. Vinton Logan with reference to the approval of the Logan Basic College of Chiropractic. Following is a brief of Dr. Peterson's report along with the discussions and comments that ensued.

(1) Dr. Peterson stated that he had, according to the instructions received at the meeting in Chicago, talked with Dr. Logan about the possible approval of the Logan College, contingent on the stipulations laid down by the Council at its meetings in Chicago. Dr. Logan, informed by Dr. Peterson, was quite reluctant to accept the stipulations and felt that he should not be expected to accept them and comply with them in order to obtain approval. He promised, however, to take the matter up with his board of directors.

(2) At this time Dr. John Nugent advised the Council that he had spent almost a week at the Logan College and had had many a meeting with Dr. Logan as well as Dr. Coggins, the Dean of the college, and also Dr. Fern Logan, who represented the college at the Chicago meeting.

According to Dr. Nugent, he was advised by Dr. Vinton Logan that he and the board of directors of the college had decided that at the present at least they did not desire to continue their efforts to obtain NCA recognition. Furthermore, Dr. Logan expressed the belief that he had been rather unfairly dealt with and that he had never practiced commercialism or separatism.

Dr. Nugent expressed the conviction that as yet Dr. Logan was still inclined to be rather hypercritical of the Council, certain of its members as well as the NCA in general. In fact, Dr. Nugent stated that Dr. Logan's attitudes in many respects were quite derogatory of both the Council and the NCA. Dr. Logan had said, that if he and the Logan College came into the NCA it would be on his own terms, and that he was not at all convinced of the sincerity of the Council's personnel and NCA program.

(3) Dr. Gardner then asked to be heard. He expressed his personal conviction that the Council had mishandled the Logan situation. He stated that he felt that the Logan people had been caused much undue chagrin and reason to question the tolerance of the Council.

Dr. Gardner asserted that the first mistake was made when the Council in Chicago invited the Logan representatives to sit in on the discussions pertaining to the Logan college as well as certain ethical elements that pertained to their method of post-graduate work, etc.

The second error, according to Dr. Gardner was made by the Council when it failed to honor the recommendation of the Committee on Educational Standards as made in Chicago relative to the Logan College.

Dr. Peterson pointed out that Dr. Gardner was in error in this point inasmuch as the Committee on Educational Standards did not recommend the approval of the Logan School either before or after the meeting with the Accrediting Committee and that they were unanimous in this matter.

It was Dr. Gardner's belief that much irreparable harm had been done. Why should the members of the Council in any way feel that they have the right to sit in judgment over any other school? Dr. Gardner felt very definitely that there should be a reconsideration of the Logan College case and a full approval status granted without delay.

(4) At this point both Drs. Peterson and Budden expressed their opinions that the members of the Council had been just and fair in their considerations of the Logan College and its representatives.

(5) Dr. T.J. Boner then asked Dr. Gardner why he maintained such attitudes in contrast to the other members of the Council. Dr. Gardner answered by saying that at the beginning Dr. Logan was willing to go along with the program of the Council and that the Council was in the position to carefully mold the attitudes of Dr. Logan in the direction that would be in conformity with the NCA program.

(6) Dr. Justin Wood expressed the belief that according to his observations the Council had offered Dr. Logan and his associates every consideration and just opportunity to affiliate themselves with the Council. Therefore, any future action in relation to this matter should originate within the desires of the Logan group.

(7) At this time Dr. Nugent injected the statement that at the time of the Chicago meeting, the Committee on educational Standards had met with the Logan representatives in private and at which time the complaints of the school men in relation to certain ethical factors aired and at which time Dr. Fern Logan especially had expressed herself as agreeing with the fact that these complaints were not unfounded but that there was a definite willingness to eventually rectify the factors that provoked them.

Dr. Nugent further stated that both in New York and St. Louis he had found Dr. Vinton Logan very inflexible and resistive to any attempt to establish an understanding.

(8) Dr. Peterson then voiced the assertion that at the beginning everyone of the now approved colleges had to correct certain discrepancies and be subject to a period of probation, consequently he could not see why Dr. Logan was so adamant to the proper requests made of him and the Logan College.

(9) Dr. Janse stated that he realized that at the Chicago meeting he had been rather determined in raising the question about the ethical elements in the Logan question, but, continued Dr. Janse, why should Dr. Logan feel that he has been unduly criticized?

(10) Dr. Hendricks called the Council's attention to his belief that the various members of the Council were over-emphasizing this matter of the Logan case. He stated that both in the Chicago meetings and the present meetings in Portland nothing had been said or done that should cause Dr. Logan to feel that his feelings had been abused. Dr. Hendricks then expressed the belief that in his opinion Dr. Logan as yet had not fully decided whether he and the Logan College actually wanted approval and NCA recognition. Certainly, according to Dr. Hendricks the Council should not be called on to beg Dr. Logan to come in. After all, to be accredited by the NCA should represent a distinction for which we should all be willing to work and make sacrifices.

(11) Dr. Nugent expressed the fact that he fully agreed with what Dr. Hendricks had said. Dr. Logan, stated Dr. Nugent, does not want it as a matter of record that he or any of his associates have ever solicited NCA recognition, therefore it might be better if we waited until Dr. Logan expressed the full desire to participate in the Council's program.

(12) After a few further but rather irrelevant discussions Dr. Peterson announced that the Logan matter was closed until further developments and decisions. He, however, drew all the members' attention to the fact that every member of both committees that constituted the Council were beholden to the Council and not just simply to their respective committee.

At this instance Dr. Boner asked the question as to what the functions of the Committee on Educational Standards are. To this question Dr. Peterson stated that it was the duty of the committee to work within the authority of the Council; that the committee was to inspect and investigate the various chiropractic colleges that sought NCA recognition, to draw up decisions of approval or non-approval, which were however, subject to the final vote of acceptance or rejection of the Council in its entirety.

Dr. Justin Wood then asked whether he correctly understood what the functioning of his committee should be, namely, to work as an accrediting agency, but that the final decision as to their conclusions rested fully upon the majority of vote of the Council. He was informed by Dr. Peterson that such were the facts of the matter.

Dr. Nugent proceeded to express his conviction that in all of their deliberations the members of the Council should not be too ready to carry the news of the same unto other persons outside of the Council. He said that it was his opinion that in the past this had been done too freely, and consequently some undue comment and criticism had evolved.

Dr. Peterson was then instructed to contact the Executive Board of the NCA and explain to them in full the exact relationship of the Council on Education to the Executive Board and vice versa, and to let them know that all matters pertaining to education and chiropractic colleges should reside in the prerogatives of the Council and should be referred to the Council for proper deliberation. This decision met with the unanimous approval of the entire Council membership.

Dr. Budden then suggested that hereafter the names of all the proponents of motions as well as those that seconded the motions not be listed along with the motions. This is recommended, he stated, so as not to make it appear that any eventual decision by the Council would represent the pet idea or peeve of any single member, but the consummate decision of the Council proper. All members of the Council approved of this suggestion, other than Dr. Gardner who refrained from voting.

Dr. Parr, as Dean of the Carver College of Chiropractic, asked for the opportunity to express his opinion in relation to the committee's report on the status of the Carver College. He stated that he felt that this institution should have received full approval by now, and that over the last year much progress had been made, and certainly the spirit and attitude of cooperation at the Carver College in relation to the NCA program was to be recognized and considered. As a result of his contentions the following discussion ensued.

(1) Dr. Peterson asked Dr. Parr if he would outline what improvements had been made at the Carver College since the Chicago meeting.

(2 In answer to this question, Dr. Parr listed the following points:

    (a) Addition of several faculty members

    (b) The redecorating of some of the college classrooms

    (c) The organization and establishment of a Carver College Alumni Association which, under the supervision of the C.R.F., represented a potential college revenue by virtue of endowments.

    (d) The procuring of certain physical aids in instruction, such as projectors, charts, etc.

(3) Dr. Nugent said that he would like to set forth his reasons why he and the Committee on Educational Standards could not as yet recommend full accreditation for the Carver College.

    (a) We have just refrained from granting the Logan College recognition, not because of deficiency in its physical plant because certainly this institution has every available physical means to represent a good school, but because of certain principles of ethics that are involved in the circumstance.

(b)   The Carver College, on the other hand, certainly expresses the right intentions and displays the proper attitude, but as yet its physical plant is not up to the standards. Certainly it would represent biased conduct on the part of the Council to play favorites.

(c)   Dr. Nugent complimented Dr. Parr on the progress that he had effected at the Carver College, but feels that as yet this progress hasn't reached the degree to realize full recognition, and he encouraged Dr. Parr to continue his efforts and assured him that as soon as they would realize the accomplishment of certain rather acute needs at the Carver College full recognition would be forthcoming.

(d)   Dr. Nugent said that he and his committee had investigated the Carver College situation and had encouraged the Oklahoma Chiropractic Association to allow their public relations man, Mr. Kueffer, to spend six months organizing a Carver College Alumni Association, and by support of Mr. MacGruder and the C.R.F. concentrated attempts be made to obtain professional support of this institution. This Kueffer-MacGruder program was to be formally instituted this coming October and there are reasons to believe that it will be very successful.

(4)   Dr. Parr asserted that he was aware of the good intentions and the attitude of the Council in relation to the Carver College, but expressed the idea that the NCA as well as the C.R.F., might be a little more conscientious and determined in rendering institutions like the Carver College more substantial and organized support so that these institutions could maintain themselves with self respect and enjoy the recognition they deserve.

(5)   In answer to this, Dr. Nugent said that if the proposed Kueffer and MacGruder program can be realized sufficient and proper help would be forthcoming.

(6)   Dr. Parr expressed the hope that such would be the case and insisted that greater consideration be afforded those institutions that have, over the years, made an effort to fully sustain the NCA program.

At this point a motion was made that the meeting be adjourned until the following afternoon. This was seconded and approved unanimously.

The third session of the Council on Education convened Tuesday afternoon, July 29th, with Dr. Thure C. Peterson presiding.

Dr. Peterson asked to have the privilege of reporting on his meeting with the Executive Board.

(1)   He informed the members of the Council that the Executive Board had agreed to instruct Dr. Emmet J. Murphy to extend every effort possible to induce federal agencies to render a favorable decision in the case of chiropractic students who are eligible for the draft.

(2)   Dr. Peterson also advised the members of the Council that he had advised the Executive Board as to just exactly what the position of the Council on Education is in relation to the Board. He said that the Board had told him that inasmuch as the Committee on Educational Standards was appointed by the Executive Board they felt that this committee is obligated to report its actions and decisions to the house of delegates, at which Dr. Peterson made the request that the Council on Education be privileged to scrutinize this report before it is presented to the house of delegates, and this request was granted.

Dr. Janse at this point, drew the attention of the members of the Council to the fact that he had received a request from the National Council of Chiropractic Examining Boards through Dr. Guy Smith, its vice president, that a closer cooperation be established between the Council on Education and the Council of Chiropractic Examining Boards. Dr. Janse stated that in conversation with several of the members of the Council of Chiropractic Examining Boards he experienced a genuine desire on their part to receive various suggestions from the Council on Education with reference to the problems of the chiropractic graduate in relation to the various chiropractic boards.

(1)   Dr. Janse was instructed by the Council to write the executive members of the National Council of Chiropractic Examining Boards and ask them for the privilege of having a joint session during the NCA convention next year.

(2)   Dr. Janse was then asked to give a report on his visit to the meetings of the National Society on Basic Science Boards that had been held in Chicago the previous winter. Dr. Janse advised the members of the Council that he had been well received by the various representatives of the basic science boards and that they had indicated their desire to next year, when the National Society on Basic Science Boards again meets in Chicago, have the chiropractic profession represented.

(a)   Resultantly, Dr. Janse was instructed, with full approval of the Council, to establish contact with the officers of this National Society of Basic Science Boards and solicit the permission to participate in their meetings this coming February in Chicago.

Dr. Walter Wolf made mention of the fact that an attempt was being made by the National Council of Chiropractic Examining Boards to establish a National Board of Chiropractic Examiners, and that this board would definitely include a basic science section in its composition.

The various members of the Council all expressed their approval of such a National Board of Chiropractic Examiners, but also voiced the opinion that it would be some years before such could be accomplished because of the heterogeneous nature of the various chiropractic boards and their individual requirements.

At this point the Carver College situation was reopened for discussion and the following deliberations and comments resulted.

(1)   Dr. Parr insisted that the Carver College situation was an emergency and that the NCA as well as the C.R.F. should certainly

clarify the program in the southwest, or else they were going to lose out.

(2) Dr. Nugent asserted that the validity of full recognition cannot be abused by granting full recognition on good intentions only, and contended that before Carver College could receive full recognition certain definite stipulations would have to be complied with.

    (a) An increase in qualified faculty members.

    (b) Definite improvement of the buildings.

    (c) Definite improvement of a college clinic and its facilities.

    (d) Definite increase in teaching equipment and classroom facilities.

(3) Dr. Janse at this point encouraged Dr. Parr to be patient and to continue his laudable efforts and assured him that the Council in general was very sympathetic toward the Carver College and its problem. He stated that in conversation with a number of prominent Carver Alumni he found that there was the attitude that the Carver College at the present time could not justify full recognition and that they would much rather see their alma mater continue its reconstructive efforts and eventually, within the next year or so, obtain recognition because of actually having qualified.

    (a)   The other members of the Council expressed similar attitudes and Dr. Parr said that he, in no way, would be adamant to these suggestions.

(4) Dr. Parr then asked Dr. Nugent whether the Kansas State College still possessed provisional recognition.

    (a)   Dr. Nugent answered by stating that the Kansas State College had received provisional approval for two years, that these two years were nearly up, and consequently he would have to make another survey of the institution and see whether during this probational period sufficient progress had been made to warrant continuation of this provisional rating.

(5) Dr. Parr encouraged the Council to make an effort to induce the C.R.F. and the NCA to make a more conscientious effort to obtain the cooperation and the understanding of the southwest states, especially Kansas, because, he maintained, the general attitude of the chiropractors in Kansas towards these organizations is one of hesitancy and consequently, inasmuch as he represents a southwest college, it is a detriment to his efforts to comply with an NCA program.

(6) In final summation of the original report by Dr. Gardner as president of the Committee on Educational Standards, it was moved and seconded that this report be accepted by the Council. All the members of the Council voted in the affirmative other than Dr. Parr.

Dr. Budden then asked Dr. Peterson, as President of the Council on Education, and Dr. Nugent as the Director of Education, as to whether or not any definite plans had been elaborated for the purpose of properly spacing as well as limiting chiropractic colleges from a geographical standpoint. In answer to this inquiry, the following comments and discussions were made.

(1) Dr. Nugent informed Dr. Budden that up to date no such plans had been effected. He said, however, that he was sympathetic to this necessity, as he realized that it would be unsatisfactory to have too many chiropractic colleges in one or another section of the country. Consequently, he expressed the idea that eventually there should be an amalgamation of the St. Louis Colleges and also probably an amalgamation between the colleges in Oklahoma and Kansas.

(2) Dr. Budden said that in his opinion a very careful territorial scrutiny should be made and an arrangement effected that would limit the aggregation of chiropractic colleges in sections of the country. The reason, he said, for this conviction of his was founded on the fact that eventually after the G.I. program runs out competition will again become very keen and if there are too many chiropractic colleges cluttered throughout the country all higher educational standards and ethical premises will be dissipated. He further suggested that there should only be one or two colleges in California.

(3) To this comment Dr. Nugent said that it was his desire to liquidate the two small, inadequate colleges in Oakland, California, and to send the prospects of that area to other chiropractic colleges. He suggested that this process of liquidation could take place right after the present crop of students in these colleges have been graduated.

(4) Dr. Martin advised the Council that the California Chiropractic Association had made the recommendation that these colleges in Oakland be closed up, and that the students be transferred to the Los Angeles College of Chiropractic for the completion of their work, or any other accredited college of their choice.

(5) Dr. Janse emphasized the necessity of allowing these students to very definitely decide as to what school they would like to be transferred.

(6) Dr. Nugent then asked the question as to what schools, in the opinion of the council, should be eliminated, and the following institutions were named.

    (a) The Ross-O'Neil College in Ft. Wayne

    (b) The Bebout College in Indianapolis

    (c) The Brooklyn College in Brooklyn

    (d) The Ratledge College in Los Angeles.

(7) In consequence to the above discussions a recommendation was made and seconded that a committee be appointed to make a careful survey of the geographical centers of population and industry that would be conducive to the full development and sustaining of accredited chiropractic institutions.

    (a)   A further motion was made and seconded that the Committee on Educational Standards be appointed to make this survey.

Dr. John Nugent then drew the Council's attention to several letters that he had received from representatives of the student bodies of some of the leading NCA recognized chiropractic colleges. The general content of those letters represented a request on the part of the student bodies to be given the permission and authority to have representative participation in the NCA house of delegates' meetings, as well as in the program of the Council on Education especially. The following discussions resulted.

(1) Dr. Hendricks said that these requests were commendable but advised the Council to be rather careful in granting any immediate concessions for the simple reason that student movements, although enthusiastic and genuine in their content were at times somewhat immature and could lead to some misunderstanding.

(2) Dr. Hendricks views were at least in part supported by Drs. Peterson, Budden, Parr, and Janse.

(3) Dr. Nugent said, however, that he felt that sooner or later the student populace of chiropractic would have to be granted greater opportunity for expressing their needs and their opinions.

(4) Attention was then drawn to the fact that in all of the accredited colleges the Junior NCA was in full organization, and that this might serve very readily as that avenue for student expression.

(5) Dr. Janse advised Dr. Nugent that in his opinion the entire official NCA family might be a little more diligent in paying visits to the accredited colleges with the intent of presenting the NCA program to the student body.

Dr. Janse then suggested that both the NCA, as well as the Council on Education, assume a more offensive attitude toward the protection of the chiropractic status and laws, and he cited the adverse circumstances that had arisen in Georgia as an example. To these comments the suggestion was made by Dr. Peterson that the representatives from Georgia, namely Drs. Livingstone and Brown, be invited to attend the next session of the Council to explain the Georgia predicament.

At this time the Council was recessed until the following afternoon.

The final meeting of the Council was held in the afternoon of Thursday, July 1st, with Dr. Thure C. Peterson presiding. Dr. Peterson, in the meantime, had contracted Drs. Livingstone and Brown, both members of the Georgia Board of Chiropractic Examiners, and resultantly these gentlemen were present at the beginning of the meeting.

In relation to the Georgia situation, the following comments and discussions ensued.

(1) Dr. Livingstone advised the Council that up until several months ago the Georgia Board of Chiropractic Examiners had only recognized and accepted the applications of graduates from chiropractic colleges who taught a course of four years of nine months each. Then, however, two of the outstanding Palmer practitioners in the state whose sons had just graduated with 18 months education from the Palmer School of Chiropractic, had approached the Board, as well as the Attorney General, and said that nowhere in the Georgia chiropractic law was mention made that a college year must be nine months. Consequently, they insisted that any college year of any tenure or duration, whether four months or nine months, must be recognized. Furthermore, they maintained that before 1939 when the law was enacted there wasn't a chiropractic college exclusively teaching a course of four years of nine months each. Consequently, how could the Board insist upon a graduate having four years of nine months education as based upon the authority of the law when the law was written at the time this circumstance did not even exist.

Furthermore, according to Dr. Livingstone, these two Palmer graduates insisted that if the Board did not grant their sons the privilege of taking the examination and obtaining their licenses, they would create such an antagonism against the use of physio-therapy by chiropractors that the Attorney General would be forced to compel all chiropractors to desist from using physio-therapy. Dr. Livingston, at this time, said that he was the only member of the Board at that time who resisted this pressure effort and that all the other members of the Board, including Dr. Brown, an NCA member and former NCA delegate from Georgia, succumbed to the pressure thus made.

(2) Dr. Brown said that his position was not an arbitrary one but it represented an attempt on his part to pacify a belligerence that might have resulted in a great deal of harm. He said that he recognized that a rather undue concession had been made to these Palmer men but that as soon as the pressure would ease off he would be willing to try and bring the standards up to their original level.

(3) To the comments of Dr. Brown, Dr. Nugent asked the question as to what side of the fence Dr. Brown was on. He wanted to know of Dr. Brown whether he realized that he had broken faith with the NCA educational program.

(4) Dr. Peterson advised Dr. Brown that as a result of this breach a very detrimental precedence had been set which may serve as the incentive for the eighteen-month proponents throughout the country.

(5) Dr. Hendricks commented that in his opinion the straight and mixer issue was but the ostensible premise for the fight; that the real cause resided, of course, in the determination to reduce the educational standards throughout the country to comply with the 18-month circumstance.

(6) Dr. Livingston reiterated the fact that he especially had been severely attacked and told that they would break him if he did not relent, and he reaffirmed his determination to resist to the end. He further advised the Council that of the five members of the Board, three were NCA members, yet they allowed this apostatizing of the NCA program to take place.

(7) Dr. Janse advised Dr. Brown that as the result of this happening the entire NCA program of higher educational standards had been compromised and if such conduct were continued the program would become futile.

(8) Dr. Hendricks said that in his opinion the concessions made by the four members of the Board as against the resistance of Dr. Livingstone represented a conduct of convenience to avoid any local trouble or pressure. He advised the Council that the 18-month element was making a supreme effort to reduce the educational standards throughout the country. He said that all 18-month schools were under terrific student pressure, and in order to appease the students efforts of this type were being made.

(9) Dr. Janse then suggested that Dr. Nugent be instructed to meet with the Georgia Board of Chiropractic Examiners as soon as possible and advise them of the jeopardy they have created, and if possible to contact the Attorney General and also advise him of what his decision has done in destroying the conscientious efforts of higher educational standards as conducted by the National Chiropractic Association.

(10) Both Drs. Brown and Livingstone consented to do all within their power to change the Board's ruling in this matter so that it would not be necessary for the Council to take action. They were told that in the event they were unsuccessful, the Council would definitely act in this matter.

At this point both Doctors Brown and Livingstone were excused and any further discussions discontinued.

Doctors Herman Schwartz and Francis I Regardie, representing the Committee on Psychology, asked for the opportunity of presenting to the Council on Education the prepared syllabus on a proposed course in psychology to serve as the guide for instruction in this subject in all of the approved schools. The Council was advised that the syllabus had been prepared by Dr. Herman Schwartz and had been approved by the Committee on Psychology.

(1) Dr. Regardie stated that it was indeed a very fine bit of work and consequently would like to recommend its approval by the Council.

(2) Dr. Schwartz said that he had worked hard on the syllabus, that in no way did he want it to represent a dictum of procedure but merely an outline to go by.

(3) Dr. Budden advised the Council that he was in favor of it because it represented another literary effort on the part of one in our own profession. He stated that he had been advised that as the result of the Baruch investigation the medical profession is going to try and prove that chiropractic is a branch of medicine because according to these investigators the majority of textbooks used in the chiropractic colleges are medical texts.

(4) Dr. Janse heartily recommended the acceptance of the syllabus as a guide but not as a mandatory outline to be followed in every aspect. He expressed deep admiration for the sincerity and efforts of Dr. Schwartz.

(5) Dr. Peterson advised the Council that the syllabus was prepared with the intention of representing a guide for the first semester of a proposed two-semester course and that if we approve of this first syllabus Dr. Schwartz will be willing to proceed with the preparation of a second syllabus for the second semester of work on the subject of psychology.

(6) Dr. Nugent complimented Dr. Schwartz on his work and advised the Council that every encouragement possible should be afforded Dr. Schwartz.

(7) It was then unanimously decided by the Council that Dr. Schwartz submit a typewritten copy of the syllabus to Dr. Janse, the Secretary of the Council, and have him arrange for the mimeographing of sufficient copies for each member of the Council, and that at the time the Minutes of the meetings are sent out a copy of the syllabus is to be included.

At this point it was unanimously decided that the mid-year meeting is again to be held in Chicago. No specific date was set because the decision was reached that the meeting should be held concomitant with or immediately before the meeting of the Executive Board, also to be held in Chicago. Dr. Peterson suggested that this time the meeting be of four days duration for the purpose of discussing a goodly number of the academic and scholastic problems of the accredited schools. This suggestion was made and approved of that the same arrangements as last year be put into effect, namely, that each accredited college as well as provisionally accredited college send a representative, and that the traveling expenses of all concerned shall be pro-rated and thus equally divide the expenses among the schoolmen.

Dr. Ralph J. Martin, President of the Board of Directors of the Los Angeles College of Chiropractic, then asked for the time and opportunity to present to the Council the program as effected by the California Chiropractic Association, in collaboration with the Administration of the Los Angeles College of Chiropractic, as it pertains to the establishment of a graduate school and specialty rating program. In consequence to this request, the following points and discussions ensued.

(1) Dr. Martin stated that this matter was brought to the Council on Education because it was the opinion of the California representatives that sooner or later all of the chiropractic colleges would have to enter into a similar program. Furthermore, he voiced the opinion that by virtue of such a program the educational efforts of Dr. Nugent and the legislative efforts of Dr. Murphy would be greatly supported and enhanced.

(2) At this point Dr. Lee H. Norcross, Dean of the Los Angeles College of Chiropractic Graduate School, was asked to detail his report. Dr. Norcross occupied approximately half an hour in the presentation of his report and covered so many important details pertaining to this program that it was decided that in order to understand it thoroughly it would be best if he would submit a typewritten outline of this program to Dr. Janse, the Secretary of the Council, who in turn would have the same multigraphed and sent out to every member of the Council for his personal and thorough study.

In substance Dr. Norcross advised the Council that much of the framework of this program had been taken from a study of the graduate schools of the Los Angeles Osteopathic College and the University of California in Los Angeles. Dr. Norcross asserted that by virtue of this program many of the chiropractors now in practice whose education had been rather meager and inefficient, would have the opportunity of augmenting their education by virtue of special classwork in the graduate school rather than having to take regular classwork in under-graduate classes. Furthermore, this program would allow the creation of chiropractic specialties such as X-ray, physio therapy, psychiatry, cardiology, etc., which, in many respects, would represent a ??? of importance comparable to the specialties existent in medicine. Dr. Norcross advised the Council that they had instituted a graduate school at the Los Angeles college, that at the present time it was functioning with success and to the benefit not only of the Los Angeles College but also the profession as a whole.

(3) Dr. Martin injected the statement that as the result of this graduate work being sponsored by the Los Angeles College a greater feeling of cooperation had been created among the California practitioners for and toward the Los Angeles College, and he expressed the belief that such would be the case in the instance of the other colleges if they were to institute a similar program. Dr. Martin stated that the California delegation felt that they would like to obtain the approval of the Council because it would give this effort more weight and importance among the California chiropractors.

(4) At this point several forms of post graduate diplomas were presented and the Council was requested to approve same. Upon questioning by Dr. Peterson, it was admitted that these diplomas were being given out already. Dr. Peterson then pointed out that they were asking for the approval of an accomplished fact and that the Council had gone on record as not approving any credentials other than Chiropractic D.C. until much further discussion was held.

(5) It was the general consensus that this indeed is a worthy program and project and consequently the expression was made that all in attendance were certainly friendly toward the idea. Dr. Janse was instructed to correspond with Dr. Norcross to obtain the detailed outline of the program and to have it multi-graphed and sent out with the Minutes.

At this point Dr. Janse advised the Council that Dr. C.O. Watkins of Sidney, Montana, and former member of the Executive Board, had submitted to him an outline and composition designed to create within all of the approved chiropractic colleges standard courses dealing with the orientation of the student in relation to the study of science, what it consists of, what its procedures are, what its methods of analysis represent, the manners it employs in the establishment of recognizable data, Dr. Watkins' contention being that by virtue of this program much of the inconsistency of scientific philosophic approach now existent in chiropractic and chiropractic education would be dissipated.

(1) The various members of the Council gave expressions of approval of this idea and some contended that this also had been a proposition that they had been thinking about for some time.

(2) Dr. Janse was instructed to have Dr. Watkins' outline mimeographed and sent out with the Minutes.

Mr. W.W. MacGruder, National Program Director of the Chiropractic Research Foundation was then invited to come into the Council meeting for the purpose of answering several questions that pertain to the Council and the C.R.F. program.

(1) Dr. Martin, representing the Los Angeles College, asked Mr. MacGruder why it was that the C.R.F. had flooded California with literature and solicitations when the C.R.F. had made a contract with the California Chiropractic Association that they would refrain from conducting a campaign in California if the California Research Foundation would turn over 15 per cent of its gross intake to the C.R.F.

(2) In answer to this inquiry Mr. MacGruder said that he realized that damage had been done, but that it was no fault of his and that the detriment had been committed by those outside of his change and without his advice. He said that the matter had been straightened out and that the original contract with California would be honored.

Minutes of the NATIONAL CHIROPRACTIC ASSOCIATION COUNCIL ON EDUCATION, Closed Meeting Afternoon Session, January 5, 1949.

This was a closed meeting and only the official members of the Council were permitted to attend, Dr. Thure C. Peterson presiding. Those in attendance included:

(A) Members of the Committee on Educational Standards: Drs. Nugent, Gardner, Wolf, and Osborne.

(B) Schoolmen: Drs. Peterson, Firth, Hendricks, Parr, Schreiber, Wolfe, Martin, and Janse.

Dr. Peterson called on Dr. Gardner as head of the Committee on Educational Standards in the accrediting of chiropractic colleges to give a report of the functions and activities of the committee since the Portland convention six months ago. Dr. Gardner advised the Council that he was very gratified with the progress that had been made. Furthermore, that Dr. Nugent, because of the many responsibilities that had evolved upon him, had not been in a position to make as many visits to the various chiropractic colleges that needed further assistance and investigation as he would have liked to have done. Consequently the status of the accredited and provisionally accredited colleges is more or less the same as reported at the Portland convention. However, Dr. Gardner advised the Council that recognition should be afforded the personnel of the provisionally accredited for the continued progressive efforts they were making in eventually qualifying their institutions for full accrediting.

Dr. Nugent then advised the Council that since Portland all of his attention had been necessitated in resolving the final issues of the change-over in California. He stated that he was most gratified with the progress that had been made in California and assured the Council that as the result of the changes effected a very commendable circumstance now existed and thus he felt free at this time to direct his efforts and attentions to other projects of importance. Dr. Nugent advised the Council that he was not unmindful or unaware of the progress that had been made since the Portland Convention in the provisionally accredited colleges, and he complemented the leaders of these institutions for their courage and determination, and the accomplishments they have realized, expressing the belief that if the same were continued it wouldn't be too long before full approval could be afforded them.

Dr. Peterson then asked Dr. Nugent whether he considered it possible that by the next meeting in Chicago in July these "out of necessity deferred" investigations of the provisionally accredited colleges could be made, and Dr. Nugent said that this was very likely.

Discussions then revolved about the disposition of the Kansas State College of Chiropractic, and it was fully acknowledged that Dr. Schreiber and his associates had made a very fine effort. Dr. Schreiber advised the Council that within the near future there was the possibility of this institution acquiring a new building in the form of a recently built small hospital which now stands empty in one of the suburbs of Wichita, and he, of course, maintained that if this could be realized many of their problems would be solved.

Dr. Peterson then asked Drs. Nugent and Gardner whether any further disposition had been made of the issues and circumstances pertaining to the accrediting of the Logan Basic Chiropractic College. A number of discussions resulted, Dr. Nugent read several letters and telegrams that had been exchanged between him and Dr. Vinton Logan, and after careful deliberation it was the full and unanimous consensus of opinion that full recognition be afforded this institution. A motion was made and passed in relation to this matter, and reads as follows:

"That the National Council on Education of the National Chiropractic Association extends full approval and recognition to the Logan Basic Chiropractic College on the basis of the telegram received by Dr. John J. Nugent, Director of Education, August 17, 1948, the contents of the telegram reading as follows:

"Received your telegram of August 7th. Indicated to you we are for doing everything that will strengthen and unify chiropractic, as per our conversation we will put Logan Basic technique in any non-profit four-year chiropractic college without cost, no contract will be required from any individual school or association, the only qualification being that the school must teach Logan Basic technic a sufficient number of hours and under properly trained and approved instructors, effective upon the return of signed acceptance by Dr. Vinton Logan."

This motion was unanimously affirmed by every voting member of the Council, and Dr. Nugent and Peterson were instructed to contact Dr. Vinton Logan and advise him of the conduct of the Council in relation to the fine institution over which he presided.

Minutes of the NATIONAL CHIROPRACTIC ASSOCIATION COUNCIL ON EDUCATION, Minutes of the mid-year meetings held in Chicago at the Sherman Hotel, January 5, 6, and 7, 1949; Dr. Thure C. Peterson presiding over all the meetings.

Those present at the meetings were:
(A) Members of the Committee on Educational Standards:
   Dr. John J. Nugent, Director of Education of the NCA, 92 Norton Street, New Haven, Connecticut
   Dr. Edward H. Gardner, Los Angeles College of Chiropractic, 920 Venice Blvd., Los Angeles, California
   Dr. Walter B. Wolf, Eureka, South Dakota
   Dr. Norman E. Osborne, Hagerstown, Maryland
(B) Members of the Committee on Educational Institutions:
   Dr. James F. Firth, Lincoln Chiropractic College, 633 N. Pennsylvania Avenue, Indianapolis, Indiana
   Dr. Thure C. Peterson, Chiropractic Institute of New York, 152 W. 42nd Street, New York 18, New York
   Dr. Ralph J. Martin, Los Angeles College of Chiropractic, 920 Venice Blvd., Los Angeles, California
   Dr. Paul O. Parr, Carver College of Chiropractic, 522 N.W. 9th Street, Oklahoma City, Oklahoma
   Dr. John B. Wolfe, Northwestern College of Chiropractic, 608 Nicolette Avenue, Minneapolis 2, Minnesota
   Dr. A.C. Hendricks, Lincoln College of Chiropractic, 633 N. Pennsylvania Avenue, Indianapolis, Indiana
   Dr. Homer C. Beatty, Denver University of Natural Therapeutics, 1075 Logan Street, Denver, Colorado
   Dr. H.C. Harring, Missouri Chiropractic Institute, 3117 Lafayette Avenue, St. Louis, Missouri
   Dr. Theodore Schreiber, Kansas State Chiropractic College, 629 N. Broadway, Wichita, Kansas
   Dr. Carl Cleveland, Jr., Cleveland College of Chiropractic, 3724 Troost, Kansas City, Missouri
   Dr. James Drain, Texas Chiropractic College, San Antonio, Texas
   Dr. J. Janse, National College of Chiropractic, 20 N. Ashland Blvd., Chicago, 7, Illinois
(C) Special guest:
   Dr. William C. Jacobs, Executive Secretary, Wisconsin Chiropractic Association, 161 W. Wisconsin Avenue, Milwaukee 3, Wisconsin

Dr. W.A. Budden, President of the Western States College of Chiropractic, 4525 S.E. 63rd Avenue, Portland, Oregon, had contemplated being in attendance but was snowbound in Wyoming. He did, however, arrive on the evening of January 7th, and had the opportunity of having several discussions with Drs. Nugent and Janse. Consequently he is fully oriented with what transpired at the regular Council meetings.

It is to be remembered that the National Council on Education consists of two intramural committees, one the Committee on Educational Standards and the Accrediting of Chiropractic Colleges, and two, the Committee on Educational Institutions. Dr. Thure C. Peterson is the elected President of the Council, with Dr. Joseph Janse serving as Secretary.

The first meeting of the Council and its guests began at 10:00 A.M. January 5th, with Dr. Peterson presiding. He designated it as an informal gathering, because as yet not all of the official members were present. The following discussions resulted.

Dr. Peterson asked those attending to voice their opinion with reference to the present issue as it relates to the drafting of chiropractic students. He advised the group that he had been informed by Dr. Neil Bishop of Denver, Colorado, that a few days previous General Hershey had been in Denver to attend some American Legion gathering. At this gathering Dr. Bishop had taken the opportunity of making the acquaintance of General Hershey and discussing the drafting of chiropractic students with him. According to the information Dr. Bishop relayed to Dr. Peterson, General Hershey said that no adverse decision was made against chiropractic but that the previous status was maintained and that it was not impossible that an alteration favorable to exemption of chiropractic students from the draft could be obtained if additional pertinent information be presented and if a uniform agreement developed between all chiropractic colleges. Furthermore, Dr. Bishop had made the suggestion to Dr. Peterson that he be sent by the NCA to Washington to continue his mediations with General Hershey. It was the final conclusion of those present that a recommendation be made to the Executive Board of the NCA that if possible Dr. Bishop be sent to Washington, but that he be accompanied by Dr. Nugent as Director of Education.

Dr. Schreiber brought up the question of whether it wouldn't be advisable to change from the hour system in estimating the chiropractic curriculum to the credit system. The ensuing discussions were pro and con and the final decision was that for the time being, at least, it would be best to leave things as they are. Dr. Firth advised the group that even in medicine the hour system is still adhered to in the majority of instances.

Dr. Peterson then presented an issue as it relates to the Connecticut Board of Chiropractic Examiners. Although the Connecticut law requires a four-year education of eight to nine months each in an approved chiropractic college, the Board had proceeded to give recognition to the Palmer School of Chiropractic on the strength of its supposed four-year course. The Palmer four-year course was then described as consisting of 18 months of classroom and laboratory work, and the rest of the time as an internship either in Dr. Palmer's private clinic, or in the Clearview Sanatorium as operated by the dean of the school. In the resultant discussion it was the consensus of opinion that this in no way represented a reputable four-year course, and certainly the recognition of the same should be discouraged whenever possible.

Dr. Firth, at this time, mentioned the fact that the reason why the Connecticut Chiropractic Board had recognized the four-year course of the Palmer School was because the Board membership was predominantly of the Palmer concept and affiliation. Dr. Peterson then made the recommendation that later on in the sessions of the Council when all the official members were present the NCA be instructed to send a resolution to all the chiropractic state boards of examiners that they recognize a chiropractic college on the strength of the composition and length of its shortest chiropractic course, not its longest. Furthermore, that all four-year courses be properly presented as to the list of subjects and material they cover. Dr. Firth then raised the question why it was that we in the chiropractic profession so ardently insisted upon a 36 months course when the majority of the medical schools only afford a 32 months medical course. He felt that an internship in a chiropractic clinic affiliated with a chiropractic school should actually not be a part of the chiropractic course. The discussions that ensued resulted in the opinion by some of the members that the reason why a 36 months course is preferable is because in chiropractic colleges the student comes to the chiropractic college with relatively little pre-professional training in essential basic science subjects, whereas in medical and even in osteopathic education many of these essential basic science subjects are obtained in the pre-professional college education, and as a result our chiropractic curriculum actually had to be somewhat heavier than those of medical schools.

Dr. Jacobs, as the Executive Secretary of the Wisconsin Chiropractic Association, was then asked to explain to the group the program that he was attempting to realize in Wisconsin with reference to the basic science law and board. Dr. Jacobs advised the group that in Wisconsin for a number of years the basic science board had permitted the giving of a special basic science examination for chiropractic applicants only. The questions of the examination related exclusively to the vertebral column and the spinal cord, although the examination, of course, was still given by the regular members of the basic science board. Now, however, he had approached the members of the Wisconsin Basic Science Board with the proposition that he be privileged to present to them a panel of professors giving instruction at chiropractic colleges and possessing degrees besides their Doctor of Chiropractic Degree, from whom a number would be chosen to prepare the questions and correct the papers for those chiropractic applicants who took the special basic science examination on the spinal cord only. Dr. Jacobs informed the group that the members of the basic science board were not untoward as far as this recommendation is concerned, but that he, Dr. Jacobs, was just a little apprehensive about it because he wondered whether the chiropractic colleges could afford him their full cooperation, and whether these proposed chiropractic examiners would propound an examination that would probably be a little more difficult than the present one, and if by chance that happened to be the case and students were failed under this new arrangement, it would certainly result in a tremendous amount of chagrin and professional disparagement.

Dr. Peterson then asked Dr. Jacobs whether the regular or the special basic science examination, as given by the regular appointed members of the board, had been unfair, and Dr. Jacobs answered that in every respect the board had conducted fair examinations. In fact, Dr. Jacobs advised the group that he and the chiropractic board in Wisconsin had received the most friendly cooperation from the basic science board in every respect. Dr. Peterson then advised the group that the primary advantage of Dr. Jacobs' proposed plan would be that of affording the profession a position of prestige and personal jurisdiction in the basic science examination in the state of Wisconsin.

Open Meeting beginning 4:15 P.M., January 5, 1949, Dr. Thure C. Peterson presiding.

As special guests of this meeting there were in attendance Dr. Wm. C. Jacobs, the Executive Secretary of the Wisconsin Chiropractic Association; Dr. James Drain, of the Texas Chiropractic College, and Dr. Carl S. Cleveland, Jr., of the Cleveland College of Chiropractic.

These gentlemen were welcomed with hearty approval by all members of the Council, and certainly the Council wishes to express its appreciation for the presence, contributions, and confidence of these people.

Dr. Nugent then asked the members of the Council, as well as the visitors, to deliberate over the proposition and program by Dr. C.O. Watkins, of Sydney, Montana. The Secretary of the Council, as well as all of the other schoolmen and Dr. Nugent, at various occasions have received rather extensive literature and communications from Dr. Watkins expressing the opinion that it is imperative that in the fundamental courses of what is ordinarily called chiropractic philosophy and principles a more exacting scientific approach should be made.

Dr. Watkins insisted that that which is ordinarily called chiropractic philosophy and taught as chiropractic concept and principles is somewhat pseudo in scientific aspect and tainted with a semi-religious approach. It is Dr. Watkins opinion that every freshman student in the recognized chiropractic colleges should receive a basic course in what is known as orientation in relation to science, what it is, what its procedures are, what it attempts to realize, and what it propounds to accomplish, and that only after this fundamental course has been taken should the chiropractic student be allowed to take a course in chiropractic principles and concept. Furthermore, that this course in chiropractic principles should be based upon fully accepted and recognized scientific data - based upon the anatomy, physiology, and pathology of the standard authorities.

A great deal of comment was made with reference to Dr. Watkins' proposition. Every schoolman of the Council recognized the merit of his program. Dr. Nugent especially emphasized the need for a more exacting clarification of chiropractic concept because according to him, so many students refuse to accept the dogma so commonly existent, and they are left befuddled and confused. The other schoolmen, including Drs. Peterson, Firth, and Schreiber, expressed the opinion that probably Dr. Watkins was not fully aware of what type of work is being taught in the courses of chiropractic principles, expressing the opinion that at least in part his program and suggestions had already found realization in some of the chiropractic colleges. They all agreed that the word "philosophy" could well be replaced by the terms concept, principles, or premise. Dr. James Drain then asked for the opportunity of expressing himself in relation to Dr. Watkins program. He frankly stated that he was very much against the idea of doing away with the chiropractic philosophy as basically and fundamentally taught by the early pioneers of chiropractic. He asserted that it was his conviction that the chiropractic profession was deviating too much from the original premise of those who pioneered its progress. Consequently he wanted to go on record in voicing a vigorous opposition to any attempt to alter or modify the original tenets of the profession. Dr. Peterson then voiced the opinion that Dr. Weiant's reply to Dr. Watkins' work should be multigraphed and sent out along with the minutes of the Council meeting. In answer to Dr. Drain, Dr. Nugent said, in substance, that he hoped that Dr. Drain will not go away with the idea that anyone is trying to destroy the chiropractic concept. All that is being done is an attempt to add to the original premise and to prove it by means of scientific investigation and deliberation.

The evening session, January 5, 1949. Dr. Thure C. Peterson presiding.

Dr. Nugent again presented the question as to what should be done with reference to the proposed program of Dr. Watkins, and after rather extensive deliberation it was concluded that Dr. Watkins should be advised that his sincerity and intent of purpose is admired, respected and acknowledged. Furthermore, that his suggested change in the manner of teaching chiropractic concepts, at least in part, already has been adopted; however, that full recommendations will be made to all schoolmen to recognize the necessity of bringing these orientation and fundamental courses in chiropractic up to standard and up to present day scientific versions.

Dr. Nugent then advised the assembled schoolmen that he honestly felt that in all of our chiropractic colleges added emphasis could be placed upon the necessity of teaching applied physics, a better training in the biological sciences, and the directing of all students to do a lot of research reading not only in college libraries but also in some of the technical and medical libraries existent in such cities as New York, Chicago, Los Angeles, etc.

Dr. Nugent advised the Council that it is becoming progressively more important for chiropractic students to be well oriented in all of the cultural and scientific subjects. He emphasized the fact that our profession no longer dares practice academic isolation and insisted that teaching in chiropractic colleges must be broad and liberal and should not be stereotyped or prejudiced.

He placed emphasis upon the need for a substantial library in every college. He emphasized the value of public classes, special classes organized by students themselves in acquiring a better understanding of basic English. He emphasized the importance that instructors in chiropractic colleges be encouraged to improve their teaching capacity and ability. In support of this premise he made reference to the fine work that is being done at the Canadian Memorial Chiropractic College in Toronto, where Major Kolbeck had put on a special course for the college faculty in the science and art of effective teaching. Dr. John B. Wolfe substantiated Dr. Nugent's comments with reference to Major Kolbeck, and advised the Council that Maj. Kolbeck had made a trip to Minneapolis and over the weekend put on a course of instruction for the faculty of that college, and immeasurable benefit had been derived from the same.

Dr. Nugent emphasized the importance of the developing of museums of pathological and anatomical specimens, the enlarging and amplifying of the college laboratories and their facilities; he stressed the need for more effective and competent clinical training. The Doctor of Chiropractic today, he said, is no longer a technician, but he is a doctor in every sense of the word, who must know the procedures of clinical and physical diagnosis, as well as all effective means of spinal analysis.

Open session, January 6, 1949, 2:00 P.M.

In the morning the entire membership of the Council, along with the members of the NCA Executive Board, attended a Jr. NCA Rally sponsored by the student body of the National College of Chiropractic. The National College administration wishes to express its sincerest appreciation to the members of the Council for their courtesy and consideration. It is certain that everyone will agree that this student body gathering contributed much toward an enthusiastic support of the NCA program by the students of this institution.

At the meeting proper, Dr. Peterson made a report on the work of Dr. August Eich, of 64 W. Randolph Street, Suite 1219, Chicago 1, Illinois. Dr. Eich for several years has been attempting to interest the NCA Council on Research in a project that he has been developing in relation to corrective manipulations of the feet, the ankle, and the knee, and the manufacturing of a specially designed shoe purported to assist greatly in the maintenance of proper postural capacity with a minimum of neuromuscular effort. Dr. Peterson advised the Council that the manipulative procedures employed by Dr. Eich were nothing too extraordinary, but that he did feel that the type of shoe designed by the doctor had distinct merit, and he recommended that the Council go on record of suggesting that Dr. Eich be encouraged to carry his proposition to the Council on Research for further study and investigation.

It might be mentioned that Dr. Eich is desirous of having the National Chiropractic Association assume the responsibility of the distribution of the shoe among practitioners who are interested for a reasonable percentage of the sales.

The matter was then brought up about the importance of chiropractic State boards, the manner in which they are administered, and the type of questions that are propounded. It was recommended by a goodly number of the members of the Council that efforts should be made to instruct some of the chiropractic state boards of examiners that many of the questions, especially in chiropractic principles, are of an obsolete and unscientific nature, and that for the sake of the profession, as well as the status that it should maintain, they should be deleted.

Dr. Nugent then proceeded to conduct a discussion about the importance of recognizing the rather ill-conditioned program conducted by the Palmer School of Chiropractic in relation to chiropractic state boards. He asserted that because of the ever-increasing educational standards in our profession the students at the Palmer School were confronting the dilemma of inadequate qualification, and as a result the administration of this institution was resorting to the falsification of their educational program to the extent where they are padding their curriculum ostensibly to represent a four-year course. Dr. Nugent mentioned that at the present time there are only three states left where Palmer graduates could fully qualify for the chiropractic board, yet as a result of political chicanery still maintain a rather exacting control of certain of the four-year states. As an example he gave the situation as it relates to the Connecticut State Board of Chiropractic Examiners. Dr. Nugent asserted that if need be he will go directly to the Governor of the State of Connecticut in order to rectify the discrepancy that now exists. Dr. Nugent asked that the Council pass a resolution in an effort to check the detriment of the policy conducted by this institution, and in consequence the following resolution was passed; namely: "Be it resolved that the National Council on Education, supported by the executive body of the National Chiropractic Association, proceed to instruct all of the chiropractic boards of examiners that the curriculum and courses of the chiropractic colleges and schools and institutions be appraised for qualification on the basis of their shortest course offers for the reception of the Doctor of Chiropractic degree rather than the longest and maximum course presented." The vote on this resolution was all in favor except one.

At this time Dr. Wm. Jacobs asked the Council to explain to him what were the circumstances pertaining to the recent trouble in Georgia. The answer to Dr. Jacobs was that the situation in Georgia is a matter of common knowledge; namely, that the Georgia law is a 4-year law of 9 months in each collegiate year, and that the Georgia Board of Chiropractic Examiners had been intimidated by representatives and supporters of the Palmer School to the extent where they had been coerced into giving several degrees to the sons of prominent Palmer practitioners in the state of Georgia who, however, only possessed an 18 month education. Dr. Jacobs advised the Council that he appreciated the explanation pertaining to his inquiry.

Dr. Schreiber advised the Council that he personally would like to advocate a two-year liberal arts education in an accredited state college as a pre-requisite requirement for entrance into a chiropractic college. Everyone present acknowledged the merit of this suggestion but felt that for the time being, at least, it was rather premature, although as Dr. Nugent insisted this eventually would be the result.

Dr. Peterson then drew the Council's attention to the necessity of recognizing the fact that in granting advanced standing to those chiropractic matriculants with a previous college background it should be limited to the basis of giving credit only for those subjects that parallel those contained within chiropractic curriculum.

Dr. Peterson then advised the Council that Dr. Clarence Weiant instructed him to advise the Council that he would like to have them pass the following resolution: namely, that the Accrediting Committee of the National Chiropractic Association should not recognize any school teaching less than 25% of its full course in specific chiropractic subjects. Dr. Nugent suggested that this resolution be tabled until a careful study can be made of the catalogues of the various chiropractic colleges. Dr. Firth at this time advised the group that at the Toronto meetings, where extended and careful study had been made of an exemplary chiropractic curriculum, this matter had been carefully studied and at that time all chiropractic colleges represented had fully complied with the essence of this resolution. Dr. Peterson expressed the idea that Dr. Weiant was fearful that if steps of this disposition were not taken there would be a detrimental encroachment upon the chiropractic subjects by adjunctive and elective courses.

Dr. Martin then brought up the subject of student screening for the purpose of eliminating the undesirables. He advised the group that at the Los Angeles College of Chiropractic this procedure had been instituted with gratifying results and that the screening examinations were based upon the estimation of the student in the following four categories - aptitude, intelligence, maturity, and emotional attitude.

Dr. Firth advised the Council that not only should the schools institute a measure of screening, but that probably the eliminating of undesirable applicants was being effected by the fact that certain state organizations, as well as chiropractic associations of foreign countries, were encouraging that the approved schools only matriculate those students who are recommended by the chiropractic society of that given state or country. He used as an example the South African Chiropractic Association who in their communications have advised the various chiropractic colleges not to matriculate anyone other than students possessing the approval of this society. Dr. Nugent then made mention of the visit to this country of Dr. Finn Christensen, the leader of the chiropractic profession in Denmark, and who, during his three months stay here in the United States, had visited all of the leading chiropractic colleges. In Denmark the chiropractic association has organized a chiropractic college designed to teach the clinical subjects only, requiring that all of the chiropractic students obtain their pre-clinical work in the regular classes of the University of Copenhagen.

Dr. Schreiber advised the Council that nationally recognized screening tests were now readily available, and Dr. Firth verified this fact by stating that at the Lincoln College various experimental procedures have been employed.

Dr. Nugent then asked the Council to pass the following resolution. At the beginning of each semester each of the accredited and provisionally accredited colleges should submit to his office, that of Director of Education, certified copies of the semester schedule, accompanied by full explanation of any of the major changes that were effected as the result of exigency. Furthermore, that the schedules for each semester must parallel the outlined curse in the college catalogue. The resolution was made and seconded and voted upon unanimously. Dr. Nugent advised the Council that this was necessary for legislative purposes. So often had he encountered the difficulty of having to debate the reason why the regular term schedule did not parallel the course presented in the catalogue of the institution.

Dr. Nugent then asked the Council to pass another resolution, the full substance of which reads as follows: "An approved college shall be incorporated as a 'non-profit' institution. Its board of trustees or directors shall be composed of chiropractors and laymen interested in the perpetuation of the chiropractic school of practice. No member of the board shall receive financial profit form the operation of the college or its associated clinic or hospital. The members of the Board should serve sufficiently long terms so that continuity of the institution's policy will be carried out without precipitate change in policy. The college shall afford to proper representatives of the Committee on Educational Standards unhampered opportunity to study and inspect the college's facilities, its faculty, and its management, including a study of its financial records, students' entrance credentials, grading, promotion, and graduation records." The resolution was made and seconded and unanimously voted upon.

A third resolution was then proposed by Dr. Nugent; namely, that all of the approved schools between now and the next meeting of the Council declare their full intention to industriously attempt to come up to the standards as laid down by the original formula of the Director of Education. However that every element of encouragement should be afforded these institutions and every measure of aid be proffered whenever possible. The resolution was passed unanimously.

The question of the Basic Science laws and boards was then carefully discussed and Dr. Nugent, as well as other members of the Council, expressed the conviction that the general approach of the profession in relation to these laws and boards was just a little ill-conditioned and ill-advised; that if any attacks were to be made they were to be made against the laws, not against the members of the boards. The belief was expressed by a number of the schoolmen that the rather vitriolic attacks made really did more harm than good because they always involved the matter of personalities and caused the members of the basic science boards to feel that their personal integrity was being attacked. It was mentioned that the personnel of a goodly number of these boards is essentially competent, honest, and straightforward.

At this time Dr. Homer Beatty made mention of the feeling that exists among some of the chiropractic leaders that certain members of the Council have been a little stubborn and resistive in always opposing any resolutions that the House of Delegates want to pass, voicing their opposition against basic science laws and boards. Dr. Beatty was advised that this opposition arose because the vindictiveness of these resolutions is always directed against the personnel of the boards rather than against the original intent of the law, and the majority of the members of the Council verified this attitude.

However, at the request of Dr. Beatty, and in support of the efforts of the Colorado chiropractors in the attempt to alter or modify or eliminate the basic science law in Colorado, the Council unanimously passed the following resolution. "It is the opinion of this Council that the enactment of Basic Science Acts does not accomplish the avowed purpose to improve the public health; that we denounce the covert purpose of these Acts - which is to destroy the chiropractic profession indirectly; that Basic Science examinations are an unnecessary duplication of those given by the chiropractic and other examining boards, and that the imposition of an exam by Basic Science Boards preliminary to examination by the chiropractic and other examining boards infers incompetency of such boards and reflects upon the integrity and citizenship of those men and women appointed by their respective Governors to such boards."

On the evening of this day the entire Council and its guests attended a dinner as given by the National College at the club of Mr. Turek, the business administrator of this institution. The secretary was instructed to include within the minutes an expression of appreciation to Mr. Turck and his associates from all of the members of the Council, as well as the others who attended this dinner.

The final meeting of the Council held Friday Morning, January 7, 1949, Dr. Thure C. Peterson, presiding.

Dr. Nugent asked for the opportunity of giving a number of instructions to the various college representatives in relation to some pressing necessities pertaining to chiropractic education. He mentioned the fact that the academic deans of the larger chiropractic colleges did find it difficult in fully and thoroughly supervising the quality of each of the classes, and in an attempt to solve this problem Dr. Nugent advised that it would be beneficial if every instructor be asked to submit at the beginning of each semester a detailed outline of the course that he intends to present. Furthermore, that competent and reliable men be appointed as heads of the various departments of instruction.

Dr. Nugent also asked the question as to whether, at the various chiropractic colleges, full advantage is being taken in the use of the available physical equipment. He mentioned that so often as the result of a lack of interest on the part of an instructor charts, visual educational instruments, etc. were being left unused. He advised the schoolmen that essentially in all of the chiropractic colleges there is a great need for more laboratory work, especially in the fields of chemistry, bacteriology, physiology, pathology, and histology.

Dr. Peterson at this time injected the opinion that as fully worthy as these suggestions were, the full realization of the same could not be accomplished without proper endowment, because college income, based upon student tuition entirely, would not be able to defray the expenses associated with such a complete program. Dr. Nugent asserted that although he realized the difficulties thus encountered, yet he felt that now when the schools are in a better financial position than ever before, a reputable percentage of the income should be expended in augmenting the laboratory facilities. He advised the group that in his defense of the chiropractic profession before educational and governmental agencies he always had to confront the accusation that the physical equipment of our chiropractic colleges, especially in the field of the laboratory, is frequently so grossly inadequate, and as an illustration he reiterated his rather distressing experience during his recent appearance in front of the Royal Commission at Ottawa, Canada.

Dr. Nugent's contentions and instruction were received with genuine appreciation by the schoolmen present, and commitments of cooperation were made.

Suggestions were then made by Drs. Schreiber, Cleveland, and others that whenever possible the instructor, as well as the students, attention should be directed toward the usage of competently written notes on the various phases of physiology and pathology.

Dr. Peterson advised the group that Dr. Herman Schwartz, of Elmhurst, New Jersey, is preparing a manual on abnormal psychology. The entire membership of the Council gave recognition to the previous constructive efforts of Dr. Schwartz in this field, and it was recommended that Dr. Schwartz be encouraged to continue his efforts, and that if his manual is completed all chiropractic colleges should be encouraged to use it.

The matter was then brought up about chiropractic colleges issuing a number of other degrees either to signify an extra amount of work or time spent, or to designate post graduate work, or to designate graduate work. The question of the Los Angeles College and its graduate school was brought in for consideration, and it was the general consensus of opinion that this matter of issuing such degrees as Master of Chiropractic Science, or degrees or certificates in chiropractic specialties such as psychiatry, proctology, ophthalmology, should not be distributed too freely. Dr. Gardner also made mention of the rather vigorous conflict that exists in California with reference to the graduate school, and how some of the leaders of this graduate school were attempting to go too far afield in teaching of various subjects that actually do not pertain to chiropractic.

The matter of some of the chiropractic colleges conducting courses and issuing degrees other than those of chiropractic was also brought into discussion. Reference was made to the National College and the course of naturopathy that it had supported. Dr. Janse proceeded to explain the circumstance under which this matter was developed. He expressed the realization that in some respects at least it represented an incompetency that should be rectified, and he advised the Council that he was appreciative of their concern and interest and that he was confident that as the result of the constructive recommendations of the Council the full membership of the college administration could be brought to realize the necessity of full differentiation in relation to the question of multiple degrees. He furthermore advised the Council that he was certain that within the near future a proper disposition would be assumed in this respect.

It is to be mentioned at this time that all of these deliberations were conducted in the spirit of frank understanding and mutual respect. Everyone present agreed that as the result of the heterogeneous picture that each of the colleges had inherited from the past immediate rectification of all the discrepancies of some form or other could not be accomplished; that with diligent effort and honest intent their eventual elimination could and should be realized. Dr. Nugent at this time gave expression to the confidence that many of these problems would be eliminated. He reviewed the rather precarious situations that originally existed in California, and how, in order to effect an amalgamation of the numerous vying groups some temporary concessions had to be made, but now that a solid front had been accomplished he felt that the various idiosyncrasies that now existed could be eliminated. The other schoolmen all expressed their full confidence in the integrity of each individual institution, and felt that the matters brought up should be left in the hands of those who confronted them as individual responsibilities; that, of course, Dr. Nugent should see to it that whenever a discrepancy could be eliminated it should be, regardless of what school it involved or what personality would be held responsible.

Dr. Nugent then advised the group that in relation to the Veterans Administration an effort should be made to bring them to realize and to acknowledge that the vacation recesses should be considered as part of the school year, and not as vacations, but as recesses.

It was suggested by Dr. Parr, and unanimously approved upon, that Dr. Janse, in preparing the minutes of the mid year meeting, should make two sets, namely, minutes for all of the schoolmen and guests of the open meetings, and that the minutes of the one closed meeting be sent to the official members of the Council only.

Dr. Peterson then expressed his pleasure and appreciation for the friendly and considerate attitude expressed by all during the course of the mid-year session. He reiterated the full confidence of the entire Council in the fine work that Dr. Nugent as director of Education, is doing. Dr. Nugent in turn expressed his sincere appreciation for the cooperation that he had received, and assured every schoolman that each institution would receive every consideration possible according to its needs and circumstances.

Minutes of the COUNCIL ON EDUCATION of the NATIONAL CHIROPRACTIC ASSOCIATION, held during the NCA convention week at the Sherman Hotel, July 24-29, 1949; Dr. Thure C. Peterson, President of the Council presided at all the meetings; Dr. Joseph Janse, Secretary

The first session was held on Monday afternoon, July 25th, and the following people were in attendance:

(A) Members of the Committee on Educational Standards:

Dr. John J. Nugent, Director of Education of the NCA, 92 Norton Street, New Haven, Connecticut

Dr. Edward H. Gardner, 2727 S. Vermont Ave., Los Angeles, Calif.

Dr. Norman E. Osborne, 2 Broadway, Hagerstown, Maryland

Dr. Walter B. Wolf, Eureka, South Dakota

Dr. George Bauer, 1608 Ball Sta., Columbia, South Carolina

(B) Members of the Committee on Educational Institutions (which consists of a representative of each one of the accredited or provisionally accredited colleges).

Dr. Thure C. Peterson, Chiropractic Institute of New York, 152 W. 42nd Street, New York 18, New York

Dr. W.A. Budden, Western States College of Chiropractic, 4525 S.E. 63rd Ave., Portland 14, Oregon

Dr. James F. Firth, Lincoln Chiropractic College Inc., 633 North Pennsylvania Ave., Indianapolis 4, Indiana

Dr. Ralph J. Martin, Los Angeles College of Chiropractic, 920 Venice Blvd., Los Angeles 15, California

Dr. Vinton F. Logan, Logan Basic College of Chiropractic, 7701 Florissant Road, St. Louis 21, Missouri

Dr. John B. Wolfe, Northwestern College of Chiropractic, 608 Nicolette Avenue, Minneapolis 2, Minnesota

Dr. Paul O. Parr, Carver College of Chiropractic, 522 N.W. 9th Street, Oklahoma City, Oklahoma

Dr. H.C. Harring, Missouri Chiropractic Institute, 3117 Lafayette Avenue, St. Louis, Missouri

Dr. Theodore Schreiber, Kansas State Chiropractic College, 629 N. Broadway, Wichita, Kansas

Dr. Rudy Mueller, Canadian Memorial Chiropractic College, 252 Blur Street West, Toronto 5, Ontario, Canada

Dr. Douglas E. Warden, Canadian Memorial Chiropractic College, 252 Bloor Street West, Toronto 5, Ontario, Canada

Dr. Joseph Janse, National College of Chiropractic, 20 North Ashland Blvd., Chicago, 7, Illinois

(C) In addition to the above the following school men and members of chiropractic state boards of examiners were in attendance.

Dr. A.G. Hendricks, Lincoln Chiropractic College, Inc.

Dr. Homer C. Beatty, Denver University of Natural Therapeutics, 1075 Logan Street, Denver, Colorado

Dr. Carl S. Cleveland, Sr., Cleveland Chiropractic College, 3724 Troost Street, Kansas City, Missouri

Dr. Carl S. Cleveland, Jr., Cleveland Chiropractic College, 3724 Troost Street, Kansas City, Missouri

Dr. William N. Coggins, Logan Basic College of Chiropractic

Dr. A.J. Darling, Board of Directors, Kansas State Chiropractic College

Dr. Guy Smith, Secretary, Arkansas Board of Chiropractic Examiners

Dr. Craig Kightlinger, Chiropractic Institute of New York

Dr. J.H. Trubenbach, Chiropractic Institute of New York

Dr. William O. Percy, Secretary, California Board of Chiropractic Examiners.

Dr. Neil Bishop, Denver University of Natural Therapeutics.

Dr. L.P. Rehberger, Missouri Chiropractic Institute.

Dr. Henry C. Schneider, Northwestern College of Chiropractic.

With Dr. Peterson presiding, the opening meeting was commenced with an invitation to those in attendance to bring up matters and problems of general importance.

Dr. John B. Wolfe asked for an opinion on a suggestion that he would like to make to the Council. He presented the suggestion that instead of the individual colleges advertising in the NCA Journal that under the auspices of the council a monthly two page spread be procured and that on this spread all the accredited and provisionally accredited colleges be properly listed in alphabetic order.

This would, according to Dr. Wolfe, avoid the element of rather inordinate competition in advertising and concurrently mitigate the expense of advertising in the Journal for some of the smaller colleges that found it rather difficult to cope with the expenses involved.

Dr. Wolfe's suggestion enjoyed the voice of approval from the majority of the college men. Dr. Logan expressed the idea that probably it would not be favored too well by the NCA because it would of course take advertisement support from the Journal. To this idea Dr. Parr voiced the opinion that it was not the responsibility of the colleges to support the Journal financially. In fact, contended Dr. Parr, it is time that the profession and all of its agencies be shown that they, instead of soliciting financial support from the colleges, should endeavor to render financial support to the colleges.

The matter was left open for further deliberation and final discussion at the mid year meeting in the coming winter months.

Dr. Peterson then called on Dr. Gardner to give the report of the Committee on Educational Standards.

Dr. Gardner stated that inasmuch as Dr. John Nugent had been involved in most of the work and that as he was the one most closely acquainted with the issues at hand, he would like to have Dr. Nugent make the report.

Dr. Nugent then proceeded to make a recommendation for full approval and accrediting of the Northwestern College of Chiropractic, with Dr. John B. Wolfe as President of the College. Dr. Nugent stated that the college had made most gratifying progress and that to date it enjoyed a very financially sound and academically substantial working basis.

A motion was then made that the Council accept the recommendation of Dr. Nugent. It was seconded and the vote was unanimous in favor of Dr. Nugent's recommendation.

Dr. Peterson then asked Dr. Nugent to make a comment with reference to the Missouri Chiropractic Institute, with Dr. H.C. Harring as President.

To this inquiry Dr. Nugent expressed the fact that at this institution gratifying progress had been made and that certainly the institution should receive the approving vote of the Council as a provisionally accredited college and that if the progress were continued full approval be afforded within proper time.

A motion was then made that the Council afford the Missouri Institute of Chiropractic a provisional rating. The motion was seconded and the vote of the Council was unanimous in favor of the recommendation.

Dr. Peterson drew the attention of the Council members to a letter that he had received from Dr. A.B. McNatt, State Commander, The Society of Military Chiropractors, 404 Apco Tower, Oklahoma City, Oklahoma. In substance, the letter contained the following cardinal inquiries:

(1) How does the Council on Education of the NCA go about determining and investigating the merit of various chiropractic colleges that wish to be accredited by the Council.

(2) Is there any possibility that credits from our chiropractic colleges will ever be recognized by those colleges that have been accredited by the North Central Association on the Accrediting of Colleges.

(3) Dr. McNatt made the suggestion that chiropractic colleges employ no instructor other than those who possess a degree from some recognized state college or university.

In answer to Dr. McNatt's letter, Dr. Peterson wrote and listed the following:

(1) The college must apply for accrediting.

(2) The college is inspected by Dr. Nugent, whether alone or accompanied by a member of the Committee on Accrediting.

(3) Dr. Nugent, with this committee, is empowered to give interim provisional approval to a college pending final action at either of the two annual meetings of the Council on Education.

(4) In these meetings the Committee on Accrediting makes its recommendations either for or against approval and action is taken following discussion and opportunity for hearing on part of an authorized representative of the college under consideration.

(5) The basis for approval is contained in the "Blue Book" issued by the National Chiropractic Association and prepared by Dr. Nugent some years ago, a copy of which you may obtain by writing directly to him.

Dr. Nugent then advised the Council that he also had received a letter from Dr. McNatt requesting that he, Dr. Nugent, send a questionnaire that might be filled out for the purpose of soliciting approval for the Carver College; Dr. Nugent advised Dr. McNatt that a personal visit and investigation would be necessary as was the case in all of the other colleges.

Dr. Nugent then asked for the opportunity of outlining to the Council members certain important and significant matters that pertained to Chiropractic education.

(1) All chiropractic colleges have been making progress and this was indeed a gratifying thing.

(2) The great influx of G.I. Students and the accompanying problems that arose were competently handled.

(3) Notwithstanding this progress and increase in educational proficiency it is now time to consider and to determine what the next step of progressive effort should be. To this effect he, as Director of Education, would like to make certain recommendations which may be listed as follows:

(a) The installation of laboratories where experimental work can be done by the students in: embryology, physics and chemistry, histology, physiology, pathology and bacteriology.

(b) That men be employed who are trained in these laboratory processes.

(c) The establishment of adequate college libraries.

(d) The acquisition of modern and proficient teaching aids and instruments.

(4) The great reason for these needed improvements, contended Dr. Nugent, was that of improving the caliber of our graduates and also because it was expected of us by all educational and governmental agencies to whom he and Dr. Murphy would eventually have to turn for support and recognition if our profession were to gain that recognition that we sought and wanted.

(5) Dr. Nugent used as example the situation in New Jersey where the composite Board of Examiners simply refused to recognize chiropractic colleges on the grounds of the deficiencies in the educational elements as mentioned above. He also cited his appearance before a Commission of the Department of Education of the Canadian Government. At which time he was very closely questioned about the laboratory facilities of the chiropractic colleges.

(6) Dr. Nugent explained to the Council how, recently, he and Dr. Murphy, in their efforts to obtain full recognition for the chiropractic profession in the proposed Truman Public Health Program, were confronted with similar questions.

Dr. Nugent explained that it was Mr. Kelly and Mr. Harman of the Dept. of Accrediting of Institutions of higher learning, as part of the Dept. of Labor, who asked for a full report on the financial, educational, and non-profit status of all the accredited chiropractic colleges. And, according to Dr. Nugent, these informations should be available if the colleges expected to be recognized by the federal government, and to place themselves in the position of being eligible for possible future educational grants.

At this point several members of the Council voiced the opinion that probably we should not be too gullible in relation to all of these matters because it might represent an effort on the part of the organized forces of medicine to obtain a lot of compromising data about the chiropractic colleges.

Dr. Nugent insisted that such was not the case and that actually it represents an opportunity rather than a hazard.

Dr. Nugent advised the Council that he was aware of the fact that all this could not be realized over night. Nor that the proposed laboratories could at the beginning be very elaborate or extensive. However, he cited the example of the efforts at the Los Angeles College of Chiropractic and how, as the result of effort and teamwork, several small laboratories were organized.

Various discussions resulted and it was a matter of opinion that conscientious efforts should be made along these lines, although it was to be remembered that because of the fact that the medical students had from 3 to 4 years of pre-professional college training, the great majority of his laboratory work in the basic sciences was obtained before he entered medical college and consequently chiropractic colleges were confronted by a problem that medical colleges avoided.

The opinion was then expressed that within a relatively short time it would become necessary to require 1 to 2 years of pre-professional college training before entering a chiropractic college.

Dr. Nugent's attention was also drawn to the fact that his demands should not be too expansive because after all, chiropractic colleges still had to defray all their expenses via their income from student tuition.

Dr. Nugent stated that he was aware of this fact. However, he contended that no one should inordinately resist these necessities because they were inevitable to our progress.

Dr. Peterson then called the council's attention to a resolution which had been received from the Oklahoma Chiropractic Association. Following is a verbatim copy.

RESOLUTION

Whereas, Carver College has been in continuous operation for 43 years; and

Whereas, it has turned out many graduates over this period of time; and

Whereas, it embodies the breadth and idea of Chiropractic in the South; and

Whereas, it has followed for three years a vigorous policy of improvement; and

Whereas, it is supported in endowment and otherwise by the Alumni Association, endorsed by the Oklahoma Chiropractic Association and declared an institution of higher learning of Chiropractic under the statues of the State of Oklahoma;

Now, Therefore, Be It Resolved:

That Carver Chiropractic College shall be declared a fully accredited institution under the concepts of the same by the NCA

Approved by the Executive Committee of the Oklahoma Chiropractic Association, July 10, 1949

S/Bera A. Smith, D.C.

Secretary

Since the meeting of the Council Dr. Peterson, as President, wrote the following answer to Dr. Smith:

Dear Dr. Smith:

The resolution relative to approval of the Carver College was presented to the Council on Education by Dr. Parr at our meeting in Chicago. This method of procedure was irregular as the Council on Education is permitted to act on approvals only if it is recommended by the Accrediting Committee.

In order to expedite approval without waiting until the next meeting, the Council authorized Dr. Nugent to give full approval upon inspection, if that would be his recommendation, and no further action by the Council will be necessary.

It is unfortunate that circumstances prevented inspection of the Carver College before our meeting in Chicago, but Dr. Nugent has assured us that he will make the inspection expeditiously.

With kindest personal regards and best wishes for continued success of the Carver Chiropractic College, I remain,

Very Sincerely yours,
S/Thure C. Peterson
Chairman

In the discussions that followed the reading of the Oklahoma resolutions the following primary comments are to be mentioned:

(1) Dr. Parr insisted that full approval be granted immediately. First, because the college was worthy of approval; and, second, because at the semi-annual meeting in Chicago held last January Dr. Nugent and the Accrediting Committee had been instructed by the Council to make an inspection of the Carver College before the coming meeting this July, and that Dr. Nugent failed to do the same and resultantly the Carver College and its sponsors felt that a breech of trust had been committed.

(2) In answer to Dr. Parr, Dr. Nugent stated that when he was ready to make the inspection Dr. Parr had asked him to wait for a

while because at that date certain improvements and pertinent matters were pending and he wanted to settle these before the inspection was made. Then, when Dr. Parr did make the invitation again, about 5 weeks before the July meeting, he, Dr. Nugent, was so involved with other very important matters he just could not make the inspection for want of time.

(3)   It was finally decided that the recommendation of the Oklahoma Chiropractic Association, although very laudable and worthy could not be responded to because it would represent a rupture of the integrity of the Accrediting Committee's authority and procedure of inspection. Dr. Peterson was then instructed to write the above listed letter to Dr. Smith. Dr. Nugent was instructed to inspect the Carver College as soon as possible and that if he and the Accrediting Committee deemed it qualified the College would receive full approval without any further necessary action of the Council.

Dr. Parr was also invited to have further discussions with Dr. Nugent and the members of the Accrediting Committee as to the most expedient date for the inspection.

This met with the full recommendation and approval of all concerned and portrayed the conscientious attitude of all.

Dr. Budden raised the question as to the portent of the resolution mentioned in the report of Dr. John Procure to the effect that no one associated with a Chiropractic College be permitted to accompany Dr. Nugent in any school inspection.

Dr. Gardner volunteered that he had caused this resolution to be introduced as he had heard that Dr. Peterson was to accompany Dr. Nugent to the Logan Basic College of Chiropractic.

Dr. Peterson took issue with Dr. Gardner and pointed out that the possible visit to the Logan College with Dr. Nugent had nothing to do with the inspection but would have been for the purpose of clarifying certain issues brought up in earlier Council meetings and that he had been empowered by the Council to hold such discussions. Dr. Peterson also indicated that the proper place for such a resolution would have been in the Council and that there was no intent on the part of anyone connected with a chiropractic college to in any way interfere with the activities of the Committee on Accrediting.

It was also decided that thereafter all Council members, whether of the Accrediting Committee or of the Committee on Educational Institutions, should not make any resolutions relative to chiropractic education and present them to the House of Counselors or the Executive Board without first consulting the membership of the Council proper.

The second session of the Council Meetings was held the afternoon of July 26, 1949, with Dr. Thure C. Peterson presiding.

The first issue that came under consideration was the matter of the United States Department of Immigration's conduct in relation to the issuance of a statement that after next November no foreign students would be allowed to enter the country on student visas for the purpose of studying chiropractic.

Dr. Nugent informed the Council that this decision of the Immigration Department was made on the fact that as yet Chiropractic Colleges were not fully recognized as institutions of higher education.

He informed the Council, however, that he had been in Washington, D.C., on this matter, and that as a result of personal good connections he had been able to contact the proper people and he felt certain that he was able to convince them that Chiropractic Colleges merit their full recognition and cooperation. It was Dr. Nugent's opinion that the matter would experience favorable resolution.

Dr. Nugent again emphasized the significance and importance of a good library in all Chiropractic Colleges. He outlined various methods that might be employed in gathering good texts for the same, including:

a.   Student book gathering campaign

b.   College Alumni Association project

c.   various federal government publications are good, and they can be listed as recognized texts.

d.   the various publishing houses are always willing to present a teacher's or desk copy of books that are ordered in numbers over 10.

e.   buying up the libraries of deceased private practitioners.

Dr. Nugent also suggested that every college subscribe to some of the better professional and scientific publications and journals. He encouraged the Council members to become members of the American Association of Science, and to subscribe to the publications of the Smithsonian Institute which come out weekly.

Dr. Peterson then made inquiry about the student questionnaire coming from student representatives of the Los Angeles College of Chiropractic. It was the general consensus that it was somewhat unqualified on the part of student organizations from any college to ask for certain vital college statistics and that such should be discouraged and that inquiries of this type should be directed directly to Dr. Nugent as Director of Education.

Dr. Nugent did insist that the accredited colleges should be more exacting in maintaining the necessary statistical data of their organization and that this should include a very concise and definite accounting system as pertaining to the college finances, the cost of instruction, etc..

Again Dr. Nugent mentioned the importance of this because of the need for the same in his and Dr. Murphy's efforts to get our colleges recognized by the federal government.

Dr. Nugent then recommended to the Council that it be determined what the standard professional color should be so that at graduations the same colors and hood be used by all accredited colleges. He was instructed by the Council to make a full investigation of this matter and to report his findings at the next meeting.

Dr. Parr then suggested that the accredited colleges also adopt a standard professional oath. Dr. Budden and others suggested that this matter of a professional oath be left up to the individual colleges, thus allowing for a certain amount of desired individuality.

Dr. Peterson then drew the Council's attention to some correspondence that he had had with Dr. Martin of the Los Angeles College pertaining to standardization of semesters or quarters, the teaching of chiropractic, and text books.

Dr. Nugent encouraged the Council members to recognize the importance of this because of the problems that had been had with the V.A. as the result of the heterogeneous manner in which the chiropractic colleges conducted their schedules. He suggested that to date the 16 week semester of 4 lunar months with 3 semesters in the year, or a total of 48 college weeks, had worked out the best for the majority of the colleges and recommended that this be adopted.

It was decided that this matter should receive further and more careful discussion at the mid-year meeting.

At this time the issues of Basic Science Boards, Chiropractic Boards of Examiners, and certain Chiropractic legal problems that had arisen in various states, were brought up for general discussion.

Dr. Norman E. Osborne, a member of the Accrediting Committee and the newly appointed Secretary of the Maryland State Board of Chiropractic Examiners, was asked to review the situation in Maryland. Dr. Osborne reported that the Board, as well as the State Association, had been beleaguered by a lot of trouble arising in the Chiropractic College in Baltimore as headed by Dr. Dean. According to Drs. Osborne and Nugent this institution had failed to qualify for approval by the accrediting committee, however had obtained a temporary recognition from the Maryland State Dept. of Education. Several months ago two of the graduates from this college had applied for examination by the Maryland Chiropractic Board and they were advised that they did not qualify. Consequently, Dr. Dean mandamused the board and that, to date, the State Supreme Court had not ruled because the judge on the case was on a foreign trip.

Dr. Osborne then reviewed the recent legislative effort of the State Assn. in Maryland. The effort pertained to including in the legal interpretation of Chiropractic the usage of physiotherapy and then to make all people using physiotherapy, other than medical physiotherapists, subject to examination and supervision by the State Board of Chiropractic Examiners. Dr. Osborne advised the Council that these efforts were bitterly fought by Dr. Dean, as well as the Palmer School of Chiropractic. However, notwithstanding this opposition, the bills went through and just recently the Governor signed them, and they have become a matter of law.

Dr. Peterson then advised the Council that on Thursday morning the House of Delegates were going to consider and air the matter of the charges made against Drs. Janse and Nugent by the International Chiropractors Association and the Palmer School of Chiropractic as they relate to the Iowa and Illinois situation.

At this time Dr. Janse was called on to explain the position of the National College in all this. Dr. Janse said that with reference to the Iowa matter the college had made no official declaration of attitude, but that under the auspices of the Student Council several telegrams were sent to the Iowa State Legislature recommending that the Iowa Basic Science Law for the time being be not repealed, for the simple reason that in Iowa the Chiropractic Law only required 18 months of resident training and that if the Basic Science Law were set aside it would flood the state with short term graduates. Another reason why these students felt that the law should not be repealed at the present time was the objective fact that the Iowa Board, of all Basic Science Boards is the easiest and affords the most extensive reciprocal privileges. Consequently, students from all chiropractic colleges, as well as osteopathic and medical schools were using the Board as a springboard into more difficult states, including Michigan, Colorado, Wisconsin, South Dakota, Oregon, and Arkansas.

Then Dr. Janse proceeded to read a letter written to him by Dr. Ben H. Peterson, Secretary of the Iowa Basic Science Board, which in substance revealed that National College students were not the only chiropractic students that had sent in telegrams, that in fact, the students from the Palmer School had also sent in telegrams requesting the maintenance of the Basic Science Law in Iowa. (Incidentally, this letter is available and contained in the files of the Secretary of the Council) The Illinois situation was then fully reviewed. Dr. Janse outlined the licensure situation in Illinois. Originally the chiropractor was licensed under the "other practitioners act", which existed up to 1927. This act provided that all practitioners other than medical men should be examined by a board consisting of 2 osteopaths, 2 chiropractors, and 2 naprapaths, and that all schools of these respective professions teaching a course of a minimum of 32 resident months would have their graduates recognized. The "other practitioners license" was a broad one even including the practice of obstetrics. However, even then in Illinois there were a goodly number of unlicensed short term practitioners and they continued to endeavor to obtain an independent board of chiropractic examiners.

Because of this constant agitation for a license, the State Department of Education eventually had the legislature revise the medical act to include the practice of chiropractic. The unlicensed practitioners were given the opportunity of qualifying by taking six months special training and taking a special board.

This of course did away with the "other practitioners act" and included chiropractic under the medical act, and Dr. Dagger was appointed as the chiropractic representative on the medical board.

At this time a goodly number of the unlicensed practitioners proceeded to qualify, others refused to do so. Since this time they have yearly proposed a bill for the purpose of establishing an independent board of chiropractic examiners.

This effort in itself was most worthy, the only fault being that each bill was of a limited and low educational standard quality, attended by such liberal "grandfather clause" privileges that it would not only have licensed the unlicensed practitioners but also given almost free entry for many people still in Chiropractic colleges.

This year the efforts of the unlicensed group because of a large political pot took on rather a formidable disposition. As a result many of the licensed chiropractors began to ask why National College, being in Illinois, and the Illinois Chiropractic Society an NCA affiliate, didn't do something about it.

Resultantly, careful considerations were made by the college administration, the board of directors of the Illinois Chiropractic

Society, and also Dr. Nugent as Director of Education NCA. It was decided to withstand the House Bill #484 on the following reasons:

(1) That the total amount of 45 minute class hours required by the Bill were not commensurate with the minimum 60 minute class hour requirements of the NCA.

(2) The interpretation of Chiropractic practice, especially the clause stating that scientific instruments could only be used for analysis (rather than diagnosis) caused the licensed group to feel that the traditional practice of Chiropractic in Illinois would be reduced and limited.

(3) The almost unlimited grandfather clause provision would not only grant licenses, on a bob-tail examination, to the unlicensed practitioners, but also to all students in Chiropractic Colleges regardless of the length of course of training. In fact, the Bill gave the specific date of Dec. 31, 1950. It is quite obvious that this date gave leeway to hundreds of 18 month students.

(4) Furthermore, the bill in no way stipulates the amount of resident months that the ostensible 4500, 45-minute hours should cover.

It was further divulged that as the result of this pending legislation nearly all of the students in short term colleges became residents of the State of Illinois within a week-end's notice.

Because of these primary reasons the Illinois Chiropractic Society and the Administration of the National College of Chiropractic saw fit to fight the passage of the Bill.

Unfortunately, these efforts were of course, subject to the criticism and displeasure of certain elements, who rather verbosely and vehemently conducted a program of severe criticism.

Dr. Budden then outlined the situation in the State of Washington. Here again, a similar element proposed a chiropractic bill and concurrently a bill to do away with the Basic Science Board. Everyone, of course, is aware of the fact that the administration of the Basic Science Board in the State of Washington has been fully under the prejudiced control of the state medical society and consequently to do away with the Board in Washington represents a prevailing desire.

However, the proposed chiropractic legislation in Washington was of the short term and limited quality. Consequently, Dr. Budden and Dr. Nugent proceeded to suggest certain amendments designed to raise the educational requirements up to the NCA standards, and for this effort they and the NCA were severely criticized by the "short term" proponents of Washington.

Dr. Nugent also gave a detailed report on the circumstances and the happenings that transpired in Nevada. In this state, for a goodly number of years, the Board was fully dominated by the short term proponents even to the extent where graduates from NCA Colleges, especially those that taught physiotherapy, found it most difficult to obtain a license.

Dr. Nugent, upon careful investigation, found that the board members had conducted rather shady measures in the process of administering the board. Such as absconding with certain moneys, and secondly, permitting students of certain chiropractic colleges to take the board after only having been in college for no more than 8 months.

In his action against the board, Dr. Nugent brought this to the attention of the State Officials. Consequently, the entire board was released and a new board appointed and given specific instructions as to how to conduct themselves.

Dr. Nugent also cited the case of the intended "squeeze play" by the short termers in the state of Georgia, but how finally this matter had been straightened. Dr. Nugent warned the members of the Council not to be taken in by the propaganda of the opposing element and advised the Council members that the NCA recognized colleges would have to stand together in the effort to defeat the attempt by the opposition to mitigate and disparage the NCA college program.

For the information of those members of the Council who did not have the chance of attending the meeting of the House of Delegates Thursday morning, Drs. Nugent and Janse were called upon to reiterate their position in relation to the Basic Science issue, the Illinois issue as well as other chiropractic licensure problems throughout the country.

Dr. Nugent, speaking first, gave a vigorous and thorough explanation of his position in relation to low standard colleges, laws, and tendencies. He recapitulated in terse terms what had transpired in Nevada, Washington, Arizona, Georgia, Connecticut, and Illinois.

Dr. Janse followed with an explanation of the National College's position on the Illinois issue as supported by the Illinois Chiropractic Society and NCA affiliate.

In relation to the Iowa situation Dr. Nugent called on Mr. Max Putnam, the Public Relations Director of the Iowa Chiropractic Association, and his assistant, a young woman who was the chairman of the State Republican Women League. Both people definitely verified Drs. Nugent and Janse's position and denounced the rather dishonest methods employed by certain elements in the profession to belittle the NCA and its representation.

It is to be mentioned that the House of Delegates proffered Drs. Nugent and Janse a rousing and unanimous vote of confidence and support.

At this time Dr. William Percy, Secretary of the California Board of Chiropractic Examiners was invited to sit in with the Council in discussion about certain problems that had arisen in California.

Essentially Dr. Nugent led the discussion and the following were the pertinent points considered:

(1) The California Board members, in order to straighten out a rather heterogeneous situation in California had a member of the Attorney General's office write an interpretation of the law which involved certain stipulations that were somewhat confounding.

(2) This interpretation insisted that the applicant for examination must show 500 hours in physiotherapy training. In fact, originally it was concluded that only colleges teaching physiotherapy would be recognized, however after carefully consulting with Dr. Nugent the board members all agreed that the physiotherapy training could be obtained by a graduate from a college teaching chiropractic exclusively at another college and still have his credit recognized by the board.

(3) It was the contention of Dr. Nugent that the distribution of required hours over certain subjects was a little inordinate and slightly beyond the possibility of expectation.

(4) Furthermore, that the wording of the interpretation was somewhat too demanding and compromising and probably would lead to some future misunderstanding.

Finally, after a great deal of discussion it was concluded that Dr. Percy would relay to his associates on the Board the matters discussed and he expressed the confidence that all issues could be properly interpreted and disposed of. And it was concluded that Dr. Nugent, at the earliest convenience should meet with the Board and go over these matters carefully. Dr. Percy expressed the confident and sincere intent of the Board, but insisted that for so many years California had been the melting pot of such a heterogeneous academic chiropractic picture that they were going to hold the line close and would not permit any digressions or deviations.

In summation the decision was derived and understood that the California Board would lend recognition to all NCA accredited colleges and that if any of these colleges did not teach physiotherapy their graduates would have to qualify in this subject by taking extra work at some recognized college that did.

Final session of the Council was held on Thursday afternoon, July 28, 1949, Dr. Thure C. Peterson presiding.

Dr. Peterson informed the members of the Council that this being the time when the election of new officers was in order he considered it necessary to proceed with this matter first.

It was unanimously agreed upon that Dr. Peterson be retained as president of the Council for the next year, and that Dr. Janse be retained as secretary.

Dr. Nugent then brought up the suggestion that efforts be made to encourage the various chiropractic and medical boards to proffer recognition to all NCA accredited colleges en masse.

Dr. Nugent also stressed the importance of continuously trying to standardize the courses of the accredited colleges so that students transferring will not be confronted with too many hazards of confusion in relation to subject mix-ups.

Dr. Nugent gave a report on the meeting that he and Dr. Janse had attended, as held by the National Society of Basic Science Boards. Dr. Nugent told the Council that both he and Dr. Janse had been well received and although neither one part participated very actively in the discussions but simply listened and observed the opinion was garnered that the majority of the Basic Science Board members were men of integrity and sincere intent.

Dr. Nugent advised the Council that he had been invited to give a paper on chiropractic education at the next meeting of the association and that he had accepted the invitation.

By this time, Dr. Walter Fischer of Fort Worth, Texas, had been introduced to the Council and he was asked by Dr. Peterson to detail the nature and disposition of the Texas situation.

Dr. Fisher advised the Council that to date in Texas there was an existing Chiropractic Law, and concurrently a rather vague and ambiguous Basic Science Law. In summation the following points of explanation were brought out:

(1) The chiropractic law that was passed proffered licensure to all chiropractors actively engaged in practice in Texas, or to those who at present were not actively engaged but had been actively engaged in practice in Texas at some past time for a period of no less than 5 years, as well as to all students in Chiropractic colleges who could prove that they had been residents of the state of Texas for the greater part of their life.

(2) The Basic Science Law requires that the applicant possess 2 years of pre-professional college education of a liberal arts or general nature.

(3) A person can be exempt from the Basic Science Law if he can show where he has obtained no less than 60 semester hours of training in the Basic Science subjects at the University of Texas or some other college or University accredited by the North Central Association on the Accrediting of Colleges and Universities.

(4) The basic science subjects in which this training must be obtained are: anatomy, physiology, bacteriology, pathology, chemistry, and public health.

(5) The future Chiropractic Board of Examiners would possess the authority to determine the qualifications of the Chiropractic college to be recognized.

(6) That the chiropractic law stipulated the requirements of 4 years of 8 months each and including in the curriculum a minimum of 120 semester hours.

Dr. Nugent advised Dr. Fischer that 120 semester hours actually only represented the equivalence of approximately 2400, 60-minute hours as ordinarily taught in a chiropractic college, and that such actually was not sufficient for a proper chiropractic education.

At this point Dr. Nugent insisted that the tendency to compare chiropractic education with an undergraduate education in the liberal arts be discontinued. He contended that the standard 4 year course in Chiropractic far extended the standard college course leading to an ordinary baccalaureate degree and consequently, the amount of semester hours for a chiropractic course should not be estimated on the basis of the standard baccalaureate college course.

It was decided that the mid-year meeting is to be held in Chicago because of the geographical conveniences.

It was unanimously concluded that much good had been accomplished and that definite ideas as to future effort and progress had been precipitated.

Minutes of the COUNCIL ON EDUCATION of the NATIONAL CHIROPRACTIC ASSOCIATION,
Minutes of the mid-year meeting held in Chicago at the Sherman Hotel,
February 1st, 2nd and 3rd, 1950, with Dr. Thure C. Peterson,
President of the Council, presiding at all of the meetings.

Those attending the meetings were:
(A) Members of the Committee on Educational Standards:
Dr. John J. Nugent, Director of Education, National Chiropractic Association, 92 Norton Street, New Haven, Connecticut
Dr. Edward H. Gardner, 2727 South Vermont Avenue, Los Angeles, California
Dr. George A. Bauer, 1608 Bull Street, Columbia, South Carolina
Dr. Walter B. Wolf, Eureka, South Dakota
Dr. Norman E. Osborne, 3 Broadway St., Hagerstown, Maryland
(B) Representatives of the accredited and professionally accredited educational institutions -
Dr. W.A. Budden, President, Western States College of Chiropractic, 4525 Southeast 63rd Avenue, Portland 6, Oregon
Drs. James N. Firth, President and Arthur Hendricks, Vice President, Lincoln Chiropractic College, Inc., 633 N. Pennsylvania Street, Indianapolis 4, Indiana
Dr. Thure C. Peterson, Chiropractic Institute of New York, 152 - 42nd Street, New York 18, N.Y.
Dr. Ralph J. Martin, President, Los Angeles College of Chiropractic, 920 Venice Boulevard, Los Angeles 15, Calif.
Dr. John B. Wolfe, President, Northwestern College of Chiropractic, 608 Nicolette Avenue, Minneapolis 2, Minnesota
Dr. Paul O. Parr, President, Carver College of Chiropractic, 522 Northwest 9th Street, Oklahoma City, Oklahoma
Dr. William N. Coggins, Dean and Rev. G. Hues, Associate, Logan Basic College of Chiropractic, 7701 Florissant Road, St. Louis 21, Missouri
Dr. A.J. Darling, Member of the Board of Directors, Kansas State Chiropractic College, 629 North Broadway, Wichita, Kansas
Dr. H.C. Harring, President and Ralph A. Power, Dean, Missouri Chiropractic Institute Inc., 3117 Lafayette Avenue, St. Louis 4, Missouri
Dr. R.O. Mueller, Dean, Canadian Memorial Chiropractic College, 252 Bloor Street West, Toronto 5, Ontario
Dr. Joseph Janse, President and Mr. Charles A. Miller, Vice President, National College of Chiropractic, 20 N. Ashland Boulevard, Chicago 7, Illinois
(C) Special invited guests:
Dr. Carl Cleveland, Jr., Dean, Cleveland College of Chiropractic, 3724 Troost Street, Kansas City, Missouri
Dr. Homer G. Beatty, University of Natural Healing Arts, 1075 Logan Street, Denver 3, Colorado
Dr. Ben L. Parker, Dean, Texas Chiropractic College, San Pedro Park, San Antonio, Texas

Morning Meeting - February 1st, 1950 (open)
The first matter of discussion was Point 3 on the published agenda and which read as follows:
Discussion of arbitrary Veterans Administration rulings as have affected the colleges during the past year.
The question arose as to whether something could not be done with reference to this matter of Chiropractic Colleges still being considered by the Veterans Administration as being little more than trade schools.
It was the consensus of opinion that the realization of a full status of being institutions of higher education would involve more time and additional effort on the part of Doctors Nugent and Murphy.
Dr. Firth advised the group that the Lincoln College, although not fully realizing its status as a corporation until February 1949, had not been made subject to Change 9 of the Veterans Administration rulings. He advised that the legal staff of the college had obtained full assurance from Washington to go ahead with the customary procedure of billing and as a result, he felt that in the instance of the Lincoln College, the Veterans Administration had been most cooperative.
Dr. Budden stated that in relation to the Western States College, the officers of the Veterans Administration in that district had been increasingly more exacting in their demands of the college. He attributed this inclination to the ever increasing tendency on the part of the Veterans Administration to cut expenses wherever possible.
Dr. Parr proffered this suggestion. He advised the Council that in Oklahoma the State Department of Education and Public Instruction, had under the prompting of the State Board of Chiropractic Examiners, granted the Carver College recognition as an institution of higher learning. Dr. Parr was certain that any of the other accredited colleges, through mediation of the State Board of Chiropractic examiners, could obtain the same clearing as institutions of higher learning for the State of Oklahoma at least.
Dr. Martin stated that the situation in California and in relation to the Los Angeles College was tough and that the institution there had been vulnerable to the inflictions of Change 9 in the Veteran's Administration rulings and consequently, the income of the institution has been rather noticeably invaded.
Dr. Peterson stated that a personal friend of his who was affiliated with the Veterans Administration advised him that there is going to be a very definite numerical cut in the personnel of the Veterans Administration and that as the result, we could all foresee greater diffi-

culty in the future because of the thus reduced proficiency.

Dr. Cleveland stated that in Kansas City, they were asked to submit and file an outline of their curriculum and that the members of the Veterans personnel told the college administration that it was most ridiculous that a chiropractic college should teach such subjects as diagnosis, etc. Resultantly, the administration of the Cleveland College invited these critics to inspect the school and also to examine the standards and necessities of the profession and in consequence, they relinquished their opposition and wholeheartedly proceeded to support the program of the college.

Dr. Firth related that in Indiana, the lobbyist, a Mr. Stump of the Indiana Medical Society, tried in every way possible to get the Lincoln College off the Veterans Administration recognized list.

Dr. Peterson then advised the group that some months ago, the administration of the Chiropractic Institute of New York had received a commission from the State of New Jersey consisting of five college professors. The general attitude of these people was of a friendly nature. Inquiry was made as to the departments of research and this commission was advised that it was not the intention of the chiropractic profession to duplicate the research done by the medical profession in various scientific and clinical phases but that the chiropractic profession was more interested in research relating to the Chiropractic concept proper. Although this commission voted 3-2 against the recognition of the Institution by the State Department of Education of New Jersey, Dr. Peterson stated that he felt that a moral victory had been won.

Dr. Janse then drew the Council's attention to a request that had been made by the Dean and Registrar of the International College of Chiropractic, 336 North Roberts Boulevard, Dayton 2, Ohio; Drs. Amos Valdiserri and Joseph Martino. This institution to date has been recognized by the Veterans Administration of the State of Ohio as well as the State Department of Education and Licensure. The student body is small and consists primarily of negro students. In a personal visit to Dr. Janse, they expressed the request that if possible, they would appreciate an official statement from the Council on Education covering the following two points -

1.   That the standard accredited course was four college years of 8-9 months each, with a minimum of 3600, 60 minute classroom hours.
2.   That a standard chiropractic curriculum necessitated a competent book list requirement, including the accepted and universally used text books, especially in the Basic Science subjects.

All members of the colleges represented were instituted to send one of their catalogs to these people and it was deemed not inordinate to have the Secretary of the Council, write an official letter to this effect. Both measures deeming to serve as verification of the degree and extent of Chiropractic education.

Dr. Firth made inquiry as to whether or not any of the other institutions had been contacted by the American Veterans Committee on discrimination against negroes. He advised that at the Lincoln College they were accepting negro students. However, that a problem had posed itself in relation to the internship of these negro people in the clinic.

Dr. Budden stated that at Western States College, they had been educating a few negro students for a goodly number of years and that at no time had any severe problems arisen.

Dr. Peterson advised the group that at the New York institution, some 9 to 14 colored students were in training and that the only difficulty that had arisen was with reference to one of the fraternities and their pledge discrimination.

Dr. Martin stated that at the Los Angeles college there were some 20 to 30 negro enrollees and that these people upon matriculating had been advised to be rather discreet and careful.

Dr. Cleveland mentioned that in his area, the problem was a rather touchy one.

Dr. Power mentioned that at the present time, they had four negro students at the Missouri college and that they had had no problems whatsoever.

Dr. Parr contended that we should frankly acknowledge and discharge properly our responsibility to the negro.

Dr. Peterson drew the Council's attention to the fact that his office had been greatly benefited by having at hand the College Blue Book, the 6th edition, 1950, prepared by Huber Wm. Hut and Christian E. Buckel; Yonkers on the Hudson, New York, price $10.00. This manual contains a brief but competent description of the National Chiropractic Association Educational Program, as well as a registry of the accredited Chiropractic institutions.

Dr. Peterson was able to obtain this inclusion in this manual and it was the consensus of opinion of the Council that he had performed an invaluable service for the profession.

Dr. Cleveland advised the group that in Missouri, the private and trade schools had organized themselves in the form of a protective association, in the meetings of which, their respective problems in relation to the Veterans Administration were aired. At one of these meetings, a decision was obtained from the Veterans Administration which made it impossible for the Veterans Administration to hold up old contracts while negotiating for new ones with the schools and colleges.

Dr. Janse made inquiry as to what the other school men, as well as the council in general, deemed advisable in relation to the G.E.D. tests. Dr. Firth proffered the information that the University of Indiana recognized these tests and that all Veterans were accepted if they possess a diploma as issued under the G.E.D. program. Dr. Budden advised the group that in his experience, many of the Veterans with G.E.D. equivalencies portrayed a superior knowledge than the average juvenile high school graduate.

Dr. Peterson made inquiry with reference to the granting of advanced standing to students transferring from other colleges. In substance, the following decisions were precipitated:

1.   In the case of a student transferring from one accredited chiropractic college to another, his work should be fully honored and he

should receive full class hour credit as long as his Semesters were complete, but should not receive any credit for a partially completed Semester or quarter, regardless of how competent his work might have been.

2. In relation to applicants for entrance into Chiropractic colleges who are immigrants and possessive of a medical degree from European schools of medicine, they should not receive more than two years credit by any of the accredited chiropractic colleges.

3. Increasing care and caution should be exhibited by the accredited colleges in granting advanced standing for work done by applicants in non-accredited and probably defunct chiropractic and medical institutions.

4. All applicants with foreign high school training should be advised to have their work evaluated by the State Department of Education. This of course would protect them when the necessity of evaluating their equivalency arose.

5. Frequent requests have been received, especially from the recognized chiropractic associations in Switzerland and Denmark, that the accredited colleges refrain from granting matriculation to foreign applicants with medical backgrounds with the intention of taking their chiropractic education back into the medical ranks. A decision was passed that in the case of applicants from Switzerland, Denmark and South Africa, they should not be accepted until a letter of approval be received from the recognized chiropractic body of that Country.

6. It was also decided that a transferee from any of the other accredited colleges and wishing to obtain a degree from the institution to which he had transferred, must spend a minimum of one college year at that institution regardless of how much previous training he might have had at the institution from which he transferred.

7. The question arose as to what to do with Palmer transferees. Dr. Peterson advised that at the New York Institute they were required to put in a full two years before they could obtain their degree. Dr. Firth stated that at Lincoln College, the Palmer graduates were accepted as postgraduates and issued a postgraduate certificate and were permitted to retain their Palmer degree. Dr. Cleveland advised the group that at the Cleveland College, the Veterans Administration had made the ruling that the Palmer graduate had obtained his initial objective and consequently could not do undergraduate work and must sign up for special postgraduate training. Dr. Parr contested this statement by this example, that in Oklahoma, a ruling was handed down that if a State requirement is more than 18 months, the Palmer graduate possessing his degree has not attained his objective for this certain State and thus may re-enter undergraduate training. Dr. Firth advised the group that the Palmer School of Chiropractic will not issue any transcript of their advanced training beyond their regular 18 months of undergraduate course and consequently it would be literally impossible to evaluate any Palmer work beyond 18 months.

8. The question was then brought up as to how much credit an individual should receive as the result of varying years of pre-medical training at recognized state universities and colleges. It was finally decided that these cases represented individual problems that should be carefully and personally considered and that it was not improper to give full credit for those subjects that found their parallel in the curriculum of the accredited chiropractic colleges.

Dr. Peterson then brought up the question as to what can be done to induce the Chiropractic State Boards to refrain from recognizing an 18 to 24 month diploma and simply a certification of additional work done at another institution when the state law requirements are beyond the 24 months level. It was Dr. Firth's opinion that very little could be done and he cited the case of the States of Connecticut and Maryland where the Attorney General had ruled that this procedure was permissible. Dr. Peterson contended that the Palmer graduate should not be permitted to use the accredited colleges simply as the vehicles of qualification when basically their allegiance and attitudes still belonged to the short term concept.

It was also suggested that the transferring of students from one accredited college to another accredited college should be discouraged as much as possible and that he should not be accepted by the school to which he wants to transfer unless his reasons are legitimate; based upon geographical, economic or familial exigency and if possible, a letter of approval from the Dean of the College from which he transfers should accompany his application. It was thought that this decorum would help to avoid misunderstandings and reduce the severity of undue competition.

Dr. Peterson then assigned the responsibility to Drs. Budden, Firth, and Martin to draw up a set of recommendations to be presented at the next meeting in relation to certain set rules of evaluation of the rating for advanced students and the conduct of transferees.

Dr. Firth made the recommendation that in the case of Postgraduate applicants, the school should be allowed to use their own judgment and that in the case of men with medical training, they should receive full credit but should be required, regardless of the amount of medical training they might have had, to put in a minimum of one year in basic chiropractic training and clinic work.

Dr. Peterson then appointed three committees -

1. A committee to serve in helping to prepare a program for the next annual NCA convention. This consisted of Drs. Budden, Firth, Peterson and Janse.

2. A committee on research for the purpose of determining what research projects could be conducted at the recognized colleges and this group included Drs. Budden, Wolfe and Muller.

3. An agenda committee to advise the Council as to the points of greatest importance and this consisted of Drs. Martin and Firth.

The meeting was adjourned until the afternoon when the closed session of the council was to be held.

Afternoon Meeting (Closed)

The accrediting committee was asked to give its report and the following was submitted by Dr. Norman Osborne, a member of this committee:

1. Those present included Dr. John J. Nugent, Director of Education, Dr. Edward H. Gardner, Dr. Walter B. Wolf, Dr. George A. Bauer, Dr. Norman E. Osborne.
2. The matter of developing a uniform transcript of credit form was thoroughly discussed and a subcommittee, consisting of Drs. Nugent and Osborne was appointed to create and present such a transcript.
3. The following resolution was adopted by the accrediting committee and to be submitted to the full membership of the Council:
    BE IT RESOLVED THAT the Council of Education of the National Chiropractic Association be recognized as the sole accrediting agency for the Chiropractic profession and that any school accepting a rating from any other alleged Chiropractic Council or Committee will automatically lose its approved membership in the Educational Council of the National Chiropractic Association.
4. Drs. Budden and Janse and Mr. Miller were to be officially invited to sit in with the committee to discuss the problem of granting the N.D. degree as well as the D.C. degree from the colleges with which they are affiliated, with the recommendation that an attempt be made to find some solution in more thoroughly differentiating the issuance of these degrees and the possible advisability of setting a time whereafter the issuance of the N.D. degree would be discontinued.
5. Dr. Nugent reported on his complete survey and inspection of the National College and has already filed his report with the Illinois commission and will file this report with the accrediting committee. Dr. Nugent has been requested by the Illinois commission to make a similar inspection and submit like reports on the other chiropractic institutions that to date are recognized by the Illinois Department of Education and Registration.
6. A long discussion followed by a statement of policy adopted by the committee resulted in asking the Council to urge the various state boards of examiners to accept the standards set up by the Council as the criteria upon which they could base their approval of chiropractic colleges.
7. Dr. Nugent gave a detailed report on the Northwestern College of Chiropractic in Minneapolis, especially with the acquiring of new school property and the solving of its many problems. This report gave evidence of the excellent progress that had been made at this institution and represented a very significant progressive step.
8. Dr. Nugent also gave a report of the final inspection of the Carver College of Chiropractic and presented his recommendations for full approval of this institution.
9. Reports were also made with reference to the progress that was being made at the Kansas State College of Chiropractic.
10. Dr. Nugent presented a report in detail pertaining to the Cleveland College of Chiropractic and voiced the opinion that remarkable progress had been made and that the administrative officers of this institution were doing everything in their power to ready this institution for accrediting.
11. Dr. Nugent also advised the committee that he had visited the Booker T. Washington College of Chiropractic for negro students at Independence, Mo. but that his impressions of the institutions were not too substantial.
12. The following discussions resulted in consequence to Dr. Osborne's report for the accrediting committee:
    A. It was moved and seconded that the Carver College of Chiropractic be recognized as a fully accredited institution and that its rating in all NCA literature and correspondence be changed from that of provisional accrediting, to fully accredited status.
    B. Dr. Janse was instructed to write the Board of Directors of the institution, advising them of this decision.
    C. Dr. Nugent advised the Council that several other Chiropractic colleges were soliciting inspection by the accrediting committee and that at the next meeting, he would have a report ready with reference to their circumstances.
    D. Dr. Nugent emphasized the significance of the proposed resolution as submitted by the accrediting committee with reference to recognizing but one accrediting agency, namely, the NCA Council on Education and punishing any provisionally or fully accredited college by dis-fellowship if the administration of this college proceeded to seek recognition by any other alleged chiropractic accrediting agency. He mentioned that if such were not done, the entire integrity and authority of the Council on Education would be undermined and would lend credence to opposing chiropractic groups. He mentioned that the International Chiropractic Association also had an accrediting agency which was attempting to usurp authority and representation of the Council on Education and that if any school recognized the authority of the ICA accrediting agency, it had no business in the membership of the council.
    E. Dr. Parr raised the question on the mechanics of the resolution, namely, what was an accredited school to do when another accrediting agency lists the school, when this institution had not solicited recognition. It was Dr. Budden's opinion that if other agencies deemed to accredit NCA accredited colleges, those colleges should repudiate or completely ignore the same. Dr. Firth verified this contention by stating that the Lincoln College had fully ignored its being listed among the accredited schools as announced by the ICA.
    F. The resolution was re-read and then its adoption was moved upon and seconded and the affirmative vote was unanimous.
    G. Dr. Martin then made the inquiry with reference to that part of Dr. Osborne's report that related to the suggested effort of encouraging the state boards of examiners to use the standards of the Council as the criterion of recognizing chiropractic colleges. Dr. Osborne said that it would be most beneficial to the Council in general if the state boards all over the country could be encouraged to accept and recognize the accrediting procedures of the Council.
Dr. Nugent mentioned that certain of the Chiropractic state boards of examiners seemed to want to remain as autonomous groups of

authority working independent of the Council or its efforts and as a result, the various chiropractic colleges are constantly being confronted by varying and heterogeneous demands and concepts as stipulated by the individual boards.

Dr. Peterson asserted that it basically revolved around two primary issues - one, the necessary effort of getting all state boards of chiropractic examiners to recognize all NCA accredited colleges and secondly, inducing all the state boards of chiropractic examiners to recognize NCA accredited colleges only.

    H.   Dr. Parr expressed the opinion that caution and care must be taken not to alienate the various boards of chiropractic examiners; that the council on state boards of chiropractic examiners was not too friendly toward this council. This opinion was verified by other members of the Council.

Then Dr. Firth made inquiry about those chiropractic boards such as California and Idaho who demanded of their examinees, qualified training in physiotherapy. It seems that the state boards of those states particularly, were rather hesitant in proffering recognition to those NCA accredited colleges that did not teach physiotherapy.

It was the unanimous consensus of opinion that those state boards should fully recognize the NCA accredited colleges that do not teach physiotherapy and that the graduates from these institutions, before taking their state boards, should be required to do extra work in those accredited institutions in the physiotherapy department.

    I.   Both Drs. Nugent and Firth asserted that there were a number of state boards that would only recognize NCA accredited colleges. Dr. Bauer stated that in South Carolina, state board recognition was only proffered those institutions that met the NCA standards, but the institutions need not belong to the Council.

    J.   Dr. Budden stated that if a chiropractic college met the full qualifications of the state requirements, it can proceed to demand and obtain recognition by that state board, regardless of what accrediting agency recognizes or does not recognize it.

    K.   Dr. Nugent said that this matter of relations with the various state boards of chiropractic examiners should be a matter of careful conditioning and education and that at no time should any effort of coercion be demonstrated.

    L.   Dr. Peterson proffered the suggestion that at the Washington convention, an informal effort be made to establish a conduct with the Council on State boards of examiners. All members of the Council felt that this effort of establishing contact should be made in a most casual manner so that in no way the members of the Council on state boards would have reason to believe that pressure was being placed on them.

    M.   Dr. Martin then made the inquiry as to what could be done to obtain a standardized and uniform conduct on the part of State boards of chiropractic examiners in relation to all chiropractic colleges. Dr. Nugent said that some of the state boards were prejudiced toward some colleges and favored others and he cited the example of the State of Utah, where the State board of examiners refused to recognize any of the colleges that taught physiotherapy.

Another matter of discussion arose with reference to the granting of credits from some of the smaller and less virile chiropractic colleges. It was the consensus of opinion that care should be exercised so as not to grant too much credit for training in these institutions.

Dr. Budden proffered the suggestion that all state boards should be encouraged to recognize the evaluations of transferees as made by the registrars of the accredited colleges.

    N.   Dr. Nugent contended that a committee should be formed to evaluate the courses of such colleges as the Palmer, The Ross O'Neil, The Columbia and the Oakland schools of Chiropractic; that this committee should submit their suggestions for evaluation to the Council for approval and thus probably standardize the advanced standing. Dr. Nugent mentioned that this would discourage the not uncommon shopping around by students from these institutions among the accredited colleges. Dr. Nugent also mentioned that the appraisal of transferees from these institutions should not be of a blank variety but that the students qualifications in each listed subject should be appraised and furthermore, that a very careful estimation be made of the number of class hours and the subject matter contained within each course. It was Dr. Peterson's contention that Dr. Nugent should be the man to make these appraisals and to set up the standard of evaluation.

    13.   Dr. Mueller asked the question as to how much latitude each individually accredited college might have in arranging their curriculum and contained courses. He advised the group that at the Canadian Memorial College, plans were in process of using what is known as the horizontal rather than the perpendicular method of teaching, namely, by studying the anatomy - gross and microscopic; the physiology, the pathology, the chemistry and diagnosis of systems of the body, in proper sequence rather than anatomy in general, etc. A rather extended discussion resulted. Dr. Muller enumerated a number of changes. On the other hand, Drs. Firth and Janse expressed the opinions that at the Lincoln and National Colleges respectively, a change like that would impose almost insurmountable problems.

Dr. Mueller also advised the group that in Canada, as an entrance requirement to the chiropractic college, they were setting a standard of five years of high school or four years of high school with one year of college and thus measuring up to the minimum entrance requirements of all professional colleges in Canada. Dr. Mueller made inquiry as to whether the Council would approve of such a move in Canada. Dr. Budden thought the Canadian College should be encouraged in this venture as it represented a pioneering experiment that might lend information to the other colleges; consequently, Dr. Nugent suggested a motion, that the Canadian Memorial College of Chiropractic be encouraged, if it desires to adopt the horizontal teaching plan and also to raise their entrance requirements as announced by Dr. Mueller.

Dr. Budden then made mention of his belief that the Council on Education should be released from any obligations to the

Chiropractic Research Foundation. Furthermore, that those in charge of the Chiropractic Research Foundation should be properly instructed and oriented as to what their prerogatives are in relation to the Council and its members and that they should desist from instructing the Council members as to what research they should or should not do. It seems that an infrequent misunderstanding has resulted between the NCA Council on Research and the Chiropractic Research Foundation to the extent where the former felt that the Chiropractic Research Foundation was stipulating suggestions and instructions that reached beyond its authority.

14. Dr. Janse then advised the members of the Council that he had received an invitation from Dr. Norman Witt, President of the American Association of Basic Science Boards, inviting Dr. Nugent and himself to attend the annual meeting of this association on February 6th, here in Chicago at the Palmer House. Dr. Janse wanted to know what the wishes of the Council were in this respect.

It was moved and seconded that Drs. Nugent and Janse be instructed to attend those meetings.

Meetings of the COUNCIL ON EDUCATION
Heard February 2nd 1950.

These meetings were open and Dr. Thure C. Peterson presided.

Points 5 and 6 of the printed agenda were the first subjects of consideration. These points being as follows:

5. Evaluation of merits of quarter and semester systems.

6. Discussion of advisability of converting to units in bulletins of the approved colleges.

The following discussions ensued -

Dr. Martin indicated that he preferred the quarter system because it did necessitate a desired Summer vacation.

Dr. Peterson stated that a conversion from the semester to the quarter system depended upon whether or not the accelerated course is to be considered.

Dr. Wolfe stated that the quarter system allowed for greater flexibility in arranging the curriculum in conforming with the necessary splitting of subjects. Furthermore, it allowed the breaking up of courses into smaller units. It allowed for the employment of part-time instructors with greater proficiency and it certainly was advantageous to the student because the quarter system was less tiresome.

Dr. Firth stated that at Lincoln College, they were on the semester system and matriculated three times per year and that each semester consisted of sixteen weeks and that it would indeed be very difficult for them to convert to the quarter system.

Dr. Janse expressed the same situation as existing at the National College.

Dr. Budden expressed his favor of the quarter system and stated that they had been using it at the Western States College for a goodly number of years.

Dr. Nugent concluded the discussion by stating that a committee should be set up to study the problem very carefully and probably make a report to the Council at the next meeting.

Dr. Peterson then drew the council members' attention to Point 6, with reference to the conversion of the 60 minute class hours into semester or quarter units. Dr. Nugent advised that most professional colleges are now on the unit system. Dr. Firth contested this statement and said that in a survey made by Dr. Koch of Pennsylvania, it was found that in the majority of the professional colleges, whether on the semester or quarter system, the procedure of registering the work in class hours was still much more common.

Dr. Budden drew attention to the fact that in our chiropractic colleges, during the average semester or quarter, more work was done than in a college of Liberal Arts for the same tenure of time and that the conversion of the clock hours into semester units would probably give a number of semester units quite a bit beyond the number that the average college student is allowed to carry. He also stated that it was also a problem of conforming with the demands of chiropractic laws and state boards because to date, all of these demand the clock hour system.

Dr. Parr made the suggestion that a formal release be attached to the copy of the minutes indicating exactly what transpired at the Basic Science Association meeting and Dr. Janse was instructed to do this very thing.

15. Dr. Peterson then drew the Council's attention to a letter which he had received from Dr. W.H. McNichols, Executive Secretary of the Chiropractic Research Foundation. Following are the two pertinent paragraphs contained within this letter -

The idea, as we understand it, is that the National Council on Education will work out an overall research program and develop it at the Council's annual meeting next January. Thereafter, the Council on Public Heath and Research, working cooperatively with the National Council on Education, will make research project assignments commensurate with the distinctive abilities of college staffs. In the final analysis, the Chiropractic Research Foundation will disburse available funds for the tools of research necessary to activate the various units of the college research program.

It is understood by CRF directors that there will be no claims made by any of the participating colleges for salaried personnel or for rentals of laboratory spaces. Furthermore, the CRF board would expect that regular monthly activity reports be filed by each unit director in the college research program.

Dr. Budden, in conjunction with this matter of research, made a report by the committee assigned in relation to proposed research work that might be done at the various accredited colleges. In substance, the resolution of his report read as follows: To the Council on Education: It is the opinion of the assigned committee on research that an informal organization, composed of those who wish to engage in research among the accredited colleges, should be set up and that said organization will welcome funds from any source to encourage and advance this program. Signed - Drs. W.A. Budden, J.B. Wolfe and R.O. Mueller.

16. Dr. Martin then drew the Council's attention to the fact that the Administration and Board of Directors of the Los Angeles College of Chiropractic indicated their intentions to initiate the stipulation of two years of pre-professional college work by September 1952. It was the consensus of opinion among the Council members that the Los Angeles College of Chiropractic should receive full encouragement and as mentioned by Dr. Parr, it might serve as the wedge which will eventually make the two years of pre-professional college training a universal prerequisite throughout the profession.

17. Dr. Budden suggested that the various school men give some consideration to the possibility of only one matriculation a year with a possible two months vacation and doing away with what is generally known as the augmented course. It was moved and seconded that meetings be adjourned for the afternoon.

Dr. Firth insisted that it was alright for those who desire it, but that certainly none of the accredited institutions should be forced into the conversion from clock hours to quarter or semester units.

Dr. Nugent then stated that the crux of the whole problem was the fact that in our chiropractic colleges, we are required to teach too many of the pre-professional subjects. He stated that the time must come when such subjects as Inorganic Chemistry, Embryology, etc., should be a pre-professional requirement of each matriculant and thus, at the chiropractic colleges proper, more time could be spent on professional subjects.

Dr. Budden in substance agreed with this and stated that during the years of training at chiropractic colleges, the student at best is confronted by the great problem of qualifying for his Boards and learning those clinical necessities upon which he is dependent for his livelihood. He contended that it would proffer the student greater opportunity to learn how to think and how to reason from a clinical standpoint. He stated that if the two year pre-professional requirement is to be set up, then we should pick those colleges to which we should send our prospects for the pre-professional education; colleges that are friendly toward Chiropractic.

Dr. Parr stated that the average high school student today was poorly educated; especially is he inept in the usage of English and his ability to express himself either in writing or verbally.

Dr. Budden, as well as Dr. Nugent agreed with this, contending that high school education as a whole was most deplorable in its deficiency.

18. Dr. Peterson drew the Council's attention to Point 8, namely; Consideration of proposal of Dr. J. Everett Clark, President of the Chiropractic Association of Nevada relative to profession sponsored scholarships in Chiropractic Colleges.

Dr. Martin mentioned that he had been in contact with Dr. Clark and that the Los Angeles College had advised Dr. Clark that they would be willing to help set up scholarships if the Nevada Chiropractic Association would meet them dollar for dollar.

Dr. Coggins stated that at the Logan College, several scholarships have been set up but that to date they had not worked out too competently.

Dr. Firth stated that no professional college dependent upon student tuition can allow itself to become too involved in too many scholarships and it was the general consensus of opinion that he was right.

19. Dr. Nugent stated that today, the medical schools were rejecting hundreds of applicants and that an effort should be made to interest these men and women in chiropractic colleges. Many of the rejections, he stated, were not based upon incompetency but because of the overcrowding at medical schools.

Then, Point 7 - came in for discussion, "preparation of standardized textbook on Chiropractic Principles and Technic."

Dr. Martin mentioned that he considered this very important because it was very necessary to do away with the teaching of personalized concepts and methods; that at the Los Angeles College, a committee had been assigned to accumulate and sift and then properly classify all literature on Chiropractic Principles and Technic.

Dr. Nugent stated that for a number of years he had thought that it would be possible to set up a commission to develop a text or a set of volumes on Chiropractic Principles and Procedures and that it was his idea to have various men prepare and write certain sections in the form of a competent encyclopedia.

Dr. Budden drew the council's attention to the text Chiropractic Principles and Technique as published by the National College of Chiropractic, stating that fundamentally and basically, this was as good a text as might possibly be found or used.

Dr. Peterson advised the Council that at the New York Institute, they had proceeded to make a very careful survey of all chiropractic concept and procedure and that within a few months, a detailed report was going to be made.

Dr. Firth expressed the opinion that everyone should be encouraged to write and to publish as much as possible because there is a great need for good chiropractic literature and that throughout the profession, there existed many substantially good clinical concepts which to date had never been prepared or published.

20. Dr. Peterson then read the letter as issued by the NCA pertaining to the high pressured procedures of certain individuals selling systems and units of colonic therapy. It was the unanimous consensus of opinion that these inordinate procedures should be discouraged and stopped and that the NCA was to be complimented on its stand.

Dr. Peterson made the suggestion that during the NCA convention in Washington, the meetings of the Council should be reduced to a minimum so as to afford the various school men more time to take care of their lectures and Symposia and to go about maintaining their public relations with the field in general. Dr. Nugent then stated that at the Washington Convention he would like to have heard a faculty member seminar, lasting for two to three days and probably the subject of Anatomy might be the one to be discussed. He said that our colleges are confronted with the danger of inbreeding and that by an exchange of opinions and methods of teaching and presentation at a Seminar, these dangers would be disputed and concurrently more qualified instruction realized.

Dr. Peterson then appointed Drs. Budden, Martin and Mueller to serve as a committee on scholarship.

Now Points numbers 11, 12 and 13 came in for some discussion, but in as much as Dr. Schreiber who proposed these points was not in attendance, it was decided to hold this in abeyance until he probably at some future date could express his personal opinions as to just what he wanted to bring out with reference to their presentation.

AFTERNOON SESSION - Dr. Thure Peterson presiding.

Dr. Budden was asked to make a report on the committee on research. Dr. Budden stated that he and Drs. Wolfe and Mueller had discussed the matter rather carefully and had come to the conclusion that all of the accredited colleges should be encouraged to establish small yet significant research projects, if at all possible. However, this should be done without any fanfare and an informal research fraternity should be established; that there should be a liberal exchange of ideas and that whenever possible, competent monograms should be written, detailing the observations made in these projects and he presented from the committee the following resolution:

It is the opinion of the committee on research that an informal organization composed of those who wish to engage in research among the accredited schools should be set up. Said organization will welcome funds from any source to encourage and advance this program. The acceptance of this resolution was moved and seconded. A rather interesting and extended discussion resulted when Dr. Peterson asked all of the college men to outline some of the research projects that had been conducted at their respective institutions and what some of the more probable future projects might be. Following is a brief resume:

1. Western States College - Blood Bile in relation to Neurasthenia.
2. Lincoln College - The establishment of mathematical proof of the vertebral subluxation by precision spinography.
3. Logan College - Establishment of proof of nerve interference by spinography in sciatic neuralgia.
4. Canadian College - The study of subluxation by spinography in Enuresis.
5. Los Angeles College - A detailed study of the percentage of anatomical short legs, as well as other structural anomalies in a controlled number of cases.
6. New York Institute - The continued work of Dr. Schwartz in dynamic psychology.
7. Northwestern College - An attempt to study the influence of subluxation as induced in small animals.
8. The Cleveland College - The effects of the adjustment on the pH of the blood.
9. The Denver College - A careful survey of the Bolus as made by the Denver Post in relation to Chiropractic.
10. National College - Because of the abundance of dissection material available, a report and continued study of the effects of faulty body mechanics and spinal subluxations upon the nervous and vascular systems as demonstrable in the cadaver.

POINTS 1, 18 and 19 of the agenda were brought up for consideration.

Point 1.   Filing of regular reports by committee on accrediting.

Point 18.   Requiring periodic reports of progress by the educational director and accrediting committee chairman in the intervals between council meetings.

Point 19.   The allotment of more of the time of the educational director to problems of the National Council or the appointment of an assistant.

Dr. Nugent mentioned that he makes as many reports as often as time will permit. Furthermore, that he considered it rather inopportune to make a written report of all of his transactions and conversations with various school men over the country. He insisted that he did not feel that it would be diplomatic nor proper to publicly announce all of the problems and difficulties that he at times has encountered in bringing the accredited and provisionally accredited colleges up to their present position.

Dr. Parr insisted, however, that the Council in general and the members comprising the Council should be more competently orientated with reference to the efforts and endeavors of Dr. Nugent; otherwise as he stated, pertinent issues arise and no proper answer is available because of a lack of information.

Dr. Mueller supported Dr. Parr in this premise because as he stated, in Canada, the college Administration had to meet once a month with the Board of Directors and unless he is Dean, or fully orientated as to the actions of Dr. Nugent and the attitudes of the committee with reference to certain important issues, he at times was left severely embarrassed and unable to properly present the NCA cause.

In final decision, it was concluded that probably a monthly bulletin should be prepared at the office of the president of the council in which there would be a brief resume contained of all of the actions of the council, the accrediting committee and the director of education during the interim between meetings. This idea was accepted with unanimous approval.

Dr. Harring then made inquiry as to why it was that very little aid was proffered the chiropractors who had been arrested in Louisiana and why it was that the ICA had been allowed to assume the lead in the defense of these practitioners. In the answer to this inquiry, Dr. Nugent stated that the Executive Board of the NCA and Mr. Holmes the senior legal counsel had concluded that there was no use fighting an injunction, that the great need in Louisiana was a legislative need, i.e., the proper sponsoring of chiropractic legislation but that in as much as there was no law regulating the practice of Chiropractic, the rest of the practitioners for the practice of medicine could not legally be defended. It was also mentioned that there was some possible thought of the NCA procuring the services of Judge Simmons to handle the cases of the unlicensed practitioners for the NCA

Then the issue of Dr. Nugent's speech at the postgraduate and homecoming course of the Cleveland College of Chiropractic at Kansas City, Missouri was brought up. It seems that certain elements of the opposition, i.e., the ICA, had misconstrued Dr. Nugent's comments with reference to chiropractic state boards of examiners to the extent that the rumor was broadcast that Dr. Nugent had insisted that it will be much better if chiropractic state boards of examiners were comprised of laymen rather than doctors of chiropractic. Dr. Carl Cleveland, Jr. then advised the council as to exactly what had transpired on this occasion and he flatly stated that the inordinate rumors about Dr. Nugent's speech were false and most improper. It should be noted that that evening, a number of the members of the Council, at the invitation of Dr. Cleveland, listened to a wire recording of Dr. Nugent's speech and all could in no way detect any statement or comment that would represent any verification for the rumor broadcast. It was concluded by the entire council and every member of the council that every member of the council should assume the personal responsibility of mitigating the spread of these improper vilifications. It was also generally concluded that the members of the council should pay less heed to the vindictive promptings of other groups and organizations and that a greater effort should be expended in the maintenance of a decorum of tolerance and understanding.

Dr. Walter Wolf stated that as long as he had been a member of the accrediting committee, Dr. Nugent had always made a competent and unbiased report with reference to all of the schools and all of his actions. It was also concluded that in many respects, Dr. Nugent had too much work to do and that every effort possible should be made to lighten his load and in an informal session by the members of the council, Dr. Janse, the secretary was advised to write an official letter directed to the Executive Board, asking them to grant Dr. Nugent several weeks vacation because of the great need for rest and also to overcome a developing illness that was making his work a most difficult task. It should also be said that Dr. Nugent received a resounding vote of appreciation and confidence.

Dr. Peterson gave a report on the program committee for the NCA convention and it was concluded that further discussions pertaining to this matter would have to be conducted with Dr. L.M. Rogers, who would meet with the council on the morrow of Friday. It was generally concluded that in as much as the convention was to be held in the nation's capitol, careful and extensive effort should be made to put on the finest program possible.

The question of faculty member seminars again arose. It was finally concluded that probably during the Washington convention, time nor distance would permit such a gathering, but that probably a project of that kind could be sponsored sometime in an area centrally located so that as many faculty members of the various institutions could attend as would be possible.

It was concluded that the idea of seminars for the various instructors in given departments would be most excellent but that they would have to be carefully supervised, otherwise they may get out of hand as far as the various college administrations being properly orientated is concerned.

Dr. Nugent re-emphasized his opinion that the seminars were greatly needed because he felt that throughout the accredited colleges there should be a greater integration of teaching and furthermore, that it is imperative that throughout the chiropractic educational system, new talent be developed. In final summation, it was decided that the matter should receive continued attention and be further investigated. There was a general feeling of readiness to cooperate, yet concurrently, an attitude of some caution; probably based upon the possible expense involved and the creation of inordinate plans and details with which no college administration at the present time would be able to successfully cope.

FRIDAY, FEBRUARY 3rd MEETINGS with Dr. Thure C. Peterson presiding.

Dr. L.M. Rogers, the Executive Secretary of the NCA was in attendance. He announced that the annual convention of the NCA was to be held in Washington, D.C. from July 30th to and including August 4th at the Statler Hotel. He was concerned and interested in having the Council present ideas and suggestions with reference to the program and after rather extensive discussion and a report by the convention committee consisting of Drs. Peterson, Budden, Firth and Janse, the following suggestions were proffered:

1. Dr. Rogers — that for two or three of the evening sessions and at the formal banquet an effort be made to obtain the speaking services of outstanding government leaders.
2. That the various councils, namely, the Councils on Psychology, Roentgenology, Physiotherapy and Public Health be assigned the specific responsibility of developing competent symposia on work relative to the subject supported by the Councils and that all lecturers should be men of reliable training and decorum so that in no way anything exiguous or untoward would be presented.
3. That Drs. Peterson, Budden and Janse be assigned the responsibility of developing respectively, panels on the distortions and subluxations of the pelvis and lumbar spine, the lumbar dorsal spine and the cervical spine and especially as they relate to visceral diseases.

Dr. Peterson was assigned the following men to work with him as his faculty, Drs. Logan, Wolfe, Parr and Trubenbach. Dr. Budden was assigned Drs. Cleveland, Mueller, Beatty and Parker and Dr. Janse was assigned to work with Drs. Hendricks, King, Martin and Power.

4. It was also suggested that not too many lecturers be invited to speak to the general assembly for the simple reason that if the program is too crowded no-one actually has a proper opportunity of presenting his material. Then Dr. Harring asked the Council to discuss POINT number 10 which reads as follows:

Point-10. Increased effort to protect status of chiropractic in states where medical society attacks are being made and discussions of situations in such states as Indiana, Louisiana, etc. and consideration of the chiropractic situation in New Jersey and report on special legislation committee.

Dr. Nugent again reiterated the NCA stand and position in relation to the issue in Louisiana. Please refer to the previous discussions on this matter.

Dr. Peterson also reiterated his previous comments with reference to the New Jersey situation and the appointed commission that visited the institute and the eventual outcome. Then Dr. Peterson also mentioned that the case with reference to the New York Institute of Chiropractic had been re-opened and that it was being taken to the State Supreme Court; that at the present time there were seven Judges presiding over this court and three of these were liberals and would very likely cast a vote in favor of the Institute and that probably it would be possible to prevail upon one of the remaining four to vote in favor of granting the institute a proper title of operation. Dr. Peterson mentioned that the whole question revolved about the issue, whether the Institute was teaching a form of medicine or whether chiropractic was singular and independent of medicine. He stated that if the State Supreme Court ruled in favor of the Institute as not being involved in the medical practice act, because it does not teach medicine; but that all of the subjects are related to the teaching of chiropractic and which is uniquely and distinctly different than medicine, it would establish a precedence for the whole State of New York. This decision would very likely render an immunity for all standing doctors of chiropractic on any further possibility of there being arrested practitioners on the charge of practicing medicine without a license. He also mentioned that if by perchance the ruling was not in favor of the institution, it would again be a matter of a stalemate and the whole procedure of going through the various courts would be begun over again.

Dr. Harring mentioned that throughout the profession there was a greater need of establishing better public relations; that it was high time that the profession as a whole get rid of the charlatans and the high pressured salesmen and that our graduates be instructed to render a competent chiropractic service unattended by any fanfare, ballyhoo and sales promotion. He expressed the opinion that greater effort should be made to instill better ethics and professionalism among our people and that greater endeavor be extended in acquainting the public with the merits of chiropractic by means of competent public lectures by penetrating the high schools; by proper radio programs as well as the conducting of children's clinics.

Dr. Janse expressed his concern about the rather serious incidents of chiropractic graduate mortality and that it was imperative that greater attention be directed toward proper placement of graduates and the geographical distribution of graduates. He emphasized the significance of penetrating the more difficult basic science states because in these states, the chiropractic population is dwindling whereas those states presided over by rather liberal chiropractic boards, the chiropractic population was becoming rather heavy.

Dr. Nugent agreed with Dr. Janse and added this point, namely, that one of the reasons for our mortality is that we do not screen our chiropractic matriculants carefully enough. Furthermore, that we should only have enough chiropractic colleges to take care of our student population and that this idea of many other and new chiropractic colleges would spread our student population altogether too thin and leave no college with sufficient economy to properly maintain the caliber of instruction.

Then Dr. Peterson drew the Council's attention to a letter he had received from Dr. Willard W. Percy, Secretary of the California Board of Chiropractic Examiners. In substance, the primary subject contained within the letter that concerned the Council was the Board's decision to classify accredited colleges according to the A.B.C. system and the sentence which read as follows:

For your information and the Council on Education; any school that is fully equipped to teach all necessary subjects required by law, also by the Board, will get an A classification. For example; a school so equipped does not have to send out any of the necessary work to another approved school such as the subjects - Dissection and Physiotherapy.

After rather extensive deliberation, the following resolution was passed - The Council on Education by resolution goes on record by requesting all State Boards to approve Chiropractic Colleges on a single standard and that this standard be not less than a minimal requirement for accrediting by the National Council on Education. It was decided that a copy of this resolution be filed with every State Board of Chiropractic Examiners. Dr. Nugent was also instructed to have a very careful discussion with the California Board on this matter as soon as possible.

Dr. Budden then mentioned how a graduate from a low standard school had been granted the privilege of taking the Board in Oregon by having received quite a bit of extra credit toward qualifying for the Board on work that he had done in some phase of the Medical Corps of the Navy. It was the full consensus of opinion of the members of the Council that all State Boards and Colleges should be encouraged to discontinue this rather inordinate practice.

Dr. Martin then drew the Council's attention to some mediations the Los Angeles College had had with a Company that made hearing aids and that would be willing to come into the chiropractic colleges and put on a course in Audiometry and then grant the thus trained Chiropractors exclusive right to the agency of their hearing aids. It was generally concluded that probably great caution should be exercised in lending ourselves to propositions of this type.

Points 4 and 9 were then brought up for discussion -

Point 4. Consideration of requirements to be met to make the Council on Education an accepted and recognized accrediting agent for the profession, and,

Point 9. Recapitulation and recognition of the very excellent attainments of chiropractic colleges in recent years.

With reference to Point 4, it was concluded that this matter was to be more a process of education and persuasion because it would not do to alienate any of the present members of the chiropractic boards of examiners.

Dr. Nugent then made a resume of the progress that had been made within the last year in the chiropractic profession as the result of the efforts of the accrediting committee, his office as director of education and the work of the council in general. Dr. Nugent's resume included the following pertinent points -

1. Admirable progress has been made at the Cleveland College of Chiropractic and Dr. Nugent feels that the administration of this institution should be complimented for lending itself to the program of the Council.

2. Great progress has been made at the Northwestern College of Chiropractic in Minneapolis; the purchase of a new building in a very fine section of the City namely, 2222 Park Avenue, which will set this college off with facilities that suit themselves admirably to education.

3. The Missouri College of Chiropractic has also purchased an adjoining building for housing a new clinic and that every effort is being made by Dr. Harring and his staff to qualify for full accrediting.

4. That progress had been made at the Carver College of Chiropractic to the extent that he was happy to be able to recommend that the Council fully accredit which incidentally, was done at a previous meeting.

5. He complimented all of the other schoolmen, stating that in all of the accredited and provisionally accredited colleges, gratifying improvements had been made which include the enlargement and the increase of physical equipment as well as the improvement in context of courses and substance matter.

6. He reiterated his hope and desire that all colleges affiliated with the Council would endeavor to augment laboratory facilities in the subjects of embryology, histology, physiology, and dissection.

7. Dr. Nugent stated that throughout the country, the council on education was becoming progressively more and more recognized and accepted as the accrediting agency for the profession.

8. Dr. Nugent mentioned that within the last ten years, 21 states had changed their chiropractic laws toward higher education and that basically, these changes were prompted by the efforts of the NCA

9. He mentioned that the following groups, organizations and agencies recognize the Council on Education as the academic and accrediting voice of the profession -

    A. The Federal Commission on Occupation and Orientation.
    B. The Federal Council on Trades, Occupations, and Professions.
    C. Teachers College of Columbia University.
    D. The new College Blue Book.
    E. The Nai Birt, Jewish Organization.
    F. All of the high schools in Cleveland and Los Angeles have asked for the NCA publication entitled "Chiropractic Career."
    G. The State Department of Education of the following states had turned to the Council for advice - California, Iowa, Illinois, Nevada, Rhode Island, Georgia, New Jersey, Maryland, and Michigan.
    H. The Census Bureau had also asked Dr. Nugent, as director of Education and member of the Council, for advice.
    I. The Bureau of War Manpower had done the same thing.
    J. That the Women's Bureau of the Department of Labor and the Department of Occupational Titles and the Post Office Department and the Department of State, the Department of Justice, as well as the Department of Veterans Affairs.

They have all indicated and given evidence that the NCA, its Director of Education and its Council on Education were accepted as the authoritative agencies of the profession.

Dr. Budden stated that the entire profession and all college men owe Dr. Nugent a hearty vote of thanks and this was moved and seconded and approved unanimously.

Further discussions were continued with reference to the teaching of the Basic Sciences and the augmentation of laboratory facilities.

Dr. Budden expressed the thought that it would not do to allow our courses and our required laboratory work to become top heavy in the basic science subjects to the extent where work both didactic and laboratory in the clinic and therapeutic subjects would be neglected and thus lessen the competence in diagnosis and clinical arts so necessary to the Doctor of Chiropractic, for his livelihood.

At the close of the meeting, the recommendation was made and seconded that the entire Council proffer Dr. Nugent a hearty vote of thanks for his untiring efforts in behalf of the council and the educational program of the National Chiropractic Association.

It was further recommended that every member of the Council be encouraged to commit himself to further and sponsor the ideals of the Council without restrictions or any element of personal misgivings. It was generally concluded that much had been accomplished by the Council and that every effort should be made in sustaining its integrity and maintaining a decorum of mutual respect and understanding.

AN APPENDAGE

A report on the meetings of the American Association of Basic Science Boards, held in Chicago at the Palmer House, February 6th, 1950.

Drs. Nugent and Janse had been invited to attend these meetings by Dr. Norman E. Witt, President of this association. Because of illness, Dr. Nugent was not able to attend and consequently Dr. Janse was instructed by the Council on Education to attend these meetings and to make a report as to the occurrence and happenings at the same.

Dr. W.A. Budden accompanied Dr. Janse during the morning sessions, but had to leave after the luncheon in order to catch his train for Portland.

Point 1. The Basic Science Boards of the following states were represented: Nebraska, Oregon, Arizona, Colorado, Rhode Island, New Mexico, Michigan, Texas, Wisconsin, Minnesota, Washington, D.C., Tennessee, South Dakota.

Point 2. Dr. Springler, the lady Chiropractic member of the Colorado Basic Science Board also was in attendance.

Point 3. Dr. Witt, in his introductory remarks emphasized the significance of the responsibilities that confronted the various basic science boards all over the country. He emphasized the necessity for as much cooperation, integration and cohesion of effort as was possible. He stated that every effort should be made to maintain the decorum of friendliness and understanding toward all groups and professional agencies, signifying the conviction that the Basic Science Boards should be as fully impartial as is possible. He took time to ask every person in attendance to stand up and introduce himself and it should be mentioned that representing the Osteopathic profession were Dr. R.C. McCaughan, Executive Secretary of the American Osteopathic Association and Mr. Lawrence W. Mills, Director of the Office of Education of the American Osteopathic Association, as well as Dr. Harney, Dean of the School of Medicine of the University of Texas who represented the National Board of Medical Examiners.

Point 4. A paper entitled "Nature and Content of a Basic Science Examination in Chemistry" by A.H. Kunz, Ph.D., head of the Department of Chemistry, University of Oregon, was read. In this paper, Dr. Kunz presented two evaluations of the topics and advantages of what are known as discussion questions and short answer questions. He also posed the question whether Basic Science Examinations in Chemistry should include questions relating to the three primary fields of Chemistry namely Inorganic, Organic, and Biological. He also stated that according to his personal experiences, one of the primary reasons why students fail in Basic Science Examinations was due to a want of ability to use proper English and to express themselves and to portray their ideas with the competence and clarity necessary.

It should be mentioned that Drs. Budden and Janse, in conversation with Dr. Kunz about the Oregon Basic Science Board, obtained the impression that the members of this Board favored the change in the Basic Science Law which would grant an examinee the privilege of taking only that subject in which he had failed over, rather than the entire five subjects if he had failed one which was the ruling. Dr. Kunz also solicited recommendations from the three professions represented with reference to the type and nature of the basic science examinations in Chemistry. Rather extensive discussions resulted and it was the final conclusion of the group that the majority of the Basic Science questions should relate to the chemistry of the body and that questions in qualitative and quantitative inorganic chemistry should be deleted. It was also recommended that questions pertaining to Pharmacology should at no time be included in the Chemistry examination of the Basic Science Boards. In as much as Chemistry was one of the primary subjects in which Basic Science Examinees failed, the question arose as to whether the examiners in Chemistry were not a little too severe in their expectations of the examinees. It was concluded that a continued study should be made with reference to those issues and a possible greater concern exhibited toward the efforts of the examinees.

Point 5. After the luncheon, Dr. McCaughan, Executive Secretary of the American Osteopathic Association read a paper entitled "Effects of Basic Science Education on the Education of Physicians." Dr. McCaughan reiterated the original intent behind the institution of Basic Science Laws, namely the medical intent of hamstringing the efforts of the Osteopathic profession (it might be significant to note that Dr. McCaughan at no time referred to the Chiropractic profession nor Doctors of Chiropractic. It seemed that he rather significantly shunned any inclination to include or rate doctors of Chiropractic along with Medical and Osteopathic physicians; this being the designation which he repeatedly used. It was quite apparent that he desired to place the Osteopathic practitioner in the same category of physician as the medical practitioner.) In his paper, he presented a series of statistics as acquired by the various deans of the Osteopathic Colleges, attempting to show that the instituting of Basic Science Laws had in no way altered the educational intention of the Osteopathic profession and that the Basic Science Laws had but very little effect upon the curriculum of Osteopathic Colleges and upon the distribution of osteopathic graduates. Dr. McCaughan voiced the concern that possible Basic Science Laws and examinations did place too much emphasis upon pre-clinical subjects. He cautioned against the inclination of becoming too pedantic in the Basic Science examinations and he expressed the personal belief that possible Basic Science examinations were superfluous.

This premise was rather acutely contested by Dr. John S. Latta, President of the Basic Science Board in Nebraska who asserted that in his experiences as head of the Department of Anatomy of the School of Medicine of the University of Nebraska, the Basic Science requirements and stipulations did much to integrate the visualization and understanding of the medical graduate. He expressed the belief that the Basic Science Laws served to control not only the Osteopathic and Chiropractic professions but also the Medical profession, making it as subservient to the Basic Science stipulations as the other two groups.

Point 6. Another matter which was rather extensively discussed was the request by the National Medical Board that all Basic Science Boards recognize their examination as a Basic Science equivalency and that if a medical graduate had passed the Basic Science subjects as given in examination by the National Medical Board, they should be exempt from any Basic Science regulation of a State in which they desire to practice. It was a unanimous decision that this request be declined and that under no circumstances should any Medical, Osteopathic, or Chiropractic examination be considered the equivalent of a Basic Science examination with the privileges of exemption.

Point 7. Dr. Clements of the Nebraska Basic Science Board made a report on the Committee of Survey and Examination of Basic Science Questions. He advised the group that in the past year, he had procured questions in the Basic Science subjects from not only the members of the Basic Science Boards, but also from the Medical, Osteopathic, and Chiropractic Boards (professional). Then he had taken these questions, had them multigraphed, had set up a chart of evaluation and had sent them out to various heads of Basic Science Boards for Evaluation; the questions being rated as Poor, Moderate, and Good. He demonstrated a series of graphs and according to this process of evaluation, the greater percentage of all questions fell in the middle category, namely, moderately good. Out of all of these, there developed a consensus of opinion that probably all Basic Science Board examiners could well afford to be a little more careful in preparing their questions. It was also suggested that every Basic Science Board member be cautioned not to allow himself to become inclined to make a fetish out of any special phase relating to his subject or to become too demanding as to theories and concepts that were his intellectual hobbies.

It was also suggested that a constant effort should be made to avoid any inclination to permit the questions to be colored by any therapeutic concept or inclination. The question arose as to whether the subject of preventive medicine or otherwise known as Public Health, or Hygiene and Sanitation was really a Basic Science Subject. However, it was the general conclusion that if examination in the subject was so compelled by the written word of the Basic Science Law, there was very little that anyone could do about it.

It was also agreed that every effort should be made to be as considerate in the possibilities of reciprocity between the states as was possible. Minnesota reiterated its intentions to maintain its reciprocal arrangements with Michigan, thus dissipating the rumor that such was going to be discontinued. Some discussion was conducted with reference to Iowa and how recently in the A.M.A. Journal, this Board had received a rather severe scolding on the assumption that it had granted Basic Science Certificates to several hundred Chiropractic Examinees without properly examining them. It was agreed that this criticism was unfounded and inordinate. It was also suggested that in making up a list of the questions for the various subjects, that the examinee be allowed a choice of for example, five out of eight, or six out of eight and furthermore, that the questions should be sufficiently general and extensive that the examinee would have an opportunity of portraying his knowledge of the whole field of the subject rather than any specific phase or aspect. It was also concluded that credit would be proffered the examinee if, although his answer was not completely correct, it did exhibit good integration of thinking and concept. It was also proposed that the papers of those who failed should be very carefully re-checked by the examiner proper and not by any person who was paid to simply read and correct the papers and that if after careful scrutiny of the paper, a passing grade could be proffered, such should be done. The example of Minnesota was utilized. After the correcting of all of the papers and the grading of the same, the Board members meet and then the papers of the failures are carefully studied by each Board member and he places his grade on that paper and then an average is made of the six grades of the six Board members for that paper. It was also suggested that for the convenience of the examinee, if he had failed in but one subject and he wished to obtain reciprocity in another state, that the subjects in which he had procured a passing grade would be honored by this state and thus allow him to make up the subject in which he had failed by writing that subject of that Board in the State in which he desired to obtain reciprocity.

All of the members of the Association were encouraged by Dr. Orin S. Madison, President of the Michigan Basic Science Board to obtain as many suggestions as well as questions from the various chiropractic, osteopathic, and medical boards, and to study them and probably to take an equal percentage from each group and thus compose his question list.

Dr. N.H. Serrer of Rhode Island Basic Science Board emphasized the significance of being as cooperative as possible, calling attention to the fact that the examinees, whether medical, osteopathic, or chiropractic in training had severe and tremendous difficulties and problems confronting them and that although the Board should represent a very careful estimation of their qualifications in the Basic Science subjects, they should not represent insurmountable hazards. It was also mentioned that the pre-professional college requirements of the three major professions: medicine, osteopathy, and chiropractic were rather noticeably different; that for example, in Chiropractic as yet, only a few states required any pre-professional college training and that consequently a chiropractic matriculant went into his professional training without having had any or relatively little pre-professional training in the Basic Sciences and although it was not the responsibility of Basic Science Boards of the American Association of Basic Science Boards to stipulate what the pre-professional requirements of a profession should be, yet every effort should be made to take cognizance of this difference and to avoid inordinately complicated and advanced questions which out of their very aspect, necessitated and compelled extensive pre-professional college work.

Dr. Madison suggested that at the next year meeting, a paper be presented by a member of the Chiropractic profession, outlining and detailing the Basic Science issue from the Chiropractic angle. He suggested the name of Dr. John J. Nugent, Director of Education of the National Chiropractic Association. It should be noted that in a subsequent business meeting and a meeting of the program committee, this suggestion of Dr. Madison was unanimously approved and it is very likely that Dr. Nugent will receive a formal invitation to prepare such a paper.

In conclusion, it should be stated that every member of the Boards represented were very tolerant and objectively fair in the consideration of their problems and especially as they related to the Chiropractic profession. Whether out of deference because of my presence, or because of genuine intent, and I am very inclined to believe the latter, the profession of Chiropractic experienced as much consideration, as much respect, and as much genuine concern as either the Osteopathic or the Medical profession did. It was quite apparent that the members of this Association were sincerely desirous of doing the best job possible.

Minutes of the meetings of the COUNCIL ON EDUCATION, Held at the Statler Hotel, Washington, D.C. during the Annual Convention of the National Chiropractic Association, July 31 through August 1, 2, 3, 4, 1950. Dr. Thure C. Peterson, President of the Council, presided over all of the meetings.

Those in attendance were:
(A) Members of the Accrediting Committee
   Dr. John J. Nugent, Director of Education, 92 Norton Street, New Haven, Connecticut
   Dr. Edward H. Gardner, 2727 South Vermont Avenue, Los Angeles, California
   Dr. George A. Bauer, 1608 Bull Street, Columbia, South Carolina

    Dr. Walter B. Wolf, Eureka, South Dakota

    Dr. Norman E. Osborne, 3 Broadway Street, Hagerstown, Maryland

(B) Representatives of the accredited and provisionally accredited chiropractic colleges:

    Dr. Thure C. Peterson, Director, Dr. Craig M. Kightlinger, President, Dr. H.L. Trubenbach, Director of   Chiropractic, Dr.

    Clarence W. Weiant, Dean, Dr. F.F. Hirsch, Departmental Head, Chiropractic Institute of New York, 152 West 42nd Street, New York 18, New York

    Dr. W.A. Budden, President, Western States College of Chiropractic, 4525 Southeast 63rd Avenue, Portland 6, Oregon

    Dr. Arthur G. Hendricks, Vice-President, Dr. Leslie M. King, Dean, Lincoln Chiropractic College, Inc., 633 N. Pennsylvania Street, Indianapolis 4, Indiana

    Dr. Ralph J. Martin, President, Los Angeles College of Chiropractic, Dr. Guy Martyn, President, California State Chiropractic Association, 920 E. Broadway, Glendale 5, California

    Dr. William N. Coggins, Dean, Dr. Frank Smutzler, Departmental Head, Logan Basic College of Chiropractic, 7701 Florissant Road, St. Louis 21, Missouri

    Dr. Ralph A. Power, Dean, Missouri Chiropractic Institute, Inc., 3117 Lafayette Avenue, St. Louis 4, Missouri

    Dr. R.O. Mueller, Dean, Canadian Memorial Chiropractic College, 252 Bloor Street West, Toronto 5, Ontario

    Dr. A.J. Darling, Member, Board of Trustees, Kansas State Chiropractic College, 629 North Broadway, Wichita, Kansas

    Dr. John B. Wolfe, President, Northwestern College of Chiropractic, 2222 Parkway Avenue, Minneapolis, Minnesota

(C) Special invited guests -

    Dr. Carl Cleveland Sr., President, Dr. Carl Cleveland Jr., Dean, Cleveland College of Chiropractic, 3724 Troost Street, Kansas City, Missouri

    Dr. Ben L. Parker, Dean, Texas Chiropractic College, San Pedro Park, San Antonio, Texas

    Dr. Homer G. Beatty, President, University of Natural Healing Arts, 1075 Logan Street, Denver 3, Colorado

The first meeting of the Council began at 10:00 A.M. July 31, 1950 with Dr. Peterson presiding. The members of the accrediting committee were not in attendance as they were in special individual session.

Dr. Peterson began the deliberations with a presentation of the situation confronting given groups in the profession in the state of Pennsylvania. Since the exposures in relation to the Philadelphia Chiropractic College a goodly number of practicing chiropractors in Pennsylvania and graduates of this defunct institution are in the unfavorable position of very likely not being able to qualify for the licensing board of chiropractic examiners if the pending chiropractic legislation in Pennsylvania were to pass.

Resultantly approaches have been made by these individuals with the inquiry as to whether the accredited colleges under the auspices of the Council could not set up some program of qualification which would result in the issuance of degrees from the accredited colleges and thus eliminate the possibility of their not being eligible for the examination if the chiropractic board in Pennsylvania be empowered to act.

Dr. Peterson further mentioned that the Administration of the Chiropractic Institute of New York had been approached by the official body of the Pennsylvania Chiropractic Society in relation to the same matter. In fact Dr. Walton Yoder, the Secretary of the Society, had been instructed to ask for the opportunity of presenting the matter to the Council.

It was also brought to the attention of the council that the Attorney General in Maryland had ruled that the Board of Chiropractic Examiners could not examine a person who was the holder of a degree and diploma from a defunct college.

At this time it was brought to the Council's attention that in Pennsylvania certain individuals had gone so far as to forge certain diplomas as issued by reputable chiropractic colleges.

Both Drs. Kightlinger and Peterson stated that such had been the case and that in cooperation with the State Society every effort was being made to ferret out these forged certifications.

It was finally decided that further discussions of the Pennsylvania matter would have to be deferred until the Accrediting Committee and Dr. Nugent, Director of Education, could sit in on the final deliberations.

Dr. Peterson next proceeded to draw the Council's attention to a proposition that Dr. Herman Schwartz, Head of the Council on Psychology, wished to have the Council discuss.

It was Dr. Schwartz's recommendation that the Council accept his proposed changes in the widely used and distributed case history chart as prepared by Burton-Shield Co., to include a definite section on the psychiatric history and colorings of the patient. After the inclusion of this modification the case history chart was to be multigraphed by the Chiropractic Research Foundation and proffer the same for distribution.

Dr. Schwartz had also obtained a gift of 500 dollars from a personal friend of his and a staunch chiropractic booster, Mr. Gray, for the purpose of running a contest of the most complete and thorough case history work including detailed data of diagnostic and clinical procedures.

The Council was also informed that Dr. Schwartz was in the process of preparing a text on general abnormal psychology in terms of the chiropractic concept, which he hoped might be adopted by the Council and prescribed in the various accredited colleges.

It was also Dr. Schwartz's intention to conduct a national research contest in the form of having students at the various accredited colleges and even faculty members seek out in authoritative psychological and psychiatric literature verifying statements and facts that substantiate the chiropractic concept in this field, and then to prepare a small publication very similar to the one issued by the New York State Chiropractic Society and prepared by Dr. C.W. Weiant, and entitled "A Case for Chiropractic In Medical Literature."

Dr. Janse, Head of the Council on Research and Public Health, asserted that Dr. Schwartz's efforts and interests should be encouraged and stated that the Public Health Council might be in a position to grant some 100 dollars to Dr. Schwartz's project. Finally it was decided to table any further discussions until Dr. Schwartz could appear before the entire Council membership. Also each college agreed to conduct contest of type suggested by Dr. Schwartz and that he should receive a letter supporting his effort.

Dr. Ralph J. Martin opened the question of possible deferments for students in chiropractic colleges. He made the inquiry as to whether it might not be possible to obtain some favorable decision from the office of General Hershey, Director of the Selective Service Department on the wording in the official statement that reads as follows, "students of the healing arts."

Because of the fact that this was such an important and significant matter it was concluded to defer any further discussions until it was possible to have Dr. Emmett J. Murphy in for an explanation of the situation as he had estimated it. Dr. Peterson was instructed to contact Dr. Murphy and to invite him to meet with the Council during their evening session.

The matter of chiropractic legislation and legislative efforts was then brought into discussion. It was the consensus that it would be very helpful, especially in orientating college men and students, if the monthly issues of the NCA Journal had a special legal section where all information pertaining to chiropractic legislation, boards, associated medical and basic science boards could appear in properly catalogued and summarized manner.

Dr. Ralph Power concurrently suggested that the legal staff of the NCA be alerted to the necessity of rendering more decisive support of or interpretation of proposed chiropractic legislation or alteration of the same. It was concluded to invite Mr. Robert Johns, Counsel for the NCA, to appear before the Council and experience these attitudes and to see whether some assistance could be obtained along these lines.

Afternoon meetings, closed to all but the representatives of the accredited or provisionally accredited colleges and the accrediting committee. Dr. Thure C. Peterson presiding.

Dr. Edward Gardner, president of the accrediting committee assigned Dr. John J. Nugent, Director of Education, to give the official report of the committee which in substance was as follows:

a. There had been a strong request made from the administration of the Texas College of Chiropractic for inspection and recognition by the accrediting committee and eventually by the Council on Education. Dr. Nugent advised the Council that the curriculum and faculty of the college had been markedly strengthened under the supervision of Dr. Ben Parker the Dean. Dr. Nugent advised the Council that an inspection would be made of the college in September and that he and the accrediting committee would be ready to submit a report to the Council at the mid-year meeting.

b. The Baltimore branch of the Columbia College of Chiropractic had been inspected by Dr. Nugent and he found that much improvement had been made. The administration had made application for approval, however because of certain problems relating to administrative policies the final decision would have to be deferred until some later date. At this point it was the expressed opinion of various members of the Council that if the Columbia College in Baltimore is to be eventually approved, such should be granted only on the stipulation that the New York division be closed because it actually represented an inadequate institution, and if the Baltimore branch were recognized it would lend credence to the New York division.

c. Dr. Nugent reported that the administrative officers of the Cleveland College of Chiropractic were very desirous to cooperate and merit approval. That there was still a matter in relation to corporate ownership that had to be worked out. Much progress had been made at the college and the administration was to be complimented.

d. Dr. Nugent next reported on the Missouri Chiropractic Institute which at the present time was provisionally approved. He commented on the progress that had been made and the diligent and cooperative attitude of the administrative staff. He advised the Council that further modifications would be continued.

e. Western States Chiropractic College had also been inspected by Dr. Nugent and certain constructive understandings had been reached with the college administration. He commented on the fine work that was being done.

At this point Dr. Nugent asked for the permission to digress and relate the efforts he and Dr. Budden had made in relation to the Washington Basic Science situation. Dr. Nugent advised the Council that the Washington Basic Science Board was becoming less adamant and resistive, and was of the opinion that with further effort the administration of the board could be conditioned to sustain a fair attitude toward qualified chiropractic students and graduates.

Dr. Nugent stated that the state of Washington was under the control of the P.S.C. and that a large group of students from this institution had taken the board with the specific intent of indicting the board. That such an effort had been made but that the Court had held this conduct as being ridiculous and had thrown the case out of court.

The Council was informed that Dr. Budden had made three definite recommendations to the board which the board had promised to thoroughly consider, these recommendations being:

(1) That the examinee be given credit for any 3 of the 6 subjects that he might pass the first time of writing. So that in a subsequent effort he would not have to take them all over.

(2) That the Governor be asked to increase the educational requirements stipulated by the chiropractic law to a minimum of 32 to 36 months, and to refrain from demanding that the applicant for the basic science board reveal his school of practice.

(3) That a conscientious effort be made that unlicensed practitioners be made to discontinue.

Dr. Nugent stated that eventually the Council had acquired the influence that should not permit or tolerate incompetence in chiropractic boards, intolerance among medical boards and bias in basic science boards.

e. Dr. Nugent then proceeded with his report on the colleges and stated that he had received an invitation from Dr. Homer G. Beatty of the Denver University of Natural Healing Arts for an inspection and stated that this invitation would be responded to as soon as possible.

f. Dr. Nugent spoke of his inspection of the National College of Chiropractic and stated that he was satisfied that diligent efforts were being experienced and that an extensive program of renovation and organization of laboratories had been initiated.

g. He stated that he had been in Los Angeles and that the L.A. College of Chiropractic had been experiencing board of directors trouble but that things were beginning to work out in good order.

Dr. Nugent had also visited the Canadian Memorial Chiropractic College, having spoken at the graduation exercises. There had also been board trouble at this college but it was but a sign of the conflicting conscientious efforts of people, which would smooth themselves out.

Again Dr. Nugent asked for the privilege of adding a digressing comment, namely that he was most grateful for the progress that had been made.

He stated that today there was not a chiropractic college in existence that had not instituted a 4 year course, although not all the colleges had been accredited.

He advised the Council that he had been privileged to establish contacts with certain prominent and authoritative officials of large Foundations and he felt that it was very possible that they could be interested in assigning certain sums of money for chiropractic colleges and other educational institutions.

He rather severely condemned the conduct of the public relations department of the ICA in their rather inordinate effort to frustrate and stymie Dr. Murphy's efforts in relation to the Bill that would have provided for chiropractic care of patients in the veterans hospitals. (It should be mentioned that at the formal banquet of the convention, Dr. Omar Ketchum legislative representative of the VFW who had vigorously supported Dr. Murphy's efforts publicly verified Dr. Nugent's criticism.)

Dr. Nugent then reported on the Kansas State Chiropractic College and stated that he was afraid that the college would not be able to continue to sustain its provisionally accredited status and that if within the rather immediate future some indications of solidification of administrative and educational effort be attained he would recommend that it be taken off the list.

Dr. A.J. Darling, a member of the Board of Directors of the college, asked if he might explain the situation of the college. Dr. Darling explained that they had just appointed a new Dean and asked for the opportunity for this new person to prove his worth. He related how the Board had planned to amalgamate the Kansas State College with the Denver College, and house this new college in the smallest of the two main buildings of the Spears Sanitarium. However, that upon further investigation the Board found out that this could only be done by a 2/3 majority vote of the Founders of the college. The vote was taken and the proposition was out voted 3 to 1. All of the members of the Board were then relieved of their positions except Dr. Darling. Since then the original site of the college had been sold, today the college was housed in a new building occupying some 5000 sq. ft. and the total Sept. enrollment would be from 60 to 70 students.

Dr. Nugent then stated that he questioned whether the college could maintain itself on the strength of such a small enrollment.

i. Dr. Nugent then mentioned that fine program that was being made at the Northwestern College of Chiropractic and he commented on the recent establishment of a well-organized Clinical Pathology Laboratory.

j. The Director of Education then drew the Council members' attention to the fact that an application for recognition had been made by the officers of the International Chiropractic College in Dayton, Ohio, which is being conducted exclusively for colored people. Drs. Amos Valdiserri and Joseph Martion being the primary executives of this institution are now teaching a 36 months course approved of by the Veteran's Administration as well as the Department of Education of the State of Ohio.

k. Dr. Nugent also mentioned the Atlantic States College of Brooklyn, New York. He stated that it merited very little consideration and that the administration of the same had exhibited a rather marked rankle because the various state boards were unwilling to offer them recognition.

Dr. Nugent asked the Council members to very carefully study the Taft-Teak Bill, especially the Section M7-513. He stated that this bill seriously reflected on the economic status of private schools and colleges as well as small professional or semi-professional colleges which ordinarily included the chiropractic colleges. Dr. Martin asked the Council to empower Dr. Nugent to contact the proper agencies and personnel and see whether or not the effects of the Taft-Teak Bill could be circumvented.

Dr. Nugent, in conclusion of his report, encouraged the school men to recognize the progress that had been made, to continually strive for greater standardization of procedure and to recognize the constant need for the improvement of the physical and educational facilities of their institutions.

The council then received Dr. Walton B. Yoder, Secretary of the Pennsylvania Chiropractic Society. He was attended by his father, Dr. Yoder, who is a director of the Pennsylvania Chiropractic Society. The younger Dr. Yoder as Secretary of the State Society asked for the privilege of presenting an explanation of the situation in the State of Pennsylvania. He explained how last year the Pennsylvania Chiropractic Society sponsored two legislative measures: One bill designed to create a Board of Chiropractic Examiners and an associated bill designed to give authority and enabling ability to the thus established Chiropractic Board. To date the result being that the bill creating a Chiropractic Board had passed, but the bill enabling the Board of officiating had been defeated by one or two votes. This year with the pending legislative session, the Pennsylvania Chiropractic Society was going to endeavor to pass the enabling bill. If such were realized, it would empower the Chiropractic Board to proceed to examine any or all of the present unlicensed practitioners in the state. Dr. Yoder then advised the group that among the unlicensed practitioners were a goodly number of men who had very little former education or who possessed degrees from the defunct and denounced Philadelphia Chiropractic College. Consequently, the Chiropractic Board was confronted by the great problems as to what to do with these individuals and what kind of a program might be established to enable these individuals to qualify for the Board.

Dr. Yoder explained that the officers and directors of the Pennsylvania Chiropractic Society were hopeful that the Council on Education of the NCA would help them in effecting a program whereby the majority of these practitioners with an unqualified college background could make themselves eligible for examination by the Board. Dr. Yoder advised the group that the officers of the State Society had thought of the possible following recommendation; namely, if a man had been in practice 20 years or more, all that would be required of him to make him eligible for the Board would be 1,000 resident class hours; if a man had been in practice 5 years, yet no more than 20 years, he would have to be able to show 2,800 class hours; if he had been in practice less than 5 years, he would have to fulfill the minimum of 3600 class hours and the 1 year of pre-professional college work in chemistry, biology, and physics.

After Dr. Yoder left the matter received further consideration and it was the general consensus that it would be impossible to set up a program which would enable these various practitioners to obtain degrees from the accredited colleges within a relative short time, that probably the best that could be done would be to make certain recommendations to the State Board stipulating a relative period of training which would be considered a qualification for the Board but unattended by any issuance of degrees.

It was finally concluded that Dr. Peterson as President of the Council should proceed to continue mediations with the Pennsylvania Chiropractic Society, call upon Dr. Leo J. Steinbach for assistance and advice and then after coming to a concise understanding, report back to the Council.. Meeting will be held in Pittsburgh September 29, 1950.

Evening Meeting July 30, 1950, Dr. Peterson presiding

Dr. Emmett J. Murphy, Legislative and Public Relations Director of the NCA, was present for the purpose of answering various questions in relation to G.I. deferment. After rather extended deliberations, it was the final realization that the deferment of Chiropractic students was essentially a matter left up to the Local Boards. Dr. Murphy advised the Council that he did not believe that at the present time a blanket deferment for all Chiropractic students could be obtained. He stated, however, that the Director of the Selective Service System, General Hershey, was very sympathetic with the matter. Dr. Murphy stated that he was confident that the majority of the Local Boards or other service personnel involved would respond to the proper solicitations from the college administrations, that in the majority of instances the Chiropractic student would experience the same in deference as students of the other professions.

Then Dr. Murphy proceeded to advise the Council of the tremendous difficulties that confronted him in relation to:

1. Student deferment
2. Obtaining commissions for Chiropractors in the various services and
3. Obtaining a status for the profession in the Veteran's Hospitals. The reasons that Dr. Martin presented in explanation of these difficulties were as follows:
    1. Service and government personnel confronted him with the argument based upon the heterogeneous picture still prevailing in chiropractic.
    2. That the methods and procedures of Chiropractic as yet were not competently standardized.
    3. That unlike the Osteopaths (who are now eligible for commissions), Chiropractors as a whole did not sustain sufficient knowledge of the orthodox diagnostic and clinical procedures to allow their integration into some of the departments of the Medical Corps.
    4. The great variance of opinion as to concept, diagnosis, and procedure still prevalent among the Chiropractors.
    5. The existence of two national organizations which in certain measures countered each others efforts.

Dr. Murphy asked the Council members for good substantial reasons why deferment and commissions should be universally offered the Chiropractors, reasons that he would present to the agencies and individuals concerned. Dr. Peterson advanced the point that Chiropractors can handle from 30 to 40 of these illnesses so common to so many people as well or more competently than any other doctor. It was concluded that continued efforts should be made by all concerned and that Dr. Murphy's position was a very difficult one and that he and his office should experience every cooperation and support possible.

Dr. Ben Parker then drew the Council's attention to Local Board memorandum No. 7, issued November 2, 1948, by General Hershey. This advised the Boards that a Healing Arts Educational Advisory Committee had been established. This committee consisting of two representatives of the medical profession, one of the dental, one of the veterinary, and one of the osteopathic. It appears that General Hershey was depending greatly upon the advice of this committee as to his recommendations to the various Local Boards in relation to deferments. Both Drs. Nugent and Murphy commanded themselves to the intent to obtain representation on this committee.

After Dr. Murphy excused himself, the council turned its attentions to making certain inquiries of Mr. Robert Johns, the legal counsel of the National Chiropractic Association. Mr. Johns was attended by Dr. Gordon Goodfellow, a member of the Executive Board of the NCA. In substance the inquiries made of Mr. Johns were as follows:

1. Whether it wouldn't be possible for the Legal Staff of the NCA to prepare an abbreviated monthly catalogue to appear in each issue of the NCA Journal listing the various legislative changes, bills, or efforts that relate to Chiropractic in the various states.
2. Whether this legal section could not also contain brief discussions on some of the more pertinent legal aspects of Chiropractic practice as they occurred in the various sections of the country.
3. Whether it wasn't possible for the Legal Staff of the NCA to penetrate the problem of necessary Chiropractic legislation in such

states as Louisiana, New York, New Jersey, Indiana, etc., and probably offer a greater measure of assistance or advice. Mr. Johns supported by the verification of Dr. Goodfellow advised the members of the Council that if the Council deemed it advisable to have such a catalogued legal advice section in the NCA Journal, such would be prepared, that as far as the Legal Staff of the NCA spearheading any efforts for Chiropractic legislation was concerned such would involve the necessities of an expenditure of money, an outlay of time and effort far beyond the point to which the present staff was authorized.

Dr. Budden and Mr. Johns then proceeded to discuss, at some length, the pro and con of the possibility of the Legal Staff of the NCA being a little less narrow in its legal interpretation of what Chiropractic is and basing its defense of malpractice cases upon rather limited interpretation. No definite conclusions were reached but not withstanding certain opinions and attitudes were aired revealing the fact that the nature of Chiropractic practice was quite sectional in its aspects.

After these brief discussions the meeting was adjourned and it was recommended that another meeting be held the following evening.

Evening Meeting August 1, 1950, Dr. Peterson presiding

Mrs. Arlene Raymond, Public Relations Director of the Iowa Chiropractors Association, at the invitation of the Council, appeared before the group with the following recommendation and request that the Council go on record of recommending to the members of the Iowa Board of Chiropractic Examiners that all futureState Board Examinations be held in some assigned public building in the State Capitol city rather than at the Palmer School of Chiropractic. She called the Council's attention to the fact that the conducts as outlined in her recommendations was that common to all other state boards and that by having the examinations given at a Chiropractic college it could possibly lead to a misinterpretation to intent. Mrs. Raymond's recommendation was heartily received and Dr. Janse, as Secretary of the Board, was instructed to contact the members of the board and made an official recommendation to this effect. Mrs. Raymond gave an enthusiastic report of the program of the organization she was affiliated with and every member of the Council expressed their admiration for the work that she was doing along with that Mr. Max Putnam, the Legal Counsel of the Iowa Chiropractors Association.

Dr. Carl Cleveland, Sr., then drew the attentions of the group to the comment made by Dr. Neal Bishop of Denver, Colorado, in relation to his acquaintanceship with General Hershey, the Director of the Selective Service System. It appeared that Dr. Bishop felt that he would be of some influence in obtaining the considerations of General Hershey in relation to Chiropractic students and their deferments and the placement of Chiropractic graduates in the Medical Corps of the armed services. It was finally concluded after some discussions to authorize Dr. Bishop to contact General Hershey and to see what could be done along those lines. However, that this effort on his part should be under the surveillance of Dr. Murphy and Dr. Nugent.

Dr. Hendricks then made inquiry about the necessity of establishing a standards for the evaluation of the credits for defunct colleges as well as those of colleges of meager educational facilities and those of colleges that do not experience approval by the NCA Council. After rather extended discussions, it was concluded that Dr. Nugent, as the Director of Education, should, as soon as possible, draw up a fundamental set of rules upon which this process of evaluation could be standardized. Dr. Nugent committed himself to this responsibility and advised the group that he would have this plan sufficiently well-organized to be able to present it at the mid-year meeting.

In continued discussions on this matter of colleges who, for some reason or other, have been caused to close their doors, the question of the disposition of certain state attorney's decisions was brought under discussion. Maryland, for example, experienced the ruling that the State Board of Chiropractic Examiners could not honor the application of any applicant who had obtained his training at an institution that was no longer in existence. The severity of this ruling was commented upon because it was obvious that it would represent a tremendous compromise to any graduates from the present accredited colleges to be rejected the privilege of taking an examination if by per chance the college was, out of economic necessity, forced to close its doors. An example was cited, namely, the Eastern College of Chiropractic which in the process of the New York amalgamation had been absorbed within the Chiropractic Institute of New York. Dr. Osborne, member of the Maryland Chiropractic Board of Examiners, was asked to comment on this issue. He stated that in his opinion the board would, under such a circumstance, honor the credits of the formerly existing Eastern College of Chiropractic. The meeting was adjourned until the following forenoon.

Forenoon and Final Meeting, August 2, 1950

At the recommendation of Dr. Homer G. Beatty a representative of the National Medical Society was invited to present the intent and program of this organization to the Council in general. The Doctor, representing the National Medical Society, advised the group that this organization was expecting a grant of some 500 acres within the vicinity of Washington, D.C., and that they intended to establish a 2.5 million dollar university which would contain a college of medicine, chiropractic, osteopathic and naturopathic toward the acquisition of a M.D. Degree. The question was asked whether the medical degree would be recognized by the various state medical boards and the gentlemen stated that as yet such privileges have not been acquired but that they were laboring under no false delusions and that they recognized the great necessity for the same. Upon his departure from the meeting it was generally concluded that as far as the Council was concerned no steps on affiliation could be established and that the matter should be allowed to run its course without any further deliberations.

The site of the mid-year meeting was rather extensively discussed and finally it was decided upon to hold it in California and Dr. Ralph J. Martin was instructed to check a likely site in the vicinity of Los Angeles, to make arrangements for the same, and to relay the information to Dr. Peterson.

Election of officers was the next order of business. Dr. Peterson handed in his resignation with expressions of appreciation for the cooperation that he had experienced but stated that his responsibility at the Chiropractic Institute of New York as well as at home demanded his resignation. He opened the meeting for nomination and Dr. Ralph J. Martin nominated Dr. W.A. Budden. Dr. Budden requested the floor and declined the nomination stating that he felt greatly honored, that it was his opinion the position as President of the Council should revolve upon the shoulders of a younger man. Dr. Janse and others spoke on behalf of Dr. Budden but the gentleman could not be prevailed upon. Every member of the Council regretted his decision, recognizing the great service that this fine person had rendered over the many years in support of better education and higher standards. Dr. Kightlinger then nominated Dr. Janse and Dr. Coggins nominated Dr. Hendricks. Dr. Janse was reluctant to accept. Dr. Hendricks was not present and thus the nominations came to a stalemate.

At this time the House of Delegates called for Dr. Nugent's report and Dr. Nugent invited every member of the Council to come into the House of Delegate meeting and listen to the report. In his report to the House of Delegates, Dr. Nugent carefully reviewed the program of the council on Education and its associated committees. He was very complimentary of the various administrative heads of the accredited colleges and advised the assembled delegates that the profession as a whole owed a debt of gratitude to those college heads for their unstinting effort and sacrifice.

After the completion of Dr. Nugent's report, the Council was quickly reassembled. Both Dr. Hendricks and Dr. Janse voiced their sincere attitude and in as much as Dr. Budden did not see fit to accept the nomination and in as much as the Council had made such competent progress under the auspices of Dr. Peterson, that Dr. Peterson should be encouraged to continue in his position at least until the mid-year meeting. Under the pressure of those attitudes, Dr. Peterson reconsidered his resignation and committed himself to the continuation of his leadership until the mid-year meeting insisting that Dr. Janse be reappointed as the Secretary.

Minutes of the COUNCIL ON EDUCATION of the National Chiropractic Association, Meetings held in conjunction with the annual convention of the National Chiropractic Association at the Statler Hotel, Detroit, Michigan , July 22-27, 1951 with Dr. Thure C. Peterson, President of the Council, presiding at all of the meetings.

Those attending the various meetings were:
(A) Members of the accrediting Committee:
    Dr. John J. Nugent, Director of Education of the National Chiropractic Association, 92 Norton Street, New Haven, Connecticut
    Dr. Edward H. Gardner, 2727 South Vermont Avenue, Los Angeles, California
    Dr. George A. Bauer, 1603 Bull Street, Columbia, South Carolina
    Dr. Walter B. Wolf, Eureka, South Dakota
    Dr. Norman E. Osborne, Hagerstown, Maryland
(B) Representatives of the accredited and provisionally accredited educational institutions:
    Dr. Thure C. Peterson, Director, Chiropractic Institute of New York, 152 W. 42nd Street, New York 13, New York
    Dr. W.A. Budden, Director, Western States College of Chiropractic, 4525 Southeast 63rd Avenue, Portland 6, Oregon
    Dr. James N. Firth, President, Lincoln Chiropractic College, 633 N. Pennsylvania St., Indianapolis 4, Indiana
    Dr. William N. Coggins, Dean, Logan Basic College of Chiropractic, 7701 Florissant Road, St. Louis 21, Missouri
    Dr. Joseph Janse, President, National College of Chiropractic, 20 North Ashland Blvd., Chicago 7, Illinois
    Dr. R.O. Mueller, Dean, Canadian Memorial Chiropractic College, 252 Bloor Street West, Toronto 5, Ontario, Canada
    Dr. Lee A. Norcross, Dean of the Graduate School of the Los Angeles College of Chiropractic, and Associate Dean of the Undergraduate school of the Los Angeles College of Chiropractic, 920 East Broadway Avenue, Glendale 5, California
    Dr. Paul O. Parr, President, Carver College of Chiropractic, 521 N.W. Ninth St., Oklahoma City 3, Oklahoma
    Dr. H.C. Schneider, representing Northwestern College of Chiropractic, 2222 Park Avenue, Minneapolis, Minnesota
    Dr. H.C. Harring, President, Dr. Ralph A. Power, Dean, Missouri Chiropractic Institute, Inc., 3117 Lafayette Avenue, St. Louis 4, Missouri
    Dr. S.W. Cole, Dean, Kansas State Chiropractic College, 629 N. Broadway Street, Wichita, Kansas
(C) Special invited guests:
    Dr. Carl S. Cleveland Jr., Dean, Cleveland Chiropractic College, 3724 Troost Avenue, Kansas City, Missouri
    Dr. Ben L. Parker, Dean, Texas Chiropractic College, San Pedro Park, San Antonio, Texas
    Dr. L.A. Bertholf, Dean, University of Natural Healing, Denver, Colorado
    Dr. Ralph J. Martin, Former President of Los Angeles College of Chiropractic, 403 W. 8th Street, Los Angeles, California

Dr. Arvis Talley, former President of the California Chiropractic Association, Delegate from California to the
National Chiropractic Association

Dr. Stuart Schillig, President of the California Chiropractic Association

Dr. Willard W. Percy, Secretary, California Board of Chiropractic Examiners, 1020 North Street, Sacramento,
California

Dr. Robert O. Mengel, President, Ohio State Chiropractic Physicians Association

Dr. Melvin I. Higgins, President, Idaho Board of Chiropractic Examiners, Coeur d'Alene, Idaho

First Meeting of the Council was held Sunday evening, July 22nd, from 8:00 to 11:00 p.m. with Dr. Thure C. Peterson presiding. Dr. Peterson called for recommendations of problems that should be discussed, for the purpose of setting up an agenda and the following matters for future discussion were submitted.

1. A discussion on the recent publications by Dr. Nugent in relation to chiropractic as a profession and the accredited chiropractic courses.
2. A discussion on effecting means of standardizing chiropractic concept and methods.
3. An analysis of the chiropractic situation in California.
4. A report by Doctors Nugent and Firth about the situation encountered while attending the convention in Alberta, Canada.
5. A study of the situation and the recent legislative measures in Minnesota.
6. A study of the present selective service situation especially as it related the passing of Senate Bill I.
7. A discussion of the issue of the appointment of non-professional men to the position of dean, president or director of any of the accredited chiropractic colleges.
8. A discussion of the European question especially as it related to Dr. Schwing of Paris, France.
9. An analysis of the possibilities of establishing scholarships in various chiropractic colleges.
10. A discussion of the proposition by Mr. Belleau of Milwaukee, Wisconsin, in relation to preparing a booklet on Chiropractic as a Career for distribution among high school and junior college students.
11. A discussion of the matter of individual school advertising in the NCA Journal.
12. Report on the talk by Dr. Orin Madison, President of the Michigan Basic Science Board.
13. Making of a small assessment to all schools participating in the Council program to help defray necessary expenses.
14. The resolution of Dr. Harring.
15. Report of the accrediting committee.
16. Passing of a resolution committing the Council to the keeping of a file on all of the official action of the Director of Education, the Accrediting Committee and the Council itself.
17. Report by Dr. Schwartz on his projects in relation to psycho-therapeutics in chiropractic.
18. Adjournment.

In order to establish proper continuity, the various subjects outlined in the agenda will be discussed individually and completely although in the course of the meetings their consideration was broken up and interceded on various occasions this being due to the fact that certain individuals concerned either had to leave, were absent or occupied with something else. The following reports however, represent an assemblage of the major discussions as they were made.

Point #1 - A discussion on the recent publications by Dr. Nugent in relation to chiropractic as a profession and the accredited chiropractic courses.

Dr. Parr expressed the opinion that it would have been better if Dr. Nugent had carefully consulted with the council as to the context of his publications. According to Dr. Parr there were certain definitions and statements that he felt portrayed misrepresentations and inasmuch as these booklets were going to experience wide distribution they probably should have been more carefully edited.

In answer to Dr. Parr's statement Dr. Nugent advised the council that he realized that the publications might contain a number of errors but that as a whole he had carefully checked the same and consequently he felt that they portrayed the picture in a very competent manner. Furthermore, because of the demanding exigencies at hand he found it necessary to prepare the same within a very limited time. He advised the council that immediately upon the passage of Senate Bill I and the signing of the same by the President, which at least in substance, placed the chiropractic student at parity with those of medicine and osteopathy in the selective service program, the department of higher education of the United States Government made inquiry as to the extent of the course in the accredited chiropractic colleges. In order to comply with this inquiry he was compelled to submit something of a standard nature and it was because of this necessity that the booklets were prepared. He advised the council that only a limited number have been published and that any future publication would be thoroughly revised.

After these discussions it was the full consensus of opinion of the entire council that a good job had been done and that an expression of appreciation should be proffered Dr. Nugent for his diligence of effort.

Point #2 - A discussion on effecting means of standardizing chiropractic concept and methods.

Both Drs. Parr and Janse voiced their conviction that some program should be initiated whereby the various definitions and concepts of chiropractic be cleared if for no other reason than to enable the various departments of chiropractic in the accredited colleges to present somewhat of a standard concept to the students.

It was the general conclusion that this was important. Drs. Firth and others drew attention to the fact that an attempt should be made to avoid making any conclusive definition of chiropractic both from a standpoint of principle and legal interpretation. It was generally consented that all school men should recommend that chiropractic as a method of adjusting the spine by hand only should be avoided.

In consequence to all of these discussions it was finally moved and seconded that from now on at the semi-annual meetings of the council a certain amount of time be set aside for a friendly discussion on some phase or aspect of chiropractic concept, probably in the form of an assignment to one of the school men to present a paper and this should be followed by a liberal and unbiased discussion.

It is to be mentioned that Dr. K.C. Robinson of Greenwich, Connecticut, appeared before the Executive Board with a proposition relating to this matter. It is also to be mentioned that Dr. Janse a year ago was appointed to head a committee on the standardization of chiropractic and that at this convention he had made a report to the House of Delegates in relation to the Council's decisions on this matter. That the House of Delegates had received this announcement with great acclaim.

Point #3 - An analysis of the chiropractic situation in California

It is to be stated that Dr. Lee A. Norcross was the official representative of the Los Angeles College of Chiropractic to the meetings of the Council on Education.

The California situation did receive attention and consideration on various occasions at different times and the following report represents a compilation of all of these discussions.

Dr. Willard W. Percy, Secretary of the California Board of Chiropractic Examiners was invited to explain to the Council, the exact nature of the various legislative measures in relation to chiropractic that had been sponsored in California during the last year. It is to be stated that Dr. Percy gave a very exacting interpretation and contributed much toward the proper orienting of the members of the Council in relation to the California matter. In substance, the following points were presented.

1. The Chiropractic Act in California, as it stands today, was one that was initiated by public vote and referendum and that any change in the present law would, of course, have to be accomplished via the same procedure.

2. The present Chiropractic act and its definition of chiropractic practice in California has been considered by a certain element in California as being inadequate and does not grant a sufficient breadth of privileges to enable the practice of certain procedures which this group considers necessary.

3. In the State of California the practice of chiropractic is very heterogeneous. Many holding chiropractic licenses and practicing under these licenses, because of ostensible necessity and personal inclination would wish to penetrate the practice of some phase of parental therapy and minor surgery. Therefore, this group proceeded to sponsor a legislative bill designed to entirely replace the present chiropractic act and by a legislative bill designed to entirely replace the present chiropractic act and by legislative vote institute a chiropractic law that would give the licentiate under this law certain privileges of allopathic practice as well as certain phases of operative minor surgery and this proposed bill was the commonly so-called Physicians and Surgeons (P&S) Bill.

4. It was considered by the members of the Board of Chiropractic Examiners, the officers of the California Chiropractic Association and the Board of Regents of the Los Angeles College of Chiropractic that such a bill would be of detriment to the profession and would eventually lead to a "back door" penetration of allopathic and surgical efforts. In order to maintain an element of unity within the professional ranks in California, the Board of Examiners, along with the California Association were willing to make a compromise with the sponsors of the P&S Bill. The compromise was to be reached by an amendment to the present chiropractic act. The amendment was to include a broader definition of chiropractic, the privilege of the usage of the word, physician and the privilege to utilize State, County and municipal laboratory facilities.

5. Unfortunately, however, although the P&S sponsors exhibited their willingness to go along with this proposed compromise, it wasn't long before the amendment became cluttered with a number of riders in the form of specialty privileges, so that eventually, the amendment and the literature of these rider amendments to the amendment simulated the demands of the original P&S Bill and would, of course have resulted in an almost unlimited type of practice privilege.

6. It was Dr. Percy's frank opinion that it was a good thing that the P&S Bill had been squelched and that the compromise Amendment Bill had been defeated for the simple reason that the whole situation had become so severely surrounded by ambiguities of effort that the whole affair had resulted in a lot of confusion and misunderstanding.

7. Dr. Percy then advised the Council group that within the next year the California Board of Chiropractic Examiners and the California Chiropractic Association were definitely going to combine efforts and sponsor an entirely new chiropractic bill. The high points of this proposition could be listed as follows:

    a. Because of the fact that the present Chiropractic Act had been a referendum act it had never been placed under the auspices of the Healing Arts Code, hence all of the privileges granted the other healing professions by this code were denied the chiropractors.

    b. This new bill would definitely afford the chiropractic profession an autonomous position under the Healing Arts Code and thus effect inclusion of the chiropractors in all of the privileges.

    c. This new bill would be carried directly to the public and because of the strength of the chiropractic vote its chances for passage would be good.

    d. This new bill would grant the broader clinical privileges and would afford the necessity of issuing two licenses.

        (1) A limited license of general chiropractic practice.

        (2) A chiropractic specialist's license granting extra clinical prerogatives especially in the specialty for which the practitioner had qualified.

    e. This new bill would require that the present licentiates in California obtain more education in order to qualify for the extra privileges of the bill.

    f. Out of state students in order to qualify for the broad privileges of the bill would have to do added work in the recognized colleges within California.

    g. Dr. Percy was asked if he would send a copy of the new bill as soon as it was drawn up to Dr. Janse, the secretary of the Council, so that he might have it multigraphed and send it to all members of the Council. Dr. Percy said that he certainly would do that, however, that such would not take place until next spring.

    h. Dr. Percy also stated that it was the intent of the C.C.A. to sponsor two campuses for the Los Angeles College of Chiropractic, one in the present Glendale site and another in Oakland, namely the McClintock college. Dr. Percy advised the group that the Oakland College had obtained new quarters of much more spacious and qualified nature and that definite concise steps had been initiated to convert this college into the northern campus of the L.A. College and to put it on a corporate rather than privately owned basis.

        (1) At this time Dr. Arvis Talley circulated a goodly number of photographs of the new facilities of this institution as evidence of Dr. Percy's descriptions.

8. Dr. Percy was also asked to explain why certain of the accredited colleges that did not teach physiotherapy had been taken off the approved list by the California Board.

He stated that such was a temporary necessity as the result of an attorney-general ruling but advised the Council that very likely within the near future this ruling would be rescinded and that full accreditation would be extended to all of the NCA accredited colleges.

Dr. Norcross was then asked to make a number of explanations in relation to his personal role in the matter as well as the role of the graduate school of the Los Angeles College of Chiropractic.

1. Dr. Norcross explained that the sponsors of the Physicians and Surgeons Bill were primarily under the auspices of Doctors Bonazza and Sayer, who at that time were members of the undergraduate faculty of the Los Angeles College. Those two individuals were encouraged in their efforts by certain elements within the profession. Unfortunately, these two faculty members utilized on various occasions, a goodly portion of their class room time in talking to students about the P&S effort. In fact, they had prompted the holding of a number of student body meetings and had procured the services of certain student groups in soliciting public support for the bill. It was Dr. Norcross' contention that it was he who had advocated the dismissal of these men from the faculty long before the then acting president and dean effected this dismissal.

2. Dr. Norcross was then asked whether he had ever been a participant in the sponsorship of the P&S movement and the answer was a vigorous no. He was then asked as to the attitude and the position of Drs. Montenegro and Taylor who are now members of the Board of Regents of the Los Angeles College, as to whether they had participated in the P&S movement. According to Dr. Norcross, to his knowledge neither of the gentlemen had ever taken an active part in the activities of the same. He did acknowledge that possibly they as well as he and others had made contributions to various chiropractic efforts in the state.

3. The direct question was put before Dr. Norcross as to whether he had sought the authority from the Board of Regents to conduct classes in pharmacology and certain phases of operative minor surgery in the graduate school. After much discussion conducted primarily between him and Dr. Nugent, Dr. Norcross stated that a number of limited classes in these subjects had been conducted and that on one occasion at an official meeting of the Board of Regents he had, out of necessity, asked for the authority to teach these subjects. Dr. Norcross qualified this commitment by stating that he was confronted by the exigency of preparing the matriculants of the graduate school for the unlimited privileges if the original P&S bill or the compromise amendment had passed. Then Dr. Norcross was asked whether or not he was in favor of the P&S bill and the subsequent compromise amendment and Dr. Norcross stated that he was because in order to obtain the right to use the term physician it would be necessary to qualify an individual in certain phases of pharmacology etc. In other words, according to Dr. Norcross, the chiropractors in California, in order to experience the privileges of public health functionaries, sick benefit insurance policies and industrial commission forms, they would have to acquire the title physician and according to him the title physician implied the necessity of the knowledge of certain of pharmacology etc. It is to be stated that this contention was somewhat questioned because in such states as Oklahoma, Oregon, Idaho, Illinois, and Michigan, the word physician can be employed by the chiropractor without possessing any knowledge of pharmacology or any privilege of pharmacology.

4. Dr. Norcross was then asked whether at any time the issue of unlimited practice under the P&S Bill or the Amendment Bill with the attached specialty practice "riders" had received support within the ranks of the administrative body of the graduate school or in any of the classes held under the auspices of the graduate school? In answer to this inquiry Dr. Norcross stated that at no time had the P&S movement received support from the graduate college. However, just as soon as the C.C.A. and the State Board of Examiners had fully approved of the compromise Amendment Bill he had been advised by Dr. Clyde Martyn, the then Pres. of the C.C.A. as well as the Board of Regents of the L.A. College that it could now become a matter of open and frank discussion

on the college campus.

5.   Dr. Norcross was asked whether he favored the broad unlimited concepts as contained within the rider amendments to the C.C.A. sponsored Amendment Bill? He stated that he did because in his opinion unless these privileges were obtained and then supported the members of the chiropractic profession in California would never experience the right of calling themselves physicians and obtain all the related prerogatives and it would never be possible for the L.A. College to be considered an institution of higher professional education.

6.   In further discussion on the subject of the teaching of pharmacology and operative minor surgery in the graduate school of the L.A. College Dr. Norcross insisted that he had received instructions from Dr. Clyde Martyn that inasmuch as the graduate school was part of the C.C.A. and the C.C.A. had sponsored the Amendment Bill and the associated specialty riders it would be necessary to teach 160 hours in pharmacology and 160 hours in Minor Surgery in order to qualify those who, if the Bill passed, wished to practice the specialties listed.

7.   It is to be stated that in all these discussions Dr. Norcross expressed the belief that he was being compromised and that those opposing him were placing words in his mouth and that he was not being allowed to display the proper picture.

8.   It is also to be stated that it was the general consensus of opinion that possibly the graduate school of the L.A. College had overextended itself in the sponsoring and teaching of the borderline specialties.

Drs. Stewart Schillig and Arvis Talley, present and past Presidents of the California Chiropractic Association were also invited in to present their viewpoint on the subject. Following were the main points brought out in the related discussions.

1.   These gentlemen felt that California should be permitted to work out its own solution to its problems.

2.   They further advised the Council that in their opinion any definite stand by the Council or the NCA in this matter would lead to a lot of resistance and probably result in a split in professional allegiance.

3.   It was the frank opinion of these men that no effort should be made by anyone on the Council to attempt to effect a reinstating of Dr. Ralph Martin as President of the L.A. College and furthermore that any attempt to place him on the Board of Regents would be met with disapproval.

4.   When asked as to what their opinion was as to where the line should be drawn on the unlimited practice issue these gentlemen simply stated that they themselves did not know and felt that the matter should be allowed to run its course, else it would result in schism and great damage to the NCA and C.C.A.

5.   When these men were asked as to whom they would approve of as the NCA representative on the Board of Regents of the L.A. College to fill the vacancy of Dr. Koer they stated that they would approve of either Dr. Clyde Martyn or Dr. Floyd Cregger but not Dr. Ralph Martin.

6.   They also signified the fact that the C.C.A. in conjunction with the Board of Chiropractic Examiners were preparing to write an entirely new chiropractic bill which would place chiropractic in a position of complete autonomy under the healing arts code. That they were going to take this bill directly to the people as an initiative bill and that if this bill goes through there will be issued two types of chiropractic licenses.

   a.   A license of general limited chiropractic practice.

   b.   A license of specialized chiropractic practice which would grant the holder the privileges prescribed under his specialty, what ever such may be.

7.   This new bill would definitely give added privileges and those now holding licenses in order to qualify for these privileges would have to take further training along prescribed lines.

8.   It should be mentioned that Drs. Schillig and Talley had previously met with Dr. Nugent and some of the members of the accrediting committee and had definitely advised them of the official C.C.A. attitude in relation to the question at hand and that essentially it was one of "hands off".

9.   Mention should also be made of the fact that in a consequent meeting the Executive Board of the NCA and a representative group of the Council on Education advised the Board that the Council recommended the appointment of Dr. Clyde Martyn as the NCA representative on the Board of Regents of the L.A. College.

Point #4. A report by Drs. Nugent and Firth about the situation encountered while attending the convention in Saskatoon, Canada.

It has been quite evident that the chiropractic body in the plain provinces of Canada has been severely anti-NCA and that definite restricting efforts had been made to keep graduates from NCA colleges to obtain licenses in these provinces and if such were obtained to confine their practice to exacting demands based upon prejudiced attitudes.

Dr. Nugent verified these observations and stated that he encountered a marked resistance toward the NCA and its educational program and that the association and the board had conducted rather severe measures of bias.

Dr. Nugent advised the Council that in one of his lectures before the group he frankly told them of his disapproval of this conduct and that if they did not desist he would with pointed intent come back to Alberta and see to it that the provincial authorities were properly alerted to the detriments that had been committed.

The Council was also advised that pressure had been placed upon the administration of the Canadian Memorial Chiropractic College to the effect that if the college did not condition its curriculum and attitudes to correspond with the wishes of this Alberta group they, the Alberta group would drop their support of the college.

It was concluded to permit this matter to boil itself out and if necessary later on have Dr. Nugent return to set the affair right.

Point #5. A study of the situation of the recent legislative measures in Minnesota.

Toward the immediate close of the legislative session in Minnesota in the forepart of June, the medical profession was able to press through a bill setting up qualifying stipulations for the practitioners of medical physical therapy.

The bill did not necessarily impose any restrictions on the use of physiotherapy by the licensed practitioners of any of the healing professions. No mention was made of the use of physiotherapy by the doctors of chiropractic.

Dr. H.C. Schneider, Dean of the Northwestern College of Chiropractic stated that although the present physiotherapy law made no mention of the use of physiotherapy by the chiropractor there was the possible inference that he might be prohibited from using the same.

Furthermore, according to Dr. Schneider, a controlling element of the chiropractic profession in Minnesota were now insisting that chiropractic be held in practice to the exact wording of the law and hence the use of physiotherapy by chiropractors was becoming severely endangered.

It seems that certain factions of the profession in Minnesota definitely favor the exclusion of physiotherapy practice by chiropractors.

Point #6. A study of the present selective service situation especially as it relates to the passing of Senate Bill I.

It was, of course, the full consensus of opinion of the Council that Drs. Murphy and Nugent had gained a wonderful advantage for the profession and especially the chiropractic colleges in being able to include the word chiropractic in the new rulings of the Selective Service Act and as contained in Senate Bill I.

The Council was advised that as yet there had not been a specific declaration of the Federal Selective Service Headquarters in relation to the chiropractic student. Furthermore, no specific directive had been sent from the National Headquarters to the State Headquarters as to the status of the chiropractic student.

Dr. Nugent advised the group that when he and Dr. Murphy made inquiry as to why a directive had not been sent out the answer was that because the inclusion of the word chiropractic in the Selective Service Act, a new precedence had been established and as yet the officials at the headquarters in Washington had not been able to agree on a proper interpretation of the chiropractic position and thus a directive had been withheld.

The Council was also advised that selective service system form #103 previously used for the deferment of professional college students had been discontinued and that all school men should obtain a supply of form #109 and then attach an explanatory letter to each one when sent in with a student's application for deferment.

It was stated that Dr. Murphy was pressing the issue as much as possible and that it was highly probable that the situation would break in the profession's favor within the next month or so.

Dr. Nugent then presented a complete resume of the efforts he and Dr. Murphy had conducted in Washington in relation to the postponement of induction of chiropractic students.

1. As soon as Dr. Nugent found out that Senate Bill I had included chiropractic students he proceeded to prepare the booklet "Educational Standards for Chiropractic Colleges." and distributed the same to all the interested federal agencies.
2. He was advised by Mrs. Wilkins of the Department of Higher Education of the Federal Government that the booklet would have to be revised in certain aspects and then it would probably be accepted by the department as the authoritative literature on chiropractic education. This would likely lead to the recognition of chiropractic colleges as institutions of higher education and thus make them eligible for all of the associated privileges and benefits.
3. Dr. Nugent stated that if such a measure were attained it would necessitate placing greater emphasis upon having the various departments headed by men who possessed pre-professional academic degrees.

Point #7. A discussion of the issue of the appointment of a non-professional man to the position of president, dean, or director of any of the accredited colleges.

This issue led to a great deal of deliberation. It was the general consensus of opinion that it would represent a hazard to permit the chiropractic educational policies of any of the chiropractic colleges fall into the hands and under the supervision of a person who did not possess a chiropractic degree or training.

It was also concluded that the position of president, dean or director if attended by the specific responsibility of supervising the teaching of chiropractic should be under the auspices of a person who might possess another therapeutic degree unless consequent to the acquisition of the same he had obtained a competent chiropractic training.

Drs. Percy and Talley speaking on certain problems that confronted the educational policies of the L.A. College stated that in California an effort was being made to obtain recognition for the college as an institution of higher learning, and in order to obtain this recognition it might be quite necessary to appoint a titular head who possessed a Ph.D. in education.

The final conclusion was that under no circumstances would the professional policies of any of the accredited chiropractic colleges come under the control of non-professional or lay persons. However, if any of the colleges wished to employ a professional educator to help conduct the mechanism of educational procedure, or employ a layman to serve as business administrator such would in no way represent a compromise of the above stated conclusion.

The following pertaining resolution was passed. Whoever holds the position, be it president, dean or director, of any of the accredited colleges, that relates to the responsibility of supervising the teaching of chiropractic principles, interpretation and procedures must be a graduate doctor of chiropractic and must not in consequence to the acquisition of his degree in chiropractic proceed to obtain another therapeutic degree. His degree in chiropractic may of course be fully supported by any extent of previous or subsequent collegiate training.

Point #8. A discussion of the European question as it relates to the proposition of Dr. Schwing and the introduction of chiropractic training into the medical colleges of France.

Several weeks previous to the Council meeting all the school men had received a multigraphed communication from Dr. Fred Illi, Geneva, Switzerland and the President of the European Chiropractic Union outlining the intents of Dr. Schwing of Paris, France, to organize a special school of instruction in chiropractic for medical practitioners and the members of the orthopedic department of certain medical colleges of France.

Dr. Illi advised the Council that Dr. Schwing was coming to the U.S.A. for the purpose of going to various chiropractic colleges and obtaining the latest developments in chiropractic and then return to France and commence his special course of instruction to the medical fraternity.

In the first part of July the European Chiropractic Union held its convention in Copenhagen, Denmark, and at that time Dr. Schwing appeared before the group and advised them of the fact that he had affected the introduction of proposal into the French legislature designed to give him the permit to conduct a special course of instruction in chiropractic to medical graduates and professors in medical schools, so that eventually chiropractic could become a specialty in medicine, and that thereafter all practitioners of chiropractic in France would first have to become medical graduates.

Dr. Schwing justified this action on the contention that such a step was necessary in order to save chiropractic from complete extinction in France. He asserted that the ministry of health in France was determined to weed out all practitioners other than those of the allopathic medical school and that already a number of French chiropractors had been arrested.

When asked as to how he the leading chiropractor in France had experienced immunity from this edict by the ministry of health, Dr. Schwing stated that he had powerful friends in the government and they had recognized him as being by far the most qualified chiropractor in France and had chosen him to introduce chiropractic into the medical fraternity.

When asked as to what would happen to the other chiropractors practicing in France if his proposition went through, Dr. Schwing flatly stated that they would be put out of practice anyway as they would not be able to qualify under the provisions of the act.

It therefore seemed to the Council that the only chiropractor who would remain in France regardless of what might happen would be Dr. Schwing. If the act did not pass the ministry of health would close up the other chiropractorsp; if the act did pass they would have to go out of practice because of lack of qualification.

A committee consisting of Drs. Mueller and Janse were assigned to meet with Dr. Schwing and hear his story. The above represents the essence of his statements to this committee.

It was finally concluded to have the secretary Dr. Janse write Dr. Illi and have him submit a formal brief of the European Chiropractic Union's complaint against Dr. Schwing. The following was what Dr. Janse received from Dr. W.J.C. Cleave, the secretary of the Union, Glasgow, Scotland:

Extracts from the minutes of the E.C.U. Conference on the French situation.

Dr. Schwing: There were only 9 chiropractors in France. The situation is very acute. The Medical Act of 1892 had many loopholes which allowed chiropractors to practice, but the medical profession has been very active and aggressive. It almost completely controls the nominations for the deputies to the Government, and as a result has been able to pass legislation which would threaten all unorthodox practitioners. Medical practitioners are forbidden to cooperate in any way with anyone outside the medical profession, the use of x-ray is confined to medical practitioners only. It would appear that the French doctors are out for a kill. Their main purpose is to destroy chiropractic and usurp it for themselves, and organize the practices of massage, physiotherapy and dentistry, etc. under their control. The 1945 Medical Act is the most drastic of any country in Europe. Every chiropractor has been on trial and fined, some many times, and we have with us today Dr. Gross, whose office has been recently sealed for a period of one year. Lectures have been given to arouse public interest, and laymen's organizations started, in addition books have been published attacking the M.D.s on their own ground. After 2 years investigation and at considerable expense Dr. Schwing has arrived at the decision that very little or nothing could be done. He had therefore made efforts to organize the medical doctors who were dissatisfied with medical affairs, and give them a course of training in chiropractic technic, by which action he hoped to deal a severe blow to the French Medical Association and (using his own words) "bust them wide open." He read a letter he had recently received from Dr. Weiant of the N.Y. School, commending this proposed scheme.

Dr. Gross: Then gave a further report and outlined some of the difficulties he and his French colleagues were working under. He also outlined his present unfortunate position of having his office sealed for the next year. He was, however, very pleased to be able to say that as a result of this persecution, patients were flocking to him in larger numbers. He closed with an earnest appeal for unity of the members, regardless of the method or technic used.

Dr. Firestorms of France. Strongly objected to the training of medical doctors.

Dr. He-man of Sweden. State that he had been invited to instruct MDs in a Swedish hospital but had refused, and he appealed to all chiropractors to do the same.

Dr. Illi of Switzerland. Appealed for the fight to be carried to the MDs and condemned the scheme outlined by Dr. Schwing.

Dr. Beyeler of Switzerland, suggested that the French and Swiss chiropractors should seek closer relations with each other, and discuss all problems. He felt that by doing so the situation would be relieved, but first the French must come to an understanding among themselves. The difficulties at present facing France had been experienced in Switzerland, but by constant spreading of the gospel of chiropractic to the public, they had gradually succeeded in changing the law. He completely disagreed with Dr. Schwing.

There was considerable discussion and many other speakers expressed similar views.

It was finally moved by Dr. Beyeler and seconded by Dr. Gross that:

"The E.C.U. is not in favor of any member of this organization individually teaching chiropractic to members of the medical profession or to any other person engaged in therapeutic work."

This motion was carried, with one dissenting vote, namely Dr. Schwing.

Copy of Report made by Dr. M.H. Brunner D.C. of France to the President of E.C.U.

Medical grasp upon chiropractic in France added by a chiropractor. On Oct. 30/50 Dr. Schwing called a meeting of his fellow practitioners and the presidents of lay organizations and announced flatly the introduction of a bill giving up chiropractic to the medical faculties, then asked for financial help to put this thru.

Here is a rough translation of this bill, introduced Nov. 7/50 by M. Duveau, Depute:

Article 1. The teaching of chiropractic is created at (in connection with) the chairs of orthopedics of the faculties of medicine.

Article 2: This matter will be taught during the transitional period by assistant lecturers holding a diploma of D.C. delivered by a foreign faculty.

Article 3. These assistant lecturers shall be allowed to practice their art in accordance with valie (existing) laws and regulations.

Dr. Schwing is the man who edited in 1947 a book "La chute d'Esculape" which is a virulent attack against medicine and which is probably at the origin of the present bad situation of French chiropractors.

In 1949, we formed a syndicate of all chiropractors in France holding an American diploma with Dr. Schwing as president. We agreed that no action should be taken concerning our profession without the consent of the majority of all members. Dr. Schwing then started a campaign in order to collect signatures for the legal recognition of chiropractic. Quite a number of petitions were handed to him by his fellow chiropractors, covered with signatures of their patients and friends. Later on we had a meeting with M. Duveau, depute, who announced the impossibility of passing a straight chiropractic bill. We made it clear that in this case, illegality was preferable to compromise with the medical authorities and let the matter dormant. But Dr. Schwing did not.

By what aberration he had this bill introduced we shall never know. He did it single-handedly and in violation of the articles of our association. Moreover, he used the petition sheets of our own patients for this project, and this without telling us beforehand.

His argument is that without this bill there would be no chance of survival for chiropractic in France and that moreover the educational standards of chiropractors is far too low for the practice of chiropractic.

Ever since No. 7/50 we endeavored to introduce a counter-project for a straight chiropractic bill. But we were unable to find a single depute willing to face the medical profession and opposition.

Finally an appointed commission adopted the following modified bill:

The teaching of chiropractic is introduced into the faculties of medicine in connection with one of the various chairs in the department of orthopedics. This teaching being reserved only for students regularly registered for obtainment of the degree of M.D.

The teaching is to be organized by the titular of the chair of rheumatology, orthopedy, or traumatology will give rise to the nomination of an assistant lecturer according to valid rules.

This of course means that chiropractic could be practiced by MDs only in France, and excluding all chiropractors, yet Dr. Schwing D.C. is still patronizing this bill. (signed) M.H. Brunner D.C. June 1951

Point #9. An analysis of the possibilities of establishing scholarships in the various chiropractic colleges.
1. It was generally admitted by the college men in attendance that attempts to initiate effective scholarship programs had not worked out too well. The reasons being as follows:
   a. Lack of sustained interest by those groups of the field sponsoring scholarships.
   b. The difficulty in actually setting up a true criterion of evaluation in any scholarship contest.
   c. Most students thus procured really weren't too well sustained in their chiropractic interests.
   d. Difficult for state associations to set up a scholarship program because individual school allegiance often made it difficult to decide which college would receive the student.
2. It was the general consensus of opinion that at least for the time being each college and state association should be permitted to make their own ventures along these lines if they wished.

Point #10. A discussion of the proposition by Mr. Wm. Belleau of Milwaukee, Wisconsin, in relation to his proposal to prepare a vocational guidance booklet on chiropractic as a career for distribution to high school and junior college students.
1. Dr. Janse advised the Council that he had been approached by Mr. Belleau with the above stated proposition. It was Mr. Belleau's plan to prepare such a booklet, have it published and then sell it to the chiropractic colleges and national organizations for so much a copy.

2. The gentleman claimed that he had done a similar job for the osteopathic profession with gratifying results.
3. Mr. Belleau professed to possess extensive entree into all of the high schools and junior colleges all over the country because of his well known work in vocational guidance.
4. Dr. Nugent advised the Council that he knew of Mr. Belleau's work, especially for the osteopathic profession and that this group were rather dissatisfied with the same and hence he recommended that the measure be shelved.
5. Such seemed the consensus of attitude and Dr. Janse was instructed to write and advise Mr. Belleau of this decision.

Point #11. A discussion of the matter of individual school advertising in the NCA Journal
1. This matter was originally taken up at the mid-year meeting in Santa Monica, California. At that time it was decided that it would be best if the various colleges discontinued their individual ads in the NCA Journal. The primary reason being that it did portray a rather severe competitive effort which might well be misinterpreted.
2. It was decided that it would be much more desirable to have a monthly full page ad simply listing the accredited colleges and their addresses alphabetically.
3. Dr. Nugent was asked to present this matter to Dr. L.M. Rogers and the executive board.
4. The Council was advised by Dr. Nugent that Dr. Rogers rather resisted the idea because it would represent quite a loss to the Journal in much needed advertising.
5. At the Detroit meeting the Council reaffirmed its belief that individual school ads should be discontinued and that the full page monthly ad listing all the colleges be instituted.
6. It was decided to inquire of Dr. Rogers just what he would consider a fair fee for such an ad. This charge was then to be prorated among the accredited colleges.
7. It was thought possibly that inasmuch as there were 12 accredited colleges each of the same could assume the payment once during the course of the year.

Point #12. Report on a talk made before the Council by Dr. Orin Madison, President of the Michigan Basic Science Board and former President of the American Association of Basic Science Boards.
1. Dr. Madison was introduced to the Council by Dr. Janse and Dr. Janse advised the group that it was his opinion that Dr. Madison had performed an invaluable service to the profession by sustaining a very democratic attitude toward chiropractic. Dr. Janse stated that it was through the deference of Dr. Madison that he and Dr. Nugent had originally received the invitation to attend the annual meetings of the American Association of Basic Science Boards.
2. Dr. Madison advised the Council that one of the happiest occasions of his life was when Dr. Janse had the opportunity of reading the paper "The Basic Science Issue in Chiropractic Education" before the American Association. He stated that the paper was very well received and would be published in the annual bulletin of the Association.
3. Dr. Madison encouraged the Council members to sense the great need to sustain an open mind in relation to the basic science program. That did not mean necessarily to condone it but to at least honestly endeavor to cope with its stipulations if for no other reason than that of helping the student who must cope with it.
4. Dr. Madison complimented the school men for the fact that chiropractic students were passing basic science boards with relative good results and that certainly chiropractic education had made remarkable strides.
5. Dr. Madison expressed his confidence in chiropractic in sincere and glowing terms. He voiced his opinion that chiropractic education in certain respects represented a greater competence than that of other professions.
6. He gave the school men some valuable hints on basic science board examinations. He encouraged the school men to sense the great need of encouraging the students to be more persevering in their studies. Our young people he stated are becoming academically soft. It is so seldom that today we find a youth who is willing to make the sacrifice of time and effort to qualify themselves for life.
7. He contended that the majority of basic science boards were quite passable if but the student would lend himself to the necessity of really studying for it.
8. He advised the Council that students of the other healing professions probably found the examinations just as difficult as did chiropractic students.
9. He gave the following as the major causes in failure in basic science examinations.
    a. Lack of literary ability and thus making the answers to questions inept in their literary portrayal.
    b. Failure to carefully read and study the question and thus not fully understanding just what the examiner wanted in the form of an answer.
    c. Inability to properly organize the work and to present it in a systematic manner.
    d. Failure to show the capacity of integrated thinking. Much of the answer material represents memorized work rather than material that is visualized and understood.
    e. Inadequacy of spelling and writing. Showing a juvenile style of writing.
    f. Lack of conciseness in answers, a great deal of irrelevant material.

Point #13. Making of an assessment to all of the representatives of the accredited colleges to help defray the expenses of the Council.
1. Both Dr. Peterson and Janse stated that their position as president and secretary of the Council involved quite a bit of expense.

Such items as the following being mentioned:

a. Preparing and multigraphing of minutes.

b. Postage, phone calls and telegrams in relation to Council affairs.

c. Expenses incurred by Dr. Janse attending the annual meeting of the American Association of Basic Science Boards.

2. At the mid-year meeting in Santa Monica an assessment of ten dollars for each of the accredited colleges was made and Dr. Janse collected some 80 dollars. He reported that he had spent some $48.01 leaving a sum of $31.99.

3. Dr. Peterson as yet had not submitted his expenses incurred during the past year.

4. It was by unanimous vote that at the time Dr. Janse sent a copy of the minutes out each of the colleges that participated in the meetings and program of the Council was to submit the assessment of ten dollars to Dr. Janse the secretary to serve as a small reserve that might be drawn upon for essential Council expenses.

Point #14. A proposition submitted by Dr. Harring.

1. Dr. H.C. Harring, President of the Missouri Chiropractic Institute asked Dr. Janse to submit the following resolution to the Council and solicited its adoption.

Whereas, chiropractic has now advanced to the point where it is recognized as the second largest healing science and whereas much of the credit for its advancement is due to its efficiency as a therapeutic measure, and whereas our increase in standards has been primarily in the academic scope of teaching pre-clinical subjects with little stress on developing the therapeutic side and whereas it is the practice of some of our Chiropractic Boards to disregard or treat very lightly the examination of an applicant in his technic but accept his word for the particular type used without actual demonstration and, whereas the government in its recognition of chiropractic in the selective service act has now entrusted us with the responsibility of supplying qualified doctors who thoroughly understand the therapeutics of the science we represent, we recommend to the Council of Chiropractic Boards of Examiners that this body urges that special consideration be given to all applicants for licensure to determine their qualifications in chiropractic therapeutic procedures in line with the fundamentals as set down by the NCA.

2. Because of the brevity of time it was concluded to table this resolution until the next meeting and then have Dr. Harring speak on the same.

Point #15. Report of the accrediting committee.

1. Dr. Edw. Gardner as president of the committee asked Dr. Nugent to make the report of the accrediting committee and to review his activities in relation to the colleges since the mid-year meeting.

2. Following is a resume of Dr. Nugent's report.

a. He had made two visits to the Lincoln College and found that everything was moving along satisfactory and that plans were being completed for new laboratory facilities in pathology, histology, etc.

b. He had not had the occasion to visit the National College but had received reports from Dr. Janse with reference to the new chemistry and histo-pathology laboratories that had been installed.

c. He had been at the Los Angeles College and had encountered a rather serious disturbance because of the divided attitudes within the Board of Regents about the P.&S. question. Felt that the matter would more or less have to find its own solution.

d. He had not been able to visit the Logan College and that it was his intent to visit the same soon. That certain commendable changes has been made in the set up of the curriculum as well as the faculty.

e. That he had been in close communication with Dr. John Wolfe of the Northwestern College. Dr. Wolfe had encountered a serious cardiac ailment and unfortunately during the tenure of his illness certain subversive elements in Minnesota had attempted to usurp control of the college. Now that Dr. Wolfe was back on his feet he felt that the situation would rectify itself. He called on all to grant as much support to Dr. Wolfe and his associates as was possible.

f. Dr. Nugent had had the occasion to speak at the graduation exercises of the Canadian Memorial Chiropractic College. That essentially, things were progressing well in this institution. There had been some tension between the elements that favored exclusive manipulative chiropractic and that element that wished adjunctive measures.

g. Dr. Nugent spoke of the progress that was being made at the Western States College in relation to the development of added laboratory facilities. He stated at this point that in his opinion the smaller chiropractic colleges might well be able to use one well equipped laboratory for most of their work in pathology, bacteriology, histology and physiology.

h. Dr. Nugent spoke of having visited the New York Institute several times. Continued progress was being made at the college. He announced the fact that Dr. Trubenbach was no longer affiliated with the college and that Drs. Peterson and Kightlinger represented the administrative authority of the college.

i. Dr. Nugent acknowledged with appreciation the presence of Dr. Ben Parker, Dean of the Texas College. He stated that it was his intent to visit the college within the near future and to make further investigation of the college. He stated that commendable changes had been made at the college in relation to the curriculum and faculty. He advised the Council that one of the snags encountered was that of the corporate set up of the college and the involvement of several high salaried officials.

(1) At this time Dr. Parker was asked to give a report on circumstances relating to the Texas College and in brief, the following represents the substance of Dr. Parker's remarks.

(a)   About a year ago, he, Dr. Parker, had resigned as Dean of the College because he felt that certain changes should be made in the college administration and he was not supported in this principle.

(b)   Since then the Texas College Alumni Association had taken over the college and had assumed the responsibility of amortizing the notes held by the former owners of the college.

(c)   That this process had progress rather well and that a good amount of the debt had been paid off.

(d)   That he had been asked by the Alumni Association to reassume his position as Dean. In the state of Texas any college to be recognized by the Department of Education must be supervised over by a person who possesses an academic degree and which Dr. Parker possesses.

(e)   That certain high salaried positions had been dissolved, although several of the individuals concerned had been retained as members of the Board of Directors as well as Officers of the college for the simple reason that they wielded an outstanding influence in the field especially among Texas College graduates.

(f)   Dr. Parker stated that the people in Texas had felt somewhat offended by the unfortunate occurrence relating to some months ago when inadvertently the NCA Journal had listed the Texas College as one of the accredited schools and then later had rescinded that listing.

(2)   Dr. Parker was assured that the Council was most anxious to reestablish relations with the Texas College. That every consideration possible would be extended in the effort to continue mediations. Dr. Nugent committed himself to a further study of the Texas College situation within the latter part of the summer or early fall.

j.   According to Dr. Nugent, conscientious efforts were being made at the Carver College. Difficulties were being encountered because of lack of reserves. He advised the Council that he would try and pay the college a visit at the same time he went to Texas.

(1)   Dr. Parr, at this time, proceeded to assert that it was a pressing necessity for the Council to endeavor to set up a program that would induce the field to come to the support of the chiropractic colleges and especially the smaller institutions, otherwise it would be impossible for any of the colleges to fully comply with all of the stipulations that were being made by the necessities of recognition confronting them.

(2)   It was the general consensus of opinion that care should be exercised by Dr. Nugent and the accrediting committee in not committing themselves too far in the direction of augmented standards of laboratory facilities, faculty members, etc., because it was obvious that all the colleges were operating on a much reduced student body and total college income.

k.   Dr. Nugent complimented Dr. Cole, Dean of the Kansas State College, for the diligent and competent efforts expended by him at this institution. He stated that it would be a difficult task to retain the program that Dr. Cole wished to carry out because of lack of support by the local field.

l.   Dr. Nugent mentioned the passing of Dr. Beatty, former president of the University of Natural Healing. He expressed his appreciation for the presence of Dr. Bertholf, the newly appointed dean of the college and stated that he would try and visit the school before the next mid-year meeting.

m.   He told about visiting the International College of Chiropractic in Dayton, Ohio operated by Drs. Valdiserri and Martino exclusively for negroes. That the college had an enrollment of some 40 students. That in his opinion it would be most difficult for this organization to retain itself and measure up to the standards of the Council.

Point #16. Passing of resolution assigning Dr. Nugent and the accrediting committee the responsibility of submitting in writing a full report of their activities and decisions, which along with the final conclusions, is to be sent to all of the members of the Council.

1.   Dr. Parr brought out the point that in his opinion, the activities, decisions, and commitments of Dr. Nugent and the accrediting committee were matters of behind the door conferences and by word of mouth dissemination and that no formal declarations or written instructions or reports reached the members of the Council, especially those persons affiliated with the institutions concerned.

2.   This matter led to a number of comments pro and con. It was generally concluded that it would be beneficial if the secretary of the Council would receive a definite report from Dr. Nugent from time to time and then have the same distributed to the Council members etc. It was, however, the consensus of attitude that certain rather intimate and personal discussions should be deleted so as to avoid embarrassment on both sides.

3.   Following was the resolution that was unanimously passed:
RESOLUTION: That the secretary of the Council keep a file and that this file should consist of a carbon copy of a letter of transmission accompanying the Educational Director's report made on the Institution or College in Question and made to the Accrediting Committee. There should also be a carbon copy in this file of the formal report made by the Director of Education or the Accrediting Committee to the Council on Education as well as a carbon copy of the final decision and report of the Council's action in relation to the institution or college in question. That the original of these three reports be sent to the best known address of the institution or college in question.

Point #17.   Report to the Council by Dr. H. Schwartz on the project in relation to his proposed year book on chiropractic verification in the literature of psychosomatic concept.

1. Dr. Schwartz advised the group that the program was bogging down because it was difficult to obtain the assistance of the various student bodies and the faculty members of the colleges were so busy that they couldn't lend themselves to this project either.
2. Dr. Schwartz advised the Council that he had just about finished a text on the subject of "psychotherapy in the home" for lay distribution and expressed the hope that the Council would support his efforts along these lines.
3. Dr. Schwartz was advised by members of the Council to develop a small but well set up book on abnormal psychology and psychotherapy from the chiropractic standpoint that could be used in the related classes in the accredited colleges.
4. It was the general opinion of the Council that such would represent a contribution of more immediate value than the year book consisting of chiropractic verifications as found in medical psychiatric literature.
5. Dr. Schwartz thanked the Council for their deference and stated that he would follow their recommendations.

Point #18 Adjournment.

1. At the close of the meetings, each member of the Council reaffirmed his confidence in the work that the Council was doing. Expressions of appreciation were proffered Drs. Nugent, Murphy and Peterson for the diligent effort in behalf of the Council.
2. It was decided to have Dr. Peterson send out a questionnaire as to where the mid-year meeting was to be held. It was the general feeling that it should be either in New York, Indianapolis, Chicago or St. Louis.

Minutes of the COUNCIL ON EDUCATION of the NATIONAL CHIROPRACTIC ASSOCIATION. Mid-year meeting held in Indianapolis, Lincoln Hotel, January 16, 17, 18 and 19th, 1952, Dr. Thure C. Peterson, President of the Council, presided at all of the meetings.

Those Attending:

(A) Members of the accrediting committee:
   Dr. John J. Nugent, Director of Education of the National Chiropractic Association, 92 Norton Street, New Haven, Connecticut.
   Dr. Edward H. Gardner, 2727 South Vermont Avenue, Los Angeles, California.
   Dr. Ralph J. Martin, 403 W. 8th Street, Los Angeles, California
   Dr. Walter B. Wolf, Eureka, South Dakota
   Dr. Norman E. Osborne, 1172 The Terrace, Hagerstown, Maryland

(B) Representatives of the accredited and provisionally accredited educational Institutions:
   Dr. Thure C. Peterson, Director, Chiropractic Institute of New York, 152 W. 42nd Street, New York 18, New York
   Dr. W.A. Budden, Director, Western States College of Chiropractic, 4525 Southeast 63rd Avenue, Portland 6, Oregon
   James N. Firth, President, Lincoln Chiropractic College, Inc., Dr. Arthur Hendricks, Treasurer, Dr. L.S. King, Dean
   Dr. William N. Coggins, Dean, Logan Basic College of Chiropractic, 7701 Florissant Road, St. Louis 21, Missouri
   Dr. H.C. Harring, President, Missouri College of Chiropractic, 3117 Lafayette Avenue, St. Louis 4, Missouri
   Dr. Paul O. Parr, President, Carver College of Chiropractic, 521 N.W. Ninth Str., Oklahoma City 3, Oklahoma
   Dr. Raymond H. Houser, Administrative Officer, Los Angeles College of Chiropractic, 920 East Broadway Avenue, Glendale 5, California; Dr. Lee A. Norcross, Dean of the Graduate School
   Dr. Joseph Janse, President, National College of Chiropractic, 20 N. Ashland Blvd., Chicago 7, Illinois
   Dr. R.O. Mueller, Dean, Canadian Memorial Chiropractic College, 252 Bloor Street, West, Toronto, Canada

(C) Special invited guests:
   Dr. Julius C. Troilo, Dean, Texas Chiropractic College, San Pedro Park, San Antonio, Texas
   Dr. Carl Cleveland, Jr., Dean, Cleveland Chiropractic College, 3724 Troost Avenue, Kansas City, Missouri

The first meeting of the Council was held Wednesday morning, January 16th, from 9:30 a.m. to 12:00 a.m. It was an open meeting and Dr. Peterson presided.

Dr. Peterson had called for recommendations of problems that should be discussed and the following agenda was prepared.

1. Discussion and final decision of composite advertising in NCA Journal for accredited schools. Also, discussion of similar advertising in various state chiropractic publications.
2. Conclusion of the matter of Dr. Schwing's program for chiropractic continuance in France. Notification of Swiss chiropractors of final decision.
3. Discussion of Council members supporting low standard legislation, contrary to Council policy.
4. Delineation of Council position in attacks on modality and supplemental manufacturers by the Better Business Bureau.

5. Review of Pennsylvania, Ohio and Illinois situation and evaluation of result of legislative efforts in those states, also discussion of Georgia situation.
6. Final clarification of California situation regarding physicians and surgeons proposed legislation, as well as evaluation of effect of such minority group concepts on the present curriculum, if any.
7. Discussion of supplemental degrees to the regular Doctorate of Chiropractic.
8. Discussion of promotion of closer relationship between state examination boards and the Council. Also consideration of resolution proposed by Dr. Harring in developing proper type of practical examinations in chiropractic.
9. Establishment of Committee on Graduate Study and Research within the National Council on Education. (This committee was abolished by the NCA Board last summer in order to bring it into the Council where it belongs)
10. Discussion of methods of developing more proficient instructors in chiropractic colleges.
11. Discussion of the written reports given out by the National Director of Education.
12. Discussion of the effects of the Minnesota physiotherapy law.
13. Discussion of methods to better prepare graduates of chiropractic colleges in proven business and practice building methods in attempt to reduce professional mortality.
14. Discussion of standardization of chiropractic principles and concepts.

Point No. 1 - Discussion and final decision of composite advertising in NCA Journal for affiliated colleges, along with discussion of similar advertising in state publications.

Dr. Peterson advised the council that Dr. L.M. Rogers editor of the NCA Journal had set up a double page middle spread for the Journal listing the affiliated colleges that might participate. Copies of this spread were distributed. It was observed that the colleges had been differentiated into the accredited, provisionally accredited and associated colleges.

Dr. Peterson advised the group that the following colleges had indicated their willingness to support this composite spread as prepared by Dr. Rogers, namely, New York, Lincoln, Western States, National, Kansas State, Los Angeles.

Dr. Harring expressed the opinion that certain elements about the descriptive narration on the advertisement would represent a detriment to the Missouri College, which as yet had not received complete accreditation. He specifically made reference to the subscription beneath each college listing, differentiating them into accredited, provisionally accredited and associated, as well as the statement "in the selection of a college choose an accredited institution."

Dr. Parr expressed the same attitude and further stated that he thought that the cost for each college was too high, maintaining that the NCA should beware of the fact that it owes the colleges something in the form of economic assistance and that it was not necessarily quite fair for the NCA to always demand payment for the college ads carried in the Journal.

Dr. Cleveland concurred with Drs. Harring and Parr in disapproving of the differentiating designation between accredited and provisionally approved colleges.

Dr. Troilo representing the Texas College as the newly appointed dean also expressed his hesitancy in support of the composite ad if a discriminating designation were employed.

Dr. Budden stated that he did not necessarily demand the differentiating designation but that the colleges participating in the advertisement should all definitely have committed themselves to the accrediting program of the Council.

Drs. Peterson, Firth and Janse all designated their readiness to support a composite ad that in its listing would not differentiate the colleges as to their state of accreditation as long as each of the colleges participating were wholly involved in the effort to retain or acquire full NCA approval.

It was then unanimously concluded to advise Dr. Rogers that all listing of accreditation in the ad be deleted and that the following heading for the ad be employed.
COLLEGES SUBSCRIBING TO THE ACCREDITING PROGRAM OF THE
COUNCIL ON EDUCATION OF THE NATIONAL CHIROPRACTIC ASSOCIATION.

It was further moved that Dr. Rogers be asked to simply list all of the accredited and provisionally accredited colleges as members of the Council on Education under the Council listing in the directory of the Journal.

It was evident that every school man present was satisfied with this conclusion. Drs. Parr and Cleveland asked for the privilege of taking this matter up with some of their constituents before they committed themselves to a participation, but they stated that they would let Dr. Peterson know within the near week.

It was also concluded that as soon as possible Dr. Peterson would advise Dr. Rogers of the final decisions of each of the schools and also as to the format of the ad. Then Dr. Rogers would bill each of the colleges on the prorated basis.

Point No. 2- Conclusion of the matter of Dr. Schwing's program for chiropractic continuance in France. Notification of Swiss chiropractors of final decision.

Dr. Janse advised the Council that transcripts of the deliberations about the Schwing matter as conducted in Detroit had been sent to Drs. Illi and Cleave, the president and secretary of the European Chiropractors Union respectively.

Dr. Janse did receive a communication from Dr. Illi thanking the Council for their consideration of the matter and advised the Council that the members of the European Chiropractors Union would vigorously resist the Schwing program. Dr. Illi was pleased with the fact that all of the NCA affiliated colleges had denied Dr. Schwing post-graduate training.

It is also to be noted that Dr. Brunner who formerly was a practitioner in France and who during the pressure of the Schwing program went into Switzerland and became connected with the Illi clinic has returned to Paris with the intent of establishing practice notwithstanding the resistance of any medical pressure.

It was decided by the Council not to do anything further about the matter unless instructed or solicited to do so by the organized chiropractic group in Europe.

Point No. 3- Discussion of Council members supporting low standard legislation contrary to Council policy.

It was the general consensus of opinion that all of the colleges affiliated with or seeking affiliation with the NCA should under no circumstance support legislative efforts supporting in any way less than the minimum set forth by the educational code of the National Chiropractic Association.

Dr. Nugent reviewed the fact that in the states of New Hampshire, Nevada, Iowa, Michigan, Kansas and South Carolina the professional requirements had been raised to those prescribed by the NCA

Dr. Nugent encouraged the Council members to wield their influence in the attempt to persuade the few remaining states to do the same.

Drs. Cleveland, Coggins and Harring were asked whether they would support the effort of increasing the educational requirements in their home state of Missouri.

The apprehension was expressed that if the law was opened up or exposed to an amendment it might give incentive to a certain group in Missouri that sought undue practice liberties.

It was also the opinion of Drs. Cleveland and Coggins that the definition of chiropractic should not be tampered with and the term physiotherapy should not be included. They insisted that the usage of conservative physiotherapy had become so traditional that it was not necessarily important to include it in the definition.

Both Drs. Coggins and Harring expressed their readiness to support an amendment to raise the requirements to the standard four years without making any change in the definition of practice.

Dr. Cleveland reserved his commitments saying that he would like to think the matter over as he was rather dubious about the matter.

It should be stated that the Council felt that all legislative measures in Missouri should be under the conditioned auspices of the three colleges housed in Missouri.

Point No. 4- Delineation of Council's position in attacks on modality and supplemental manufacturers by the Better Business Bureau.

The example of the conduct of the Better Business Bureau in Ohio, Indiana, Texas and California gave evidence of the fact that essentially they were biased toward the chiropractic profession and that their conduct against the profession was being financed by moneys from indirect medical sources.

Furthermore, the B.B.B. did not fully attempt to differentiate between the acceptable diagnostic and clinical elements in chiropractic and those of a less definite and probably of a more questionable nature.

For example, in Ohio not only did the usage of the radionic units come under attack but simultaneously the usage of supplemental foods also experienced a severe scrutiny and interpretation to the extent where their usage had been severely curbed.

Consequently, it was concluded that mediation with the B.B.B. should be careful and guarded and that this organization should be made to understand that if certain matters were to be rectified in our profession, we of the profession are well qualified to do so.

It was generally decided that the Council or its members should not permit themselves public involvement or expression of opinion in relation to the efficacy or lack of efficacy or certain common instruments of analysis, diagnosis or treatment.

Dr. Firth expressed the fact that the attack on the radionic users by the newspapers and B.B.B. in Cleveland, Detroit, and Chicago did definitely hurt the profession and mitigate its reputation.

Dr. Gardner pleaded for tolerance in the profession's attitude toward the radionic users. He stated that he was one and that he could verify the effectiveness of the principle.

Dr. Martin advised that none of the colleges teach the usage of the principle in either the undergraduate, post graduate or graduate schools.

Dr. Budden advised the group that the Council on Physiotherapy proposes to make a survey of the clinical claims of the radionists. The plan includes the proper classification and tabulation of all information and then to make a formal declaration of the findings.

Dr. Nugent asked why the Council on Physiotherapy did not proceed with this study as soon as possible? In answer, Dr. Budden stated that the Council wished to be assured that its investigation would not be disrupted because of the Executive Board's fear that it might incur the disapproval of the radionists many of whom are NCA members.

In summation, a motion was made, seconded and passed that read as follows: All matters pertaining to usage of modalities, radionics and supplemental foods be referred to the Council on Physiotherapy.

Point No. 5- Review of Pennsylvania, Ohio and Illinois situation and evaluation of result of legislative efforts in those states. Also discussion of Georgia situation.

It was generally concluded that the new legislative situation in Pennsylvania was working out satisfactorily and that full support should be proffered the new licensing mechanism.

Dr. Nugent said that he wanted to correct a misrepresentation of fact that had been disseminated in relation to the Pennsylvania situation. He said that he had been accused by certain parties that he had stipulated the pre-professional requirements and had influenced the Governor through Senator Andrew J. Sordoni not to condone the Bill unless these requirements were met.

The pre-professional college requirements of one year of chemistry, biology and physics, stated Dr. Nugent, were the insistent stipulations of the medical board, who formerly had the licensing of chiropractors under their auspices, and who advised the Governor that they would not resist the independent chiropractic legislation if these pre-professional reservations were included.

Dr. Nugent advised the Council that the original literature of the chiropractic bill in Pennsylvania contained all together too many grandfather clause privileges and would have left so many loopholes for the short term graduates that it constituted a definite compromise of all NCA standards. That was the reason why, when he was asked by Senator Sordoni to study the bill he advised the Senator of those hazards and as a result Senator Sordoni advised the proponents of the bill that he would not support it and would advise the Governor against it unless these inordinate grandfather clause loopholes were deleted.

Although rather reluctantly, the proponents of the bill conceded to the Senator's insistence, rewrote the bill and, under the supporting auspices of the Senator it was passed to become a law.

Because of the necessary alterations, Dr. Nugent felt that possibly certain feelings were hurt, but expressed the belief that all in all benefit for the profession was accrued and asked the Council to help mitigate any misunderstandings that might still exist.

Dr. Nugent then reviewed the past legislative efforts in Ohio. He outlined the contents of the bill sponsored by the licensed group in Ohio and then the one sponsored by the unlicensed. He flatly stated that the latter was a short term bill and furthermore that it contained numerous grandfather clause loopholes that would have privileged licenses to numbers of short term graduates and reduce the standards of the profession in Ohio to a marked detrimental degree.

Because of the deadlock that ensued both bills were defeated but definite penetrations had been made by the licensed group and it was Dr. Nugent's opinion that within the next year there might be sustained good promise for independent chiropractic legislation.

Dr. Nugent then outlined the fact that in Illinois, a rather similar effort was made by the unlicensed group to pass a low standard bill and that is the reason why he and the Illinois Chiropractic Society resisted its passage. According to Dr. Nugent we dare not reduce our standards in the effort to get from under the control of medical boards.

According to Dr. Nugent it was no coincidence that the original bills in these three states were of the same literature in every respect and certainly must have been prompted in their low standard tendency by a certain segment within our profession.

He stated that he felt that it was inherently unfair to the graduates from the four year colleges to permit such type of legislation to pass because it would put them in direct competition with short term graduates and make the higher standard program of the NCA ineffective.

A brief discussion was made of the recent situation in Georgia where there had been a great deal of intramural dissension on the chiropractic board resulting in a failing of 26 out of 27 applicants. This consequence had caused much resentment among the members of the state society and eventually the entire board was strictly reprimanded by the Governor and the board of directors of the state society. The papers were re-examined and in finality all but one of the examinees were issued licenses.

This circumstance represented but an example of the severity of differences of opinion that still existed in the profession.

Point No. 6- Discussion relating to the distribution of the Spears Sanigram among the students of the colleges.

Dr. Peterson presented this matter stating that he felt rather hesitant in distributing the same among the members of the students of the New York Institute because of the nature of the contained claims.

Recently Dr. Spears had made the request that issues of the publication be distributed. It was finally concluded that the various colleges should make their individual decisions on the matter.

Point No. 7- A discussion of the proposition by various state associations or societies to organize another school men's council for the claimed purpose of talking over school matters but with the intent of remaining unaffiliated with any of the national organizations.

It is to be stated that this discussion did extend in part into various sessions of the meeting but the following is a general summation of all.

The Council's attention was drawn to a letter prepared by Dr. Parr and released from his office on December 28, 1951, following being a reproduction of the same.

CARVER CHIROPRACTIC COLLEGE
521 Northwest Ninth Street
Oklahoma City 3, Oklahoma
December 28, 1951
TO ALL CHIROPRACTIC SCHOOLS AND COLLEGES ON THE NORTH AMERICAN CONTINENT

After considerable discussion with the heads of other schools at the last several State Association meetings and much correspondence in the last sixty days, it seems to have fallen my lot to extend to you an invitation to attend a meeting, the date for which is tentatively set as March 8, 1952, the location for which is tentatively set for Chicago, since it is centrally located and has excellent transportation possibilities.

The purpose of this meeting is the discussion of school problems by school men. You are cordially invited to be represented by any or all bona fide representatives of your school. We urge that you be represented by at least one of your clear-thinking, forward-looking authorities.

In recent correspondence with deans and presidents of chiropractic colleges I have made many suggestions as to possibilities of organization of schools, etc. I had thought at first that I would include in this invitation a proposed outline for a school organization. I had even thought of stating my position as to having another accrediting association, but I have been advised by the president of one of the chiropractic colleges that this might be taken on the part of some of you as meaning that decisions have been made, when they have not. I should like to quote three sentences from this great educator's letter to me:

"I feel the only thing that is needed is an invitation to the schools to attend a called meeting, which would contain a designated place and time to consider mutual problems for the benefit of all. At the conclusion of such a meeting an association of chiropractic schools and colleges might be formed if that was the consensus of opinion of those in attendance. By this I mean that any action that might be taken and the nature of any association that might be formed would entirely depend upon those attending the meeting."

It is a little difficult for me to inculcate in this letter the urgency I feel without discussing some of the problems of endangering the proposition by giving the impression that conclusions have already been formed. So, again let me invite you and even strongly urge you that in the interest of unity and advancement of our profession and toward the goal of a better health service for our people, please, let us once get the brains of the school business into a close-harmony meeting.

Sincerely yours
(signed) Paul O. Parr
President

Attention was then drawn to letters sent out by state society groups in Massachusetts, Texas, Louisiana, and New Mexico. Following being a copy of the one sent out from the Massachusetts Chiropractic Association.

MASSACHUSETTS CHIROPRACTIC ASSOCIATION
1139 Beacon Street, Brookline, Massachusetts

Therefore, we the Massachusetts Chiropractic Association, duly assembled in annual convention in Boston, Massachusetts, December 2, 1951, suggest and recommend that chiropractic schools give serious consideration to the formation of a North American Association of Chiropractic Schools and Colleges for the purposes herein stated, to the end that:

(a) The Association undertake such programs as are feasible for the mutual benefit of all...to the end that the integrity of Chiropractic be preserved at its source.
   1. That it encourage enrollment of qualified prospective students in Chiropractic Schools.
   2. That at least once each year it sponsor a symposium for instructors to exchange ideas.
   3. That it provide information, development and instruction in the field of education, with special emphasis on methods and curriculum.
   4. That it provide facilities for faculty exchange and/or student exchange.
   5. That it make available an opportunity for friendly relations between respective student bodies.
   6. That it maintain such office and personnel as are necessary to effect its objectives.
(b) That it (THE ASSOCIATION OF SCHOOLS AND COLLEGES) act as the recognized and official accrediting agency for all Chiropractic institutions; that the accrediting program be divorced from Professional Association and placed where it belongs, namely, the association of the schools themselves.

Allyn H. Winkler, D.C., President
Leo Shilts, D.C., Secretary

Dr. Janse, in relation to the matter asked the question whether something is wrong with the Council and its intent or whether it was a definite effort on the part of those opposing the NCA to create a counter organization.

Dr. Nugent contended that all of the state letters came from societies that were ICA and PSC affiliates and therefore he felt that the primary incentive had arisen in the influences of the ICA rather than unassociated individuals or groups.

Dr. Parr stated that he wanted to clarify his conduct in the whole matter. He related his observations at the last Oklahoma State Convention where Drs. Hender of the PSC. Firth of the Lincoln, Logan of the Logan, and he, Parr, of the Carver Colleges had put on the educational program and how the entire state group had commended on the apparent unity of attitude sustained by these school men.

Dr. Parr insisted that there is need for a school men's council that has no national organization affiliation. He stated that the people of the profession were demanding that the school men get together irrespective of their concepts or national affiliation.

He insisted that the Council was failing in its purpose and that the conduct of the Director of Education and the Accrediting Committee was too free handed and independent. He claimed that neither the Council nor the NCA had done anything to help the smaller schools in their economic struggle.

It was his contention that the Council had snubbed and derogated those school men who did not belong to the Council and that the

Council was not fully representative of the educational needs and wishes of the profession.

It was Dr. Parr's frank declaration that he was going to continue to seek the establishment of another council.

At this time Dr. Firth stated that he had talked to Drs. Hender, Logan and Parr in Oklahoma City about this and had said that he would be willing to participate in a school men's gathering for the purpose of discussion of general school problems but he would not in any way participate in any gathering or effort with the intent of establishing another accrediting agency.

It was Dr. Nugent's belief that the real intent behind this movement was exactly that of establishing a new accrediting agency and stated that such would lead to a lot of competitive detriment.

Following are some of Dr. Parr's direct statements on the matter.

a. The people of our profession want all school men to get together and not affiliate themselves with national organizations.
b. At the present time there is a group of renegades in Michigan who have been driven from the state society by unfair duress and now find their only support in the PSC.
c. We incriminate against each other and belittle each other's attitudes and concepts.
d. Can we not as school men meet together and talk about our problems without the politics of organizations.
e. The NCA group is being accused of a lot by the PSC group because they have never met together.
f. Such men of the PSC as Chance, Dave Palmer and Hender are willing to help mitigate the tensions that exist.
g. I personally, am not in favor of a new accrediting agency and I have advised Dr. Palmer of this attitude of mine.
h. The school men outside the Council wish a school men's council uncolored by NCA policies.
i. I do not believe that the state resolutions asking for the establishment of a new council with an accrediting agency are PSC inspired. Yet I feel that this attitude can be controlled.

Dr. Budden then stated that the very fact that these states had passed these resolutions calling for a school men's council and an accrediting agency was an evidence that what the present Council had done was correct and must be worthy.

Dr. Budden asked why it was that the school men outside the Council did not seek to obtain membership in the Council? The doctor expressed the opinion that we should sit tight and that the progress and compulsion of events would eventually bring all factions together. To try and force all vying and competing factions into the same organization at the present time would but result in further misunderstandings.

Dr. Peterson then asked Dr. Parr whether he didn't realize that at one time the individuals sponsoring this move other than he had promised him that they did not seek to establish another accrediting agency, yet that the various state resolutions calling for such an agency was a direct disclaim of their sincerity.

According to Dr. Peterson, if the newer personnel at the PSC wished to seek affiliation with the Council they certainly may do so and would experience every proper consideration.

In answer, Dr. Parr stated that such would cause the PSC to lose from 40 to 50% of its support, because of the severe anti-NCA feeling among its proponents.

If that is the case, contended Dr. Peterson you should then realize that you are being used as the front for a spearhead to effect a council that would permit the PSC to maintain its autonomy and still experience the advantages of a council.

Dr. Parr contended that he would be willing to take his chances on being used for that purpose. He claimed that if the Council humiliated the young leading personnel of the PSC by asking them to set aside the ICA and become NCA affiliates, it would drag the chiropractic profession into another 15 years of strife and intra-mural contention.

Dr. Peterson countered by stating that by the same token, he Dr. Parr and the PSC leaders were asking the Council to set aside all of its past accomplishments and permit its entity to become absorbed in this new Council in which certainly the control of vote would be against the segment that now constituted the membership of the present Council. It would be we who would have to make the concessions and sacrifice all our accomplishments and permit the control of federal, state and national influence to pass into the hands of others who, up to the present, have resisted every measure of progress that has been initiated. Such does really represent a rather unfair and inordinate demand.

Dr. Peterson then mentioned the list of some chiropractic colleges that Dr. Parr had listed as being possible candidates for membership in the proposed new schoolmen's group. Some of the schools listed certainly did not and could not in any measure, represent an integrity of scholastic competence as measured not only by the standards of the NCA but also those of any other group. Therefore, why should we or anyone else be asked to lend them credence and voice of expression.

Dr. Firth stated that there have been times when the Council or members of the Council have said and done things that had alienated certain professional individuals and had placed the non-accredited schools on the defensive. He then proceeded to read an original letter received from Dr. Wolfe of Abilene, Texas, following being a copy of the answer to the same.

October 19, 1951
Dr. J.A. Wolfe
760 Orange Street
Abilene, Texas
Dear Dr. Wolfe:

Your letter of October 2nd was on my desk upon my return from the Florida State Convention.

It is my opinion that any special meeting of representatives from the various Chiropractic schools and state organizations for the single purpose of adopting a definition of the practice of Chiropractic, either in Washington or Texas, would not be well attended. The Educational Council of the NCA, which is composed of school men, discussed this problem at the last meeting held in Detroit during the month of July. It was agreed that all give the matter some thought until the next meeting which will be held early the 2nd week of January at Miami Beach and at that time, it was agreed that such a definition will be adopted.

I am enclosing herewith a copy of the Lincoln Bulletin, under date of February 1950, which contains an article bearing on the subject. This will, at least, give you my views on the subject.

I feel that if representatives of every Chiropractic school in the country, and every state association, could agree upon a definition, it would be highly beneficial; but any definition agreed upon by a hand-picked group, that would not meet the approval of those not in attendance, would be of no value whatever.

Sincerely,
LINCOLN CHIROPRACTIC COLLEGE, INC.
J.N. Firth, D.C.

The Council members will recall that the letter by Dr. Wolfe had been sent to all of the school men and Dr. Peterson, president of the Council sent out an inquiry as to what the reaction of the Council members was in relation to the letter. Following is a copy of Dr. Firth's letter to Dr. Peterson and which, in general, portrayed the opinion of the majority of the Council members.

October 26, 1951
Dr. Thure C. Peterson
152 West 42nd Street
New York 18, New York
Dear Doctor Peterson:

Your letter of October 24th was received this morning. In reply to same, will state that we will send one representative of the Lincoln College to the meeting if it is held in Miami, January 9th to 13th. If it is held in Chicago or St. Louis at the same time we will send two representatives. In answer to Questions 3 and 4, I am enclosing herewith copy of my reply to a letter from Dr. J.A. Wolfe of Abilene, Texas. At the time I wrote this letter, I had not read Page 16 of the ICA Journal and did not have the background pertaining to Dr. Wolfe's inquiry; however, I believe my answer would have been the same as stated in my letter of October 19th.

I have no knowledge of the attitude of the other schools, but I do believe that such a meeting, called by a representative of the Texas Association, would result in a very few schools attending. It undoubtedly would be attended by all non-NCA approved schools. If a few of the NCA approved schools decided to attend, it would accomplish nothing more than to break down the foundation that has thus far been achieved by the NCA. Personally, I do not think any NCA approved school should attend until first our resolution - stating that the Education Council is the only recognized accrediting agency of the Chiropractic profession - is repealed, and naturally that would not be repealed until such time as there was either a majority or unanimous decision to make a change. I do not have a mature opinion on the advisability of making a change at this time, but I do have a few thoughts that relate to Dr. Wolfe's project as follows:

First; There is still a reasonable amount of clamor for unity in the Chiropractic profession. I think it emanates largely from the ICA members, whose officers have already demonstrated that they are unwilling to cooperate.

Secondly, it emanates from those Chiropractors who are not members of any national association.

Thirdly, it emanates, to some extent from NCA members.

The above three groups of chiropractors are to be found in nearly every state in the union. They have been living with one another and endeavoring to participate jointly in the activities of their state chiropractic organization. They seem to feel there is a great gulf fixed between them as the result of the two national associations. Yet, they know they must live together and jointly participate in chiropractic affairs in their respective states. Many things have been published by both organizations that make each group distrust the other. They have proven that individually they can live with one another and accomplish some constructive things individually. The same can be said of the schools. I can say for the Lincoln College that individually, we are on a friendly basis with every other Chiropractic school in the country, yet, professionally, because of our organization setup, there is a barrier that causes a coolness in some of our contacts. The same may be true of some, or all, of the other schools. The men in the field see different school men, belonging to different national organizations, who attend as speakers at their conventions, and who exchange ideas and mingle with one another in a friendly manner. Naturally, they can not understand why there can not be the same unity and friendliness between the schools and the organizations of which they are a part, as is apparently existing between the individual school men attending their meetings. Anything said or done by one national organization, that exhibits intolerance toward the other, constitutes the breeze that fans the flame in the field, and cause a state association to pass such a resolution as was passed in Texas and Louisiana. I believe this to be true from my contacts with field men and if true, then an exhibition of a little more tolerance of those on the other side becomes a breeze that fans the popularity of that organization.

Therefore, I do believe that in the near future, some degree of cooperation must be forthcoming from both national organizations, schools belonging to each, and the men representing those schools.

Sincerely
LINCOLN CHIROPRACTIC COLLEGE, INC.

J.N. Firth, D.C.

cc: Dr. Harry McIlroy

Dr. Firth also read a letter received from a general practitioner in New Mexico, one of the states that had passed the resolution advocating the organizing of a new council of chiropractic colleges. Following is a copy of this letter.

NEW MEXICO CHIROPRACTIC ASSOCIATION
"A Non Profit Organization" Incorporated Albuquerque, New Mexico
1606 E. Central Avenue
Albuquerque, N.M
December 28, 1951.

Dr. James N. Firth
633 N. Penn. St.
Indianapolis, Indiana

Dear Dr. Firth,

Sure glad to hear from you — will attempt to answer the questions you have asked regarding the Louisiana school resolution.

I think an Association of Schools and Colleges would be a fine thing. I believe it would be a beginning toward solving some of the problems that are facing the profession today.

I sincerely believe the biggest danger to Chiropractic today is the lack of unity among the chiropractors themselves. Chiropractic students generally believe and practice what they are taught at school. When a fellow graduates from school and believes that whatever technic his school teaches is the answer as far as Chiropractic is concerned, I maintain that in 95 percent of the cases that is the fault of the school and not of the student. Even (we will suppose) if one school had by far the best technic, it seems to me the school heads would realize that it would be to their advantage for financial reasons if nothing else, to send their students into the field thoroughly indoctrinated with the idea of working with their fellow chiropractors.

In the main, I think some chiropractors are too straight and radical in their belief and practice. On the other hand, I feel that a percentage of the mixers are going to the other extreme. Again I maintain that a good portion of this originates in the schools. The "exchange of ideas" sounds like a good proposal especially in the field of technic. I have seen quite a few chiropractors who were actually amazed that good adjustive "moves" were taught by other schools and when instructed in these moves, were glad to add that technic to their own. I think if the schools could work out a general outline to follow in chiropractic analysis and general adjustive procedure, it would reduce the number of patients who drift from one office to the other, looking for the kind of adjustment they had from the first chiropractor they ever went to or the chiropractor that treated them in the last town where they lived. The doctor could use his special technics in addition to the above. If we ever get into VA hospitals such a thing as the above would almost be a necessity.

In my opinion the schools missed a golden opportunity during and at the close of World War II. If during the war, the schools could have been unified along the lines suggested in the resolution, they could have graduated thousands of men who would have given our science the biggest boost since Chiropractic was discovered, merely by working together instead of as is so often the case, being divided into factions.

I realize that putting such a resolution into effect would present many problems and the biggest obstacle would be the school heads who put "I" in front of Chiropractic instead of behind it.

Dr. Firth, the men who attended our state convention were unanimously behind the resolution. Of the chiropractors in our state who did not attend the convention, I feel they fell into four categories -

1.   Those who couldn't attend for valid reason, just opening an office, illness, etc. These would have voted for the resolution.
2.   Those who have a good practice and feel they are "set" so let the other worry about the future of Chiropractic.
3.   Those who have been plodding along in the same rut for years and don't give a damn one way or the other.
4.   Those who at one time had been active in state and national organization and finally said the hell with all of it until the NCA and ICA and the schools make definite progress toward settling their differences. I believe these men would be for the resolution.

I hope I don't sound too caustic or pessimistic. I believe the schools, almost without exception are doing a good job of teaching their students and have many times operated under terrific handicaps. I realize we owe a lot to the school men and that we chiropractors in the field are oftentimes guilty of not giving the schools the support they merit.

With best wishes for the new year,

Sincerely,

S/Bill Held

In conclusion Dr. Parr stated that he would continue his endeavors to bring all the school heads together under the auspices of another council and that a meeting had been proposed for March 2 and 3, in Chicago.

At a later time in the final session of the Council it was the general consensus of opinion that none of the school men subscribing to the accrediting program of the NCA should attend this proposed meeting for the simple reason that it would lead to nothing other than a frustration of the fine program that had been initiated and possibly dissipate the advantages that had been accrued.

Point No. 8- Discussion of supplemental degrees to the regular Doctorate of Chiropractic.

Inquiry was made as to whether any of the colleges represented issued any other degree in chiropractic in the undergradute school other than that of Doctor of Chiropractic. All colleges declared that the undergraduate degree had been restricted to one, namely Doctor of Chiropractic. Some of the colleges did offer the Cum Laude to those students having a high scholastic rating. One or two of the colleges also issued certificates and honorary certificates but which in no way represented a degree.

After considerable discussion it was concluded that definite undergraduate credit should be given for work done at the PSC and that it was no longer desirable to withhold recognition of PSC credits and permit PSC graduates to proceed to work for his degree at one of the accredited colleges and do so on the basis of advanced standing enjoyed because of his PSC training.

In the past it had been the usual custom to accept a PSC student as a P.G. and then simply issue a statement of credit earned but deny him a degree.

It was recommended that in the instance of any short term graduate or transferee from any school the credits should be carefully scrutinized and evaluated and then a special program set up for the individual on the basis of what he has had and what he should have in order to earn his degree.

It was decided that no credit should ever be given for an incomplete semester or quarter.

In relation to osteopathic and medical students full credit should be given but under any circumstances a minimum of three semesters should be insisted upon in order to fully acquaint him with the chiropractic concept and procedures.
Credit could also be given to people with pre-professional college work if this work contained subjects germane to the chiropractic course.

Applicants from foreign countries having had schooling in medical schools of Europe should be asked to obtain as thorough a description of their work as possible and then a careful estimation should be made.

It was unanimously concluded that a standard transcript form for all of the colleges be prepared. Drs. Raymond Houser and Lester King were appointed to assume this responsibility and all school heads were instructed to have their school office send a copy of the form now used by the college to each of these men for the purpose of their study.

Point No. 9- Discussion of promotion of closer relationship between state examining boards and the council. Also, consideration of resolution proposed by Dr. Harring in the developing proper type of practical examinations in chiropractic.

Dr. Harring's resolution as presented to the Council at Detroit was reiterated. In substance it encouraged the affiliated college heads to encourage the members of the chiropractic examining boards to pay more careful attention to the study of the examinee's ability as a chiropractic clinician and his grasp of diversified technic.

It was the full consensus of opinion that the recommendation of Dr. Harring should be followed out.

It was also concluded that every conscientious effort should be made to cooperate with the various state boards and to encourage the chiropractic students to properly qualify themselves for the examinations.

Dr. Cleveland recommended that the various schools exchange final examination questions.

Dr. Troilo stated that the Council should set a committee to develop typical state board questions and send them to the boards.

It was concluded that an effort should be made to encourage the state board members to avoid questions that were obsolete and incongruous especially in chiropractic philosophy and principles.

Point No. 10- Establishment of committee on graduate study and research within the Council.

The original committee on chiropractic specialties organized by the executive board of the NCA had never really functioned to any marked capacity. Hence, last summer in Detroit it was deemed advisable by the Board to dissolve it. Unfortunately, this was done without having fully advised the various members of the committee of this conclusion.

Dr. Norcross presented the Council with the idea that possibly it might be of value to create such a committee within the Council.

The majority of the Council members, however, concluded that inasmuch as graduate and specialty education had not been established to any noticeable degree at any of the colleges other than the Los Angeles College it might be best to refrain from organizing such an elaborate program until the objective need for one actually existed. Therefore the matter was tabled until further necessity arose.

Point No. 11- Consideration of letter from the General Practitioners Society of the California Chiropractic Association.

Dr. Norcross attending the Council meetings as the Dean of the Graduate School of the Los Angeles College of Chiropractic presented to the Council, a letter as signed by the president and secretary of the General Practitioners Society of the California Chiropractic Association. Following being a copy of the same.

CALIFORNIA CHIROPRACTIC EDUCATIONAL AND SPECIALTY SOCIETIES
CALIFORNIA CHIROPRACTIC ASSOCIATION
BY THE GENERAL PRACTITIONERS SOCIETY
January 12, 1952

In order to help facilitate the National Educational Program, and to help increase the unit memberships, and since the difference between Chiropractic and any other healing art is the philosophy and technic, and since the more technic we have the better Chiropractic service we can give to the public; THEREFORE, be it resolved that the California Society of Chiropractic General Practitioners sponsor the following resolution to the National Council on Education:

1. That the National Council of Education, through the Research Foundation, have moving picture films made of the different technics as taught in the various approved NCA Chiropractic Colleges.
2. That these films be produced with sound.
3. That the National Council on Education correlate the technics filmed to prevent duplication.
4. That also, x-ray films be shown and explained, as well as gaits, etc., as a practical aid in diagnosis of seldom-seen cases.
5. The cost of production of these films be assumed by the National Council on Education, and film to be rented to State or national units, providing the schools will not donate the film to the National Council of Education at the school's expense.
6. Since the California Society of General Practitioners has indicated that this Society is desirous that the National Council of Education assist in this project, and because the project seems worthwhile, that if the National Council of Education feels unable to assist this program, the California Society of General Practitioners will continue to develop this project.

Signed, G.I. Harmon, D.C., President
M.L. Holmes, D.C., Secretary

After some discussion it was concluded that the program sustained merit but that at the present time the necessary amount of time and money expenditure would make its adoption prohibitive.

It was unanimously agreed that the General Practitioners Society of the C.C.A. should be encouraged to endeavor to affect as much of the proposed program as it possibly can.

Point No. 12- Consideration of suggestion to organize a committee on postgraduate and graduate instruction in the NCA affiliated colleges.

Dr. Ralph J. Martin advanced the idea that it might be of benefit to set up a program and a committee for the purpose of systematizing postgraduate and graduate instruction in the affiliated colleges.

Dr. Nugent stated that he realized that at the present time most of the colleges are primarily occupied with undergraduate instruction, however, we should set up an outline of graduate instruction and the conduct of all graduate schools.

Dr. Nugent stated that we should develop a general pattern so that any ventures along these lines could be properly guided.

Dr. Martin recommended that no post graduate or graduate work at any of the affiliated colleges should include studies that are foreign to the chiropractic concept.

Finally it was moved that Dr. Nugent be instructed to prepare an outline for graduate and post graduate study and submit it to the Council at the next meeting.

Point No. 13- Discussion of methods to better prepare graduates of Chiropractic Colleges in proven business and practice building methods in the attempt to reduce professional mortality.

Dr. Martin stated that he had proposed this matter for discussion because he considered it of great importance. We must see to it that a greater effort be made to acquaint the student with the technics of public relations and proper professional sales approach.

Dr. Peterson advised the group that in New York much benefit had been derived by inviting a number of successful practitioners in to speak to the senior class.

Dr. Budden claimed that the mortality of chiropractic graduates was not too severe and certainly all professions had some degree of mortality.

Dr. Firth outlined the program that had been instituted at the Lincoln College which included (1) How to serve the patient; (2) Practice in the clinic; (3) Art of practice; (4) Public relations, which included public speaking, jurisprudence, and ethics.

Dr. Hendricks expressed the conviction that we should attempt to develop a keener sense of business acumen and then he gave a very concise and informative outline of the course that he taught in relation to this necessity.

Dr. Nugent asked Dr. Hendricks to prepare an outline on his course and to submit it to the Secretary of the Council and have him multigraph the same and send it out to the Council members.

Dr. Janse recommended that the students be encouraged to incorporate the interests of their wives and other family members in their professional futures. Stating that he was of the opinion that some of the graduates had their problems augmented by the fact that the other family members were not fully convinced of the chiropractic principle.

Dr. Troilo advised that competent statistics be developed in chiropractic success and clinical results which may be used as convincing evidence of chiropractic merit.

Dr. Nugent related the fine work that had been done by Dr. John Wolfe at the Northwestern College in relation to the cultivating of ethical consciousness among the members of the student body of the college.

Student placement was encouraged and it was concluded that greater effort would be made in carefully estimating every graduate and the potentials he portrayed and what practice circumstances best suited the same.

Point No. 14- Matter of academic endeavor at chiropractic colleges.

Dr. Nugent stated that in his mediations with state board and basic science board members he had encountered the general opinion that within the average chiropractic college there was too much academic leniency, that the examinations were too easy and that the grading was too high and hence the students in general were given a false sense of security.

According to Dr. Nugent the state board examiners had one common criticism of the average chiropractic college graduate, namely that the graduate did not organize his answers very competently, that he portrayed rather fuzzy comprehension of certain subjects, that his written work was not too well outlined and that his general grasp of the use of English was poor.

It was generally conceded that these criticisms were warranted and that the college faculties should be encouraged to carefully observe these deficiencies and attempt to rectify them.

Dr. Janse reminded the Council that the process of education at chiropractic colleges was charged with responsibilities and difficulties that did not reside in other professional colleges, especially medicine, for the simple reason that in other professions pre-professional requirements brought into the professional colleges students who are fully conditioned in attitude and standardized in background and hence as a group other professional student bodies were more homogeneous.

Point No. 15- Consideration of Dr. Houser's effort to compile comparative statistics on the subject content of the various curricula of the colleges represented in the Council.

Dr. Houser distributed prepared sheets portraying an effort to set up a comparative picture of the amount of hours each of the colleges are lending to each of the basic science, and clinical subjects.

Dr. Houser had taken the information from the various catalogs of the colleges but acknowledged that possibly changes had been made since then at the colleges and invited all of the school men to take the copies home and correct them and then, if they wished to return them.

This is primarily being done for the purpose of enabling Drs. Houser and King to set up a competent standard transcript form, and every member of the Council was asked to respond to this necessity.

Point No. 16- Final clarification of the California situation regarding physicians and surgeons proposed legislation, as well as evaluation of effect of such a minority group concept on the present curriculum of the L.A. College.

Dr. Peterson restated the fact that Dr. L.A. Norcross was attending the Council meetings as Dean of the graduate school of the L.A. College and that he had been assigned to attend the meetings by the Board of Regents of the college and that Dr. Milbank, the president of the board, had written Dr. Peterson to this effect.

Dr. Peterson asked Dr. Norcross whether he had anything he desired to state in relation to the circumstances in California or in relation to his meeting with the Council last summer in Detroit. Dr. Norcross stated that he did not and that he was happy in being able to meet with the Council.

Dr. Nugent then stated that it was the consensus of opinion of the accrediting committee that the Council should go on record advising the profession against the teaching of any subject that related to standard medical and surgical procedures, whether this be in undergraduate or graduate classes. He especially emphasized such subjects as pharmacology, aperture surgery and the usage of the antibiotics.

Dr. Nugent claimed that the teaching of these parental subjects in the graduate courses of the L.A. College had caused considerable trouble and annoyance throughout the profession and he and the other members of the committee felt that such should be fully avoided.

It is a fact that in the graduate school of the L.A. College courses in these borderline subjects were taught in the anticipation that the new enactments in relation to the chiropractic law would grant these liberties. Such is borrowing trouble because it precipitates illegal practitioners.

Dr. Nugent advised Dr. Norcross that the accrediting committee had never approved of the teaching of these subjects in the graduate school. He further stated that an accredited college was an accredited college and that both the undergraduate and graduate departments of that college were subject to the rules of the Council.

Dr. Norcross then asked the question, whether the officers of the undergraduate and graduate schools of the L.A. College were to be subject to the instructions of the Council or the Board of Regents in the event that the C.C.A. were able to effect the change in the chiropractic law and that would permit the practice of some of these questionable subjects?

Dr. Norcross further explained that last summer in Detroit he had been instructed by the Board of Regents to advise the Council that the graduate school would have to teach these subjects because the C.C.A. had gone on record of approving these subjects.

Dr. Norcross informed the Council that within the last few days the original P&S group had recognized themselves and this is quite likely that the C.C.A. and the Board of Examiners would approve of the proposed new amendments. Now the question is whether the officers of the college, including both the graduate and undergraduate schools should follow the instructions of the Council or the Board of Regents if the request is made from the C.C.A. to teach these subjects?

Dr. Norcross wanted to know whether the Council would be willing to commit itself as to what the conduct should be of the L.A. College officers.

Dr. Budden proffered the advice that the L.A. College should sever its relations with the graduate school and permit the latter to operate fully under the auspices of the C.C.A.

Dr. Nugent stated that the C.C.A. had the right to instruct the members of the Board of Regents that were appointed by the C.C.A.

but that they had no right to control the other members of the Board.

Dr. Nugent again expressed the hope that the Council would advise the Board of Regents that they should not lend themselves to condoning the teaching of these borderline subjects in anticipation of changes in the law.

Dr. Janse expressed the opinion that some of the difficulty was arising out of the fact that chiropractic practice does not lend itself to a great deal of specialization, simply because the basis of the chiropractic concept is that of systemic correction. Therefore, as soon as a great deal of specialization is indulged in it will lead to an over lapping onto other fields.

After some further discussion Drs. Budden and Martin were appointed to draw up resolution, the following being the unanimously adopted wording of the same.

The Council will look with disfavor upon schools which offer courses which represent changes in the principles or objectives of the standard approved curriculum, or include subjects relating to the practice of medicine or surgery unless required by law in the state in which the school is located.

Point No. 17- Discussion of the effects of the Minnesota Physio-therapy law.

Dr. Martin expressed the opinion that the recent physiotherapy legislation in Minnesota was a rather sinister omen.

Dr. Wolfe explained that in his conversations with leading members of the profession in this state he obtained the information that the legislation did not have any effect upon the chiropractors. That law was sponsored by the medical profession with the intent of regulating the conduct and practice of those graduating from medical course in physiotherapy and wishing to practice as medical physiotherapists.

Dr. Budden drew the Council's attention to the clause contained within the writings of the law, namely "nothing shall be misinterpreted as interfering with the conduct of practitioners practicing under another license."

Point No. 18- Discussions in relation to the new NCA News Letter.

Dr. Nugent pointed out that he had attempted to keep the writings in this medium factual and dispassionate. It was the intent of the NCA through these News Letters to acquaint the entire profession with the actual happenings of important events that conditioned the future of the profession.

The meetings of the Council came to a conclusion in the late forenoon of Saturday, January 19th. There was a unanimous reaffirmation of good will and intent.

Dr. Janse expressed the conviction that every member of the Council should at all times seek to maintain the decorum of understanding and friendliness in all professional mediations. All elements and groups in our profession should experience thoughtful consideration. Our position as a Council should be maintained in the dignity of friendly relations. We should seek to mitigate involvements by avoiding argumentations and differentiations. As a Council of the NCA we should seek to portray the full premise of professional democracy upon which the national association was founded.

Closed Meeting. Attended only by the members of the Accrediting Committee and the representatives of the accredited or provisionally accredited colleges.

Dr. Peterson asked for the report of the Accrediting Committee.

Dr. Gardner the outgoing president of the Committee advised the Council that Dr. Nugent as Director of Education would give the report.

Dr. Nugent stated that in Detroit the Executive Board had instructed him to devote all of his time to the circumstances relating to the Texas College of Chiropractic. Therefore, since the Council meeting in Detroit, the greater percentage of his time and efforts had been directed toward this project.

a. According to Dr. Nugent in Texas there is the potential and definite basis for a very fine college and faculty.
b. There are certain aspects of the physical plant that should be altered.
c. There is need for extended laboratory facilities and Dr. Troilo and his associates were affecting plans along these lines.
d. In consultation with the officers of the college, the board of directors as well as members of the college alumni association it was decided that no recommendation would be made at the present time in relation to the status of the college as pertaining to accreditation. The Texas College would fully participate with the Council as an Associated College.
e. The Texas College Alumni Association has exhibited definite desire to effect all of the changes and alterations suggested by the Director of Education.
f. The Texas Chiropractic Association is not in the full position to render complete support for the simple reason that there are members of the state association who are the alumnae of other colleges and hence they feel that they cannot commit themselves to exclusively support the Texas College.
g. The new dean, Dr. Troilo sees eye to eye with the Council program and has given the accrediting committee every cooperation and assistance.
h. All circumstances point to the happy probability that the Texas College of Chiropractic will within a reasonable amount of time become fully accredited and affiliated with the Council.
i. Dr. Nugent advised the Council that in a clarification of its stipulation the Texas Basic Science board has stated that the two years of pre-professional college requirements need not be procured before one enters a chiropractic but can be obtained concur-

rent to the professional training.

j.   Dr. Nugent stated that he intended to return to San Antonio within the near future and to remain there until a definite program of qualification had been set up and instituted.

Dr. Nugent then advised the Council that he and the accrediting committee had had a long conference with Dr. Carl Cleveland Jr. Certain misunderstandings had been corrected and Dr. Cleveland now definitely knew what the accrediting committee would expect of the Cleveland College in its program of qualifying for full accreditation.

The Missouri College according to Dr. Nugent was continuing to sustain its program of....

Minutes of the COUNCIL ON EDUCATION of the NATIONAL CHIROPRACTIC ASSOCIATION, Annual meeting held in conjunction with the annual convention of the National Chiropractic Association in Miami Beach, Florida, Saxony Hotel, June 23, 24, 25 and 26th. 1952; Dr. Thure C. Peterson, President of the Council, presided at all of the meetings.

Those Attending:

(A) Members of the Accrediting Committee

   Dr. John J. Nugent, Director of Education of the National Chiropractic Association, 92 Norton Street, New Haven, Connecticut.

   Dr. Walter B. Wolf, President of the Accrediting Committee, Eureka, South Dakota

   Dr. Norman E. Osborne, Secretary of the Accrediting Committee, 1172 The Terrace, Hagerstown, Maryland

   Dr. Ralph J. Martin, 28 W. Sierra Madre Blvd., Sierra Madre, California

   Dr. Edward H. Gardner, 2727 South Vermont Avenue, Los Angeles, California

(B) Representatives of the accredited and provisionally accredited educational institutions.

   Dr. Thure C. Peterson, Director, Chiropractic Institute of New York, 152 W. 42nd Street, New York 18, New York

   Dr. W.A. Budden , Director, Western States College of Chiropractic, 4525 Southeast 63rd Street, Portland 6, Oregon

   Dr. William H. Coggins, Dean, Logan Basic College of Chiropractic, 7701 Florissant Road, St. Louis 21, Missouri

   Dr. Ralph J. Power, Dean, Missouri College of Chiropractic, 3117 Lafayette Avenue, St. Louis 4, Missouri

   Dr. Raymond H. Houser, Dean, Los Angeles College of Chiropractic, 920 East Broadway Avenue, Glendale 5, California

   Lester M. King, Dean, Lincoln Chiropractic College, Inc., 633 N. Pennsylvania Ave., Indianapolis, Indiana

   Dr. Paul O. Parr, President, Carver College of Chiropractic, 521 N.W. Ninth Street, Oklahoma City 3, Oklahoma.

   Dr. William Cole, Dean, Kansas State Chiropractic College, 629 N. Broadway, Wichita, Kansas

   Dr. Julius C. Troilo, Dean, Texas Chiropractic College, San Pedro Park, San Antonio, Texas.

   Dr. Joseph Janse, President, National College of Chiropractic, 20 N. Ashland Blvd., Chicago 7, Illinois

(C) Other representative and faculty members of chiropractic colleges

   Drs. Henry C. Schneider and J. LaMoine DeRusha, faculty members of the Northwestern College of Chiropractic, 2222 Park Avenue, Minneapolis, Minnesota. These gentlemen sat in on the open council meetings unofficially.

   Dr. A.E. Homewood, faculty member of the Canadian Memorial Chiropractic College, 252 Bloor Street, West, Toronto 5, Canada. Dr. Homewood also sat in on some of the open meetings unofficially.

   Dr. L.A. Bertholf, Dean of the University of Natural Healing Arts, 1075 Logan Ave., Denver, Colorado. This college seeking affiliation with the Council.

The first session of the Council was an open one and was held in the evening of June 22, 1952 with Dr. Peterson presiding.

1.   Discussions were initiated with reference to various scholarship plans and programs. Various members of the Council outlined some of the procedures that had been attempted in their respective colleges. It was the general consensus of opinion that as yet nothing greatly beneficial had been realized through any one of these programs.

   a. Probably the most effective program was the one sustained by the Health Research Foundation in support of the Western States College of Chiropractic in Portland, Oregon, and with Dr. W.A. Budden as Director.

   b. Dr. Peterson voiced the opinion that most students procured under scholarship programs did not sustain too substantial of an interest in Chiropractic and hence they frequently dropped out in the course of their studies.

   c. It was, therefore, concluded that the individual colleges would simply have to determine the programs that they wish to pursue.

2.   Dr. Peterson advised the council that he and Dr. Janse had been invited into a meeting of the executive board of the NCA, wherein the official body stated that they had set aside a goodly sum of money for the purpose of assisting the affiliated colleges for

some scholarship program.

   a. It was the original idea that each of the affiliated colleges offer a complete scholarship of four years defraying all tuition and laboratory fees. The NCA would advertise these scholarships and would offer to each of the winners $1,000 to help defray the other expenses.

   b. Both Doctors Peterson and Janse stated that they had advised the executive board that such a program would probably be of relative advantage. If, however, the NCA could obtain high school and Jr. college graduation lists from the primary cities in which the chiropractic colleges were located and then circularize these graduates, possibly a great deal of good might be realized.

   c. The executive board expressed the readiness to investigate and follow through with this recommendation. In fact, further unofficial deliberations with members of the board lead to the understanding that if the economy of the NCA would permit, a program of this type might well experience yearly renewal and support.

   d. The entire council membership expressed an appreciation for this helpful attitude of the executive board. It was the consensus of opinion that a program of circularizing high school and Jr. college graduates with competent literature via lists and brochures would be of distinct benefit to the colleges and if this program could be continued over a number of years the accumulated effect might bring students into the colleges for a given number of years.

   e. Drs. Peterson and Janse were instructed to advise the executives accordingly.

3. The need of student procurement was further discussed and following were the primary matters brought out.

   a. Dr. Peterson advised that in New York they had provided to procure thousands of names of high school graduates of the greater New York area, from the National Scholastic Lists Company. This company makes such a business of obtaining the names and addresses of the tentative graduates of high school, Jr. colleges and colleges. For a certain fee they will send informative literature to these students.

   b. Dr. Peterson stated that this program was working out well for them in New York.

   c. Dr. Budden recommended that the affiliated colleges match the NCA proposal dollar for dollar. Discussions were conducted but no conclusions were arrived at in relation to this recommendation.

   d. Dr. Martin suggested that more interest be exhibited in approaching Jr. college students. He emphasized the opinion that the chiropractic colleges should raise our pre-professional entrance requirements to two years of college work. It was his belief that if the chiropractic colleges had a pre-professional college requirement it would raise the reputation of the colleges and attract a better caliber of students.

4. Dr. Nugent next proceeded to initiate a discussion on the raising of the tuition for all of the colleges.

   a. It was his opinion that all of the colleges should have the same tuition rate in order to avoid commercial competition among the chiropractic colleges.

   b. He states that it was his opinion that the tuition should be $1,800 for the course, such as including laboratory fees and book expenses.

   c. Dr. Troilo expressed the opinion that if the affiliated colleges were to adopt a uniform tuition rate it might be possible that a more substantial relation could be sustained with the Veterans Administration.

   d. Dr. Janse maintained that the geographical differences of locations of the various colleges wielded a definite influence in the determining of the tuition rates and he felt that the colleges should be permitted to set their own tuition.

   e. Dr. Peterson advised that at the New York institute they had raised their tuition to $200 a semester (16 weeks) and that no detrimental effects had been experienced.

   f. Dr. Budden recommended that the tuition rates be guided by the fees charged by the non-state supported colleges.

5. A discussion relative to the spread on chiropractic colleges in the ICA Journal was then initiated.

   a. Dr. Nugent expressed the conviction that the recent invitation of the Public Relations Department of the ICA to participate in the spread on chiropractic colleges in the ICA Journal was an attempt to woo allegiance from the NCA to ICA.

   b. Dr. Nugent recommended that the chairman, the secretary and another member of the council be empowered to serve as a board of clearance for issues of this type.

   c. That a final veto in relation to such matters be made by mail.

6. Dr. Janse made a report on the financial outlay of the council.

   a. He advised the group that the last assessment for all of the affiliated colleges have been made in Detroit. A year ago since then, expenses encountered such as, stenciling and mimeographing of the minutes, postage, phone calls and telegraphs, fee for council room in the Indianapolis meeting as well as rental of a recorder had completely exhausted the treasury.

   b. Dr. Peterson advised that in the instance of himself and Dr. Janse the barest expenditures had been covered by defrayments out of the council's treasury.

   c. Dr. King recommended that another assessment of $10 be made and that this was to involve every one of the colleges that was desirous of participating in the program of the council regardless of their status in the accrediting program.

The second session of the Council was held in the evening of June 23, 1952 at 8:00 P.M. with Dr. Peterson presiding:

   I. Dr. Parr recommended that the two page NCA Journal advertisement on the chiropractic colleges definitely carry the inscription of being a paid advertisement.

a. This recommendation was acknowledged and the chairman of the council was instructed to advise Dr. Rogers of the same.

II. Dr. Power expressed his conviction that the membership of the NCA throughout the country should be enlisted in campaigns of student procurement. He expressed the opinion that all NCA delegates should be instructed to go home and campaign for a program of this type.

III. Dr. Peterson stated that the readiness of the executive board in establishing a student program was most laudable. He recommended that the president of the NCA in his monthly letter to the field might well emphasize the need for chiropractic matriculants.

IV. Dr. Nugent emphasized the conviction that student procurement primarily centered about the activities of a well organized alumni association.

V. Dr. Budden expressed the desire to have Dr. Houser detail the program of the Los Angeles college in relation to the two year pre-professional college requirements and Dr. Houser responded with the following major comment.

a. In September 1952 the Los Angeles College of Chiropractic will initiate its program requiring two years of pre-professional college work.

b. These two years must have included a semester grade in Inorganic Chemistry, Organic Chemistry and Physics.

c. Dr. Houser stated that the administration of the Los Angeles college recognized the fact that for the first year or so the enrollment under this program would be relatively small, however, he explained that it had been a similar circumstance in case of the osteopathic, optometry and chiropody colleges.

d. Dr. Houser advised that they had conducted a special program of approach to the deans and counselors of some 16 to 20 Jr. colleges in southern California for this purpose. They had prepared a special built portfolio which was left with these college people. This format was designed to place the counselors' immediate service all of the information pertaining to chiropractic education and practice.

e. Dr. Houser stated that this program had worked without fail, that they had been well received by the administrative personnel of the Jr. colleges, that these individuals had been especially impressed with Dr. Houser's outline of the pre-chiropractic course. According to Dr. Houser some of the Jr. colleges had expressed the readiness to carry the prescribed pre-chiropractic course in the college catalogue as well as list the Los Angeles College of Chiropractic for further reference.

VI. Dr. Coggins was then asked to inform the council about the plans at the Logan College with reference to the organizing of a Jr. college on the campus and following are the comments made by Dr. Coggins.

a. The intent is to operate a separate and distinct Jr. college.

b. Full approval has been obtained from the Department of Higher Education of the State of Missouri.

c. It has been the intention to commence the course September 1952 but in order to effect a more conclusive program a date has been deferred to September 1953.

d. The Jr. college faculty must be separate from that of the chiropractic college faculty and be approved by the University of Missouri.

e. The beginning class not to exceed 35 and the students cannot concurrently be occupied with any other course, for example, such as the chiropractic course.

VII. Dr. Bertholf of the University of Natural Healing, stated that they had a five year course and that they did allow one year of advanced standing for ??? years of Jr. college.

If a high school student wishes to matriculate in the college, the first year is preparatory to the chiropractic course.

VIII. Dr. Budden expressed the opinion that all the chiropractic colleges should desist from conducting summer school or semester. Dr. Nugent concurred with this idea, stating that the all year round grind is too difficult both for students and faculty.

IX. Dr. DeRusha inquired whether something could not be done about correcting the faculty statistics in relation to the basic science board examiners that were periodically put out by the medical profession.

a. The conclusion was that we should be more diligent in the accumulation of our statistics and these should be more frequently published.

The third session of the council was held on Wednesday morning at 9:30 a.m. with Dr. Peterson presiding.

1. Dr. Peterson read a letter from Dr. Milbank, President, Los Angeles College of Chiropractic and the following three major points were to be noted.

a. That Dr. Lee A. Norcross had been relieved of his position as Dean of the Los Angeles College of Chiropractic.

b. That the accrediting committee and the director of education have been encouraged to make a thorough inspection of the Oakland College of Chiropractic. That Mr. McClintock, Dean and holder of the college was ready to effect an agreement with the California Chiropractic Educational Foundation to turn the college over to the foundation so that it might become a co-op organization and thus qualify for the council's approval.

c. Dr. Milbank asked that if any criticism should be made of the Los Angeles college, that from now on, instead of allowing the same to become rumors, that they should be relayed directly to him for deliberation and discussion.

II. Dr. Peterson also read a letter from Dr. Harring, President, of the Missouri College expressing greetings and best wishes and an excuse for not being able to be present.

III. Dr. Peterson then read a letter from a Dr. Steven L. Fielder, head of non-affiliated group called the Council on Manipulated

Surgery. It was a request to investigate and approve a new technic.

    a. It was eventually concluded that these new technic measures should be investigated and evaluated by the college of the area in which it arose and then later a report submitted to the council.

IV. Dr. Peterson read a letter addressed to the council by Dr. Carl Cleveland, Jr. expressing his regret and that he would not be able to attend and proffered his best wishes for a successful gathering.

V. Dr. Peterson, next, proceeded to bring up the matter of the licensure problem confronting the newly appointed Pennsylvania Board of Chiropractic Examiners and following are the pertinent matters brought forth in the discussion.

    a. Since the realization of an independent chiropractic act ??? board of examiners in Pennsylvania a harassing and difficult problem has arisen.

    b. There are some 150 to 200 unlicensed practitioners in the state of Pennsylvania who have sustained practice for a given number of years now wishing to qualify for the chiropractic board.

    c. Unfortunately these practitioners hold diplomas from colleges that have long closed their doors and who scholastic conducts, at least, under certain circumstances might have been questioned.

    d. These individuals would, of course, like to obtain a blanket privilege of taking a short term qualifying course at any one of the accredited colleges and then obtain from that college a certificate of qualification for the Pennsylvania board and also a diploma from that college.

    e. On various occasions members of this group as well as officers of the Pennsylvania Chiropractic Societies have approached the officers of the council seeking a solution to this problem.

    f. Dr. Peterson submitted a letter as written to him by the chairman of board the following being a direct copy of the same.

COMMONWEALTH OF PENNSYLVANIA, DEPARTMENT OF PUBLIC INSTRUCTION
Bureau of Professional Licensing, State Board of Chiropractic Examiners
898 Park Avenue, Meadville, Pa.

June 23rd, 1952
Dr. Thure C. Peterson
Saxony Hotel
Miami Beach, Fla.
Dear Dr. Peterson,

In reply to your letter of June 16th, regarding special classes being set up at your school for the benefit of Pennsylvania Chiropractors, I herewith give you the Board action on this matter that you may take it up with the Educational Council while at the Convention.

The Board did not approve the plan as suggested by Dr. Yocum or Dr. Ritchie and since the Penna. law requires graduation from a Recognized School, nothing else can be accepted, therefore, the following was established as the policy of the Board in this matter.

"To meet professional educational requirements for admission to an examination for licensure to practice Chiropractic in Pennsylvania, persons who were graduated from a school or college of Chiropractic not legally incorporated and reputable at the time of their graduation, must submit their credentials to a legally incorporated and reputable school or college of Chiropractic for evaluation and must make up any deficiency to graduate. Persons having their credentials evaluated and attending a legally incorporated and reputable school or college of Chiropractic to make up any deficiency to graduate therefrom must be in regular attendance at such school or college of chiropractic at least one year."

The above means one full college year at least, not six months, and a certificate of graduation to be issued. If you can work out such a program for this group and if they will accept it, the Board will approve it.

Thanking you for your cooperation and consideration of our problems, I remain,
Sincerely yours
Kenfield K. Lane, D.C., Chairman
State Board of Chiropractic Examiners

After much discussion Dr. Janse was instructed to write the chairman of the Pennsylvania State Board and advise him of the continued resolution that was unanimously passed by the council. Letter as follows:

June 28, 1952
Dr. Kenfield K. Lane, Chairman,
State Board of Chiropractic Examiners,
Commonwealth of Pennsylvania,
898 Park Avenue,
Meadville, Pennsylvania
Dear Doctor Lane,

The Council on Education of the National Chiropractic Association in session instructed us to advise you of the following resolution in answer to your letter to Dr. Peterson, dated June 23rd.

"The Council on Education of the National Chiropractic Association will authorize any of its affiliated colleges to arrange for such special courses as the Pennsylvania State Board of Chiropractic Examiners will stipulate, with the approval of the Department of Education of the Commonwealth of Pennsylvania, and will issue certificates of attendance."

"The colleges will not evaluate, accept or certify the professional credentials possessed by the candidates, nor will these credits be acceptable toward the completion of the regular professional course."

This resolution was passed with the unanimous vote and may we ask you to submit the same to the other members of the Board and all other individuals concerned.

We shall be happy to comply with any likely program that may be established in keeping with the conditions of this resolution.

With every good wish we beg to remain,

Sincerely yours,

Thure C. Peterson, President

Joseph Janse, Secretary

VI. Dr. Peterson then asked Drs. Houser and King to submit their report and ideas on their assignment in relation to the Standardization of the Curriculum and Transcript Forms of the various colleges.
   a. Dr. Houser advised the council that since the Indianapolis meeting he had not gone any further with the then submitted program on the Standardization of Curricula, the reasons being:
      1. The difference in the semester quarter and summer term programs of the various colleges.
      2. The obvious difference of the curricula of those schools not including physiotherapy in their courses and those including physiotherapy.
   b. Both Drs. Houser and King were agreed on the following points in relation to this matter of student transcripts.
      1. Transcripts should not be handed out to students at random because experience has proven that some graduates will falsify the same.
      2. Whenever possible the transcripts should be sent to all requesting colleges on state board directory rather than turning it over to the graduate.
      3. Every college should have two transcript forms.
         1. One for the various state boards which usually necessitate the abbreviation into departmental divisions.
         2. Transcript forms to be given out when a student transfers to one college from another or when he wishes to do graduate work or P.G. work.
   c. The latter transcript should be most thorough and complete and should include the following.
      1. Information relating to the pre-professional secondary in college education.
      2. The number of 60 minute hours, grade hours, and his grades in each of the subjects taken.
      3. A definite indication of any failure or necessary make-up.
      4. A departmental summation of the courses.
      5. Transcripts should also indicate the number of clinic and intern hours.
   d. Dr. Houser recommended that each school improvise a photo-copy box, hereby, transcripts could be prepared from the original on photo-sensitive paper, to which the college seal and signature could be applied and this could avoid any possibility of falsifying the record.
   e. It was recommended that all colleges obtain the transcripts forms of the other colleges and proceed to renovate each necessary and present forms and methods.
   f. It was also recommended that the permanent student record cards [which] have folders be brought up to date and be made a little more complete as far as the pertinent informations are concerned.
   g. Every college should have within the files of the registrar's office a complete library of the transcript forms of the other colleges as well as the catalog for the purpose of being able to more completely interpret the records of student transferees.
VII. Dr. Budden brought out a point that resulted in rather an extended discussion and conclusion.
   a. He expressed the idea that in Dr. Nugent's outline of the chiropractic course in his manual on Chiropractic Education that Dermatology and Syphilology was a rather hazardous misrepresentation.
   b. According to Dr. Budden a number of occasions had arisen where he had been confronted by the inordinate claim that in as much as syphilology were now a special designation in chiropractic courses a chiropractor might proceed to treat the venereal diseases by means of the standard methods measures.
   c. Dr. Budden expressed the apprehension that this would lead to a lot of contentious discussion.
   d. Dr. Nugent insisted that the only reason he included the term syphilology was because throughout the state the Public Health Departments insisted upon such a designation and on various occasions it had been questioned whether Drs. of Chiropractic knew anything about the proper diagnosis of the social diseases.
   e. It was finally concluded that the term syphilology would be dropped and inference would be made that in chiropractic colleges the social diseases were studied thoroughly on a diagnostic basis.

The fourth session of the council meetings was held on Wednesday afternoon at 2:00 P.M. June 25th with Dr. Peterson presiding. This session was a closed meeting with the full members of the Council only being in attendance, those present being: Drs. Nugent, Wolf, Osborne, Martin, Gardner, Peterson, Budden, Coggins, Houser, King, Cole, Troilo, and Janse.

Dr. Peterson called for the report of the accrediting committee. Dr. Nugent advised the Council that the accrediting committee had organized itself with Dr. Walter B. Wolf as the president, and Dr. Norman E. Osborne as the secretary.

Dr. Wolf called on Dr. Osborne as the secretary to make the report. Following were the essential points presented in Dr. Osborne's prepared report.

(1) Dr. Nugent in his mediations in Washington had found out that the Federal Government had gone out of the business of conducting a department of higher education, and hence his efforts to acquire recognition by this agency for the chiropractic colleges would have to be channeled into other directions.

In speaking on this point, Dr. Nugent advised the council that he had already established connections with the scholastic agency that had come to assume this work and that he was personally acquainted with several of the individuals in key positions in this agency. Dr. Nugent did express the opinion that recognition from this body will be more difficult to obtain than had the government retained its bureau on higher education.

(2) Brief reference was made to the Columbia College of Chiropractic in Baltimore. The college was making progress and it was the full opinion of the accrediting committee that Dr. Dean the president of the college was sincerely desirous of attempting to qualify for approval of the council.

(3) Drs. Martin and Gardner had inspected the University of Natural Healing, Denver, Colorado. At this visit they had been informed by Drs. Bishop and Bertholf that a full chair of chiropractic had been organized and established in the college.

Drs. Martin and Gardner had reported to the committee that the state of the college had undergone no change and consequently it was the unanimous opinion of the committee not to do anything about the status of the college at the present time.

(4) After the midyear meeting in Indianapolis Drs. Martin and Gardner had visited the Carver College of Chiropractic and had concluded that it was impossible for the administration of the college to fulfill its commitments to the accrediting committee on certain assigned changes, improvements and renovations.

For these reasons the accrediting committee recommended that the Carver College be tentatively dropped from the approved list of the Council on Education.

(5) It was the general opinion of the accrediting committee that Dr. Vinton F. Logan, President of the Logan Basic College of Chiropractic, had through his attitudes and dispositions portrayed an opposition to the policies of the NCA hence it was the unanimous recommendation of the accrediting committee to the Council on Education that the Logan Basic College of Chiropractic be asked to resign from the Council on Education.

(6) Dr. Nugent had spent a considerable amount of time during the last year in San Antonio, mediating with the administration of the Texas Chiropractic College. Dr. Martin had also visited the college for the purpose of verifying Dr. Nugent's opinions.

These gentlemen had reported to the accrediting committee that decided improvements had been affected in the Texas College both in the manner of setting up a competent non-profit corporation and in relation to the academic standards to be maintained.

Dr. Troilo the dean of the college had proceeded to establish a competent curriculum, supported by a well conditioned faculty and class schedule.

For these reasons it was the recommendation of the accrediting committee that the Texas College of Chiropractic be offered a full approval status for one year, based upon certain stipulations which would have to be fulfilled within the coming year.

(7) Mention was made of the fact that Dr. William Cole had been reappointed as Dean of the Kansas State College of Chiropractic and Dr. Cole had asked for another year to endeavor to bring about certain changes at the college and it was the recommendation of the committee that the Council proffer such a deference.

A motion was made that the report of the accrediting committee as made by Dr. Osborne be unanimously accepted, with the reservation that each point could be talked upon and discussed.

Dr. William Coggins, Dean of the Logan Basic College of Chiropractic asked for the opportunity of voiding the standard of the Logan College in the issues that confronted it. In resume the following were his assertions.

(1) The Logan College does support the NCA
   a. We use NCA Literature
   b. We support the educational tenets of the NCA
   c. We have sustained a four year course for a long time.

(2) We do differ with Dr. Nugent and the element supported by Dr. Power of the Missouri College in the legislature issues in Missouri. We feel that we have a right to do so.

(3) We do oppose the control of Chiropractic by medical acts, as for example in Illinois and we shall continue to strive for independent chiropractic legislation.

(4) We do not feel that we should be obligated to subscribe to every attitude of the NCA or Dr. Nugent in order to retain our position on the Council.

(5) It was Dr. Coggins' opinion that the Logan issue was very much the result of the personal animosity that existed between Drs.

Nugent and Logan.

Dr. Nugent in rebuttal to Dr. Coggins made the following assertion.

(1) We have tried but cannot find agreement with Dr. Logan.

(2) Dr. Logan has personally done much more to further the cause of the other national organization than the NCA.

(3) There has been a planned campaign of indoctrinating students and field members against the policies of the NCA and the efforts of the Council and his position as Director of Education.

(4) That Dr. Logan had failed to support the college's position on the Council by his presence, yet he had always found time to attend the meetings and conventions of the other national groups as well as the newly founded schoolmen's group.

(5) That both Drs. Logan and Cleveland had resisted the raising of the professional standards to four years in the state of Missouri, although such was one of the standards of the council.

Dr. Wolf then advised the group that the opinions expressed by Dr. Nugent represented the consensus of opinion of the entire accrediting committee and that the executive board of the NCA had been consulted with and they concurred.

It was also mentioned that at the Indianapolis meeting there had been a gentlemen's agreement that no member of the Council should participate in other affiliations, especially representing a competitive school group.

At this time both Drs. Coggins and Troilo were asked to leave the room until the remaining members of the Council officially voted on the Council's disposition with reference to the status of the colleges they represented. It should be stated that Dr. Parr was no longer in attendance having not appeared for the meetings of the 25th.

Dr. Troilo was invited to come in first and he was advised that it had been the unanimous decision of the Council to respond to the recommendation of the Accrediting Committee in extending to the Texas College of Chiropractic full approval for one year and following is a copy of the official statement that the president and secretary of the Council were instructed to send to the Board of Trustees of the college thru Dr. Troilo:

June 28, 1952
Dr. Julius C. Troilo, Dean
Texas Chiropractic College
San Pedro Park
San Antonio, Texas
Dear Doctor Troilo:

We are pleased to advise you that the National Council on Education of the National Chiropractic Association by unanimous vote accepted the recommendation of the Accrediting Committee of the Council to grant the Texas Chiropractic College full approval.

This approval is to extend, without reservations, for one year at which time its continuance will depend upon the fulfillment of several conditions with which the Accrediting Committee has acquainted you.

The entire membership of the Council wishes to congratulate the Texas Chiropractic College. We acknowledge our respect and admiration for the fine work that you have done.

Your attendance at the Council meetings has been a pleasant experience for all of us. May we ask you to inform the Board of Trustees of the College of the Council's designation.

With every good wish we wish to remain,
Sincerely yours,
Thure C. Peterson, President
Joseph Janse, Secretary

Dr. Troilo expressed his appreciation and happiness and advised the Council of his undivided readiness to support the Council and to seek their understanding and cooperation.

Dr. Coggins was then asked to come in and he was advised of the unanimous conclusion of the Council as expressed in the following official letter that the president and secretary of the Council were instructed to send Dr. Logan.

June 28, 1952
Dr. Vinton F. Logan, President
Logan Basic College of Chiropractic
7701 Florissant Road
St. Louis 21, Missouri
Dear Doctor Logan:

We have been instructed by the Council on Education of the National Chiropractic Association to advise you of the following recommendation of the Accrediting Committee of the Council.

"The Accrediting Committee recommends that the Logan Basic College of Chiropractic resign from the Council on Education for the reason that the Council considers its actions to have been incompatible with the policy of the National Chiropractic Association."

This recommendation was moved upon, seconded and unanimously accepted by the Council.

We sincerely regret the necessity of this responsibility.
Sincerely yours,
Thure C. Peterson, President
Joseph Janse, Secretary

The president and secretary of the Council were then instructed to send the following decision to Dr. Parr as president of the Carver College of Chiropractic.
June 28, 1952
Dr. Paul O. Parr, President
Carver College of Chiropractic
521 N.W. Ninth Street
Oklahoma City 3, Oklahoma
Dear Doctor Parr:

We have been instructed by the Council on Education of the National Chiropractic Association while in session on June 24th. of the following recommendation submitted to the Council by the Accrediting Committee:

"It was the unanimous decision of the Accrediting Committee that we recommend the removal of the Carver College of Chiropractic from the provisionally approved college list for the reason that the above named institution has not been able to comply with the scholastic stipulations laid down by the Committee."

This recommendation was moved upon and seconded and accepted by unanimous vote of the Council.

We wish to express our sincere regret in the discharge of this necessity, with every good wish,

Sincerely yours,
Thure C. Peterson, President
Joseph Janse, Secretary

The fifth session of the Council was held on Thursday morning of July 26th at 9 P.M. with Dr. Peterson presiding.

Dr. King expressed the desire to relay to the Council the greetings and best wishes of Drs. Firth and Hendricks of the Lincoln College, emphasizing their wholehearted support of the Council and the NCA program.

Dr. Janse made a financial report of the Council treasury reiterating the conclusion that had been reached in Santa Monica, namely that each college participating in the meetings of the Council yearly submit 10 dollars to help cover the expenses of the Council. To date the following college have paid their dues:

> Chiropractic Institute of New York
> Western States College of Chiropractic
> Lincoln Chiropractic College
> Texas Chiropractic College
> National College of Chiropractic
> Los Angeles College of Chiropractic
> Kansas State College of Chiropractic
> University of Natural Healing

The secretary would request that the other college upon receipt of the minutes submit their dues and thus mitigate the chagrin of having to solicit the same.

Dr. Budden made inquiry as to what the experience the other school men had had with reference to the intra-mural administrative set up of the colleges. This inquiry was made in interest of the rather unfortunate happenings that had occurred at several of the colleges when the administrative staffs had been vulnerable to an unstable dictatorial board of trustees.

(1) Dr. Peterson voiced the opinion that it was detrimental to permit the authority over a college to fall into the hands of a vacillating board of trustees.

He recommended that the colleges be supported by an administration possessive of perpetuating authority supported by an advisory board and the college alumni association.

Experience had shown that where the college was too completely under the supervision of professional groups it became the football of pressure groups and politics.

(2) Dr. Cole stated that at the Kansas State College they had had a classical example of a professionally owned and controlled college and the great hazard that resulted.

(3) Dr. Budden voiced the strong opinion that the Council should go on record recommending that no college be so changed in its administrative policies that it become the scapegoat of pressure groups of the profession.

Dr. Peterson then advised the council that he had been in conference with Dr. Claude Henderson, president of the Council on Chiropractic State Boards of Examiners that they had set up an accrediting program and sought the cooperation of the Council on Education.

Both Drs. Peterson and Nugent expressed the belief that as the result of this action there would be a reduplication of effort.

Dr. Peterson recommended that whenever an inspection or request for information be made from the Council or Examining Board they be advised of the inspection that had been made by Dr. Nugent under the auspices of the accrediting committee.

After careful deliberation it was the unanimous conclusion of the Council to ask Drs. Peterson and Janse to retain their positions as president and secretary of the Council respectively.

Because of the fact that several of the Council members had reports to give before the House of Delegates the meeting was adjourned until after luncheon.

The sixth and final session of the Council meetings was held on Thursday afternoon at 2 P.M. June 26th with Dr. Peterson presiding.

1. After rather extensive discussions the final conclusions were reached with reference to the Pennsylvania situation and the afore-recorded letter that the secretary of the Council was instructed to draw up and send to the Dr. Kane, chairman of the Board of Examiners was unanimously decided upon.

2. Dr. Osborne then presented a request from Dr. Leo Klein. Dr. Klein in working for his degree in psychology has asked the various colleges to cooperate with him in obtaining certain information from students in chiropractic colleges in relation to their social, psychological and personality dispositions. It was concluded that it would be entirely a voluntary thing for the various college heads to decide upon. It was to be encouraged that cooperation be proffered Dr. Klein in the completion of his project.

3. The final session was adjourned with everyone expressing the desire and determination to continue the program that the council had initiated. The program of raising professional standards, augmenting the educational facilities of the colleges, and acquiring governmental and public recognition for the educational institutions has accrued for the profession a tremendous benefit and progress that must be continued and expanded.

Minutes of the NATIONAL COUNCIL ON EDUCATION, Annual meetings of the Council held in conjunction with the annual convention of the National Chiropractic Association, held July 26 to 31, 1953, inclusive at the Statler Hotel, Los Angeles, California; Dr. Thure C. Peterson, Chairman of the Council, presided at all of the Meetings.

Those attending:

(A) Members of the Accrediting Committee

Dr. John J. Nugent, Director of Education of the National Chiropractic Association, 92 Norton Street, New Haven, Connecticut

Dr. Walter B. Wolf, President of the Accrediting Committee, Eureka, South Dakota

Dr. Norman E. Osborne, Secretary of the Accrediting Committee, 1172 The Terrace, Hagerstown, Maryland

Dr. Ralph J. Martin, 28 W. Sierra Madre Blvd., Sierra Madre, California

Dr. Edward H. Gardner, 2727 South Vermont Avenue, Los Angeles, California

(B) Representatives of the accredited, provisionally accredited, and subscribing educational institutions.

Dr. Thure C. Peterson, President, Chiropractic Institute of New York, 152 W. 42nd Street, New York 18, New York

Dr. W.A. Budden, Director, Western States College of Chiropractic, 4525 Southeast 63rd Street, Portland 6, Oregon

Dr. Arthur G. Hendricks, Treasurer, Lincoln Chiropractic College, Inc., 633 N. Pennsylvania Avenue, Indianapolis, Indiana

Dr. Joseph Janse, President, National College of Chiropractic, 20 North Ashland Blvd., Chicago 7, Illinois

Dr. George H. Haynes, Dean, Los Angeles College of Chiropractic, 920 East Broadway Avenue, Glendale 5, California

Dr. Julius C. Troilo, Dean, Texas Chiropractic College, San Pedro Park, San Antonio, Texas

Dr. John B. Wolfe, President, Northwestern College of Chiropractic, 2222 Park Avenue, Minneapolis, Minnesota

Dr. A. Earl Homewood, Dean, Canadian Memorial Chiropractic College, 252 Bloor Street West, Toronto, Canada

Dr. H.C. Harring, President, Missouri Chiropractic College, 3117 Lafayette Avenue, St. Louis 4, Missouri

Dr. Bera A. Smith, President, Carver College of Chiropractic, 521 N.W. 9th Street, Oklahoma City, Oklahoma

Dr. L.A. Bertholf, Dean, University of Natural Healing Arts, 1075 Logan Avenue, Denver, Colorado

(C) Other representatives and faculty members of chiropractic colleges.

Dr. R.O. McClintock, President, Oakland College of Chiropractic

Dr. E.G. Christensen, Faculty member of the Oakland College of Chiropractic

Dr. Raymond H. Houser, former Administrative Dean, Los Angeles College of Chiropractic and now newly appointed President of the Board of Directors of this college.

Dr. Vierling Kersey, Administrative Director of the Los Angeles College of Chiropractic.

Dr. Sidney Milbank, retiring President of the Los Angeles College of Chiropractic and its Board of Directors.

Dr. J.D. Walp, retiring president of the California Chiropractic Association.

The first session of the Council was an open meeting and held on the morning on Monday July 27th, 1953 with Dr. Peterson presiding.

1. An agenda was set up for progressive consideration.

2. The first topic of discussion was the recently developed situation in Pennsylvania.

   a. As the result of recently passed amendments to the chiropractic act the Pennsylvania Board of Chiropractic Examiners have been authorized to set up a qualifying program for those in chiropractic practice, but without a license and possessing degrees from colleges that were now defunct.

   b. Recent communication with Dr. Yoder the secretary of the Board advises the Council that the Penn. Board has stipulated a total of 936 sixty minute hours to be procured at one of the accredited colleges.

   c. To date this stipulation carries no further instruction as to whether the total amount of hours are to be procured at one tenure or whether it can be obtained in piece meal manner for the convenience of the practitioner.

   d. Because their colleges would be the one primarily involved, Drs. Peterson, Hendricks and ??? were instructed by the Council to hold a special conclave to determine what conduct the accredited colleges should sustain in relation to this matter. Following are the major points concluded upon:

       (1) No attempt should be made by any of the colleges to define or prescribe but all colleges should simply wait until the Board had reached its own conclusions.

       (2) Unless some 20 or more of these practitioners are in a position to take their work simultaneously it would be economically impossible to put on special work and classes, and they would have to be absorbed in the regular undergraduate classes.

       (3) It was deemed inadvisable to permit these practitioners to accumulate their hours faster than 10 hours a day, it being academically impossible to absorb work beyond this daily hour schedule.

       (4) Upon the completion of his work the practitioner would simply receive a certification of the hours put in and nothing else.

       (5) Because of the difference in class and clinic time each college should be privileged to handle the problem as they see fit, other than that some standard agreement should be reached on the tuition rate.

   e. Dr. Peterson further advised the Council that in corresponding with some of the people in Penn. he had advised them that the Chiropractic Institute would be willing to send members of their faculty to Philadelphia over the week-ends to put on special work for these practitioners. To date no further opinions had been received with reference to this recommendation.

   f. Dr. Peterson had also corresponded with Dr. Stokes and made the following recommendations as to the course and the tuition.

       Anatomy review   120 hours.
       Physiology   120 hours.
       Public Health   80 hours.
       X.ray pathology   80 hours.
       X.ray interpretation   40 hours.
       Diag. & Symptomatology   200 hours.
       Lab. diagnosis   80 hours.
       Principles 120 hours.
       Practice   96 hours.

       making a total of 936 hrs., 60 min. With an approximate cost of 468 dollars per graduate student.

2. Discussion in relation to the Virginia State Board issue.

   a. Recent communications from Virginia advised the Council that this Board, a mixed board, had recently deliberated two questions;

       (1) Whether in the definition of chiropractic as contained within the literature of the medical act the word therapeutics should be deleted?

       (2) Whether it was congruous for the Board to recognize the accredited college lists of both the NCA and the ICA, or whether the one or the other should be deleted?

            (a) In answer to the first question it was the emphatic conclusion that this word should be retained in the defining literature of the Act. It appears that by virtue of this word the practitioners of chiropractic in the state of Virginia maintain the privilege the generic adjunctive therapeutic measures.

            (b) Dr. Nugent was instructed to seek consultation with the Virginia Board and submit the case of the Council's accrediting program in the anticipation that such would obtain a solution to the second question.

3. Dr. Nugent's report on the progress of his efforts to get the accrediting program recognized by the Federal Government.

   a. Several years ago he Dr. Nugent had contacted the Department of Education of the Federal Security Agency with the intent of obtaining recognition of the accreditation program of the Council. Progress had been made but then this department was dissolved and hence the efforts were of little avail.

b. Within the last year extended contact had been made with the newly established Department of Health, Education and Welfare under Secretary of Health Evelyn C. Hobby. In mediating with the department Dr. Nugent had been instructed as to what the Department wishes to know about an accrediting agency.

   (1) There can only be one accrediting agency for each profession.

   (2) The nature of the organization supporting the accrediting agency.

   (3) The nature of the governing mechanism employed by the accrediting agency and the methods and technics employed in the processes of inspection and accreditation.

   (4) Completeness of files, inspection records and accumulated informations.

   (5) The background, history precedence and qualifications of the accrediting agency as well as the budget available to it for the conduct of its official work.

c. Dr. Nugent advised the Council that he had submitted a complete file on all of the accredited colleges as well as the function of the accrediting committee along with copies of the recently prepared publications entitled:

   (1) Educational Standards for Chiropractic Colleges.

   (2)

   (3)

d. Dr. Nugent also advised the Council that the recent cut in the Federal Budget had reduced the activity of the office of the Mr. Armstrong in Washington to whom this material had been submitted and hence the final conclusions had been delayed.

e. It was of course the full consensus of opinion that if this effort on the part of Dr. Nugent could be realized the entire accrediting program would receive a tremendous verification and strength of authority.

f. Dr. Nugent encouraged all of the school men to fill out the prepared and submitted questionnaire as soon as possible and to be as exacting as possible in preparing the answers and entries. His reasons being that he would like to have as complete up to date detailed information on the accredited colleges as available so that he could continue to present a competent case to the government.

g. At this time an extended discussion arose between Drs. Nugent, Walp and Milbank in relation to the trip that Dr. Lee Norcross made at the instruction of the California Chiropractic Association for the purpose of attempting to get federal accreditation for the Los Angeles College.

   (1) Dr. Nugent insisted that such had frustrated the integrity of the program he had initiated and felt that Dr. Norcross' efforts had been rather compromising.

   (2) Both Drs. Walp and Milbank expressed their regret about the entire matter and insisted that it had arisen out of misunderstanding and lack of proper informations. They expressed the conviction that such interventions would not occur again.

   (3) It was the consensus of the council that the ambivalence of attitude in California of the past was being rectified.

   (4) Proposition in relation to a budget for the Council and the expenses incurred.

      a. The report was made that the Council had $25 in its treasury.

      b. Dr. Homewood of the Canadian Memorial College paid Dr. Budden $10 in back dues for the college.

      c. Dr. Janse made the recommendation that the Executive Committee be approached and asked to set up a $1000/year budget for the Council because of the importance of its position and the extent of its activities.

      d. Drs. Budden and Troilo were appointed to meet with the executive board about this proposition.

      e. In due time those gentlemen reported that the executive board felt that the NCA could not at the present time extend itself to this amount but did commit the executive-secretary to accept vouchers of expense of the Council and pay accordingly.

      g. It was then suggested by Dr. Nugent that the remaining $35 in the treasury be used to pay any past expenses and then simply turn in a requisition on expenses after each semi-annual meeting to Dr. Rogers the NCA secretary.

Evening Session, July 27th, 1953, Dr. Peterson presiding.

1. Dr. Nugent rather severely criticized the competitive advertising that was being done by the accredited colleges in the various state publications as well as their own.

a. He insisted that some of the claims and contentions of the various colleges were altogether too competitive and that all colleges should desist from such practices.

b. He further commented on the neglect of the accredited colleges to mention their source of accreditation. Such statements as universally accredited, etc. were somewhat of a subterfuge and misleading.

c. He recommended that all colleges in their advertisements employ the statement, "accredited by the Council on Education of the National Chiropractic Association."

2. Dr. Harring was called on to advise the Council as to the issue that had caused so much talk in Missouri.

a. The doctor stated that the anti-Nugent comments and literature coming out of Missouri had no basis and was instigated by the anti-NCA forces in Missouri.

b. He stated that the two colleges in Missouri other than the Missouri College and their representatives had severely resisted any attempt to increase the latitude of chiropractic definition as well as the raising of the educational standards.

c. Dr. Harring also outlined for the Council the newly established mechanism of basic science training that the students at the Missouri College of Chiropractic might obtain at the St. Louis University.

    (1) The plan simply consisted of a permit granted by St. Louis University to students of the Missouri College of Chiropractic to obtain training in such subjects as chemistry, bacteriology and physiology at the University for which they would get credit toward their degrees in chiropractic at the Missouri College.

    (2) The entire plan, however, is voluntary and to date only several students had entered into the function of the plan. Thus the necessity for basic science classes and training still remained the full responsibility of the Missouri College.

d. Doctor Harring expressed the opinion that the Council had been too lenient in its attitudes toward the other chiropractic colleges in Missouri, who had actually conducted NCA activities, and hence the position of the Missouri College had been severely compromised.

3. Dr. Troilo was then invited to report on the progress of the concurrent two years of college program initiated at the Texas College of Chiropractic.

a. The doctor advised the Council that the plan was working out very well, resulting in much success, progress and growth at the Texas College.

b. He stated that the authorities of both the Texas University and the San Antonio Junior College had been more cooperative in their efforts in this respect.

c. He declared that the students were enthused about the entire program as well as the entire body of the profession in Texas.

d. The doctor mentioned that inasmuch as all the students having entered into the program spend only part of their daily school time at the junior college it permits the Texas Chiropractic College staff to keep them under daily surveillance and to see to it that they are properly chiropractically indoctrinated.

4. Dr. Margaret Schmidt, representing the Council of Women Chiropractors appeared before the Council to advise them that a full scholarship had been set up by this group for some young woman interested in chiropractic as a career.

a. She sought advice as to just how this scholarship might be announced to the field.

b. Several suggestions were made and it was finally concluded that she should consult with the executive board to determine just what the NCA could do in the form of sustaining publicity.

c. In a consequent meeting Dr. Schmidt advised the Council that Dr. Rogers and the executive board had committed themselves to running a full page spread on the scholarship in both the NCA Journal and Healthways.

5. Dr. Janse explained to the Council that Dr. Orin E. Madison, a member of the Michigan Basic Science Board had sought the support of the Council in seeking a reappointment to the Board. The following is a letter that the secretary was instructed to prepare and send to Governor Williams.

Honorable G. Mennen Williams
State Capitol Building
Lansing, Michigan
Dear Governor:

    Our attentions have been drawn to the fact that within the next few months the reappointment of Dr. Orin E. Madison as a member of the Michigan Basic Science Board will be a matter for consideration within your office.

    It has been the privilege of this Council to know Dr. Madison in an official capacity and we have been impressed by his integrity and fair-mindedness in dealing with each of the healing professions.

    Furthermore, his pioneering efforts helped to organize the American Association of Basic Science Boards which has been of great assistance in creating uniformity in the policies and attitudes of the various boards throughout the country. This of course is a distinct advantage to all chiropractic, medical and osteopathic students seeking licensure qualification.

    We as a Council of chiropractic educators wish to assure you of our continued desire to seek the best for the healing professions in the state of Michigan and hence may we solicit your consideration of the reappointment of Dr. Madison.

    With every good wish we seek to remain
    Respectfully yours,
    Thure C. Peterson, President
    Joseph Janse, Secretary

6. Dr. Haynes the newly appointed dean of the Los Angeles College of Chiropractic was then asked to inform the Council on the experiences encountered since the institution of the two year pre-professional requirement at the Los Angeles College.

a. Dr. Haynes advised the group that the Sept. Matriculation would be light. However, that such had been expected and that it would take about two years for the results to level off and show benefit.

b. The doctor did state the fact that the other two colleges in Los Angeles had not instituted the pre-professional stipulation had mitigated the effectiveness of the program.

c. Rather extended discussions ensued. Dr. Budden insisted that the colleges of the East and Midwest should also fall in line. In general, however, it was the consensus of opinion that caution should be exercised and probably in the long run the entire event might be best served if the various states gradually and progressively initiated the program.

d. This led to the information that both Maryland and Maine had enacted the two year ruling, although both states so arranged it that the college work could be obtained concurrent with the professional training.

Tuesday morning, July 28th, 1953 session, Dr. Peterson presiding.

1. The first subject of discussion was school economics.

   a. Dr. Nugent asserted that all of the schools should raise their tuition to a standard comparative level insisting that 200 dollars a semester was not too high.

   b. It was concluded that some geographical variance should be allowed.

   c. It was Dr. Nugent's opinion that if recognition could be obtained for the NCA accrediting program from the department of health it would serve to eliminate the borderline colleges and thus improve the economic advantages of the accredited colleges.

2. Dr. Nugent advised the Council that in his consultation with Mr. Armstrong of the department of health he committed himself to obtaining a complete up to date file on all of the accredited colleges.

   a. It was requested that all accredited colleges fill out as quickly and completely as possible the new set of questions as contained within the green backed prepared booklet.

   b. An up to date roster of the students in school, and number matriculated in the last class, the total enrollment and the amount in each class year.

   c. According to Mr. Armstrong each college should have at least 6 full time teachers of professorial rank.

3. Dr. Peterson stated that a more careful standardization should be attained in relation to students seeking advanced standing.

   a. It was the conclusions that too many prospective students with pre-professional college work were shopping to determine where they could obtain the most advanced standing.

4. The recently released text by Weiant and Verner entitled Rational Bacteriology was discussed. It was highly recommended as a reference book because it portrayed the principle of infection in light of the chiropractic concept. All school men were encouraged to recommend its distribution.

   a. It was a common consensus that it was not sufficient as a text for basic science instruction.

5. Both Drs. Nugent and Budden encouraged the usage of the texts written and distributed by members of the chiropractic profession, mention being made of the publications of Houser, Firth and the National College, and Dr. Verner.

6. By unanimous vote a resolution was passed forming a committee on the study and recommendation of chiropractic textbooks. Dr. Budden was appointed to head this committee and Drs. Haynes and Martin were instructed to assist him.

7. Dr. Nugent then emphasized the importance of attempting to standardize the teaching of chiropractic principles. He contended that much of the ambivalence of attitude among the members of the profession arose out of the heterogeneous concepts of chiropractic taught within the colleges.

   a. As a beginning he recommended that all instructors in chiropractic principles seek to accumulate all of the better written monograms on chiropractic.

   b. He asked all school men present to permit a free exchange of college literature in this respect.

Wednesday sessions, July 29th, 1953, Dr. Peterson presiding.

A. Morning session at the Los Angeles College of Chiropractic, 920 East Broadway, Glendale 5, Los Angeles.

   1. Upon arriving at the college the entire group made an inspection of the college plant and everyone remarked about the fine physical equipment and establishment that was observed.

   2. Dr. Henry C. Higley, faculty member of the L.A.C.C. and head of the college's department of research gave a very interesting talk upon the importance and advantages of doing research in the Laboratories of the accredited colleges.

      a. He contended that this research could be profit producing if done for companies that wished certain research products conducted. It was his contention that the research may extend into any field. He contended that any of the college staffs possessed more than enough technical know how to do this type of work and for which the average producer or manufacturer would be willing to pay. He cited several instances of how in the laboratories of the college research projects had been conducted for various concerns and for which the department had been paid.

      b. Each member of the Council was presented with a handsome monogram on research by Dr. Higley.

      c. Dr. Budden made the recommendation that Dr. Higley be appointed to head a research committee and that the first activity of this committee be that of gathering all the descriptive literature of the research projects that had already been conducted under the auspices of the various professional agencies.

   3. Miss Heycock the librarian of the Los Angeles college of Chiropractic then conducted a seminar on library procedures.

      a. Miss Heycock advised the group that she was a registered medical librarian and as such she had the privilege of contacts that enabled her to obtain information and publications by exchange and subscription that augmented the reading facilities of the library.

      b. She made the following recommendations.

(1) If possible each college should endeavor to have its librarian join the Specialists Librarian Association. The membership fee being 10 dollars a year. Application should be made for the Biological Science Division. The contact could be made through Mrs. Kathryn Stebbens executive secretary, 31 East 10th Street, New York 3, New York.

(2) She also recommended membership in the American Library Association, the yearly dues being 7 dollars and the address being 50 Huron Street, Chicago 11, Illinois. For $1.20 more one can obtain literature on the classification and cataloging of textbooks and periodicals for scientific libraries.

(3) Another contact that might be important is Miss Helen Woelfel, Treasurer Medical Library Association, 4802 3rd Street, Louisville, Kentucky.

(4) Following are the standards for an acceptable library.
   a. The library must contain a minimum of 1000 volumes that have been published within the last 10 years.
   b. The library should contain a minimum of 3000 volumes of all age.
   c. In 1953 the stipulation was that each library should have a minimum of subscription or access to 25 periodicals.
   d. Nearness to another library of national reputation emphasizes the qualification of the local library.
   e. Encyclopedias are counted as volumes.
   f. Each library should possess the text entitled Dictionary of Signs and Symbols, by Allen.
   g. Each library should possess an unabridged dictionary.
   h. A German-English dictionary should reside in the library, as well as a French-English and Latin-English, and Spanish-English.

(5) Methods of cataloging.
   a. The Boston Medical Classification is the method of preference, information being available at the Boston Medical Library, Boston, Mass. The books related are the Boston Medical Library Classification 2 volumes, $2.50 each, and printed by the Fenway Press, Boston, Mass.
   b. The manual Simple Library Cataloging, by Susan Gray Ackers, obtained from the American Library Association, 50 East Huron Street, Chicago is probably the simplest and possibly most effective for small libraries.

(6) Miss Heycock stated the American Library Assn. stipulated that every library should have a minimum budget of 300 dollars to start with and that 150 to 300 dollars a year should be spent for the procuring of added volumes and subscription to periodicals.

(7) It is recommended that there be from 1 to 3 new books on the library shelves for each of the subjects listed in the catalogs of the college.

4. After the discussions by Miss Heycock the entire visiting personnel was invited to a buffet luncheon prepared by the college staff and served in one of the class rooms. Dr. Vierling Kersey the newly appointed administrative director of the college served as host.

B. The afternoon session was held at the Statler Hotel upon the return of the Council from the Los Angeles College visit.
   1. Dr. Nugent emphasized the need for improving the library facilities at the accredited colleges. He stated that one of the first inquiry made by all departments of education and federal higher education agencies was about the library.
   2. Dr. Nugent encouraged assigning the librarian the responsibility of carefully culling out all articles related to the chiropractic concept from all of the available periodicals and texts, make a cataloged listing of them for student and faculty reference.
   3. Dr. Nugent advised the Council that he had been preparing a new booklet entitled "The Profession of Chiropractic," which should be ready for distribution within a couple of months.
   4. The Council was also advised that each college librarian could write to the congressional library and ask them to send catalogued cards on all of the standard medical texts that have been and will be published. These cards can be used in the regular college library indexed file.
   5. The Council was also advised that the congressional library had been accumulating a lot of texts from veterans who had discontinued their training and that these were being sold for ridiculously low prices.
   6. The Council next received Dr. Gordon Pefley, representing the American Society of Military Chiropractors. Dr. Pefley stated that the likelihood of chiropractic being included in the privileges of the Veteran might not be too distant and hence the Society felt that plans should be effected whereby courses could be set up at the various accredited colleges in hospital procedures etc.
      a. It was concluded that Dr. Pefley's recommendations were good but would necessitate very careful study and organization before such could be realized.
   7. Dr. Earl Homewood, the newly appointed Dean of the Canadian Memorial Chiropractic College made a report on the professional circumstances in Canada.
      a. The chiropractic bill sponsored by the Maritime Province of Nova Scotia had been killed.
      b. A chiropractic bill is pending in the Province of Quebec. The literature of the same is such that anyone in practice at

the time of the passage of the Bill would obtain licensure without any further effort.

In consequence to this lenience there at the present time over 30 Canadians taking the short term course at the Bebout College so that they may get under the "grandfather clause" wire.

    c.   Some of these individuals have now approached the Canadian College with the request that they be given full credit for their Bebout College training toward a four year degree at the Canadian College. This the Council frowned upon severely.

    d.   The situation in Ontario had become so complicated since about a year ago when an independent Board of Chiropractic Examiners had been established. Prior to this the mixed Drugless Therapy Board had granted the Doctor of Chiropractic liberal practice. The present law has a limited chiropractic definition and hence the Canadian Memorial Chiropractic College now issues Doctors of Drugless Therapy degrees so as to allow its graduates to get a naturopathic license from the Drugless Therapy Board.

    e.   In the Province of Alberta they have done away with written examinations necessitating only a degree from a college recognized by the Chiropractic Board.

    f.   In Manitoba the basic science law has been repealed.

    g.   Dr. Homewood advised the school men that if they wished their colleges to be recognized by the Ontario Board they would have to make an application for recognition every year, such being a written stipulation of the Board.

8. Dr. E.J. Wohlschlager, President of the Wisconsin Board of Chiropractic Examiners, and member of the National Council of Chiropractic Boards of Examiners, asked for the opportunity of consulting with the Council. Following are the major resultant discussions.

    a.   The doctor stated that the majority of the Board felt that the average run of applicants were weak in their understanding of x-ray, both in the field of technic and interpretation.

    b.   There is a strong trend among the members of the various boards to favor the two years of college requirement. It was however, the consensus of opinion among the board members that the initiative should come from the states rather than the colleges.

    c.   Dr. Peterson took time to brief Dr. Wohlschlager on the position of the Council on the two years college issue as decided upon at the mid-year meeting of the Council in Chicago.

    d.   Dr. Wohlschlager advised the Council that he and Dr. Cecil Martin, and Dr. Edward Poulsen had been appointed by the Council of Examining Boards to set up a file of questionnaires in the form of an accrediting survey.

He told the Council that the various boards were planning to make a yearly survey of the various chiropractic colleges.

The question immediately arose as to whether these surveys would be in the form of personal visits to the colleges by board members and who would be expected to pay for these visits.

The doctor stated that the Council realized that financially it would be prohibitive for either the state boards or the colleges to make or invite such personal visits and inspections and hence the surveys would be in the form of an extensive questionnaire to be filled out by the colleges every year.

He then asked Dr. Nugent whether his group might have the privilege of studying the book of questions prepared by Dr. Nugent for the surveys that the Accrediting Committee is going to make. Later questionnaires should be sent to Dr. Wohlschlager if for no other reason than a gesture of help.

Dr. Wohlschlager stated that the Council of Examining Boards did not wish to go into competition with the accrediting program of the NCA but because of the split in the profession and because the ICA was also entering into the field of the accrediting of chiropractic colleges, they, the Council of Examining Boards, could in no way tie themselves to any single one of the national organizations.

    e.   Dr. Wohlschlager sought in behalf of his Council the privilege of consulting with the Council on Education so that as little counter effort as is possible would result. This was granted and the Council concluded to maintain a working liaison with the other group.

9. The Council then received three members of the California State Board of Chiropractic Examiners, namely Drs. Walker, Poulson and Simons. The discussions primarily related to the situation of the three chiropractic colleges in Los Angeles. The Council was advised that the Ratledge and Hollywood Colleges had obtained a court decision of merit and hence they the Board of Examiners were compelled to give them approval equal to that of the L.A.C.C.

The three gentlemen expressed the hope that Dr. Nugent, as well as the Council as a body would be a little more diligent in keeping them acquainted with the policies of the Council.

10. Dr. Cecil Martin the chiropractic member of the New Jersey Board of Medical Examiners, was asked to present to the Council informations about the New Jersey situation. Following is a resume of the subsequent discussions.

    a.   Assembly Bill No. 456 was passed and signed by the Governor. This Bill was sponsored by one faction of the chiropractic profession in the state of New Jersey. Although it does not create an independent Chiropractic Board it makes specific arrangements for the possible licensing of a goodly number of the new unlicensed practitioners in the state, and also sets up a mechanism of inspecting chiropractic colleges for the possibility of their being accredited by the Board of Examiners.

        (1) The governor is to appoint two chiropractors to the board, these are to be licensed men, and to serve for a term of 3 years.

(2) The definition of chiropractic is as follows, "A licensed chiropractor shall have the right in the examination of patients to use the neurocalometer, x-ray, and other necessary instruments solely for the purpose of diagnosis and analysis. No licensed chiropractor shall use endoscopic, or cutting instruments, or prescribe, administer, or dispense drugs or medicine for the purpose whatsoever, or perform surgical operations excepting adjustment of the articulations of the spinal column."

(3) "No person licensed as a chiropractor shall sign any certificate required by law or the State Sanitary Code concerning reportable diseases, or birth, marriage or death certificates."

(4) Any person who prior to July 31st, 1944, and graduated from a legally incorporated chiropractic college, and who holds a license to practice chiropractic in any state of the Union and which was obtained thru written examination, and who has been a resident in the state of New Jersey before 1944 and in active practice since then and up to an including Dec. 31st, 1952 may obtain a license without examination.

(5) Any person who fills the foregoing stipulations but does not possess a license by examination in any other state, may within 90 days make application to the board for examination in the subjects of anatomy, physiology, hygiene, chiropractic diagnosis and the therapeutics of chiropractic and upon passing receive a license to practice.

(6) Any person who subsequent to July 31st, 1944, was a graduate of a chiropractic college teaching no less than 4 years of 7 months each, and who has been a registered resident in the state of New Jersey since then but who has served in the armed forces since Dec. 7, 1941, and who holds a license by examination in another state, may make application for a license without examination.

(7) Any person, who subsequent to July 31st, 1944, and prior to Jan. 1st., 1953, and who graduated from a chiropractic college with no less than 4 years of 7 months each, and who has been a resident in the state of New Jersey for no less than 4 years, and who holds a license by examination in any other state, as well as a basic science certificate, may make application for a license in the state of New Jersey without examination.

(8) Any person who subsequent to July 31st, 1944, and prior to Jan. 1st, 1953, and having graduated from an incorporated chiropractic college in a course of no less than 4 years of 7 months each, and who has been a continuous resident of the state for 4 years and in active practice, may make application for examination in the subjects of anatomy, physiology, pathology, hygiene, chiropractic diagnosis, and the therapeutics of chiropractic, and successfully passing the same will receive a license.

(9) Anyone who subsequent to Dec. 31st, 1952, and who has graduated from a chiropractic college teaching a course of 4 years of 9 months each, and who graduated after the 13th of June, 1953, may make application for examination in the subjects of anatomy, physiology, pathology, bacteriology, non-surgical diagnosis, chemistry, hygiene, and the therapeutics of chiropractic, and if successful in passing the same will receive a license.

(10) Any one making application for the board after 1954 must possess one year of pre-professional college education.

(11) Anyone making application to the board after 1957 must possess two years of pre-professional college education.

b. Dr. Martin reminded the Council that all matriculants from New Jersey should be advised by the registrar's offices of the colleges that the 4 years of 9 months each must be spread over 4 calendar years. It was estimated that if New Jersey matriculants would only enter college either in May or Sept. and avoid a Jan. matriculation they could go right through and still have one semester of their 36 months extend into the 4th calendar year.

c. Any communication with the Board should be directed to Dr. Cecil Martin, New Jersey State Board of Medical Examiners, Trenton Trust Bldg. Trenton, New Jersey.

d. Dr. Martin advised the Council that inasmuch as the present Bill had been severely fought by a certain segment of the profession in New Jersey they would not tolerate any intervention from that group and advised the college to direct their influences in support of the group under whose auspices the Bill had passed.

Closed Meeting, July 31st, 1953, Friday Morning.

1. Dr. Norman E. Osborne the secretary of the Accrediting Committee made the following report and recommendations.

   a. That a new designation be listed, namely colleges that subscribe to the program of the Council on Education. This recommendation was made because the term provisionally approved was rather inflexible and not fully correct.

   b. That the Carver College of Chiropractic be dropped from the approved list and placed on the list that subscribe to the program of the Council.

   c. That the Kansas State Chiropractic College be dropped from the provisionally approved list and placed on the list of those colleges that subscribe to the program of the Council.

   d. The same for the Missouri Chiropractic College. It should be stated that the Accrediting Committee had had a long session with Dr. Harring of the Missouri College and a very satisfactory understanding had been reached and effort was going to be made to help in every possible manner to enhance the position of the college.

e. That the University of Natural Healing be placed on the list of those colleges subscribing to the program of the Council.
f. That the Drs. Cleveland of the Cleveland Chiropractic College in Kansas City, and the Ratledge Chiropractic College of Los Angeles had given no indication of their desire to continue their affiliations with the Council.
g. That the Oakland College of Chiropractic be placed on the list of the subscribing colleges.
h. That the Logan Basic College of Chiropractic be dropped from the accredited list and membership in the Council for the following reasons.
   (1) Attitudes incompatible with the policies of the Council and the NCA.
   (2) Refusal to grant the Director of Education the privilege of making a full inspection of the college.
   (3) The failure to participate in the activities and program of the Council.
   (4) Drs. Peterson and Janse were instructed to write the following letter to Dr. Logan, as President of the College.

Dr. Vinton Logan,
Logan Basic College of Chiropractic
7701 Florissant Road
St. Louis 21, Missouri
Dear Doctor Logan:
   The recommendation of the Committee of Accreditation that the Logan Basic College of Chiropractic be removed from the list of the approved schools has been accepted by the Council on Education of the National Chiropractic Association.
   According to the rules and regulations of the Council, you have the privilege of appealing this action by requesting a hearing before the entire Council or appealing its decision to the House of Delegates.
   You have thirty days from the date of this notice to request a hearing.
   Very truly yours,
   Thure C. Peterson, Chairman
   Joseph Janse, Secretary

2. After due discussion the recommendations and substance of the report of the Accrediting Committee was unanimously accepted.
3. Dr. Julius Troilo invited the Council to hold its mid-year meetings in San Antonio, Texas, and this invitation was accepte

Minutes of the Semi-Annual Meeting of the NATIONAL COUNCIL ON EDUCATION OF THE NATIONAL CHIROPRACTIC ASSOCIATION, Gunter Hotel, February 11-12-13, 1954 , San Antonio, Texas

The semi-annual meeting of the National Council on Education of the NCA was held in San Antonio, Texas, at the Gunter Hotel, February 11, 12, and 13, 1954. Dr. Thure C. Peterson, Chairman of the Council, presided at all of the meetings. Those attending:
A. Members of the Accrediting Committee:
   Dr. John J. Nugent, Director of Education of the National Chiropractic Association, 92 Norton Street, New Haven, Connecticut.
   Dr. Walter B. Wolf, President of the Accrediting Committee, Eureka, South Dakota.
   Dr. Norman E. Osborne, Secretary of the Accrediting Committee, 1172 The Terrace, Hagerstown, Maryland
   Dr. Ralph J. Martin, 28 W. Sierra Madre Blvd., Sierra Madre, California.
   Dr. Edward E. Gardner, 1655 N. Normandie Avenue, Hollywood 27, California
B. Representatives of the accredited educational institutions and those institutions subscribing to the program of the Council.
   Dr. Thure C. Peterson, Chairman of the Council and President, Chiropractic Institute of New York, 1252 W. 42nd Street, New York 18, New York
   Dr. Joseph Janse, Secretary of the Council, and President, National College of Chiropractic, 20 N. Ashland Blvd., Chicago 7, Illinois.
   Dr. W.A. Budden, Director, Western States College of Chiropractic, 4525 Southeast 63rd Street, Portland 6, Oregon.
   Dr. Arthur G. Hendricks, Treasurer, Lincoln Chiropractic College, Inc., 633 N. Pennsylvania Avenue, Indianapolis, Indiana.
   Dr. Julius C. Troilo, Dean, Texas Chiropractic College, San Pedro Park, San Antonio, Texas.
   Dr. George Haynes, Dean, Los Angeles College of Chiropractic, 920 East Broadway, Glendale 5, California.
   Dr. Earl Homewood, Dean, Canadian Memorial College of Chiropractic, 252 Bloor Street, West, Toronto 5, Ontario, Canada.

Dr. Bera A. Smith, President, Carver Chiropractic College, 521 N.W. 9th Street, Oklahoma City 3, Oklahoma.
C.   Special guest and officials of the NCA
Dr. L.M. Rogers, Executive Secretary of the National Chiropractic Association, Webster City, Iowa.
Mr. Robert Johns, Legal Counsel of the National Chiropractic Association, La Crosse, Wisconsin.
Dr. Hugh Warren, President of the Alumni Association of the Texas Chiropractic College.
Dr. H.E. Turley, Head of Department of Neurology of the Texas Chiropractic College
Dr. Wm. D. Harper, Jr., Head of Department of Pathology of the Texas Chiropractic College.

First meeting, morning of February 11, 1954, beginning at 9:00 A.M.

Dr. Peterson read letters of greetings from Drs. S.W. Cole, Dean of the Kansas State Chiropractic College, John B. Wolfe, President of the Northwestern College of Chiropractic and H.C. Harring, President of the Missouri Chiropractic College. These men were unable to be in attendance.

Dr. Peterson also read a letter from Dr. J.N. Firth, President of the Lincoln Chiropractic College, Inc. Sincerest greetings were conveyed to the Council. Dr. Firth also drew the Council's attention to the fact that in the instance of a student with pre-professional college background and receiving credit for several courses in physiology, the V.A. deducted a prorated amount from the G.I.'s subsistence as well as the college's billing. When the student offered to take the courses over in order to obtain a full subsistence, the V.A. denied him the privilege.

The whole matter was referred to because several of the state boards had insisted that no advanced standing or credit be given for college courses that paralleled those in the course at a chiropractic college.

Dr. Peterson then read a letter received from a Mr. Russell W. Gibbons, a student at Northern Ohio University and who had been interested in chiropractic as a career. The letter, well written and presented in content, drew attention to the competitive literature of advertising that some of the accredited colleges are employing in the effort of student procurement.

Dr. Nugent, as well as members of the Accrediting Committee, expressed the opinion that all competitive claims of the various colleges should be deleted from the catalogs and literature prepared by them.

Mr. Gibbons also drew attention to the lack of standard format of the catalogs issued by the various colleges, stating that such unconformity simply led to faulty impressions and lack of respect by investigating lay people.

Mr. Gibbons also asked why it was that a goodly number of the non-accredited colleges were listed in the College Blue Book and why several of the accredited colleges were not listed? Dr. Nugent promised to look into the matter.

At this point the matter of two years of pre-professional college requirement was brought into discussion and following are the pertinent points of reference.

1.   All students who contemplate matriculating at any one of the accredited colleges and come from states demanding one or two years of pre-professional college training, yet who do not possess the same, must not be permitted to matriculate until the pre-professional education is obtained.

2.   Dr. Nugent stated that the accredited colleges that as yet had not instituted the two year pre-professional requirement were conducting a delaying action and he personally felt that they should come to a definite conclusion of instituting this requirement setting as early a deadline as possible.

3.   Dr. Nugent also emphasized the possibility of the accredited colleges establishing contact with undergraduate colleges in the city of domicile with the intent of having the students take a goodly number of their pre-clinical subjects at these colleges. The affiliation between the San Antonio Junior College and the Texas Chiropractic College was cited as an example.

4.   Both Drs. Peterson and Janse expressed the opinion that in the instance of the respective colleges they represented this would not be desirable or practical.

5.   Dr. Budden insisted that all of the accredited colleges should institute the two years of pre-professional requirements by this coming September enrollment, insisting that they should make a direct clean cut decision.

6.   Dr. Haynes of the Los Angeles College of Chiropractic was asked how the program was working out at the college. He stated that it had cut down the enrollment quite noticeably and it had represented a definite economic compromise. However, that ever since the pre-professional requirement was instituted every subsequent enrollment had progressively increased, and as a result they of the Los Angeles College were hopeful that the severity of the situation had passed.

7.   Dr. Janse asked Dr. Haynes to interpret their policy with reference to transfer students without pre-professional college background. Dr. Haynes answered by stating that the time of the student's original matriculation was compared with the date when the L.A. College instituted the program and if his matriculation had preceded this deadline he was eligible for continuing his education at the L.A. College.

8.   Dr. Homewood advised the Council that at the Canadian Memorial College they were planning an extra year of education, e.g., a course of five years rather than four. Thus permitting added income and at the same time more or less paralleling the two years pre-professional college requirement program which seems to be setting a precedent in the States.

9.   Dr. Budden made a motion, namely that the Council re-endorse the recommendation of two years of pre-professional requirement and that all of the accredited colleges not having instituted this program begin making definite preparations to institute such

a program.
10. Dr. Hendricks stated that he thought the two year program was a little premature and that if caution and care were not exercised it might serve to compromise the economy of all of the colleges and hence he was against the motion.
11. Dr. Wolfe stated that he could not see any possible harm in the motion because it did not contain any specific stipulations and was but a simple reiteration of the conclusions reached at the last two sessions of the Council.
12. Dr. Janse insisted that the motion was unnecessary because all of the colleges were well aware of the ever increasing tendency of the various states to introduce the requirement and hence the colleges would automatically have to devise mechanisms of adaptation.
13. Dr. Peterson advised the Council that both the States of Wisconsin and North Carolina were contemplating the move. He read a letter he had written the President of the North Carolina State Chiropractic Society in answer to his inquiry as to what the school men's opinion was in relation to this matter. Following being a reprint of Dr. Peterson's answer.

January 27, 1954; Dr. L.G. Harrison; 614 North Main Street; High Point, North Carolina
Dear Dr. Harrison:
Replying to your letter of January 25th relating to the inclusion of two years of pre-professional studies for chiropractic qualifications, may I state that it is our opinion that such requirement is an excellent one, provided it is not instituted with undue haste. May I make the following recommendations, based upon our experience.
1. That the requirement not be circumscribed as to content, so that a student may take the two years in Liberal Arts or Science as he sees fit.
2. That the effective date of the legislation be four to five years from the date of enactment to permit students in school to qualify without retroactive effect.
3. That in the beginning, it not be mandatory that the work be all completed prior to entrance into chiropractic school, so that a student who may lack a few credits will have some leeway to complete these credits, even after he has started his chiropractic studies.
Until such time as the great majority of states institute the two-year pre-chiropractic requirement, the Chiropractic Institute of New York will not institute it as an absolute requirement, but, of course, will require it from those students who intend to qualify in states that have already, or proposed to institute this requirement.
I hope the above gives you the information you desire. At the next meeting of the National Council on Education, which takes place in February, this matter will again come up for discussion and if there is any change, I shall write you again at that time. Very truly yours, Thure C. Peterson, President

14. Dr. Budden withdrew his motion and the matter was set aside for further discussion during some subsequent meeting.
The meeting was adjourned at 12 p.m.

Second meeting of the Council, held in the afternoon of Thursday, February 11, 1954.
This was a closed meeting. Only members of the accrediting committee and the immediate representatives of the accredited colleges were permitted to attend, with Dr. L.M. Rogers and Attorney Robert Johns having received special invitations to attend as representing the executive board of the National Chiropractic Association.
Dr. William N. Coggins, Dean of the Logan Basic College of Chiropractic and Mr. Robert Evans, Legal Counsel for the Logan College, were in attendance and were the official representatives of the college.
This special closed meeting had been set at the written request of Dr. Logan for a "hearing" before the Council in relation to its decision to remove the Logan Basic College of Chiropractic from the accredited list.
Dr. Coggins and Mr. Evans advised the Council that Dr. Logan could not be in attendance because of the serious illness of one of his children.
Mr. Evans advised the Council that he thought that it was making a serious mistake in removing the Logan College from the accredited list. He insisted that it would further the breach between the primary factions in chiropractic and that the Council should not judge the merits of a college by the personal attitudes one of its administrative officers might have toward the Council and the NCA.
Both Mr. Evans and Dr. Coggins insisted that they in no way spoke for Dr. Logan as far as the latter's attitude and conduct were concerned. That it was unwise to take accreditation from the Logan College on the basis of the incompatibility of Dr. Logan's attitude and conduct.
Mr. Evans further stated that the whole difficulty had arisen out of the physiotherapy issue in Missouri and because the Logan College had not supported Dr. Nugent's efforts in this direction it had come to stand in disfavor. According to Mr. Evans, the Logan College had never attempted to influence legislative efforts anywhere; furthermore, that its faculty and employees had always been permitted to free agency maintaining those professional affiliations and interpretations they considered to be correct.
It should be noted here that the entire membership of the Council wondered why Mr. Evans even made either of these points a matter of concern or emphasis, as certainly neither had come into any consideration as far as reasons for the disaccreditation was concerned.

Mr. Evans further contended that disaccreditation would be damaging to the college and would constitute a basis of slander and libel and an infringement of Sherman anti-trust act. Here again the entire Council as well as Mr. Johns the Counsel for the NCA, questioned the premise of this contention.

Mr. Evans recognized the fact that the accrediting program of the NCA had received much approval and recognition in certain quarters of the profession as well as the government and hence disaccreditation of the Logan College would redound in great detriment to the college. He referred to the refusal of the Idaho Board of Chiropractic Examiners to accept recent Logan graduates for examination.

According to Mr. Evans, accreditation should be estimated on standards of education and physical facilities rather than upon the policies and attitudes of the administration. Again the Council expressed their disagreement.

Mr. Evans asked the question, "Why should the dissenter of an association be asked to resign?" He continued by stating that throughout the profession we should change the attitude of maligning and desist from vindictive conducts or else we would destroy ourselves. The entire Council agreed to this premise and asked whether the administration of the Logan College would commit itself to such a premise.

Mr. Evans then asked for the permission of reading a "brief". Following is a duplication of the same:

Dr. Logan has asked us to convey to you his regrets in his inability to be here today. I know he would like to be with you and discuss the question now before us, but certain imperative demands on his time prevented his attendance. Logan Basic College of Chiropractic is therefore represented in this matter by Dr. William N. Coggins, Dean of the school, and by myself as its counsel.

We are here as a result of the action of the Accrediting Committee of the Educational Council, first suggesting that Logan College withdraw from the Council because it considered it incompatible with the policies of the NCA; and upon the failure of the College to so resign, the Accrediting Committee then recommended that Logan College be removed from the list of accredited schools and colleges because of this so-called "incompatibility" between the college and the policies of the NCA. The school has appealed this matter to the Council and we are present today on this invitation of Dr. Peterson, Chairman of the Council. Our purpose in appearing here is to ask you to reject this recommendation as we believe it is a mistake that would be damaging to all, not just to the college, but the chiropractic and to this Association itself.

While the letter from the Accrediting Committee did not disclose just what constituted the incompatibility, we all know that the basis of the matter is the physiotherapy question, and perhaps what precipitated the action was the failure of the Missouri Legislature last spring to enact legislation which included physiotherapy in the definition of chiropractic.

While this legislation was opposed by Dr. Logan and Dr. Coggins and other chiropractors, all of which was perhaps the catalyst for the action of the Accrediting Committee — I want to point out, and very particularly so, Logan Basic College of Chiropractic does not engage in legislature activities — has not and will not take any position with respect to any legislation. Moreover, the College and its Board of Trustees have not, nor will they attempt to dictate to the College employees what their position should be on any subject — physiotherapy or otherwise. Academic freedom demands no less, and as citizens of the country they are guaranteed that right.

Having made myself as clear as I know how on this, I want to pass on to another matter, but in passing, I might say that it should be obvious that incompatibility is a rather impossible charge to be leveled against the college, and while it might be charged against others, it would be rather an anomaly to attempt to punish or damage the college because of its president or other employee exercised their constitutional and academic right of free speech.

But to return to the question of damage, it goes without saying that the disaccreditation of any institution of learning by any accrediting body is damaging to the institution. In law, it is a form of slander and libel. Indeed, Logan College has already felt the first twinge of such injury. Through possibly a misadvertancy, the disaccreditation of Logan College, as if it were then already an accomplished fact, was communicated to one of the State Chiropractic Boards, who denied one of our students the right to take the State Board Examination. While this matter has not as yet been completely ironed out, I will say that your Chairman, when we called the matter to his attention, took prompt action to advise that Board that such was not a fact.

While this example is but one small instance, it is a clear indication that disaccreditation would cost any college many thousands of dollars of damage. There is no question but that the College would be hurt by such action, and while Logan Basic College is one of the larger colleges and relatively of considerable financial means as chiropractic colleges go, this fact would not ameliorate the damage, but would undoubtedly increase it.

It is easy to comprehend the injury done the college, by such action, but what of the injury to this Association and to Chiropractic itself?

The NCA has for some time been recognized by many as a qualified accrediting agency and your accreditation has been accepted in many quarters. I am sure that such recognition and acceptance is, and can be, based only on the fact that your accreditation has heretofore been based solely on academic standards and not on questions of policy. These standards used to judge chiropractic colleges have been accepted not only by Chiropractic Boards, but more important by State Departments of Education. This latter is much more important as the general well-being of chiropractic and its acceptance is in a great measure dependent on the recognition of its educational standards, not by Chiropractic Boards, but by the general educational department of the State, and for that matter, the Federal Government.

In this connection, it is important to remember that the forward progress of chiropractic and its increasing recognition requires the approval of schools of chiropractic by the United States Department of Education to a much fuller degree than has heretofore obtained. Because of this greater opportunity for chiropractic service in or through instrumentalities of the Federal Government, Federal acceptance of State accreditation of chiropractic colleges no longer suffices so that the United States Department of Education is approving its own accrediting agencies. I am informed that the NCA has applied for approval as such an approved accrediting agency.

I am informed also that for the determination as to whether or not you are a qualified accrediting agency, it was necessary for you to supply the basis of your accreditation. And I am sure that you supplied the U.S. Department of Education a full statement of the academic standards used by you.

I hardly think that you also stated in your application that your accreditation was also based on whether or not the school being tested, or its officers, were compatible with the policies of your association — or that you might not grant, or might disaccredit a school who, though meeting the highest academic standards, was incompatible with the policies of the association.

Had you done so, there is little question but that you would not be acceptable as a qualified accrediting agency.

That this would hurt the association is obvious, but the injury to chiropractic goes much further. The disapproval of the Association's accrediting function by the U.S. Department of Education would hurt all chiropractic schools now accredited by you. It would cast doubt on whether the accreditation was based on academic standards or merely on adherence to association policy. It might lend credence to some of the claims of the enemies of chiropractic. In any event, it would supply ammunition for their attacks on chiropractic. The increasing acceptance of chiropractic by Federal agencies and by the general public would indeed receive a setback were this difference between us to be followed to its logical conclusion.

Let us consider for a moment the accreditation of Logan Basic College of Chiropractic. It has been accredited by every accrediting agency who has examined it. Besides the NCA, it has been examined and approved by the Missouri Department of Education, the ICA, the North American Association of Chiropractic Colleges, the Veterans Administration, the State Departments of Education of the several states who make their own examinations, and it has also been accredited by the remaining states whose accreditation is based on the examination by others.

What about its physical plant? It has a campus covering 17 acres, a new clinic, x-ray and administration building as finely equipped as is possible. It has a laboratory and physics building, classrooms buildings, library, dormitories and other auxiliary buildings, in all a total of 22 buildings, all modernly equipped.

It has a faculty who are all graduate chiropractors, several of whom have other degrees, and of the rest, all of them are presently enrolled in their spare time in a local liberal arts college and working towards their B.S. degrees. This latter fact has received much approbation from educators and heads of state departments of education.

Last but not least, the college's academic standards. Logan College was the first to teach a four-year chiropractic course exclusively. For that matter, since its inception it has been a four-year chiropractic college. The subjects and hours of instruction meet the standards set up by this and every other accrediting agency. It is believed that Logan Basic College of Chiropractic would stand high in any impartial test or rating of all of the chiropractic colleges.

Should it then be disaccredited on a question of compatibility rather than on the basis of its academic merit? — Particularly so without any examination or testing against academic standards. The question, of course, answers itself.

That brings me to another matter, and that is: Why should the dissenters or members who may not concur in the policies of the Association resign or be forced from membership in the Association? I can find no parallel to such a situation in any modern American Institution. Our system requires that dissenters and minorities, as well as majorities, have the right to speak their thoughts and to disagree without fear of retaliation. Are differences between chiropractors in some way different than differences between lawyers, MDs or other professional men?

The very fact that differences between chiropractors at times engender such extreme heat, would seem to indicate that chiropractic has not yet reached the stage of maturity we all claim for it. When we can only compose our differences by what practically amounts to internecine warfare, we can hardly expect any great segment of the public to rally to our cause. I am not trying to point the finger of blame at anyone. All of us are at fault. But certainly it is time that we changed our method of approach and sought a more reasonable method for the determination of our differences than by the attempt to destroy one another.

If we look back at the history of chiropractic for the last 30 years in a detached manner, we see a rather obvious picture of the old conformity fight that has plagued nearly every religion, every government, every profession and many associations such as this. The conformity fight in England founded the Episcopal church, drove the Puritans to this country, and they in turn became as bad. You all recall how the non-conformists in the early days of our history were burned at the stake. Religion and religious leaders have since matured and the various denomination, churches and religions, all worship the same God in their own manner to the betterment of all.

With respect to governments, it is a queer thing, but if you look at it you will find that the attempt to enforce conformity occurs generally when the governments are young or when they are on their last legs. Russia is one example. The extreme brutality of the Czarist government in punishing non-conformists in its last years of existence compared with the same brutality of the communists today. The history of Spain and its fight on the non-conformist, known as the Inquisition, in the fading years of Spain's international leadership, and Franco's extreme brutality in attempting to force conformity today.

In our own early history and the beginning of our government, the extreme bitterness engendered in the attempts of the Whigs and the Tories to make the others conform to the ideas each held resulted in bloodshed and extreme measures, including the Sedition laws used by the Party in power to jail the non-conformists, is all recalled. Maturity, however, soon overcame these extremes and our country prospered and today, while we may have our arguments on politics and policy, we do not try to destroy each other.

I hope that chiropractic has reached that maturity and that we can compose our differences in a manner beneficial to all.

I would like at this point to try to analyze this incompatibility which apparently lies between us. Now of course, it all stems back to the old straight vs. mixer fight, but I want to discuss only the Missouri phase of the situation. At the last session of the Missouri legislature, several bills were introduced which affected chiropractic in one way or another. One bill increased the educational requirements from three to four years. All chiropractors supported this bill. Then there was a bill which would have included physiotherapy in the definition of chiropractic. There was some other proposed legislation, not important here, and there was also the threat of a basic science bill. The four year education bill, though supported by practically all chiropractors and not opposed by the medical lobby, failed because it was held up by the fight over the physiotherapy bill.

The physiotherapy bill had an unfortunate start in that letters were written asking for a $20,000 fund to support the bill, and intimating that the Governor would sign it. The Governor was incensed and the newspapers and some legislators described the $20,000 fund as a slush fund. This bill had been proposed by a Missouri physiotherapy group and it was opposed by the Missouri State Chiropractic Association, the Medical and Osteopathic lobbies. Unfortunately again, the first bill proposed, because of some flaws, was replaced by a second and very different bill. It defined chiropractic as including physiotherapy and defined physiotherapy so broadly that during the course of the hearing the Senator offering it, found it necessary to amend the definition. Dr. Coggins and other members of the State Association spoke in opposition to it. Dr. Nugent was one of the speakers for the bill, and he gave an excellent and informative talk.

The bill failed — in fact it really had very little, if any, chance because of the bad publicity — the necessity of changing bills in midstream, and then the damage that was done when the sponsoring senator had to withdraw the bill and delete certain parts of it which apparently permitted surgery by electricity. Of course, the fact that the chiropractic profession was not united behind the bill left it little chance of passage in the face of united medical and osteopathic forces. That in brief is the history of the matter.

While I realize that personalities and feelings from away back have perhaps clouded the matter, I believe, however, that we should push past animosities aside and forget them if we can — they are prejudices doing no one any good. Chiropractors who have felt the unreasoned prejudices from medical men for so long should be the first to recognize the danger of letting our prejudices guide us.

Dr. Nugent, Educational Director of the NCA, and Dr. Logan, were on opposite sides in this matter, and in a sense might be said to have been incompatible — that is, in disagreement with each other. But that is hardly a reason to disaccredit a school of which Dr. Logan is an officer. The NCA may believe that physiotherapy is a very valuable adjunct in connection with chiropractic, while Dr. Logan and others may believe that straight chiropractic is to be preferred. And there may be other areas of disagreement about manners and methods, but in the last analysis, you are all chiropractors and working for the advancement of chiropractic, so though you may differ in many things, in truth you have but a single goal; that is, the advancement and improvement of chiropractic and chiropractors for the benefit and improved care of the sick and the prevention of illness through the precepts of chiropractic. So, if I may, on my own account, I would offer a suggestion that the two sides of this difference see if it isn't possible for you to work together instead of trying to force the other to conform to your own ideas.

It isn't a very new approach, but I don't believe you have ever tried it. There is a very good possibility that it might work for the benefit of all.

For example, let us examine the proposal in the light of the physiotherapy question. Last year when the attempt was made to pass a physiotherapy law, the proponents prepared the bill and offered it to the rest of the State Chiropractic Association on a "take-it-or-leave-it" basis. The Association and a majority of its members left it and opposed it. In fact, the bill was so defective that the proponents had to leave it and prepare a new bill which, because of the shortness of time, was hastily prepared and as a result faulty in some respects. This bill also was offered on a take-it-or-leave-it basis with similar results. Now, I will say that when Dr. Nugent came to Missouri he was met with the problem of having to support this bill as it was, so it was on a take-it-or-leave-it basis for him also.

Now, suppose that instead of this take-it-or-leave-it approach, those who felt they needed protection in connection with their use of physiotherapy as a part or adjunct of their practice, had gone to those who did not, and said, "We want a bill. Let us see if we can work one out that is acceptable to both sides." It is entirely possible that a common ground could be found. At that same session of the legislature I handled a bill for the licensing of practical nurses, who for years have fought and been fought by the registered nurses. We did just exactly what I propose here, and as a result we today have a licensing bill obtained at that session of the legislature.

It seems to me as a lawyer with some experience in legislature matters that the crux of the trouble is the attempt on one side to include physiotherapy in the statutory definition of chiropractic, while the attempt on the other side is to try and hold to a statutory definition that is too restrictive. Actually, both your positions are too restrictive, and I believe you are both wrong. You are both attempting to encompass in the definition of the science of chiropractic what you can and cannot do in the practice of chiropractic, which from the angle of statutory draftsmanship, is an impossibility unless your definition is to be so long as to be meaningless.

To me a proper chiropractic act would define the science of chiropractic in as simple language as was possible, and would then define the practice of chiropractic as following that science. As an example, and only as an example, it could run something like this: "The system, method and science of treating disease and abnormalities of the human body known as chiropractic and which teaches that disease and abnormalities of the human body occur because of impingement of the spinal nerves and generally resulting from displacement of the vertebrae."

The practice of chiropractic, then, might be defined somewhat like this: "The practice of chiropractic is the use of the chiropractic art for the purpose of removing nerve pressure in the treatment of disease and abnormalities of the human body as is taught in chiropractic schools and colleges. The practice of chiropractic is hereby declared not to be the practice of medicine, surgery and osteopathy."

I want to make clear that this is but a mere suggestion to indicate that generality of the defining language is to be preferred and is not an attempt on my part to write a satisfactory definition.

Under such a type of definition it is clear that the straight chiropractors could practice purely by adjustments, while the physiotherapist could use what adjuncts he cared to use to aid him in his adjustments as he was taught by his school of chiropractic. There might still be arguments as to which method was superior, but there would be no reason for two groups of chiropractors to be at each other's throats and everyone would be secure in his right to practice chiropractic in his own school method.

In this connection, I want to tell you how the medical and osteopathy statutes in Missouri take care of this matter.

Medicine is not defined. The statute merely uses the term "the practice of medicine." The statute merely provides that anyone practicing medicine must be licensed. There are no limitations whatsoever. Not a bad idea, is it?

Osteopathy, which was born in Missouri, is defined as "that system, method or science of treating disease of the human body known as osteopathy and as taught and practiced by the American School of Osteopathy of Kirksville, Missouri." How simple and for that matter, expedient. When the practice of osteopathy had grown to where it was felt necessary to include drugs and surgery, the teaching at the American School of Osteopathy was enlarged to encompass those things, and they thus became the practice of osteopathy.

Neither of these healing professions have attempted to proscribe themselves as chiropractic has done and as it is apparently still trying to do. You see, when you try to define the science or its practice too exactly, you effectively proscribe growth and progress.

The only point I try to make here is that perhaps by being more general it will be much easier for both sides to agree and for both sides to obtain to a reasonable degree what each seeks.

Now, if you prefer not to try and handle your problems in the manner that the other healing arts have handled it, and although in the long run I am firmly convinced that it is by far the wisest course, there still may be other methods where by consulting each other you might find common grounds. For example, perhaps a law permitting the use of physiotherapy but not defining it as chiropractic might be worked out acceptable to all chiropractors whether they use and believe in physiotherapy or not.

In any event, gentlemen, some approach other than the one chiropractic has been following is worth trying, and to my mind it is necessary.

Just one more thing — in such a new approach, it is not only important but absolutely essential that both sides attempt it with an open mind and with the idea of trying to work something out beneficial for chiropractic, and not to get concessions or promises as to action out of the other.

To me as a layman, chiropractic is such a wonderful thing, I can't begin to tell you what it has done for me, and I want it to continue to grow and to prosper so that we will always have the benefits of chiropractic and not just a few of its attainments under the guise of physical medicine.

I want to thank you for your very gracious attention to this somewhat lengthy discourse, and trust and hope that some good for all of us will result, and particularly for chiropractic.

Upon the completion of the reading of the brief Dr. Peterson, chairman of the Council, advised Mr. Evans that the claim that physiotherapy and the issue of "straight" versus "mixer" was the basis for disaccreditation was an evasion of the real issue and had never constituted a matter of discussion.

Dr. Walter B. Wolf, President of the Accrediting Committee, was asked to review the reasons why the committee had recommended to the Council that the Logan College be removed from the accredited list and following are Dr. Wolf's references:

(1) Upon making a visit to the Logan Basic College of Chiropractic with the intent of making an inspection Dr. John J. Nugent, Director of Education was denied the privilege of making the inspection.

(2) Dr. Logan personally had violated the rules and resolutions of the Council, adopted without objection while a representative of the Logan Basic College of Chiropractic was present, particularly a resolution prohibiting any member of the Council from participating in any other accrediting organization, particularly referred to being the North American Association of Chiropractic Schools and Colleges. Direct reference was made to the contents of the Council minutes of the mid-year meeting held in Chicago, February 1, 2 and 3, 1950, and at which Dr. Wm. H. Coggins, and Rev. G. Hussar representing the Logan College were present.

The following quotes from pages 8 and 9 were read: "Be it resolved that the Council on Education of the National Chiropractic Association be recognized as the sole accrediting agency for the chiropractic profession and that any school accepting a rating from any other alleged Chiropractic Council or Committee will automatically lose its approved membership in the Educational Council of the National Chiropractic Association."

Dr. Nugent emphasized the significance of the proposed resolution as submitted by the accrediting committee with reference to recognizing but one accrediting agency, namely the NCA Council on Education and punishing any provisionally or fully accredited college with disfellowship if the administration of this college proceeded to seek recognition by any other alleged chiropractic accrediting agency."

(3) That Dr. Logan had continued to practice separatism amongst his followers and had spoken against the policies and program of the NCA.

(4) That Dr. Logan had consistently avoided attending the meetings of the Council, notwithstanding constantly being encouraged to attend.

At this point Dr. Nugent, Director of Education, asked for the privilege of advising Mr. Evans on a number of points in relation to the issue which possibly Mr. Evans had not been alerted on.

(1) Dr. Logan in public and private has disparaged and belittled the NCA, its program and the efforts of the Council.

(2) That on various occasions maligning comments and falsifications had been indulged in to belittle and hamstring the efforts of the Director of Education and the Accrediting Committee.

(3) That Dr. Logan, knowingly and with intent had aligned himself with anti-NCA forces in various states to hinder legislative programs that would maintain or raise the professional standards.

(4) That the issue of "physiotherapy" injected into the brief as the primary issue of contention was but a "smoke screen" to cover the real facts of the issue, namely Dr. Logan's frank disinclination to make himself a part of the Council.

(5) That Dr. Logan had permitted his name to be placed on the membership committee of the International Chiropractic Association, and that he had always found time for the activities of this organization but certainly not for that of the Council.

(6) That at the beginning when accreditation of the Logan College was first considered Dr. Logan in telegram had committed himself to the policies of the Council and its program.

(7) That Dr. Logan had attempted to control the politics of state associations with detrimental effect to the NCA and its program in those respective states.

Dr. Budden advised Mr. Evans that from the beginning it had been a question whether Dr. Logan would lend himself to the policies of the Council. Now it was quite evident that he had not and did apparently have no intentions to do so.

Dr. Budden then asked the question of the Accrediting Committee if the Council conclusively decided to persist in its decision of the Los Angeles meetings whether the administration of the Logan College would have the privilege if they desired to re-apply for accreditation?

Dr. Wolf, as president of the committee, stated that such would be the privilege of the Logan College and the Accrediting Committee would then proceed to inspect the college and make its recommendations to the Council.

Dr. Coggins and Mr. Evans then excused themselves. They were advised that Dr. Logan, as President of the College, would be advised within a few days as to the final conclusion of the Council.

In subsequent discussions it was concluded that Mr. Evans as a person was a very fine and worthy gentleman but that he evidently had not been fully advised by his client as to the exact nature of the case and the reasons behind the same. Hence both his brief and verbal efforts were outside the point of the real issue.

All members of the Council expressed their disappointment in Dr. Logan for not appearing himself because certainly he must have known that the issue of his personal activities represented the primary reason for removing the Logan College from the accredited list.

Drs. Peterson and Janse were instructed to send a letter to Dr. Logan and advise him of the decision of the Council to sustain its previous decision to remove the college from the accredited list.

(The consequent letter to Dr. Logan in copy has been appended to these minutes.)

Meeting of the evening of February 11, 1954

Dr. Nugent was asked to bring the Council up to date on the progress of his efforts in Washington to get the accrediting program of the NCA established as the official accrediting agency for the Chiropractic Profession by the Federal Department of Education.

Following were the primary comments of Dr. Nugent:

1. In 1953 the Council authorized him, Dr. Nugent, to go to Washington for the purpose of submitting an application for accreditation by the Federal Department of Education.

2. Upon initiating his efforts he found a rather severe state of confusion in the Department of Education because of the advent of the new Eisenhower administration. However, he did establish contact with a Mr. Armstrong who was very friendly and cooperative. At that time Mr. Armstrong requested a brief on all of the accredited colleges. He, Dr. Nugent, hesitated in giving him the same because he felt that the majority of the colleges were still too weak in their over all picture to make a substantial impression and hence he rather hesitated to precipitate action and delayed further efforts until after the Los Angeles convention when once again he was instructed by the Council to proceed.

3. In the meantime the whole picture had become badly clouded because of two visits to Washington by Dr. Norcross of Los Angeles first in behalf of the Los Angeles College and at the insistence of the California Chiropractic Association and later in behalf of the "Specialty Societies." Furthermore, Mr. Evans the Counsel for the Logan College had also appeared before Mr. Armstrong possibly in behalf of the North American Association of Chiropractic Colleges and Schools. Direct representatives of the International Chiropractors Association had also made inquiries and submitted application. Consequently the Washington officials became quite dubious and simply asked why it was that so many different elements of the chiropractic profession sought to assert itself as the dominating and authoritative body.

4. To further complicate the matter the government decided to discontinue the accrediting program of its Department of Education maintaining that such should be done by a private academic agency of national scope. Consequently the entire original effort had to be set aside and a new program decided upon.

5. That from now on the approach would have to be made to the National Commission on Accrediting, with Chancellor R.G. Gustavson of the University of Nebraska as the Chairman.

6. It is evident that the Commission under Dr. Gustavson would be much more critical of the facilities of the chiropractic colleges.

This Dr. Nugent had already found out by the interrogation he had experienced at the hands of Mr. Goldthorpe of the Federal Department of Education and who had taken over the responsibilities of Mr. Armstrong.

7. If such application were rejected would it compromise the Council position and influence and might it in any way alter the readiness of the V.A. to approve the chiropractic colleges for G.I. training?

Following were the subsequent discussions and final conclusion of the Council in relation to this important issue:

1. Dr. Budden expressed the opinion that the Council should proceed carefully as any hasty application for accreditation and possible resultant refusal might jeopardize our position with the V.A.

2. Dr. Hendricks was of similar position and contended that any loss of V.A. recognition would mark the demise of some of the accredited colleges.

3. Dr. Peterson felt that care must be exercised but that the entire effort should not be scuttled, and that the program should be kept alive.

4. Finally a motion was passed as follows: Dr. Nugent was instructed to investigate whether the continuance of the Council's application for accreditation by the National Commission on Accrediting would in any way compromise the colleges' present relations with the V.A. Furthermore, whether accreditation by the Commission would result in a listing of the chiropractic colleges as institutions of higher learning with the V.A. and this privilege them to an increase of benefit and privilege or whether it would result in the individual chiropractic colleges losing their status with the V.A. Upon obtaining this information Dr. Nugent was to report to the Council.

5. The motion also included the instruction that if the findings of Dr. Nugent assured the possibility of having the chiropractic colleges listed as institutions of higher learning and yet if the rejection of this application would not compromise the present relations with the V.A. he was to proceed with the program already initiated. If, on the other hand, a continuation of the application for recognition as accredited institutions by the newly appointed National Commission on Accrediting would in any way jeopardize the present relations with the V.A. no further action should be taken until the next meeting.

6. It was also concluded that this whole program should be kept confidential so that no undue gossip or ill-conditioned propaganda material might result from it.

Dr. Janse recommended that the Council extend an invitation to the National Council of Chiropractic Examining Boards to attend one of the sessions of the Council during its meetings in conjunction with the annual convention of the National Chiropractic Association, to be held next July in St. Louis. This recommendation was unanimously passed and Dr. Peterson as Chairman of the Council directed a letter to Dr. Adam Baer the Chairman of the Council on Examining Boards to this effect.

Dr. Nugent reminded the Council that the final purpose of the accrediting program of the NCA was to persuade the Boards of Chiropractic Examiners to fully recognize this program as the official accreditation mechanism for the chiropractic profession

Dr. Peterson made inquiry of Dr. Nugent whether he still wanted the colleges to fill out his prepared "School Survey"? Dr. Peterson felt that probably it was rather unwise to have the colleges sit in decision on their own facilities.

Dr. Nugent persisted in his request that the survey be filled out as soon as possible.

It was the consensus of the Council members that Dr. Nugent should visit and inspect every one of the accredited colleges at least once a year and Dr. Nugent committed himself to this assignment.

Dr. Nugent advised the Council that he would like to repeat the decision in Los Angeles to have a new listing for the colleges, namely those that are accredited and those that subscribe to the program of the NCA but are not accredited.

A discussion ensued as to whether the "subscribing colleges" should be listed on the NCA Journal spread listing the colleges. Dr. Nugent felt that they should not unless the qualified statement "those colleges as yet not fully accredited but subscribing" head that particular portion of the listing.

Dr. Bera Smith, a representative of the subscribing colleges, was asked about this matter and he stated that possibly such a listing would probably be satisfactory to the Board of Directors of the college he represented. He felt that the line of differentiating should not be too severe, otherwise it might be looked upon as mitigating and alienate the subscribing colleges rather than gain their efforts of cooperation.

On Friday morning all the members of the Council were taken out to the San Antonio Junior College and the Texas Chiropractic College.

As is understood the Texas Chiropractic College, under the auspices of the dean, Dr. Julius C. Troilo, has established a very agreeable and advantageous connection with the administration of the San Antonio College. The students of the Texas Chiropractic College take much of their basic science work at the San Antonio Junior College concurrent with their training at the Texas College and thus simultaneously qualify for their basic science certificate.

Mr. Loftin and Dr. Brown, the president and dean of the San Antonio College, respectively, were most considerate in their readiness to show the splendid facilities of their institution. It was the consensus of opinion of the Council membership that the Texas Chiropractic College was most fortunate in being able to experience this connection.

The Council then inspected the Texas Chiropractic College proper and had the opportunity of attending a general assembly of the student body at which Dr. Troilo asked every Council member as well as Dr. Rogers to speak briefly to the students.

It was evident that a commendable and diligent effort was being expended at the college and the Council was unanimous in its attitude of respect and admiration for the accomplishments of the college administration.

At the noon hour Drs. Nugent and Troilo appeared on television and made a most commendable presentation of the functions of the Council and the educational standards of the accredited college.

Friday afternoon meeting, February 12, 1954

The issue of the recommended two years of pre-professional college education as entrance requirement to the accredited colleges was again brought under consideration and following were the primary points of discussion.

1. Dr. Nugent stated that it was inevitable that the program would have to be instituted sooner or later and recommended that those colleges who as yet had not committed themselves proceed to make all necessary preparations to set a deadline.
2. Both Drs. Hendricks and Janse insisted that any decision to set a deadline would be premature and might represent a compromise from which some of the colleges would not be able to recuperate.
3. Dr. Wolf stated that in his opinion the idea of two years of pre-professional college requirement would continue to be instituted by the various states and that within a short time it would be more or less national.
4. Dr. Nugent recommended that the various colleges investigate the possibility of establishing contact with some adjoining state or city college with the purpose of having certain of the classes and laboratory courses in the basic sciences taught to the chiropractic matriculants at these colleges rather than at the chiropractic college, asserting that this would cut down on expenses and overhead and also permit the student to probably enjoy the privileges of better laboratory facilities.
5. Drs. Peterson, Hendricks and Janse felt that in the instance of the respective colleges with which they were affiliated, such a program would not be possible or desirable.
6. Dr. Nugent also emphasized the necessity of making objective preparations for the eventual institution of the two year pre-professional college requirement, and made the following recommendation to this effect.
   (1) Increasing the tuition.
   (2) Seeking contributions from the alumni.
   (3) Establishing new and increased sources of added income, including better clinics, writing and selling of text books, doing laboratory work for practitioners, etc.
   (4) Seeking endowments.
7. It was finally concluded that the decisions of the Council at the Los Angeles meetings, namely to withhold any definite commitment on the two year pre-professional requirement program, should stand.

The matter of the individual colleges advertising in the various state Journals was brought into discussion.
1. Dr. Nugent felt that this tendency should be stopped immediately claiming that it was high time that the state societies start supporting the colleges rather than constantly imposing financial demands on the colleges.
2. Dr. Peterson maintained that in most instances it was a matter of diplomacy and done for the purpose of retaining the approval of the alumnae followings.
3. Dr. Janse recommended that all the accredited colleges pool a yearly contribution and then have a format prepared listing all of the colleges and then send it to the editors of the various state journals with a check out of the general pool prorated on the basis of the state association membership.
4. Dr. Rogers then recommended that he be permitted to prepare such a format and send it to the various editors of the state journals and invite them to publish the same as a service to the colleges and without charge, the same as the NCA Journal is doing. It was the unanimous decision to have Dr. Rogers do this.

Dr. Budden asked for a frank and open discussion on the Naturopathic issue.
1. Dr. Nugent reminded Dr. Budden that the Western States College was the only remaining school on the accredited list that still conducted a course in Naturopathy.
2. Dr. Budden maintained that it was his opinion that it is better to, at least for the time being, sustain a reputable school of naturopathy so that any illegitimate effort to institute naturopathic legislation could be blocked by pointing to a school whose standards in naturopathy could not tolerate such a procedure of legislative effort.

Dr. Budden referred to the situation that had existed both in Idaho and South Dakota; in both instances unqualified naturopaths had attempted to sponsor legislation and possibly the same would have been passed if attention had not been drawn to the naturopathic course at Western States College and the standards insisted upon.

At this time the meetings were adjourned and the above matter was referred for further discussion for the following morning meeting.

On Friday evening the entire membership of the Council were guests of the Texas Chiropractic College at a Rodeo held at the City Arena. An annual event of national repute and certainly it was an evening of much pleasure and interest.

Saturday morning meeting, February 13, 1954
Continuation of discussion on the issue of naturopathic education.

1. Dr. Budden gave a complete review of the history of naturopathy and asked the Council to give him concise opinions and expression of decision so that he and the Board of Directors of the Health Research Foundation under whose auspices the Western States College and its schools of Chiropractic and Naturopathy are conducted, might come to a conclusion upon which the future policies of Western States College could be determined.
2. Dr. Wolf reminded Dr. Budden that in 1950 at the mid-year meeting in Chicago he and Dr. Janse and Mr. Miller of the National College had agreed to discontinue the courses of naturopathy in the colleges they represented.
3. Dr. Homewood inquired as to what the attitude of the Council would be if a course of naturopathy would be instituted at the Canadian Memorial College of Chiropractic in order to accommodate those Provinces in Canada that sustained naturopathic laws.
4. Dr. Budden inquired whether the Council had the right to remove a college from the accredited list if it continued to conduct a naturopathic course.
5. To the above discussions and inquiries the following conclusions were made:
   (1) The Council would frown upon any attempt on part of the Canadian Memorial College of Chiropractic to institute a course in naturopathy either in part or entirety.
   (2) The Council advised Dr. Budden to inform the Board of Directors of the Health Research Foundation that they recommended that the course and school of naturopathy as conducted at the Western States College be discontinued as soon as obligations and commitments can be fulfilled or terminated.
   (3) That the Council does have the right to remove any college from the accredited list for teaching a course in naturopathy if the college facilities, faculty and administrative talents were employed for this purpose concurrent in time with the teaching of chiropractic.

Dr. Ralph Martin asked the various schoolmen to be somewhat more diligent in the efforts to cooperate with Dr. George Higley of the Los Angeles College and to whom had been assigned the responsibility of collecting and cataloging all the data on the research projects that had been conducted by the various colleges and their staffs.

Dr. Haynes insisted that the Council be more diligent in its efforts of public relations and establish more competent contact with the various state boards of examiners as well as state association officers so that progressively they would be prevailed upon to lend themselves more fully to the accrediting program of the Council.

Dr. Nugent asked that all the schoolmen upon returning to the colleges of their affiliation alert the members of the student body to the functions of the Council and its importance to the overall progress of the profession.

He wanted to know whether it would be possible for the various accredited colleges in their journals to make mention of the Council meetings and emphasize the importance of its program. Also whether in the new issues of their catalogs a definite paragraph describing the accreditation by the Council be carried.

Dr. Janse was instructed to write a letter to the management of the Gunter Hotel to thank and compliment them for the excellent services experience by the Council.

Dr. Peterson voiced the genuine appreciation of the entire Council to Dr. Troilo and the other representatives of the Texas Chiropractic College for the most considerate hospitalities experienced at their hands.

Dr. Peterson then submitted his resignation as Chairman of the Council which was followed by that of Dr. Janse as secretary.

A short discussion revealed the inclination on part of the Council to have Dr. Peterson continue as chairman until at least the St. Louis meeting. Dr. Peterson expressed his willingness to do so if Dr. Janse would remain as secretary and unanimous assent was expressed.

It was the consensus of opinion that the meetings had been most advantageous and constructive. Certainly a general feeling of cooperation and friendly understanding had permeated and sustained all the meetings.

Following are copies of letters written by the chairman and secretary of the Council subsequent to the decision of the Council:

February 15, 1954, Dr. Vinton Logan, President, Logan Basic College of Chiropractic, 7701 Florissant Road, St. Louis 21, Missouri
Dear Doctor Logan:

Following the appearance before the Council on Education, Thursday, February 11, of Mr. Robert Evans, Counsel, and Dr. William Coggins, Dean, appealing the action of the Council removing the Logan Basic College of Chiropractic from the list of accredited schools, the following was the result of the afternoon's discussion.

Inasmuch as Mr. Evans' statement completely ignored the matters which led up to the removal of the accreditation and that he failed to refute any of these matters, but sought to introduce an extraneous subject, that of physiotherapy, which has never been a matter of contention in the Council, and inasmuch as Mr. Evans was unable to give any assurances that your actions contrary to the rules of the Council would cease, it was unanimously voted to deny the appeal and to sustain the action of the Council taken in Los Angeles last July.

The principle points on which the accreditation of the Logan Basic College was removed were restated to Mr. Evans as follows:
1. Dr. Vinton Logan had refused to permit an inspection of the school by the National Director of Education.
2. Dr. Logan had violated the rules and regulations of the Council, adopted without objection while a representative of the Logan Basic College of Chiropractic was present, particularly a resolution prohibiting any member of the Council from participating in

any other accrediting organization, particularly referred to being the North American Association of Chiropractic Schools and Colleges.

3.   The continued separatism in the actions of Dr. Vinton Logan.

4.   The fact that Dr. Logan had attended only one portion of one session of the meetings of the National Council on Education since becoming a member thereof.

Hence, the Logan Basic College of Chiropractic, from this date, is no longer an accredited institution under the program of the National Council on Education. According to the rules and regulations of the Council, the Logan Basic College of Chiropractic may reapply for accreditation, should it so desire.

Very truly yours, Thure C. Peterson, Chairman, Joseph Janse, Secretary

Minutes of the Annual Meeting of the NATIONAL COUNCIL ON EDUCATION of the NATIONAL CHIROPRACTIC ASSOCIATION, Hotel Claridge, July 4-5-6-7-8, 1955, Atlantic City, New Jersey

The annual meeting of the National Council on Education of the NCA was held at the Hotel Claridge, in Atlantic City, New Jersey, July 4, 5, 6, 7, and 8, 1955. Dr. Thure C. Peterson, Chairman of the Council on Education, presided at all of the meetings. Those in attendance included:

A.   Accrediting Committee:

Dr. Ralph J. Martin, Chairman, Accrediting Committee, 28 W. Sierra Madre Blvd., Sierra Madre, California

Dr. Edward H. Gardner, Secretary, Accrediting Committee, 1655 N. Normandie, Hollywood 27, California

Dr. Walter B. Wolf, Eureka, South Dakota

Dr. Norman E. Osborne, Longmeadows Extended, R.D. 5, Hagerstown, Maryland

Dr. John J. Nugent, Director of Education of the NCA, 92 Norton Street, New Haven, Connecticut

B.   Representatives of the accredited educational institutions and those institutions subscribing to the program of the Council.

Dr. Thure C. Peterson, Chairman of the Council and President, Chiropractic Institute of New York, 325 East 38th Street, New York 16, New York

Dr. Joseph Janse, President, National College of Chiropractic, 20 N. Ashland Blvd., Chicago, Illinois

Dr. Arthur G. Hendricks, President, Lincoln Chiropractic College, Inc., 633 N. Pennsylvania Avenue, Indianapolis 3, Indiana

Dr. Julius C. Troilo, Dean, Texas Chiropractic College, San Pedro Park, San Antonio, Texas

Dr. Earl A. Homewood, Dean, Canadian Memorial Chiropractic College, 252 Bloor Street West, Toronto 5, Canada

Dr. John B. Wolfe, President, Northwestern College of Chiropractic, 2222 Park Avenue, Minneapolis, Minnesota

Dr. Ralph W. Failor, President, Western States College of Chiropractic, 4525 S.E. 63rd Street, Portland 5, Oregon

In addition to the foregoing school heads the following representatives of various accredited colleges were also in attendance:

Dr. Clarence W. Weiant, Dean of the Chiropractic Institute of N.Y.

Dr. F.F. Hirsch, Faculty member of the Chiropractic Institute of N.Y.

Dr. J. LaMoine DeRusha, Dean of Northwestern College of Chiropractic

Dr. John Glason, Officer of the Texas Chiropractic College Alumni Association

Dr. Wm. D. Harper, Jr., Faculty member, Texas College of Chiropractic

The first meeting of the Council was called for 10 A.M. July 5, 1955, with Dr. Peterson presiding.

Dr. Peterson called the meeting to order and advised the group that he had received a letter from Dr. Margaret Schmidt of Seattle, Washington, Vice-president of the Council on Public Health, in which she recommended the following two points:

(1)   That the various accredited colleges of chiropractic seek to include in their curricula various pre-professional subjects the total credit of which would be equivalent to those obtainable in the first two years of college work leading to a baccalaureate degree. The reason being that such would provide more income for the colleges and while at the same time providing for the ever increasing two years of pre-professional college requirements it would permit the student to obtain the same yet under the auspices and influence of those who were chiropractically minded.

(2)   The institution of an "office assistant" course. Dr. Schmidt insisting that there was an ever-increasing need for well trained office assistants throughout the profession.

The conclusions of the Council were that the introduction of pre-professional courses into our chiropractic colleges would not meet the demands of the various departments of education and state board requirements. That to date "office assistants" courses hadn't worked out too profitably.

Dr. Peterson next presented to the Council a resolution presented by Dr. J.E. Clark, Delegate from Nevada relating to "Scholarships", which read as follows:

Whereas the Convention held two years ago in Los Angeles, California, passed a motion to appoint a national committee for scholarships, and

Whereas it is generally agreed that something should be done about a state and national promotion of scholarship, and

Whereas it has been proven more or less successful wherever it has been developed; such as Nevada, and

Whereas the colleges need students and a progressive plan for more students in the years to follow and will cooperate, and

Whereas the other methods of scholarship — such as federal and the G.I. Bill of Rights — will soon be extinct,

Be It Resolved that the incoming President of the National Chiropractic Association shall appoint for confirmation a committee of at least five to be known as the National Committee on Scholarships. They will serve as a permanent committee for at least five years — to do research and promote scholarships. Two members of this committee shall be the Chairman of the National Education Committee in 1955 and the author of this resolution. Offered For Consideration by Dr. J.E. Clark, Delegate from Nevada

After rather extended discussion the following conclusions were reached:
a. That scholarships were not the answer to the economic problem of the colleges as a whole, because usually more scholarships required certain concessions from the already overtaxed colleges.
b. That too many scholarships might lead people to form the idea that "chiropractic education" can't even be given away.

The resolution was approved in principle.

Dr. Janse then advised the Council that he had been approached by Dr. Frank Keller of Zurich, Switzerland, over here on an educational tour, about the fact that several people now practicing chiropractic in Switzerland had obtained degrees from the defunct O'Neil-Ross College in Fort Wayne, Indiana. Dr. Keller wanted to know whether the Council would present to the Swiss Chiropractic Association an official statement that these degrees were obtained under false circumstances. The conclusion was that if Dr. Keller in his visit to Fort Wayne could produce definite evidence such a statement from the Council would be presented.

The next matter brought into consideration was that of the ever increasing inquiry from European medical students and graduates who are desirous of obtaining training in chiropractic. The following were the main decisions reached.
a. The credits of all European medical students should be carefully evaluated and credit given only for the basic science and possibly some for the diagnostic subjects. However, the total credit should not exceed that of two college years.
b. That if the European applicant is a graduate in medicine he should be required to put in a minimum of two school years, regardless of the extent of his previous training.
c. That European graduates in medicine should not be permitted to take short one or two months courses at the various accredited colleges.

Dr. Peterson further recommended that all colleges do what they do at the Chiropractic Institute, namely, that of requiring a payment of all tuition before matriculating and this would reduce the tendency for the individual to "run out" before the prescribed time had been put in.

It was the consensus of opinion that the colleges could not deny chiropractic training to European medical graduates if they were willing to put in the prescribed time.

Dr. Peterson next drew the Council's attention to the correspondence he had had with Dr. L.R. Getchell, Secretary of the Montana State Board of Chiropractic Examiners, relating to the information that had been received about the fact that the new legislation sponsored by the State Association and supported by the Examining Board stipulated that all matriculants for examination by March 1959 would have to be graduates from colleges that required two years of pre-professional college training as entrance requirement.

Following are direct copies of the ensuing correspondence:

"Montana State Chiropractic Association   April 11, 1955
Gentlemen: This letter was sent to Dr. M.J. Klette, President of the Board

It has come to our attention that legislation has been enacted requiring that, in order to qualify for licensure in the State of Montana, a student must be a graduate of a chiropractic college that has, as an entrance requirement for all students, two years of pre-professional education.

I sincerely hope that this is not so, as you undoubtedly realize that this would restrict any further licentiate of the State of Montana to graduates of the Los Angeles College of Chiropractic or the Western States College of Chiropractic. We of the National Council on Education, vigorously oppose such discriminatory action which would affect the very fine accredited colleges that are members of our Council.

The Council on Education is not opposed to a two year pre-professional requirement, but has gone on record as opposing the administration of this as a universal requisite until such time as all, or the greater majority of the states, have enacted such law.

Certainly, we do not present any objection to the State of Montana requiring this pre-professional work, which, we understand, goes into effect in 1959, but we do object to requiring that, in order to be approved by the State of Montana, a school must now immediately set forth this requirement for all of its entering students.

The chiropractic colleges of the country have been doing heroic wok in building up not only the quality and depth of their courses, but also their physical plants and facilities. We think the profession should realize that chiropractic colleges are not, in essence, professionally supported and are dependent almost exclusively upon income from student tuition for their very existence.

The enforcement of a regulation such as is referred to in this letter would have very serious restrictive effects upon the profession in Montana for many years to come, aside from being unfair to graduates of the accredited colleges whose geographic location does not, as yet, justify the universal acceptance of the two-year pre-professional training.

We of the National Council on Education respectfully request that this action be considered and modified in line with the practical picture in chiropractic education.

Very truly yours, Thure C. Peterson, Chairman

Dr. Thure C. Peterson, Chairman   (4/25/55)
National Council on Education of the
National Chiropractic Association, Inc., 325 East 38th Street, New York 6, New York
Dear Doctor Peterson:

We have waited until after a meeting of our board before answering your letter of April 11th to Dr. M.J. Klette of Havre.

The change in our law reads as follows: "Each applicant shall be a graduate of a college of chiropractic approved by said board of chiropractic examiners in which he shall have attended a course of study of four school years of not less than nine months each, and after March 15, 1959 shall present evidence of showing completion of two full academic years of college or university work acceptable to the Montana State Board of Education".

Our Board realizes it is not in a position to personally visit and inspect all chiropractic colleges; therefore, it will accept for approval all colleges accredited by the National Council on Education of the National Chiropractic Association, Inc., it being the only accrediting agency within our profession that has a code and facilities for accrediting chiropractic colleges that is acceptable to the Montana Board of Chiropractic Examiners.

I trust this satisfactorily answers your letter, and I shall be pleased to send you a copy of the law and regulations as soon as we can have them printed.

Most sincerely yours,   L.R. Getchell, D.C., Secretary

Dr. L.R. Getchell, Secretary
Montana State Board of Chiropractic Examiners
Strand Theatre Building
Livingston, Montana
Dear Doctor Getchell:

Thank you very much for your letter of April 25th, which clears up a number of points. As so frequently happens when information is transmitted, there are errors of construction which is apparently what occurred in this situation.

I feel sure that the change in law that you have enacted will be considered fair and equitable by all the members of the Council.

If it is possible for you to obtain the information as to what the Montana State Board of Education will consider the content of two full academic years of college or university work, such information would be very helpful to us in guiding the pre-professional education of beginning students.

Again, many thanks for your courtesy, Cordially yours, Thure C. Peterson, Chairman

Dr. Thure C. Peterson, Chairman
National Council on Education of the National Chiropractic Association, Inc.
325 East 38th Street, New York 6, New York
Dear Doctor Peterson:

In the hustle of things following our board meeting I failed, in my letter of April 25th to accurately quote the change in our law. It should have read as follows:

"Each applicant shall be a graduate of a college of chiropractic approved by said board of chiropractic examiners in which he shall have attended a course of study of four school years of not less than nine months each, and after March 15, 1959, shall present evidence showing completion of two full academic years of college or university training from an institution acceptable to the Montana State Board of Education; provided, however, that those who are now duly licensed to practice chiropractic under the laws of the State of Montana shall not be affected by this provision."

You will note that the above wording does not give the State Board of Education authority to pick the subjects of pre-chiropractic training. This is left to the discretion of our own board and we have made no decision regarding the matter. I might state that the board would probably demand a fair percentage of liberal arts.

Schools and colleges acceptable to the State Board of Education are generally those acceptable for listing in the College Blue Book when those institutions have been approved by a recognized state or regional agency.

Very truly yours, L.R. Getchell, D.C., Secretary

The Council extended their expression of compliment and appreciation to Drs. Peterson and Janse in correcting the Montana matter and concluded that it was time that the Council proper seek to voice its dispositions more directly in all state legislative measures.

Dr. Failor, President of the Western State College in Portland, Oregon, was then asked to explain the legislation that had recently been passed in Oregon. Following were Dr. Failor's statements in substance:

(1) After March 1, 1958 all applicants for examination must present to the Board of Chiropractic Examiners evidence of having completed 2 years of liberal arts or science education which has been approved by the Northwestern Association of Secondary and College Education or like Associations, prior to entering chiropractic college.

(2) That the applicant for examination must be a graduate of a chiropractic college requiring the 2 years pre-professional college education as a prerequisite and entrance requirement.

(3) The Board of Chiropractic Examiners has passed a ruling that the chiropractic education must be obtained in 4 separate calendar years.

Dr. Peterson asked Dr. Ralph J. Martin as to whether it was so that the Los Angeles College of Chiropractic, because of the severity of reduced enrollment, had been compelled to matriculate students without pre-professional college education in their May matriculation? Dr. Martin advised the Council that such was so. That because of economic pressure the two year pre-professional college entrance requirement had been temporarily rescinded and that possibly the same would have to be done for the September enrollment.

The recent legislative enactment in Delaware was next discussed with the following informations detailed:

(1) All students entering chiropractic college after September 1st, 1955, must possess two years of pre-professional college education prior to having entered chiropractic college.

(2) These two years of pre-professional college education must contain 8 credits each in the following subjects: physics, chemistry and biology.

Dr. Peterson then proceeded to explain the pending legislation in Connecticut, which in substance pertained to the following informations:

(1) Broadening the definition which if legislation is passed will read as follows: "The practice of Chiropractic shall be understood to be a system or method of diagnosing, except by methods which include drugs or surgery in any form, and treating human ailments by means of manipulation of structures of the body, by hygienic, dietary and physiotherapeutic measures as taught in chiropractic schools, but shall not include the use of drugs, surgery or osteopathy nor the use of roentgen ray or radium for therapeutic purposes."

(2) After July 1st, 1955, the educational requirements would be increased to a total of 4,000 sixty-minute hours.

(3) By 1960 the applicant for examination by the Board of Examiners would give evidence of 2 years of pre-professional college education, but which may be obtained in part concurrent to the chiropractic education.

Dr. Peterson was asked to review the New Jersey requirements and he presented the following informations:

(1) That after Dec. 1st, 1957, all applicants for examination would have to give evidence of having obtained prior to entering chiropractic college one year of accredited pre-professional college training.

(2) That after Dec. 1st, 1958, the pre-professional college requirements prior to entering chiropractic college would be increased to 2 years and would have to include a total of 8 college credits each in physics, chemistry and biology.

(3) That he, Dr. Peterson, as Chairman of Council, was going to present the following outline for the two years of pre-professional college education to the Board and Department of Education in the hope that it would be accepted and thus reduce the severity of the specific subject stipulation.

First Year

1st Semester	Credit	2nd Semester	Credit
English	3	English	3
Biology	3 or 4	Biology	3 or 4
Foreign lang.	3 or 4	Foreign lang.	3 or 4
Electives	6 or 4	Electives	6 or 4
	15 - 15		15 - 15

Second Year

1st Semester	Credit	2nd Semester	Credit
English	3	English	3
Chemistry	3 or 4	Biology	3 or 4

Electives	9 or 8	Electives	9 or 8
	15 - 15		15 - 15

Total
English   12
Biology   6 or 8
Chemistry   6 or 8
Foreign lang. 6 or 8
Electives   30 or 24
               60 - 60

Dr. Failor advised the Council that in the state of Washington, the ICA had rescinded its low educational standard policy and was permitting its followers to sponsor a four year chiropractic law.

He also advised that the recent passage of a bill has forced the basic science board to open considerations for reciprocity and that within the next month the board should announce with what states the Board would extend reciprocity.

Dr. Hendricks was then asked to review the recent legislation in Indiana. Dr. Hendricks advised the Council that for years the unlicensed as well as the licensed practitioners had sought an independent chiropractic bill in Indiana but to no avail.

Finally it was concluded by the Lincoln College Administration and the membership of the Indiana Chiropractic Association to seek legislation that would enable and instruct the Indiana State Medical Board to re-evaluate the status of the unlicensed practitioners in the state and also inspect existing chiropractic colleges.

For the last three years both the Lincoln College and the National College had been in mediation with the medical board and each school had experienced two inspections by commissions from the board.

Both the department of education and the medical board were contacted and it was observed that they also were anxious to do something about the garbled existing situation. Hence on various occasions, committees from both sides met in council to determine the nature of the possible legislation. The Director of Education, Dr. John J. Nugent, was called in for further consultation and advice. Dr. Harry McIlroy, as well as Dr. Davidson, the chiropractic member of the medical board, also lent great and extended service.

Finally a bill was decided upon possessing a rather liberal and well determined definition and certain arrangements for the eventual licensing of the unlicensed practitioners.

Dr. Beneville, a doctor of Chiropractic and State Legislator sponsored the bill. At this time the unlicensed ICA element threatened to have the bill thrown out if certain reductions in the definition as well as certain extra grants for the unlicensed men were not included. Dr. Beneville, for fear that their opposition would kill the bill, permitted these changes to be made.

Dr. Hendricks voiced the opinion that this was a mistake because the original bill had the full sanction and support of the medical board, department of education, as well as the medical profession.

The bill was passed almost unanimously. Its prescriptions and stipulations, however, had been rather severely garbled and hence its initiation has been rather difficult.

It is agreed by all that in certain respects the present legislation has been somewhat unfair in giving undue privileges to those who flaunted the law and practiced without license in the state and afforded no licensure privilege for those who in deference to the law left the state to practice elsewhere.

Both the Lincoln College and the National College have been approved by the Department and the Board and very likely within the next year all of the other accredited schools would be inspected.

Dr. Hendricks advised the Council that the requirements were 4,000 sixty-minute hours involved in four years of eight months each. By April 1st, 1959, anyone entering chiropractic college and wishing to qualify for the Indiana Board will have to present evidence of having had two years of pre-professional college work.

Second meeting of the Council morning of Wednesday, July 6, 1955, with Dr. Peterson presiding.

Dr. Clarence Weiant was asked to review his observations on his recent trip to Europe. Following were his major observations:

1. He had found Dr. Illi's work most interesting and revealing. That the work did accomplish a great deal. However, it involved procedures and mechanical adjuncts that would make its application in general practice most difficult and limited.

2. That Dr. Illi was hopeful of getting his mechanical aids marketed and installed in the offices and clinics of the practitioners and schools here in the U.S.

3. Dr. Illi had held a reception and at this he had met a German medical practitioner by the name of Biederman who advised him that in Germany medical research groups on chiropractic had been organized throughout the country. That nearly every week current publications presented articles on chiropractic. That probably some 3,000 German medical practitioners were anxious to study chiropractic.

4. That since the war German medical practitioners had found competition very severe and hence were turning to chiropractic as another means of practice and gaining patient attention.

5. That Dr. Werner Peper of Hamburg, graduate of the P.S.C., had during the war become a personal friend of an outstanding

German orthopedist. Dr. Peper had interested him in chiropractic and had possibly given him some instruction. That Dr. Peper had on occasions made demonstrations before medical groups. Peper had published a pictorial book on chiropractic which appeared to be a copy with Peper as the model of the text published by the National College of Chiropractic.

6. That the Chiropractor Bielefeld had been the individual who had gone to the clinic of Dr. Sell, the medical practitioner, who had held the lectures on chiropractic in Stuttgart, during the summer of 1954, and adjusted many of Sell's patients and possibly it was by means of this procedure that Sell had picked up some adjusting technics.

7. The Swede, Dr. Sanberg, periodically flies from city to city in Germany and holds clinics at which he adjust hundreds of patients of medical practitioners, although he has always maintained that he has never taught his work to any of these practitioners.

8. In Germany there is legislation defining the practice of "irregular practitioners" and that there is a school of two years length for these "irregulars" that gives so many hours in chiropractic.

9. In Switzerland 9 out of the 22 Cantons have legislation regulating the practice of chiropractic. That at Illi's reception were Swiss medical practitioners who frankly acknowledged the merit of chiropractic and encouraged its application and study.

The Council received Dr. Leo E. Wunsch, President of the National Council on Roentgenology, who presented the following two Council decisions and recommendations.

1. "To the Educational Council of the National Chiropractic Association and House of Delegates:

We, the officers of the National Council on Chiropractic Roentgenologists, in meeting have discussed the college situation regarding two years pre-college requirements before entering same to obtain a degree of Doctor of Chiropractic.

We are of the opinion that the schools should control entrance requirements until such a time that they are in position to meet same or said higher educational requirements.

In lieu of the financial conditions surrounding the various schools and colleges we feel it is not to the best interests of these colleges in operation to add additional burdens for at least five to seven years.

We feel by that time an over all endorsement can be made by the colleges and the NCA Educational Council.

We are sure the heads of the various Councils realize the existing circumstances that now exist in some of the colleges and surely we do not want to close the doors to the future of chiropractic and her students.

Respectfully submitted, Leo E. Wunsch, President of N.C.C.R.

2. Dr. Wunsch then advised the Council that the Council on Roentgenology felt that they should seek to inspect the X-ray departments of all the accredited colleges. That due to the very technical nature of the subject of X-ray those of the Roentgenological Council should have the privilege of inspecting and accrediting the departments of X-ray of the colleges.

He then submitted to the Council the following resolution and prescription as prepared by the Council on Roentgenology along with the recommended list of text books in X-ray that should be in the departmental library of each college:

(Material from Dr. Wunsch not received.)

Dr. Nugent inquired of Dr. Wunsch as to what the objective of the recommendation was? Whether it was the intent of the X-ray Council to establish two types of classification of X-ray users in chiropractic: a Roentgenologists

b. Spinographers.

Dr. Nugent further advised Dr. Wunsch that the Council on X-ray should remember that the departments of X-ray in the various colleges were designed for undergraduate study, not for graduate study.

Dr. Nugent recommended that the considerations of the Council on X-ray should be clearly divided into a program of undergraduate education and graduate education and that the Council should primarily busy itself with the former.

At this time Dr. Nugent, who had just arrived from Connecticut where he had been in counsel with the Governor, advised the group that the pending legislation in the state would very likely be passed. He stated that in one of the bills pending certain reciprocal privileges were being set forth; namely, if a person was a graduate of an accredited college and possessed his high school as well as a basic science certificate by examination and had been in practice some 5 years, he could seek reciprocity into Connecticut without further examination.

Dr. Peterson then asked Dr. Nugent to narrate for the Council his observations on his recent trip to New Zealand, Australia and Hawaii.

Dr. Nugent told the group that while in California attending to the situation at the Los Angeles College in the spring of the year he received an urgent call from a New Zealand practitioner, who was a Lincoln graduate, inviting him to come over to help formulate a legislative program. They of New Zealand providing solely for his transportation. He decided to go and inasmuch as he was going that far he concluded to make a trip to Australia and a stop-over in Hawaii on his own expense.

Upon his arrival in New Zealand he found the practitioners divided into two groups: those sponsoring the concept of the P.S.C. and the ICA and those primarily Lincoln graduates sponsoring the concepts of the NCA However, all practitioners in New Zealand practice straight chiropractic; hence, it was not an issue of physiotherapy.

It appeared that under the prompting of the ICA group letters and communications had preceded him derogating the NCA educational program and advising the ICA followers to have nothing to do with him, Dr. Nugent, and not to permit him to contact any of the governmental officials.

While in New Zealand he met with the various groups and was received with great warmth of hospitality. Sought to maintain a reserve of observation rather than stipulation. He had the occasion of speaking to a number of civic organizations and throughout his tour found the practitioners interested but markedly uninformed of the NCA program. He, Dr. Nugent, felt that the trip from a standpoint of public relations was very successful.

Upon his departure the entire group voted him, Dr. Nugent, a unanimous expression of appreciation but simultaneously expressed a lack of confidence in the NCA program.

His next step was Melbourne, Australia. He was received by the entire professional group at the airport, along with members of the press and government.

While in Australia and making a tour of the major cities he was constantly occupied with luncheons, receptions, press conferences, public addresses and was treated with royal deference. However, as per always the split between the NCA and ICA was fully apparent and in influence. On various occasions he was called on to differentiate the intents and programs of the two.

As in New Zealand the need for a more thorough understanding of the NCA program was very much needed. Dr. Nugent felt that he left a good impression and that the Australian practitioners would be much more receptive to the NCA program from now on.

His visit to Hawaii was pleasant but brief. The chiropractic situation there is well established and rather wholesome. That pending legislation was asking for two years of pre-professional college education, a broadening of the law and requiring one year's residence before being permitted to write the board. However, the ICA element was again in obvious effort to mitigate any extension of NCA influence.

Dr. Nugent concluded that he had helped to formulate plans for a straight manipulative law in New Zealand. That the practitioners of all schools did not wish to include physiotherapy. That more than likely legislation would be passed within the year.

Dr. Peterson then presented to the Council a communication from Dr. Nugent to all the accredited colleges and it was recommended that the same be included in the Council minutes.
"To: All NCA Accredited Schools
"Subject: Annual Convention, American Association of Junior Colleges.
Gentlemen:

You will remember that last year the NCA had an exhibition booth at the American Association of Vocational and Guidance Personnel Convention at which it distributed career information. We thought that this was a success and that eventually it would help the schools.

In line with this thought and as another effort on the part of the NCA to help our accredited schools, we also had a booth at the Annual Convention of the American Association of Junior Colleges which was held at the Hotel Sherman, Chicago, on March 1-4, 1955. This was attended by some 320 presidents and deans of Junior Colleges across the country. Because of the location of the convention there was, of course, a heavier attendance from the Middle Western States.

We had a nice booth and had samples of all our career information and catalogs of each of your schools with blank forms for requests for this material to be sent to them. I was able to talk to between 40 and 50 gentlemen participating and was able to correct some mistakes and misconceptions regarding our educational program. All expressed interest and assured me that we were taking the right steps to achieve acceptance for our schools.

Attached you will find a list of those who made particular requests for your catalog. I was fortunate in being able to obtain a complete list of those attending the convention and, since it is rather lengthy, I will not recopy it but send it to you each in turn and ask that you forward it to the next school indicated at your earliest convenience. I would like you to look over this list and determine for yourself whether you consider it worthwhile to send your catalog to those schools in your areas.

If you do so I suggest that you do not send any illustrative material or pictorial supplements with the catalog. I have very good reason for making this suggestion and I will discuss it with you at our next meeting.

We are faced with a number of hard facts and we must deal with them realistically. First the decrease in our enrollments consequent to the closing of the G.I. program and secondly the swift rush of the states to amend their acts requiring two years of college as a prerequisite for licensure.

With the passage of the new law in Indiana and the action of the California Board of Chiropractic Examiners we now have 16 states which require college education. Eleven other states are seriously considering it, or already have introduced such legislation, so that by the end of this June we may have 20 to 27 states requiring two years of college.

The program theme of the American Association of Junior Colleges was: "Planning in Junior Colleges to Meet the Impending Tidal Wave of Students." This convention spent four days trying to decide what to do about the coming influx of students.

In view of these facts, it ought to be evident that in a very short time two years of college is going to be a national standard, that the average young man and woman of tomorrow will have at least two years of college education, in fact the V.A. administration statistics show that the Korean veteran has an average of two years college. Therefore, we must bend every effort toward informing the junior college student that chiropractic presents an opportunity for a career in a non-crowded field. The older professions will not be able to absorb these great numbers and the situation will present a golden opportunity if we seize it.

Important as it may be to bring our message to the junior college student, it is my opinion even more important to bring it to the high school student before he graduates. If he is given the proper vocational and career information he will make his decision before entering the junior colleges and thus be prepared for entrance into our schools. The very future of our institutions depends upon getting this message across to these students.

I would, therefore, suggest that the administration of each school appoint someone, either an employee, a faculty member, or some student whose background or experience is equipped to do the job, to act as vocational counselor for the school and to prepare and follow up an active and aggressive program. It is no longer possible for us to sit back and wait for students to be sent to us. We must now carry on an active campaign for candidates. I further suggest that each school, even at the expense of sacrificing in other directions, must make a substantial provision in its budget for such a program.

If I can be of any assistance in this matter, please feel free to call upon me.

Fraternally yours, John J. Nugent, D.C., Director of Education

Dr. Peterson advised the group that he had received a communication from Dr. Joseph S. Hoyt the secretary of the Vermont Board of Chiropractic Examiners detailing certain alterations in their methods of examination and Dr. Peterson recommended that the following letter be included in the minutes.

Special Meeting Held February 20, 1955

A special meeting of the Vermont Board was held February 20, 1955 at the office of Dr. Joseph S. Hoyt in Burlington, Vermont with the following doctors present: Dr. S.N. Olson, Dr. R.T. Smith, Dr. Joseph S. Hoyt

The meeting was called to order by Dr. Olson at 11:00 A.M.

It was unanimously decided to add the following provisions to the Board ruling governing the issue of license by endorsement.

"Applicants for licensure by endorsement, who graduated after January 1, 1945, must have completed a college course of not less than 3,600 sixty (60) minute hours."

Dr. Hoyt gave an extensive report on the recent meeting of the NCA Council on Education and the Council of State Examining Boards, held in New York City.

It was unanimously decided that the Board should meet to adjudicate the applicants and their examination papers following the regular semi-annual meetings.

Following is a list of subjects to be contained in the examinations, together with the examining doctor:

Doctor Olson - Anatomy;   Histology, Neurology; Physiology; Chemistry; Physiotherapy (optional)

Doctor Smith - Pathology; Orthopedy; Diagnosis; X-ray, Symptomatology

Dr. Hoyt — Hygiene-Sanitation-Bacteriology; Chiropractic therapy; Principles and Practice, Nerve Tracing, Adjusting

Meeting adjourned at 1:30 P.M.

The Council then received Dr. J. Dawson Walp, National and International Coordinator of the "We Walk Again" International Foundation, Inc.

Dr. Walp advised the Council that the above designated foundation was seeking the full support of the NCA and that it was going to ask the accredited colleges to permit the foundation to introduce its program to the students by conducting a yearly course at the colleges.

Dr. Walp advised the Council further that the foundation contemplated staging its second annual polio conference in Chicago, Sept. 13-17 of this year and sought the assurance from the school men that they and their schools would participate if invited. He presented the following aims of this conference.

Aims

1. To arrive at a conclusive standardization of treatment in the management of the acute, post-polio and the chronic polio victim.
2. To prepare to teach, as a result of this conference, the standardized technics as shall be formulated.
3. To simultaneously, from the materials presented, develop a list of problems requiring specific research.
4. To record, to screen, to publish the results of this conference, in the name of chiropractic and to make this material available to members of the chiropractic profession ONLY through established educational enterprises as shall be promulgated by WWA and to sponsor symposia.
5. To prepare, upon conclusion of this conference, materials for use in brochures for public information.
6. To promote a field of free exchange of ideas from the profession which shall in some instances be placed into the hands of specific committees for further consideration prior to release to general conference business.
7. To so conduct our activities that in no instance shall we lose sight of the fact that our prime consideration is the victim of polio and not a matter of argument regarding therapy.
8. To accumulate statistical record on forms (case histories) as shall be prepared by WWA on all cases of polio that are treated through WWA.
9. To sponsor a Polio Prevention Program as shall be prepared and supervised by WWA, as a result of the activities of this conference.
10. To reaffirm the necessity of establishing chiropractic treating centers under WWA and to augment the present programs of the new established acceptable polio treating centers and to incur their favor of the program of the WWA.
11. To prepare to certify all graduates who complete the prescribed course of study as shall be developed and approved as a result of

this conference.

The matter was left for further discussion and deliberations.

Dr. Homewood of the Canadian College advised the Council that their school had spent a lot of effort and quite a bit of money in preparing a set of colored slides on the educational facilities of the college and which were now being shown in high schools with commendable results. He stated that the set of slides could be obtained by any doctor in the field to show to his local high school students.

Dr. Troilo advised the Council that in Texas under the sponsorship of the state association weekly television programs were being sponsored and that once a month such a program was dedicated to chiropractic education and especially designed to attract students to the Texas College. This program was costing the state society $750 a week.

Dr. Wolf of South Dakota advised the Council that the film "The Chiropractic Story" was being shown in all of the high schools of that state.

Dr. Ralph J. Martin then drew the Council's attention to the possibility of obtaining the cooperation of the various special technic itinerant instructors to put their courses on at the various chiropractic colleges on a percentage basis.

Dr. Martin related his interests in the new organization called the "Neurological Research Society" which had done a lot of work in developing the new "stretch reflex technic." He, because of this personal interest, had been in contact with the leaders of this society and felt that they would be more than ready to put the work on in the accredited colleges and permit the colleges to retain a certain percent of the income from these special courses.

Dr. Martin further recommended that in each of the accredited colleges there be organized a special screening committee for these special technics and therapy measures. In fact he felt that the Council should have such a committee.

It was concluded after thorough discussion that the matter should experience some more deliberation by all the schools and that in the meantime the colleges should handle the matter as they individually saw fit.

Meeting of Thursday morning July 7, 1955, convening at 9:00 A.M., with Dr. Peterson presiding.

Dr. Peterson called for a discussion on the reevaluation of the two year pre-professional college education program and the impact of concern that it was representing to all of the accredited colleges.

Dr. Janse insisted that the Council should be more active in lending advice and instruction to both state board officials and state associations in their considerations of this matter. That recent events had shown that many states were contemplating the introduction of the program or had already instituted it with but little deference to the hazard they were so rapidly creating for the accredited colleges. According to Dr. Janse in a number of instances it was quite evident that the entire program was being encouraged and sponsored by those who simply wished to use it as a vehicle of public impression in order to obtain added licensure privileges or added public relations recognition, or even to reduce the number of new entrees into the state.

Dr. Hendricks felt that it was high time that the Council step in and seek to call a halt to the "mad rush." That he had foreseen the dangers and he expressed the conviction that the Council, the Accrediting Committee and everyone concerned had made a mistake in not controlling the "wildfire" of the situation more closely.

Dr. Janse insisted that the "tail was wagging the dog," that the profession and all of its representatives and organizations were constantly instructing the schools what to do but no one or no group ever sought to assist the schools in the problems that confronted them.

It was after further discussion the unanimous resolution of the Council to have its resolution of the mid-year meeting in New York printed up in the form of a brochure along with explanatory literature of the terms and intent (as prepared by Drs. Wolf and Troilo) and then sent out to every state board member, as well as the officers of all the state associations, along with the legislative representatives and all other influential members of the profession, regardless of their affiliations, associations and interests.

The original resolution of the February, 1955, New York meeting read as follows:

"The National Council on Education of the National Chiropractic Association on several occasions has announced its policy in relation to the program of extra or pre-professional education now so commonly considered throughout the profession. In substance this policy may be stated as follows:

The Council on Education is not opposed to the institution of extra-professional college requirements but is concerned with the mechanism by which this program might be instituted and operated. Therefore, the following recommendations are offered to guide and advise state organizations and examining boards who may be contemplating the adoption of such requirements.

1. There should be no stipulation of required subjects except that the courses taken must lead to a baccalaureate degree.
2. That the maximum supplemental educational requirement not be in excess of two years.
3. That this extra-professional college education for the present not be made a matriculation requirement but rather licensure.
4. That at least six years elapse between its enactment date and the date of enforcement.
5. If by virtue of state requirements it becomes necessary to stipulate content we recommend that they not exceed the ordinary requirement which is necessary in the pursuance of the first two years of the course leading to a baccalaureate degree.

It was further recommended that the above resolution be printed in all of the college journals and field publications.

Dr. Peterson then asked the Council members to suggest an agenda for the afternoon meeting with the Council of Chiropractic Examining Boards. The following recommendations were made:

1. A discussion on and evaluation of the recent California developments so far as pending legislation and board ruling is concerned.
2. Announcing the resolution and intent of the Council on Education in relation to the pre-professional college education program.
3. Expression of congratulation and compliment to the Council of Examining Boards on the progress and foresight portrayed by them.
4. Recommending that all Boards seek to employ a standard and accepted terminology in the basic sciences and also the clinical subjects, especially chiropractic.
5. Seeking to obtain the cooperation of the Boards to set their examination dates to those compatible with the following recommendations so as to more closely conform to graduation dates: Early part of February, the latter part of June and the early part of October.
6. Recommending that all Boards seek to avoid the dictating influence of any single school or group in the profession.
7. Discussion of the increasing interests exhibited by state boards in the objective type of state board questions and prepared by State Board Question Service Organizations.

Joint Meeting of the NATIONAL COUNCIL ON EDUCATION and the NATIONAL COUNCIL OF CHIROPRACTIC EXAMINING BOARDS, Hotel Claridge, Atlantic City, New Jersey, Thursday Afternoon, July 7, 1955

Drs. Thure C. Peterson, Chairman of the Educational Council, and Adam Baer, President of the Examining Board Council, presiding.
Mrs. Beulah Hayse, assistant to Dr. Peterson at the Chiropractic Institute, was present to take the minutes in shorthand.
Those in attendance included:

A. Of the Council on Education:
    Dr. Thure C. Peterson, Chairman — Chiropractic Institute of New York
    Dr. Joseph Janse, Secretary — National College of Chiropractic
    Dr. Ralph J. Martin, Chairman of the accrediting committee
    Dr. John J. Nugent, Director of Education
    Dr. Arthur G. Hendricks — Lincoln Chiropractic College, Inc.
    Dr. Julius C. Troilo — Texas Chiropractic College
    Dr. John B. Wolfe — Northwestern College of Chiropractic
    Dr. Earl A. Homewood — Canadian Memorial Chiropractic College
    Dr. Ralph W. Failor — Western States College of Chiropractic
    Dr. J. LaMoine DeRusha — Northwestern College of Chiropractic
    Dr. Walter B. Wolf — Accrediting Committee
    Dr. Norman E. Osborne — Accrediting Committee
    Dr. Edward H. Gardner — Accrediting Committee
    Dr. Clarence W. Weiant — Chiropractic Institute of New York
    Dr. William Harper — Texas Chiropractic College
    Dr. F.F. Hirsch — Chiropractic Institute of New York

B. Of the Council of Chiropractic Examining Boards
    Dr. L.R. Getchell - Montana; Dr. C.H. Peters — North Carolina; Dr. Guy Smith - Arkansas; Dr. L.S. Tawney - Maryland; Dr. E.M. Cardell - Wisconsin; Dr. J.A. Ohlson - Kentucky; Dr. E.C. Poulsen - California; Dr. E.E. Gruening — New Jersey; Dr. G.E. Hariman — North Dakota; Dr. A.W. Bradley - Delaware; Dr. J.A. Glasin - Texas; Dr. R.U. Sierra — Puerto Rico; Dr. F.L. LeBaron - Wyoming; Dr. H.L. Ramsay - Indiana; Dr. S.H. Cane - Michigan; Dr. J.S. Hoyt - Vermont; Dr. Adam Baer - Maryland; Dr. H.T. Opsahl - Ohio;   Dr. D.R. McDowell — South Dakota; Dr. O.A. Ohlson - Colorado;   Dr. W.B. Yoder - Pennsylvania

Dr. Peterson suggested that the joint proceedings follow the pattern of the previous joint meeting of the two Councils at which there were opening remarks of each of the co-chairmen followed by a discussion of the points contained within the agenda of each of the Councils.

Dr. Baer, in his opening remarks, stated that the Examining Boards at their meeting during this convention had considered three categories for discussion, viz., Accreditation, Examination, and Education. That there had been a very friendly and constructive interchange of information between the various boards, which was expected to bring about a standardization of subjects of examination, methods of examination as well as standards of qualification for examination. Dr. Baer emphasized the conviction that cooperation between the two Councils would serve to eliminate many avenues of misunderstanding.

Dr. Peterson in his opening remarks stressed that the combined body forming the National Council on Education consisted of the Committee on Accreditation composed of four members of the profession not associated with any school plus the Director of Education and the Administrative Officers of the accredited colleges constituting the other component of the Council. These two groups thus forming an intramural body each part of which possessed equal voting strength regardless of numerical differences.

Dr. Peterson emphasized the fact that the members of the two Councils owe a great responsibility, first to the public in providing properly trained members of the profession to serve society, secondly to the young chiropractic graduate to assist him in his entrance into the profession, and thirdly to the schools seeking to aid them in acquiring new students and thus maintain the volume of their student bodies.

He stressed the problem confronting the schools today. He maintained that the school men represented on the Council on Education were performing difficult and extended tasks for modest remuneration and that they are all salaried employees of non-profit institutions and that none of them profit from the respective schools which incidentally exist solely on student tuition and what might be accrued from clinic operation.

Continuing, Dr. Peterson pointed out that the very structure of the two Councils required that they be and remain separate bodies but that they perforce of their responsibilities must function in harmonious cooperation for the good of the public and the profession.

The profession of chiropractic needs numerical strengthening and it should be a mandate to both the schools and the examining boards to provide this strength.

Dr. Peterson further pointed out that all schools have and graduate students of excellent academic capacity, some of average capacity and others of under average capacity and that it is not prudent for anyone, whether it is the Accrediting Committee or the Council of Examining Boards, to use the above average student and his record as the full criterion for all applicants to Boards, but rather that the average student and his accomplishments be used as the basis for evaluation.

In conclusion Dr. Peterson appealed to the Examining Boards that they not be swayed in their judgment by allegiances to any one school or to their Alma Maters but that they be unbiased in the administration of their duties.

The agenda of the National Council on Education was then considered and Dr. Janse, secretary of the Council, directed the first matter to Dr. Edward Poulsen, secretary of the California Board of Chiropractic Examiners.

Dr. Poulsen was asked to elaborate on the proposed changes in the pre-professional requirements for the state of California. Dr. Poulsen advised that there would be a meeting on August 27th, at which final decision would be reached by the California Examining Board as to what dispositions would be conducted in relation to this matter. It was Dr. Poulsen's opinion that at this meeting the Examining Board would very likely ratify the following stipulations:

(1) That beginning January 1st, 1956, the California Board of Chiropractic Examiners will only recognize NCA accredited schools.

(2) As of the same date students entering accredited chiropractic colleges and intending to practice in California must have two years of pre-professional college work in an accredited college of arts and science.

(3) Students in accredited colleges and who have been in process of their education before January 1st, 1956, will be permitted to complete their courses and qualify for the Board without further pre-professional requirements.

(4) Night school students will not be eligible.

(5) Students desiring to qualify for the Board must be graduates of professionally or publicly (non-profit) owned schools.

(6) There will be two groups of schools, first the fully approved and second the provisionally approved. The provisionally approved schools will be given a grace of two years in which to meet qualifying requirements.

(7) The two year pre-professional requirement will not be required to be a school entrance requirement for all students but only for those intending to qualify in California.

The next item on the Council on Education agenda was the reading of the resolution regarding the Council position in the matter of pre-professional requirements. This resolution having been unanimously passed at the Council's mid-year meeting in New York. The resolution reading as follows:

"The National Council on Education of the National Chiropractic Association on several occasions has announced its policy in relation to the program of extra or pre-professional education now so commonly considered throughout the profession. In substance this policy may be stated as follows:

(a) The Council on Education is not opposed to the institution of extra or pre-professional college requirements but is concerned with the mechanism by which this program might be instituted and operated. Therefore, the following recommendations are offered to guide and advise state organizations and examining boards who may be contemplating the adoption of such requirements.

(1) There should be no stipulation of required subjects except that the courses taken must lead to a baccalaureate degree.

(2) That the maximum supplemental educational requirement not be in excess of two years.

(3) That this extra-professional college education for the present not be made a matriculation requirement but rather licensure.

(4) That at least six years elapse between its enactment date and the date of enforcement.

(5) If by virtue of state requirements it becomes necessary to stipulate content we recommend that they not exceed to ordinary requirement which is necessary in the pursuance of the first two years of the course leading to a baccalaureate degree.

Dr. Janse noted that this resolution with explanatory literature would be sent in pamphlet form to all the members of all Boards of Chiropractic Examiners, to officers of all state associations and to all association legislative representatives.

Dr. Peterson in elaborating on the reasons for this resolution pointed out the problems and hardships faced by the schools and the students in the schools when requirements are suddenly changed without adequate periods of adjustment.

Dr. Nugent supported the position of the schools in this matter. He advised the group that as long as the schools were entirely dependent upon student tuition for their economy, care should be exercised in setting up measures that would compromise their economy.

Dr. Ohlson of the Colorado Board expressed the opinion that he could not understand why chiropractic schools could not give advance standing for paralleling credits obtained in state colleges and universities, etc. The conclusion was that such was being done whenever possible but at certain instances state boards would not permit the student to have obtained or to receive credit for any of his work done elsewhere. Hence it was concluded that the matter would still have to experience individual interpretation.

Continuing the agenda Dr. Janse stated that the Council on Education had passed a resolution commending the Council of Examining Boards for their cooperation, farsighted attitudes and for the splendid results that had already been effected.

The next recommendation from the Educational Council was that old and obsolete terminology be no longer used and the B.N.A. nomenclature be resorted to entirely. It was further recommended that whenever possible the clinical terminology of chiropractic subjects be standardized and all "pet" and "vernacular" terms be avoided.

The representatives of the Texas Chiropractic College (Drs. Troilo and Harper) urged that the Examining Boards avoid using the names of persons when designating anatomical, physiological, pathological as well as disease states. They also suggested that questions be slanted toward fundamentals of the subjects rather than isolated and rare conditions which did not give the applicant the opportunity to disclose his basic knowledge.

The next request or recommendation made by the Council on Education was that wherever possible state board examinations be held close after graduation dates. A survey of the schools showed that the most desirable dates from the school standpoint to be: the early part of February; the latter part of June; and the early part of October.

The final item of the Council on Education was a request for a more thorough study of the use of the mechanized examinations and examinations prepared by independent services which are being used by some boards. It was the consensus of the schools that care should be taken in the selection of such services and that the schools be informed when such services are contemplated.

Dr. Poulsen of California expressed the conviction that these examination services might well represent a distinct aid to the examining boards as well as the applicants to the boards. His contact with these services lead him to believe that they would be able to set up unbiased and strictly objective examinations which would help to eliminate the personal element of preferences, etc.

Dr. Baer, Chairman of the Council on Examining Boards, was then asked as to what matters his Council would like to bring into discussion.

Dr. Baer stated that a survey by the Examining Board Council showed that in 36 states whose Boards were represented on the Council a total variation of 35 subjects were being examined in. That the Council on Examining Boards had come to realize that this placed a tremendous burden on the chiropractic colleges and hence it felt that it would be highly desirable either to reduce or combine subjects under a general listing.

Dr. Baer made further comment with reference to the usage of questions prepared by these various state board examination services, contending that it was the consensus of opinion among the members of his Council that especially in the basic sciences the average chiropractic state board member was not always too well qualified in preparing questions, setting up examinations and grading the papers.

Other professions were using these "services" with benefit and expedience and that they had found that the angle of personal bias and possible discrimination was thus reduced.

Dr. Janse asked whether these special agencies of examination preparation would slant their questions along the lines typifying chiropractic thinking. Dr. Poulsen, as well as others, stated that contact with such agencies afforded them the assurance that the personnel of these agencies would sit in extended counsel with our professional representatives to estimate the nature of this essential slanting.

Dr. Baer maintained that the chief complaint against these prepared examinations was the prohibitive cost.

Dr. E.M. Cardell, Secretary of the Wisconsin Board, stated that the Wisconsin Board to date had confined itself to the essay type of examination and he wanted to know whether such type of examination would now be looked upon with misgiving. All school men attending assured him that fundamentally this was still the most effective and legitimate type of examination. Dr. Peterson stated that possibly a combination of the essay and discussion type along with the objective type of examination could be developed. Probably in the basic science subjects the latter type might be quite frequently applicable and in the clinical subjects the discussion type of examination would predominate.

Dr. Nugent made further explanation of the objective examination when he stated that they were first prepared by experts from standard textbooks, then they are checked for any regional prejudices, then a psychologist goes over them for ambiguity and clarity and reframes the questions where he finds weakness. Then the questions are again submitted to the experts.

Dr. Baer expressed the opinion that the school men could possibly help the examining boards if they would possibly submit sample examination questions of the work covered by the schools in the various subjects of their curricula.

Dr. Baer, in behalf of the Examining Board Council, sought the advice and recommendations of the school men in the effort to reduce the amount of subjects given on state boards. Dr. Joseph S. Hoyt, Secretary of the Vermont Board, advised the group that recently in Vermont certain secondary subjects had been grouped under one major. He gave as example anatomy, stating that in Vermont the once independent subjects of histology and neurology were now included under anatomy. He stated, however, that a goodly number of the examinees found this inclusion of subjects under one major designation as confusing.

Dr. Janse contended that such was the consequence of the not infrequent tendency in all chiropractic colleges to conduct what is known as segmented education. Too often he contended the need for integrating anatomy with physiology, etc., is left out of consideration. He encouraged all the Boards to do what Vermont had done and alerted the school men to the needs that would thus arise.

Dr. Janse drew the groups' attention to the fact that one of the primary criticisms of all state board members, whether of chiropractic boards, composite boards, of basic science boards of the average chiropractic examinee, was the fact that he often was too brief in his answers, that he frequently failed to interpret the questions, and that often he neglected the importance of proper conjugation of sentences and spelling. He suggested that most applicants are under tremendous tension and he sought the cooperation of the various state boards in giving a little friendly talk before the examination and seeking to place the applicant at ease and remind him of some of these common mistakes.

Dr. Peterson endorsed Dr. Janse's comments and then spoke of the feeling of many applicants in being first examined in the basic science subjects by basic science examining boards and then being re-examined in the basic sciences when appearing before chiropractic examining boards. The feeling is that this is needless repetition.

Dr. Cardell asserted that in Wisconsin it was not too uncommon to find that although an examinee had passed the basic science board he still failed in one or two of the basic science subjects when given on the chiropractic board. He maintained that his board felt that they owed an obligation to society and that anyone had a right to demand to look at the examination papers and his board was not going to be found wanting or remiss in their duty and thus this re-examination in the basic sciences by his board was a safeguard.

Dr. Nugent expressed the opinion that in states where such procedure is a matter of law it originated out of the circumstance that the chiropractic law and the subjects to be examined stipulated before the institution of a basic science law and when the latter was introduced there was of course this natural overlapping.

Dr. Janse thought that possibly in case of this circumstance the chiropractic board could seek to slant the questions in the basic sciences along lines that are explanatory of the chiropractic principle. He realized that this would put added work on the faculty of the colleges, yet if the state boards would seek to advise the various schools of this intent it probably would contribute to better doctors of chiropractic.

Dr. Baer thought we should have a system to help schools eliminate students not qualified or prepared to take state board examinations. He expressed the belief that a two year pre-professional requirement would bring a better type of student into our colleges who would in general find it much less difficult to pass state boards.

Dr. Peters, Secretary of the North Carolina State Board, and the newly elected Chairman of the Council of Examining Boards, stated that his board had given this matter much thought. Their concern was that graduates going into the profession did not have the qualifications of professional people and so a two year college requirement was instituted in North Carolina as a Board decision. He advised the group that the state association was sending out letters to all high school students to notify them that if they contemplated entering chiropractic college they would first have to obtain the required two years pre-professional college work. He encouraged the school men to consider a similar program of contacting high school graduates with the instruction to obtain pre-professional college work before contemplating chiropractic education.

Dr. Troilo, Dean of the Texas Chiropractic College, said that they had found that since the institution of college requirements at the Texas College the average student was more able to pass his state boards and as a whole exhibited a higher threshold of moral and professional competence.

Dr. Nugent then spoke to the state board members and pointed out that they are leaders in their individual states and in some cases their leadership went even further than that. He advised the board members that as leaders of their profession it is important that they be cognizant of the problems confronting the schools.

In order to have an income for survival, each school must have sufficient enrollment for student tuition to cover operating expenses. In order to have such an enrollment the schools must enroll some poorer students, by the law of averages. He pointed out that the upper one-third of the students are usually very good and the school is proud of that group. The next one-third must be classed as fairly good and are still a credit; however, the lower one-third must be considered as an "endowment." If the profession could provide the schools with the needed "endowment" then the enrollment could be curtailed and screened to a much greater degree. The schools would be much happier if this could be done.

Dr. George Hariman, President of the North Dakota Board, maintained that the two year pre-professional college requirement had served to eliminate not only the poorer students but would also help to eliminate the poorer schools.

Dr. Ralph Failor, President of the Western States College, said that the faculty of this college had seen the difference in the student's ability to grasp the subject matter since they instituted the two year pre-professional college program.

Dr. Peterson ended the meeting by inviting a continuation of these conjoint meetings. He advised the Council of Examining Boards that the Educational Council meetings will be next February 12th in Toronto and invited the Examining Board Council to send their representatives to attend a joint meeting.

Meeting adjourned at 4:30 P.M.

Closed meeting of the National Council on Education, Hotel Claridge, Atlantic City, New Jersey, July 7, 1955, held in afternoon after the joint meeting with the Council of Examining Boards, Dr. Peterson presiding and Mrs. Hayse taking the minutes.

The meeting was called to order at 4:45 P.M. All schools were represented with the exception of the Los Angeles College of Chiropractic.

Dr. Ralph J. Martin, Chairman of the Accrediting Committee, was called upon to give a report of the Accrediting Committee to the

Council in general.

He stated that Mr. Otto J. Turek, Chairman of the Board of Trustees of the National College of Chiropractic had taken the position that he does not care to meet with the Accrediting Committee of the NCA and had referred the matter of issue between the National College and the Accrediting Committee to the Executive Board of the NCA.

The Executive Board, after deliberating the matter, felt that they are not in a position to dispose of the matter and that it should be referred to the National Council on Education.

Dr. Wolf stated that in a personal visit to Mr. Turek in Chicago, Mr. Turek had invited the Committee on Accreditation to meet with him in Chicago. That Mr. Turek had been invited to meet with the Committee in Atlantic City. That although Mr. Turek at first had committed himself to meet with them in Toronto, (the convention having been transferred to Atlantic city) for some reason had later declined to come to Atlantic City.

Dr. Martin then asked Dr. Peterson as the chairman of the Council to write Mr. Turek to try and resolve the matter before the mid-year meeting.

Dr. Janse interceded and stated that he was certain that Mr. Turek would be willing to meet with the Committee or any other assigned group of the Council in Chicago and that Mr. Turek hesitated coming to Atlantic City for fear of further squabbling.

Dr. Nugent pointed out that it is most inconvenient for the Committee members to go to Chicago for a special meeting with Mr. Turek. It would entail a lot of expense whereas if Mr. Turek would meet with the Committee during one of the regular meetings this would be avoided.

Both Drs. Martin and Peterson stated that Mr. Turek would have to seek solution to the issue through mediation with the Council on Education and the Accrediting Committee.

The Accrediting Committee had nothing further to present to the Board.

Dr. Nugent expressed his appreciation for the cooperation and sympathetic treatment he had received from the Council in the past. He also wondered if the group would like to send a note of recognition to Mrs. Budden as this was the first NCA Convention that Dr. Budden had not attended since its inception.

Dr. Peterson made a few closing remarks and also stated that he believed the combined meeting of the Council on Education and the Council of Examining Boards was a most constructive one. He acknowledged Dr. Janse's good judgment for having inspired the inviting of these men.

The meeting was adjourned at 5:15 P.M.

Minutes of the Mid-Year Meeting of the NATIONAL COUNCIL ON EDUCATION OF THE NATIONAL CHIROPRACTIC ASSOCIATION,
Hotel Royal York, February 15, 16, 17, 1956, Toronto, Canada

Dr. Thure C. Peterson, Chairman of the Council on Education, presided at all of the meetings. Those in attendance included:

A. Accrediting Committee.
    Dr. Ralph J. Martin, Chairman of the Accrediting Committee, 28 W. Sierra Madre Blvd., Sierra Madre, California
    Dr. Edward H. Gardner, Secretary of the Accrediting Committee, 1655 N. Normandie, Hollywood 27, California
    Dr. Walter B. Wolf, Eureka, South Dakota
    Dr. Norman E. Osborne, Longmeadows Extended, R.D. 5, Hagerstown, Maryland
    Dr. John J. Nugent, Director of Education of the National Chiropractic Association, 92 Norton Street, New Haven, Connecticut

B. Representatives of the accredited educational institutions of the National Chiropractic Association.
    Dr. Thure C. Peterson, Chairman of the Council and President of the Chiropractic Institute of New York, 325 East 38th Street, New York 16, New York
    Dr. Joseph Janse, Secretary of the Council and President of the National College of Chiropractic, 20 N. Ashland Blvd., Chicago 7, Illinois
    Dr. Arthur G. Hendricks, President of the Lincoln Chiropractic College, Inc., 633 N. Pennsylvania Ave., Indianapolis 3, Indiana
    Dr. Earl A. Homewood, Dean of the Canadian Memorial Chiropractic College, 252 Bloor Street, West, Toronto 5, Canada
    Dr. John B. Wolfe, President of the Northwestern College of Chiropractic, 2222 Park Avenue, Minneapolis, Minnesota
    Dr. George H. Haynes, Dean of the Los Angeles College of Chiropractic, 920 East Broadway, Glendale, California
    Dr. Julius C. Troilo, Dean of the Texas Chiropractic College, San Pedro Park, San Antonio, Texas
    Mr. Charles A. Miller, Vice-president of the National College of Chiropractic, 20 N. Ashland Blvd., Chicago 7, Illinois
    Dr. Ralph M. Failor, President of the Western States College of Chiropractic, 4525 S.E. 63rd Ave., Portland 6,

Oregon, sent his greetings to the Council and expressed regret in not being able to attend because of pressing responsibilities at the college.

C. Special Guests.

Dr. Justin C. Wood, Member of the Executive Board of the National Chiropractic Association, Salisbury, Maryland.

Dr. C.H. Peters, Chairman of the National Council of Chiropractic Examining Boards, Rocky Mount, North Carolina.

Dr. James E. Ellison, Secretary of the Ontario Board of Examiners, in Chiropractic, Toronto, Canada.

The first session was called for 9:30 a.m. Wednesday, February 15, 1956 with Dr. Peterson presiding.

The first point of consideration placed before the Council from the prepared agenda was the matter of the Western States College in Portland, Oregon still conducting a course in naturopathy.

Dr. Peterson asked for the opportunity of reading an extended statement as prepared by Dr. Nugent, as Director of Education, and sent to Dr. M.I. Higgens, Chairman of the Board of Trustees of the Western States College, in relation to the matter.

The brief related to the board of trustees the position of the council as pertaining to the naturopathic issue; namely, that the council considers it inopportune for any of the accredited colleges to seek to sustain a naturopathic course.

The brief also encouraged the board to consider the necessity of discontinuing the course as soon as possible, even at cost and sacrifice of certain advantages that it might represent.

Dr. Hendricks expressed the conviction that it was time that the Western States College discontinue its affiliations with the naturopathic profession as the National and Los Angeles College had done. That a continuation of the naturopathic course at the Western States College would constitute an embarrassment to the council.

Dr. Nugent sought to advise the council that relinquishing the naturopathic course by Western States College would impose on the college and its board of trustees tremendous economic problems and rob it of certain significant allegiances, yet in conversation with Dr. Higgens he had been advised that the college and the board of trustees stood ready to make these sacrifices.

Dr. Nugent stated that Dr. Higgens for years had been most generous in his support of the Western States College, because of his intimate friendship with Dr. Budden. That upon the death of Dr. Budden, he had been asked by Dr. Higgens to help manage the Western States and to help solve the naturopathic situation. The council was advised that Dr. Higgens, personally, had invested thousands of dollars in the Western States College, yet he was ready to sacrifice the same if the naturopathic problem could be resolved; that he, Dr. Higgens, was anxious to have the Western States College sever its association with naturopathic education.

While attending the mid-year meetings of the Executive Board, of which Dr. Higgens is a member, he, Dr. Nugent, had thoroughly discussed the matter with Dr. Higgens and both had concluded that if possible it would be best to accept no further naturopathic enrollees after September 1, 1956.

The council was then advised by Dr. Nugent that he was expecting a phone call from both Dr. Higgens as chairman of the board and Dr. Failor, president of the college, in relation to the matter and that by the time the accrediting committee would be ready to make its report more than likely something definite would have been resolved at the college.

It was the conviction of Dr. Nugent that a decision by the Western States College to discontinue the naturopathic course would deal a severe blow to naturopathy and that unless the profession is able to organize its own school it might well represent the demise of the profession.

With Western States College out of the picture of naturopathic education only two schools would be left that issued naturopathic degrees and these were institutions of minor quality and influence; namely, the Great Lakes College of Mechanotherapy in Dayton, Ohio and the Spitler College of Naturopathy in Eaton, Ohio.

Dr. Peterson read a four page statement as prepared by the Committee on Educational Standards of the NCA entitled, "A Statement on the Control and Objectives of the Western States College."

In this brief the problems confronting Western States College were fully presented and the recommendation of the accrediting committee exactingly stated. It was evident that thru the death of Dr. Budden, former president of the Western States College, the present administration and board of trustees of the college had inherited many compromising and not readily solved problems.

It was the general disposition of the council that patience should be exercised in relation to the circumstances of Western States College. Dr. Nugent assured the council members that a conscientious effort was being made by the college administration as well as the Board of Trustees in solving the matter and that he was certain that before the conclusion of the council meetings he would obtain word from Drs. Higgens and Failor that a definite decision to eliminate the naturopathic course at Western States had been consummated.

The second point of consideration placed before the council was the matter of standardizing the procedure of evaluating credits from non-NCA accredited colleges.

Dr. Nugent advised the council that in his opinion it was time the council came to a definite decision as to how much credit should be granted for education in non-accredited colleges. He encouraged the schoolmen of the council to make up their minds to grant as little credit as possible, contending that any undue generosity in this matter would but reduce the effectiveness of the council's own accrediting program.

Dr. Nugent further voiced the opinion that colleges like the Bebout College, the Atlantic States College and the newly founded LaFayette College, in Brooklyn, New York, should not be dignified by enjoying any recognition of the work given by them.

Dr. Peterson expressed the fact that among the non-accredited colleges a tremendous range of variance existed within their educational programs; hence, it would be almost impossible to set a single criterion.

It was further drawn to the attention of the Council that such non-accredited chiropractic colleges as the Palmer School and the Logan College enjoyed a rather broad and extensive influence and following throughout the profession and with a number of chiropractic boards of examiners. Furthermore, their physical plants as well as depth of curriculum merited consideration. A number of states and their departments of education as well as boards of examination afforded these schools recognition equal to that of NCA accredited colleges.

It was, therefore, concluded by everyone in attendance that the matter needed extended and most careful evaluation. Dr. Peterson cited the example of the manner in which the problem was handled at the Chiropractic Institute. The graduate from a non-accredited college was advised that it would involve too much of his time to obtain a degree from the Institute and he was encouraged to simply take post-graduate work for which he would receive a certification of clock hours put in, no more. On the other hand if a student transferred from a non-accredited college, a careful estimation would be made of the quality of the school from which he came, his transcript would be carefully studied to determine just how the work already done would parallel to the sequence of the course in the Institute, and then the transfer student advised as to how much advanced standing he might receive. That student who transferred from a non-accredited college at an early period of his professional education might probably receive more credit than one who transferred when well along in his program of education. Never, however, was more than 80% credit given for the total amount of work done.

Dr. Haynes then made inquiry about the past tendency of granting credit for work done in colleges of massage and physiotherapy. The subject was further investigated by drawing attention to the fact that work done in the various short term schools of massage and physiotherapy throughout the country could not receive much, if any, recognition. On the other hand, work done toward a degree in physical education or medical physical therapy could certainly experience a careful evaluation for the possibility of providing the person in question with advanced standing.

A rather extended discussion was next conducted about the transfer of students from one accredited college to another. The following major points being carefully emphasized.

(1) The transferring of students from one accredited college to another should be discouraged as much as possible, and the administration of the college to which the student seeks to transfer should do all possible to advise the student to remain where he or she is.

(2) The dean or registrar of the school to which the student seeks to transfer whenever possible without compromise of the student or the institution in question should seek to advise the dean of the other school of the student's intentions.

(3) Care should be exercised not to permit a student or a possible candidate for chiropractic education to play one school against the other for certain advantages, privileges and concessions.

(4) It was acknowledged that under certain circumstances of geographical, economic and social significance there might be occasions when it is advisable for a student to transfer and these cases should be respected.

(5) If in case of a student who has academically or morally failed to conform to the standards of one college and seeks to transfer to another, the transcript should certainly contain some information in relation to these deficiencies. It was conceded that at times a change in college environment might provide the delinquent student with the incentive necessary.

The discussions relating to the matter were closed with a recommendation from Dr. Nugent that a committee be appointed by the chairman of the council, from amongst the school men, to carefully study the issue and to present to the council a thorough analysis with recommendations.

The third matter of discussion related to the extension graduate course that was being conducted by the Specialty Societies of the California Chiropractic Association, and accredited by the Los Angeles College of Chiropractic, in Michigan.

Dr. Haynes advised the council that some months ago he had been visited by representatives from a small group in Michigan who sought graduate training in certain diagnostic and clinical phases. After careful estimation of their desires they were directed to contact the Specialties Society of the California Chiropractic Association. Eventually an extension program was set up by the Specialties Society, and the Los Angeles College was requested to accredit the same.

Dr. Haynes stated that he had directed the Michigan representatives to the fact that the National College was much closer and they should seek to get the National to set up such a program.

Dr. Janse advised the council that he had been approached by the Michigan people, but when he found out the nature of work they were primarily interested in he had to advise them that the National College could not be interested in considering their request.

He, Dr. Janse, had an opportunity of finding out that for the past several months this graduate work had been going on. That essentially the local group had procured the services of doctors in osteopathy, medicine, and psychology to conduct the classes. That although good and informative work in certain phases of diagnosis had been taught, there had also been classes in fundamental pharmacology, proctology, ambulant minor surgery and other borderline subjects.

It was Dr. Janse's opinion that such procedure constituted a hazard and danger that would provoke division of professional concept in Michigan and result in possibly much misunderstanding.

Dr. Hendricks expressed the opinion that the teaching of the specialties in chiropractic represented a hazard for the simple reason that their full clinical comprehension and handling does definitely necessitate the eventual usage of anodynes, antibiotics, and the participation in minor surgery measures.

Dr. Peterson expressed the feeling that if the Los Angeles College accredited such an extension program it would make it appear as if the council were sanctioning the teaching of borderline subjects.

Dr. Nugent felt that no school should seek to conduct extension courses beyond the limits of its geographical interests. Furthermore, that no extension program or graduate program should be conducted by instructors who did not represent members of the faculty of an accredited college and over whom the college administration has no control.

Dr. Haynes contended that if the Los Angeles College were now asked to reject the Michigan Internist Course it would constitute a severe threat to the unity that he and his associates had been able to establish in relation to the college, among the various factions in California.

The matter was tabled so that the accrediting committee might have an opportunity to study the matter more completely.

The fourth matter presented for discussion was that of the foreign student and the possibility of interesting him in entering one of the accredited colleges.

Dr. Janse drew the council's attention to the fact that the large majority of students from foreign countries matriculated at the Palmer School of Chiropractic; that at present the P.S.C. had a colony of some 60 to 70 foreign students; that the ICA was seeking the aid of its members in providing affidavits of responsibility. Dr. Janse felt that Dr. Peterson, who had been invited to attend the annual convention of the European Chiropractors Union this coming July, might be commissioned to make it a special point to meet with the members of the E.C.U. and encourage them to center their interests about NCA accredited colleges and encourage them to send their students to these schools. Dr. Peterson stated that he would do his utmost in directing the attentions of the European chiropractors to the advantage of referring prospective students to the colleges represented by the council.

Dr. Nugent advised the council that, if at all possible, he was also going to Europe with the intent of evaluating the situation and sponsoring the NCA program of accreditation wherever possible.

A thorough discussion was then conducted in relation to foreign credits and the manners in which they might be evaluated, the following primary points being rather definitely concluded upon.

a. That all foreign medical graduates seeking a degree in chiropractic should be required to put in a minimum of two scholastic years. It was further recommended that they be asked to pay the entire tuition and related fees at the beginning so as to reduce the possible tendency for them to drop out before completing the prescribed time.

b. Dr. Peterson advised the council that on several occasions the registrar's office of the Chiropractic Institute had accepted the matriculation application of a foreign applicant on the strength of character and personal reference affidavits, as prepared by leading citizens and professional people, whenever it was impossible for the applicant to produce regular academic transcripts because of their destruction during the war, or because the territories are now under Russian control.

It was conceded that this might be a proper disposition inasmuch as statements of credentials by such persons as the mayor, local physician, or head of the high school, or a university professor over in Europe usually represented a most substantial verification of a person's background and qualification.

It was decided, however, that when foreign applicants in this circumstance were accepted they should specifically be advised that they would not qualify and should not seek qualification for any of the state boards in the States.

c. It was also concluded that possibly some credit might be given for the education received in such schools as those teaching medical gymnastics, because in Europe they represented a rather competent degree of education and were frequently associated with the medical school of that section.

The fifth matter of discussion related to the program of "We Walk Again" and its desire to have the accredited colleges institute special classes in the management of "acute polio" cases.

This foundation organized by two lay women seeks to simulate the Polio Foundation program, but with the intent of emphasizing the chiropractic management of acute polio cases. The intent and purpose of the "We Walk Again" Foundation has received the sanction of the executive board of the NCA and has received a moderate amount of financial support in sponsoring its program.

The annual convention had been held in Chicago. The attendance had been small. Dr. Levine of the Chiropractic Institute, Dr. DeRusha of the Northwestern College, Dr. Nielson of the Los Angeles College, and Dr. Janse of the National College appeared on the program. During the evening of the final session of the conference the officers of the foundation submitted a program that would seek to induce all the accredited colleges to add to their curricula an extended number of hours in the management of the acute polio case chiropractically.

Dr. Janse advised the council that all the school men attending the conference immediately sought to advise the individuals concerned that such would really be impossible and that they should not seek to make this specialty a part of undergraduate education.

The council in conclusion emphasized the fact that the chiropractic management of the acute chiropractic patient was really not something that the average practitioner might consider doing as a general routine of management. That this clinical practice should be considered and taught as a specialty to select special groups in graduate courses.

The sixth matter brought up for discussion related to the request by the officers of the American Association of Manipulative Surgery to have their graduate course approved by the council.

Dr. Janse advised the council that he had been visited last fall in Chicago by Dr. W.H. Pyott, of 720 E. 1st South, Salt Lake City, Utah, the secretary of the American Institute of Manipulative Surgery, and requested to submit to the council this organization's application for accreditation as a specialist organization in graduate education in manipulative surgery.

Upon being asked by Dr. Janse why the organization sought accreditation by the council, Dr. Pyott gave the following reasons.

(1) The science and art of manipulative surgery is of such significance that it should not experience demise for want of recognition and accreditation by the chiropractic profession.

(2) That in contacting Dr. Rogers, as editor of the NCA Journal with the intent of running ads pertaining to the course and the related books and manuscripts, they had been advised that the NCA Journal could not accept their ads unless the Council on Education approved of the work that they were seeking to represent.

(3) That by obtaining accreditation it would offer the work a protection and sanction, safeguarding it from exploitation.

Dr. Pyott advised Dr. Janse that the course consisted of 120 sixty-minute clock hours of technical training, and some 500 sixty-minute clock hours of clinical training with patients provided out of the practice of the doctor who is taking the course.

The entire cost of the course is $500. There is no desire on the part of the organization to enter their work into undergraduate education, but they would like to see it taught in the graduate schools of the various accredited colleges. If such an arrangement were possible they would provide an instructor at 8 dollars an hour.

Dr. Pyott stated that he felt that failure of recognition of the course would represent a disservice to the men in the field because it would prohibit them from acquiring a method of much merit in clinical practice.

Dr. Pyott stated that the American Institute of Manipulative Surgery had been organized in 1948 and defined manipulative surgery as "A specific manipulative technic designed to accomplish the detachment of adhesions, existing between fascial and muscle planes, and the walls of internal organs."

After some extended discussion the council unanimously concluded that it was not in a position to offer accreditation to the course of the American Institute of Manipulative Therapy and instructed Dr. Janse as secretary of the council to write Dr. Pyott and advise him accordingly. See the attached copy of the letter written to Dr. Pyott.

The seventh matter brought up for study and discussion was that of the accredited colleges seeking to set up a program of collective advertising in state journals; the preparation of a booth display for conventions that would represent all of the accredited colleges.

Dr. Peterson drew attention to the recent solicitation from the advertising editor of the Journal of the New York Chiropractic Society. He expressed the opinion that, if at all possible, individual schools should seek to discourage running ads in various state journals and recommended that all the accredited colleges advise the editor of the New York State Society Journal that it was the council's policy to discourage individual school advertising in state journals.

The council proceeded to make the following recommendations:

(1) That all state Journal advertising and convention exhibit booth space be on a collective basis and so arranged that all the accredited colleges are listed and represented.

(2) That appointed members of the council at the next NCA convention meet with the council of editors of state journals to discourage the soliciting of individual ads from individual accredited schools.

(3) Contact Dr. Rogers and see whether or not a proper attractive ad could be designed. Then have the advertising managers of all state journals write to Dr. Rogers and have him, at his discretion, place the ad or reject the solicitation and then at the end of the year prorate the expenses for the various participating accredited colleges.

(4) That a similar set be arranged if possible for convention exhibit booth space.

As an eighth point of discussion, the matter of dual situation of an NCA and ICA accrediting program was brought up for observation.

Dr. Nugent asserted that the accrediting program of the NCA had been brought into effect long before the ICA had ever thought of an accreditation program. In fact, that the ICA accrediting program was very much a "Johnny Come Lately" and actually represented but very little of an actual attempt to accredit.

He reminded the council of the fact that other than the P.S.C., the schools now recognized under the accrediting program by the ICA had at one time or another sought recognition by the accrediting agency of the NCA.

It was Dr. Nugent's insistence that the council should employ every possible measure to induce state boards and other accrediting authorities to adopt (if not recognize) the NCA accrediting standards and program. To this end he as Director of Education had done the following:

a. Sending specially prepared copies of the booklet "Educational Standards for Chiropractic Schools" to all state boards. With intent any reference to NCA association had been deleted, hoping that the personnel of the state boards would accept the contained standards and prescriptions if not recognize the source and authority as being the NCA.

b. On several occasions has been able to prevail upon attorney generals to submit opinions in favor of the NCA accrediting program.

c. Has been able to induce the state boards of the states of California, Oregon, Montana, Wyoming, Maine, Connecticut, Maryland, and Ontario to accept the NCA standards of accreditation, and of recent date, Delaware also.

A ninth matter for discussion related to various changes in state legislation, especially as pertaining to pre-professional college requirements.

As pertaining to the state of New Jersey, Dr. Peterson submitted the following information. Any student presenting him or herself to the New Jersey Board before Dec. 31, 1957 does not have to have any specific subject material in the one year pre-professional requirement. After December 31, 1958 the following is required.

As prepared by: Chiropractic Institute of New York
Pre-matriculation College Requirements for the State of New Jersey
1st Year

1st Semester	Credit	2nd Semester	Credit	Total
English	3	English	3	6
Biology	3 or 4	Biology	3 or 4	6 or 8
Foreign Language	3 or 4	Foreign Language	3 or 4	6 or 8
Electives	6 or 4	Electives	6 or 4	12 or 8
	15 - 15		15 - 15	30 - 30

2nd Year

3rd Semester	Credit	4th Semester	Credit	Total
English	3	English	3	6
Chemistry	3 or 4	Chemistry	3 or 4	6 or 8
Electives	9 or 8	Electives	9 or 8	18 or 16
	15 - 15		15 - 15	15 - 15

Total Semester hours for the 2 years.

English	12
Biology	6 or 8
Foreign Language	6 or 8
Chemistry	6 or 8
Electives	30 or 24
Grand Total	60 Semester Hours.

The above is the recommended schedule, but it is not required that the subjects be taken in the exact sequence, e.g., the foreign language could be taken in the second year, or the biology and chemistry could be interchanged as to the year in which the subject is taken.

Reference was then made to the changing circumstances in California and the following informations detailed. A letter from the secretary of the California Board.

To: Chiropractic Schools and Colleges
From: Emmett V. Silent, D.C., Secretary, California Board of Chiropractic Examiners
Re: Article 4 — Rules and Regulations

We wish to advise that all students enrolled in a recognized or approved college prior to March 1, 1956, will be acceptable for examination in the State of California when they finish their chiropractic education and meet all of our legal requirements.

The rule changes that become effective on December 3, 1955, affect only those students who enroll in a chiropractic college after March 1, 1956.

If a school is approved at the time a student is enrolled and subsequently is disapproved, the same rule applies as above for enrollment. A graduate will be accepted if he meets all legal requirements if the school from which he graduates was during the time of his attendance at one of our approved schools.

The tenth matter to be brought into consideration was mention of the fact by Dr. Peterson that he was able to secure general hospital care and service under the Blue Cross and Blue Shield auspices at a special group rate for the faculty and clinic staffs of the Chiropractic Institute. Each faculty and clinic staff member paying for the service at a reduced rate and of course designating or declining his desire to participate.

Dr. Peterson gave the address of Blue Cross and Blue Shield, One Hanson Place, Brooklyn 17, New York, if any of the other accredited colleges were interested.

As the eleventh matter for discussion, Dr. Janse read the following letter as received from Dr. Demos Quarry, Secretary of the South African Manipulators Society.

Dear Sir,

A few years back we approached accredited colleges and requested their aid in accepting only those South African students who had passed the necessary higher educational qualifications. This request was made so as to conform to the professional entrance educational standards which prevail in this country; namely, that students entering any of the professions must have a South African Matriculation Certificate as the minimum entrance requirement. A Matriculation Certificate in South Africa means the successful completion of a higher school education, and is the necessary entrance qualification to our universities.

It has come to our notice that some prospective students bypass screening by our Association and apply direct to overseas colleges for acceptance as chiropractic students. Appreciating how difficult it is for you to investigate educational claims of prospective students, my Association would be very pleased to act as your appointed accrediting agents for South Africa. We make this a very special and urgent appeal, because it has been brought to our notice that a prospective student has been accepted as a student by an accredited college, although he does not possess the South African Matriculation Certificate. This embarrasses our position here very greatly, as we have built our case for statutory recognition on the basis that the higher school Matriculation Certificate is a necessary minimum requirement to study chiropractic.

Lincoln College has ruled that prospective South African students must possess a South African Matriculation Certificate, or proof of its equivalent educational standard, before being accepted for study.

Yours faithfully, Demos Quarry, Foreign Correspondent.

After careful deliberation, the council unanimously instructed Dr. Janse to write Dr. Quarry a letter agreeing to the principle of his request. Following is a copy of the communication sent.

Dr. Demos Qually, Foreign Correspondent
South African Manipulative Practitioners' Association, 902 Bree Street, Johannesburg, South Africa
Dear Doctor Qually:

Your communication to all the accredited colleges of October past was carefully reviewed at the recent February mid-year meeting of the Council on Education. In consequence to the discussions conducted I was instructed to advise you that the Council agrees fully with the principle of your recommendation.

There is some question as to what might constitute the best procedure to follow. It is the consensus of opinion that each of the accredited colleges should receive a formal statement from your association, detailing and clarifying what is specifically meant by a South African Matriculating Certificate. This deposition could then be referred to the Registrar of each college and used as the criterion by which all South African applications are estimated.

May we expect to hear from you at your earliest convenience in relation to this matter. The entire membership of the council seek to join me in all good wishes and expressions of respect to you and your associates.

Sincerely yours, J. Janse, D.C., Secretary, National Council on Education of the National Chiropractic Association

On Wednesday evening the entire council membership were the guests of the Canadian Memorial Chiropractic College and its Board of Management and Directors at a major sports event, an occasion that offered much enjoyment and pleasure and certainly representing a most generous and inviting expression of hospitality.

Thursday morning meeting, February 17, 1956, Dr. Thure C. Peterson, Presiding.

Dr. Peterson introduced to the council membership Dr. James E. Ellison, secretary of the Ontario Board of Chiropractic Examiners. Dr. Ellison was then asked to direct a few words to the council. Following are the primary comments as made by Dr. Ellison.

   a.   The council was advised that the Ontario Board of Chiropractic Examiners sustains a reasonable period of grace in that it permits a senior of good standing (as verified by the college) to take the examination several weeks prior to the time his diploma is received if waiting until the next session of the board would exercise an undue hardship on him.

   b.   Dr. Ellison sought the cooperation of all the schools in carefully scrutinizing the transcripts of transfer students especially those who left the original school with a bad record.

   c.   The council was further advised by Dr. Ellison that the Ontario Board would only accept applications for examination from graduates of those colleges accredited by the NCA.

   d.   He complimented the council and stated that the accrediting program was a definite service to all state boards and that the Ontario Board would be willing to pay for these services by paying a yearly honorarium to the council.

Dr. Ellison was unanimously thanked for these expressions of confidence and compliments and asked to convey appreciation to the entire membership of the Board.

The twelfth point brought up for brief consideration was the scholarship program as sponsored by Dr. J. Everett Clark of Las Vegas, Nevada.

Dr. Haynes advised the group that the Clark scholarship program didn't sustain much integrity or capacity and would recommend that very little if any attention be afforded it.

Dr. Peterson voiced the opinion that scholarships as a whole were of little benefit for the simple reason that they benefited students and not the colleges.

Dr. Nugent emphasized the idea that alumni groups should be encouraged to underwrite school projects rather than to seek to sponsor scholarships.

The thirteenth matter for council consideration were a series of recommendations by Dr. Nugent.

   a.   In the future issues of the various school catalogs, the terms, freshman, sophomore, etc. should be deleted and replaced by the designations, first, second, third and fourth year students.

   b.   The term neurology should not be used to represent neuro-anatomy in the various school bulletins.

   c.   An attempt should be made by all the schools to pattern their catalogs after an accepted format.

   d.   Have a cut made up listing the National Council on Education of the National Chiropractic Association and place on the front page of the school catalog.

    e.   Send NCA prepared literature to all prospective students.

    f.   The council was advised that he, Dr. Nugent, was preparing a special bulletin listing all states with pre-professional requirements and exact prescription of these requirements. This bulletin is to be included in all Vocational Guidance Portfolios.

    g.   The word "chiropractic" has been used rather than "chiropractic" because grammatically it is more correct.

    h.   All make-up examination grades should be low; otherwise, this measure might degenerate into becoming a farce.

    i.   Conducting a college year round constitutes a faculty and scholastic hardship.

    j.   There should be a closer standardization of tuition and fees. A resentment is arising between school men because of competitive tuition rates.

    k.   College accrediting agencies might be induced to recognize credits from chiropractic schools if we can progressively get men with academic degrees on our faculties.

    l.   We should encourage the younger elements of our faculties to matriculate part time or by means of extension courses at colleges and universities and work toward their academic degrees.

The Executive Board of the NCA has been approached asking for a yearly $1000 grant to each of the accredited colleges to help defray the expenses that the afore designated program would entail.

The participating faculty member would have to sign a three year contract with the college to avoid any "run out" after the privileges had been enjoyed.

The fourteenth point presented for deliberation was a reference to the extended questionnaire that each of the accredited colleges had received from a Mr. Victor Presale in relation to the recommended facilities and arrangements that might be included in a new college building plant. It appears that the gentleman is interested in chiropractic and working toward his master's degree in architecture and had chosen this project. Dr. Nugent was asked to answer the questionnaire as thoroughly as possible.

As the fifteenth point, reference was made to the Illinois situation.

Dr. Janse advised the council of the recent happenings that had created such a reaction in all of the major newspapers of the state. It appears that the lobbying firm that had been employed by the unlicensed group to sponsor their bill had sought to conduct a suit against the unlicensed group because of failure to meet their financial obligations to them. The newspaper quoted this lobby concern as maintaining that a "war chest" of $150,000 had been collected to help put the unlicensed bill through. Apparently after the bill failed the unlicensed group reneged on their obligations to the lobby organization; hence, the suit.

Since then a graduate of the P.S.C. had instituted an injunction suit against the medical board and compelled them to permit him to take the state board examination notwithstanding the fact that the P.S.C. was not accredited by the state department of education.

Dr. Nugent then advised that he had been in Chicago and had been asked by officers of the Illinois Chiropractic Society to consult with them upon the matter. He met with Judge (Miss) Bionics, the Director of the Department of Registration, and had sought to impress upon her the seriousness of the situation. Judge Bionics had advised him and the ICS officers that the unlicensed problem was actually not the concern of her department but a matter for the attorney-general and his law enforcement agents.

Judge Bionics had invited him to meet with the Board at its next meeting. It might be added that since the council meetings he, Dr. Nugent, did meet with members of the board and he had made the following recommendation to the board, that an interim committee of two medical men, two chiropractors and he meet for the purpose of studying the unlicensed situation and if possible come up with some kind of solution.

Afternoon meeting, Thursday, February 17th, 1956, Dr. Thure C. Peterson, presiding.

This meeting had been set aside for the purpose of meeting with representatives of the National Council of Chiropractic Examining Boards. Drs. G.H. Peters, Adam Baer, and Joseph Hoyt had been expected to attend but only Dr. Peters was able to attend, he being the chairman of the council.

Dr. Peterson drew Dr. Peters' attention to the fact that graduates of the accredited colleges were at times put to a rather severe economic hazard by being required to wait 4 to 6 months before they are able to take boards. He recommended that all boards make it a policy to conduct three examinations a year, designating the months of February, June and October as the most favorable months for boards to meet as they represent the months after college graduation.

A discussion was then conducted in relation to the matter of accreditation. Reference was made to the questions posed by Dr. Hoyt in the Bulletin of the Council of Chiropractic Examining Boards; namely, what accrediting agency should be recognized and awarded deference. Dr. Peters commented by stating that it appeared as if there existed a three sided struggle between the NCA and ICA and the state boards proper and as a result the entire profession was in a state of confusion and division.

Dr. Peterson then stated that the NCA accredited colleges were making extended sacrifices for the sake of an ideal. He used the example of Dr. Ellison, the secretary of the Ontario Board, and his comments about the great service that the council was rendering.

To this comment Dr. Peters directed the question as to whether the council recommended that the Council of Chiropractic Examining Boards only recognize NCA approved colleges.

Dr. Nugent interjected the comment that wherever possible boards should seek to award recognition to the NCA accrediting program, but if that is not possible the educational standards and policies of the accrediting committee should be acknowledged.

It was concluded that the Council on Education could not expect all boards to recognize the NCA accredited list only but possibly the boards might be induced to accept the NCA standards.

Dr. Peters then asked the council's aid in discouraging the sponsoring of various professional "salesmanship" courses which, in his opinion, were converting chiropractic into a sales seduction procedure. He mentioned that the North Carolina State Association had ruled against the teaching of these courses in the state.

Dr. Peters then inquired whether it wouldn't be possible to have a composite accrediting committee, consisting of representatives of the NCA, ICA, Canadian Chiropractic Assn. and the Council of Chiropractic Examining Boards.

Dr. Nugent advised Dr. Peters that such would be impossible for the simple reason that the ideological differences between the NCA and ICA would not permit such an amalgamation of effort.

Dr. Walter Wolf of the accrediting committee then advised the council that he had attended the recent meetings of the American Association of Basic Science Boards in Chicago. He stated that certain segments of the medical profession were seeking the repeal of basic science legislation. He also advised that the following basic science boards had indicated their possible readiness to honor the certifications of national medical, osteopathic and chiropractic boards. The boards included Alaska, District of Columbia, Connecticut, Iowa, Minnesota, Oklahoma, Tennessee, Texas and Wisconsin.

It was the consensus of opinion that a careful study should be made to determine whether the council might not be the agent through which a competent National Board of Chiropractic Examiners could be organized so that if this opportunity did arise advantage could be taken of it.

Dr. Justin C. Wood, member of the Executive Board was then asked to detail certain matters that he wanted to present to the council. Following are the major points of his discussion:

    a.   He expressed his pleasure in the efforts of the council and voiced the conviction that every member of the council was a strong supporter of the NCA program.

    b.   In order for our profession to succeed it must become a fully disciplined profession.

    c.   Might it be that we have failed to sell NCA to our students? We should be more militant and enthusiastic in presenting the NCA program to the members of the student bodies of the accredited colleges.

    d.   Every student in the accredited colleges should be a Jr. NCA member.

    e.   Every faculty member of the accredited colleges should be a member of the NCA.

    f.   There should be a faculty advisor for the Jr. NCA.

At this time the hour was late and it was time to adjourn.

That evening the council membership were guests at a reception as conducted by the personnel of the Canadian Memorial Chiropractic College and its board of management. After the reception a most delightful dinner was had, Japanese style, at which Dr. Homewood, Dean of the college, presided. He called on various members of the council, as well as the Canadian College and Board of Control, to make some friendly comments.

Friday morning, February 18, the entire council membership visited the Canadian Memorial Chiropractic College. After a tour through the entire plant during which a number of classes in session were observed and laboratories visited, a general assembly of the student body was called and a friendly, interesting program was conducted. Dr. Homewood, dean, led the assembly and he called on every member of the council to say a few words.

Following are copies of the letters written by Dr. Janse to Dr. Homewood, Dean of the college, and Dr. Price, President of the Board of Control.

Dr. Earl A. Homewood, Dean, Canadian Memorial Chiropractic College, 252 Bloor Street, West, Toronto, Canada
Dear Doctor Homewood:

It is my pleasant responsibility to express the appreciation of all the members of the council for the hospitalities enjoyed during the Toronto meetings. Certainly you and your associates were most considerate hosts and provided us with a warm and genuine feeling of "welcome".

We especially enjoyed our visit to the college and the privilege of visiting with your student body in assembly. We were impressed with the well integrated program that is being conducted and were pleased with the student spirit in general.

Certainly it was an evidence of good management and instruction. Be assured of our pleasure in having Canadian Memorial Chiropractic College as a participating member of the council and may we express the hope that such will always be the mutual privilege enjoyed by us of the States and you of Canada.

With expressions of personal admiration and appreciation I seek to remain Very truly yours,   J. Janse, Secretary

Dr. James A. Price, President
Board of Control, Canadian Memorial Chiropractic College, 141 Danforth Avenue, Toronto, Canada
Dear Doctor Price:

It gives me a genuine pleasure to express the heartfelt appreciation of the members of the council for the most hospitable considerations that we experienced during the meetings in Toronto. Your kindness and that of your associates was gracious and abundant. Permit us to express our sincerest respect and admiration.   All of us enjoyed the social functions very much, they serving to relax the pressures of work and to augment the friendliness that must attend any group effort if it is to be successful.

Our visit to the college was a pleasant one. Certainly there was every evidence to show good management, student control and instruction. I am confident that every member of the council was impressed and would like to extend compliments.

We are proud that Canadian Memorial is a full participating member of the council and we hope that this relationship between the colleges of our sister countries might continue with benefit to all.

Might I personally express my pride and admiration for the grand job that you are doing, I seek to remain with every good wish Sincerely yours, J. Janse, Secretary.

Friday afternoon meetings, February 18, 1956, Dr. Peterson presiding.

Dr. Justin C. Wood of the Executive Board was again in attendance and Dr. Peterson asked whether the council might submit to Dr. Wood a number of recommendations to be carried back to the board for their deliberation.

(1) It is the desire of the council to have the NCA executive secretary set up an ad listing all of the accredited colleges. That this ad should be announced to all the editors of the various state journals with the advice that it is the wish of the schools participating in the council program not to advertise individually but to have this collective ad serve the purpose of representing the council schools in any and all professional publications.

(2) That a similar effort be made in relation to a display for convention booths. That this display should be so arranged that it emphasizes the collective standards of the NCA accredited colleges.

(3) That because of previous commitments nothing should be done on the above until the July convention in Chicago.

(4) That Bulletins number one and two (as prepared by the Committee on Educational Standards) be sent to all educational agencies, libraries, as well as leading figures in the profession at large.

(5) That bulletin number one be inserted in the folder sent out to vocational guidance directors.

(6) That the latest issue of "Educational Standards For Chiropractic Schools" be included to all sendings to libraries, etc.

(7) The possibility of providing each of the accredited colleges with a grant of $1000 annually for the purpose of helping to send one or more of the faculty members to a state or city college or university for further training in his major of teaching.

(8) That it was the general consensus of opinion on the part of most of the schoolmen that it might be best to include Jr. NCA membership in the matriculation fee, or yearly student body activity fee. The idea of a flat rate of $5 Jr. NCA membership fee for the total of the four years at college was recommended.

(9) There should be some reduction in the general membership fee for members of the faculties of the accredited colleges, possibly half rate.

Dr. Homewood advised the council that because of the fact that the Canadian College was heavily subsidized by the field and a goodly number of these people were ICA members it would be impossible for the Canadian Memorial to sustain a 100% Jr. NCA program.

Dr. Peterson then advised the council that he and Mrs. Peterson were contemplating a trip to Europe this coming summer. These plans would not permit him to attend the council meetings at the annual NCA convention to be held in Chicago. Furthermore, the staggering amount of work confronting him at the Chiropractic Institute prompts him to deem it necessary to submit his resignation as Chairman of the Council.

Every member of the council expressed his regret at this decision. Sincere and heartfelt comments of appreciation were directed to Dr. Peterson for the wise and prudent service that he had rendered.

Dr. Peterson turned the meeting over to Dr. Janse, secretary who called for nominations for the office of chairman. The name of Dr. Arthur G. Hendricks, President of the Lincoln Chiropractic College, was presented. This nomination was seconded and then it was recommended that the nominations be closed and Dr. Hendricks elected by acclamation. This recommendation was seconded and Dr. Hendricks was unanimously elected by acclamation to the chairmanship of the council.

Dr. Hendricks then took the chair and Dr. Janse submitted his resignation as secretary of the council. It was recommended by both Drs. Peterson and Hendricks that Dr. Janse remain as secretary. This recommendation was unanimously carried.

Drs. Peterson and Janse then expressed their appreciation to the council for the cooperation that they had been privileged to experience. Each voiced admiration and respect for each other and complimented the council on the wise choice in electing Dr. Hendricks. Dr. Hendricks then expressed his appreciation for the confidence placed in him and committed himself to the desire to seek the cooperation and support of everyone.

Drs. Nugent and Martin both spoke with appreciation about the fine work that Dr. Peterson had done and expressed the hope that the council would be always aware of the same.

Dr. Peterson in his final remarks stated that he felt rather sentimental about the fact that some of the former associates of the council were no longer present and hoped that possibly some of the institutions who had pulled away from the council might be induced to come back as subscribing participants.

Closed meeting, Friday afternoon, February 10, 1956 - Dr. A.G. Hendricks, presiding.

Dr. Hendricks called for a report of the accrediting committee. Dr. Ralph J. Martin, chairman of the committee made the following statements.

(1) Dr. Nugent, as the Director of Education had made an extensive report to the committee and hence the committee was well informed as to the circumstances existing throughout the profession in relation to chiropractic education.

(2) The Committee on Educational Standards (Accrediting Committee) wished to submit a resolution which in substance instructed

the Western States College of Portland, Oregon, that beginning September 1, 1956, it should seek to discontinue matriculating students for training in naturopathy. That the school should continue to progressively terminate its obligations to those naturo-pathic students already enrolled as competently as time and circumstance would permit.

    a. Dr. Nugent advised the council that he had been in almost constant contact with both Drs. Higgens and Failor in relation to this matter and that both had agreed that this step was necessary, although it would involve extended financial loss and result in a severe economic compromise that the college might not be able to survive.

    b. Dr. Nugent further stated that Drs. Higgens and Failor had advised him by telephone that they had just had a Jr. NCA day at which they had announced the decision to discontinue the naturopathic course, and that although a marked disturbance had been sensed among the students and constituents the entire matter had been consummated without any untoward reaction.

    c. Since the council meetings, the following announcement has been received from the Western States College:

A STATEMENT OF POLICY ON WESTERN STATES COLLEGE

After lengthy deliberation by the various segments of the profession interested in this college, an important decision has been made.

For a number of years Western States College has maintained a School of Naturopathy and a School of Chiropractic. The National Chiropractic Association and the American Association of Naturopathic Physicians, through their school accrediting agencies, had agreed to this co-educational cooperation. Circumstances and legislative actions now indicate that this alliance is no longer necessary.

This letter is intended to inform the profession that we will accept no more applicants for matriculation in the School of Naturopathy. All students of Naturopathy now matriculated are assured that classes will continue until they receive their degrees. The graduates in the field may rest assured their diplomas will remain valid. The School of Naturopathy is not being dissolved. There will merely be a suspension of matriculation. The organization, charter and records will remain active and current at all times.

This action has not been done in haste or by the demand of any profession or organization. The leaders of Chiropractic and Naturopathy have been helpful and considerate in bringing this about. The many necessary details pertaining to this action have not been fully understood by persons not directly interested in Western States College. Doctors of Chiropractic and Naturopathic profession who have not kept abreast of this development have received much misinformation and this notice is to inform you that Western States College will continue to maintain the highest possible scholastic standards. It will concentrate its efforts on the School of Chiropractic.

Yours very truly, WESTERN STATES COLLEGE,   R.M. Failor, D.C., N.D., President.

Following is a copy of the letter that Dr. Janse as secretary of the council had been instructed in substance to write.

Dr. Ralph M. Failor, President, Western States College of Chiropractic, 4525 S.E. 63rd Ave., Portland 6, Oregon
Dear Doctor Failor:

The entire membership of the National Council on Education of the National Chiropractic Association wishes to express their greatest respect for the decision that Western States College has made in announcing its discontinuance of naturopathic matriculation.

Such we know has represented a difficult and financially compromising thing to do. We have been aware, at least in part, of the varying and overlapping circumstances that have confronted the institution. Certainly the courage and integrity that this commanded is to be respected by all.

We wish to express our warmest greetings to you personally and hope that you will be able to be with us at the next meeting.

Please convey this message of appreciation and admiration to the entire college family.

With every good wish for a most competent and satisfying future for Western States College, we seek to remain as a council
Yours sincerely, J. Janse, Secretary

    (3) Dr. Martin then presented the matter of the Internists or Extension Course that was being conducted by the Specialties Societies of the California Chiropractic Association, and being accredited by the Los Angeles College of Chiropractic.

    a. Dr. Nugent expressed the opinion that it was bad policy to teach an extension course conducted by instructors who were not part of the regular college faculty and over whose teaching and subject material there apparently was little control.

    b. Dr. Peterson expressed the opinion that apparently the course entailed the teaching of subjects which the local (territorial) chiropractic colleges did not desire to teach.

    c. Dr. Haynes advised the council that if he were to be asked to go back to California with instruction that the Los Angeles College should step away from this venture entirely it would severely disturb the unity that he and his associates had been able to affect between the vying elements out in California and whose support the school needed.

    d. After further deliberation it was unanimously concluded that a committee consisting of Drs. Nugent, Martin and Gardner should seek to consult with the related individuals and determine whether a proper solution could not be found.

    (4) Dr. Martin then asked that a resolution be passed that would ask the chairman of the council to appoint a committee which would bring in recommendations as to how graduate and post-graduate education might be most competently conducted in the accredited colleges.

    (5) Dr. Martin then submitted the following recommendation in relation to the procedure to be followed by the Director of Education when making an official inspection of a school.

"It has been agreed within the Committee on Educational Standards (accrediting committee) that school inspections by the Director of Education shall be filed with the committee before a bill of particulars and recommendations shall be given the school."

This was unanimously passed as a resolution by the council.

(6) The next matter for report was that pertaining to the problem of the National College of Chiropractic. Dr. Martin advised the council that he and his associates on the accrediting committee had been in frequent conference with Mr. Miller and Dr. Janse who were at the meetings representing the National College. That after extended deliberations an amicable and fully acceptable solution to the problem had been reached, which fully satisfied the accrediting committee and represented conformity with the educational code of the committee. Following were the mutual agreements attained:

a. That a doctor of chiropractic will be placed on the Board of Trustees of the National College of Chiropractic. That this person will be a leading personality in the profession and the National College alumni faculty.

b. That the accrediting committee is to receive annually a statement of the net worth of the college.

c. That the National College in fulfilling these agreements would then fully conform to the educational code of the committee and experience all the consideration and deference that related thereto.

Dr. Nugent stated that he was glad that a conclusion to the problem had been attained. He expressed the opinion that the members of the accrediting committee, as well as the council in general, had been more than patient with the situation and that Mr. Turek in his hesitancies to conform had necessitated added work and sacrifice on the part of certain council members. He expressed the hope that the chiropractic member of the Board of Trustees of the National College would find it possible to attend some of the council meetings to evaluate the importance of the council's work.

Mr. Miller expressed his satisfaction in the understanding that had been reached but expressed the hope that the accrediting committee would instruct the Director of Education to refrain from talking about the intimate details and problems of one school to representatives of another school or to the field in general, and to refrain from being unduly hypercritical of any school when in conversation with students or the alumni of that school.

This was acknowledged by the council as being essential in all instances.

Dr. Janse then expressed his appreciation for the fact that an understanding had been reached. He stated that on no occasion had Mr. Turek thought of being inconsiderate of the council or its ideals, but that he, in his own singular way, had made outstanding contributions to the profession of chiropractic and the program of the NCA and the council.

Dr. Martin then stated with emphasis that all feelings of the past, delinquents of disposition, and accusations must be entirely forgotten and buried.

Dr. Nugent then asked for the privilege of referring to a subject of previous discussion; namely, the one relating to Dr. Wolf's announcement that certain of the basic science boards were contemplating extending recognition to the National medical and osteopathic boards. This according to Dr. Nugent should prompt the council into the effort of creating a National Board of Chiropractic Examiners, consisting of the finest talent in the profession. The board should be patterned after the National Medical Board and should be conducted with the strictest decorum. Dr. Hendricks expressed the opinion that the National Board should be set up by the council. In conclusion, it was the consensus of opinion that much had been attained in this session of the council.

Schoolmen expenses were prorated.

Subsequent occurrences.

While Dr. Janse was in Switzerland he had been approached by the officers of the Swiss Chiropractic Association in relation to a problem that confronted the doctors of chiropractic in the Canton of Zurich. Two men are practicing chiropractic in this Canton who claim to possess degrees from the Ross-O'Neil College, Fort Wayne, Indiana. Investigation proved that they had obtained these degrees in no more than six months' residence time. Furthermore, that during these six months not too much scholastic and clinical participation had been obtained. The medical society in the Canton of Zurich is now using these two men as an example of the low educational standards sustained by chiropractic as a whole and thus seeking to eliminate legislation permitting the practice of chiropractic in the Canton.

Since then Dr. Janse has received an official communication from Dr. Frank Keller, of Zurich, Switzerland, requesting that the council submit a deposition detailing the accepted standards in chiropractic and also the circumstances surrounding the Ross-O'Neil College. Dr. Janse consulted with Dr. Hendricks, chairman of the council, by telephone. The following brief was prepared and sent to the chairman for approval and then relayed to Dr. Keller.

TO WHOM IT MAY CONCERN:

This deposition has been prepared at the request of the Swiss Chiropractic Association the official representative of the chiropractic profession in Switzerland.

In order that the statements contained herein may be interpreted as coming from an authoritative source the following brief informations are pertinent.

1. The National Council on Education is the Accrediting Agency of the National Chiropractic Association.

2. The council has been in existence since 1945 and from that time on has recognized nothing less than a course in chiropractic of four collegiate years of nine months each.

3. Since its inception the council through its committee of accreditation and the director of education of the National Chiropractic Association has sought to maintain the standards as defined in the accompanying bulletin: "Educational Standards For

Chiropractic Schools," as prepared by John J. Nugent, D.C., Director of Education, National Chiropractic Association.

It has been drawn to the council's attention that there are several individuals now occupied in the practice of chiropractic in Switzerland who because of unqualified training stand to compromise and jeopardize the professional integrity of those who constitute the legitimate element of the profession in Switzerland.

We understand that these people claim to have obtained their training at the former Ross-O'Neil Chiropractic College of Fort Wayne, Indiana.

The circumstances surrounding this claim, along with the deficiencies both in the academic and administrative aspects of this college prompt us to set for the following reasons why these people in question, should not be privileged the status of being recognized as qualified representatives and practitioners of chiropractic.

1. Reputable evidence cause us to know that their degree, doctor of chiropractic was procured by these individuals within a resident time of six months. Such a tenure of training being ridiculously brief and certainly wholly inadequate.
2. The Ross-O'Neil Chiropractic College, because of its low standard program never enjoyed accreditation by the National Council on Education.
3. The Ross-O'Neil Chiropractic College, long before its demise in 1952 had operated on a very limited and wholly inadequate budget and scholastic program.
4. During the latter years of its existence this college did not sustain a proper curriculum, students were accepted for enrollment at any time and beginning and advanced students were received in the same classes.
5. The college was finally forced to close in October 1952, for the following reasons.
   a. Lack of operating funds.
   b. Lack of sustaining enrollment.
   c. Refusal on the part of State Boards of Chiropractic Examiners throughout the country to further accept graduates of the college for examination.
   d. Loss of accreditation by the Department of Veterans Affairs of the State of Indiana.

We, therefore, strongly urge that the Swiss Chiropractic Association be sustained in its insistence that the court deter the individuals in question from any further privileges to represent themselves and to practice as chiropractors or as doctors of chiropractic. Anything less than this would represent a compromise of justice and a disrespect of public safe-guard.

Joseph Janse, D.C., Secretary, National Council on Education of the National Chiropractic Association

Subscribed and sworn to and before me this 17th day of March 1956. My commission expires April 26, 1956.

Minutes of the COUNCIL ON EDUCATION of the NATIONAL CHIROPRACTIC ASSOCIATION, Morrison Hotel, July 1-6, 1956, Chicago, Illinois

The annual meeting of the Council on Education was held in conjunction with the convention of the NCA July 1, 2, 3, 4, 5 and 6 at the Morrison Hotel in Chicago. Dr. Arthur G. Hendricks, Chairman of the Council, presided at all the meetings.

Those attending included:
A. Members of the Committee on Educational Standards:
   Dr. Ralph J. Martin, Chairman of the Committee, 30 W. Sierra Madre Blvd., Sierra Madre, California
   Dr. Edw. H. Gardner, Secretary of Committee, 1655 N. Normandie, Hollywood, California
   Dr. John J. Nugent, Director of Education, 92 Norton Street, New Haven, Connecticut
   Dr. Walter B. Wolf, 207 W. Main Street, Eureka, South Dakota
   Dr. Norman E. Osborne, Long Meadows Extension, Hagerstown, Maryland
B. Representatives of the accredited colleges:
   Dr. Arthur G. Hendricks, Chairman of the Council, President of the Lincoln Chiropractic College, Inc., 633 N. Pennsylvania Ave., Indianapolis 5, Indiana
   Dr. Joseph Janse, Secretary of the Council, President of the National College of Chiropractic, 20 N. Ashland Blvd., Chicago 7, Illinois
   Dr. Clarence W. Weiant, Dean, Chiropractic Institute of New York, 325 E. 38th Street, New York 16, New York
   Dr. Julius C. Troilo, Dean, Texas Chiropractic College, San Pedro Park, San Antonio, Texas
   Dr. John B. Wolfe, President, Northwestern College of Chiropractic, 2222 Park Avenue, Minneapolis 2, Minnesota
   Dr. Earl A. Homewood, Dean, Canadian Memorial Chiropractic College, 252 Bloor Street, West, Toronto, Canada
   Dr. George E. Haynes, Dean, Los Angeles College of Chiropractic, 920 E. Broadway, Glendale 5, California
C. Others in attendance included:
   Mr. Charles A. Miller, Vice President, National College of Chiropractic; Dr. A.H. Barmen, Dean, Lincoln Chiropractic College, Inc.; Dr. Sol Goldschmidt, Member of Board of Directors, Chiropractic Institute of New York; Dr. J. Lamoine DeRusha, Dean, Northwestern College of Chiropractic; Dr. H.C. Harring, President, Missouri Chiropractic College, Inc., St. Louis, Missouri; Dr. Louis G. Gearhart, President, University of Natural Healing Arts, Denver, Colorado; Dr. Edw. G.

Hearn, President, Texas Chiropractic College; Dr. Bernard Levine, Faculty Member, Chiropractic Institute of New York; Dr. Henry C. Schneider, Faculty Member, Northwestern College of Chiropractic

Dr. Thure C. Peterson, President of the Chiropractic Institute of New York, vacationing in Europe and attending the Annual Convention of the European Chiropractors Union, in Zurich, Switzerland, sent his greetings and best wishes to the Council.

The Western States College of Chiropractic did not have representation at the meeting.

FIRST SESSION

At the first order of procedure Dr. Hendricks, chairman of the Council, read a letter of appreciation from Dr. Peterson, for the plaque that had been sent to him by the Council in honor and gratitude for the great service he had rendered during his tenure as chairman of the Council. The prorated expense of the plaque was covered by the various accredited colleges and submitted to the Council Secretary.

Another letter was read from Dr. Peterson relaying his greetings to the Council and extending his best wishes.

Dr. Hendricks then called on Dr. Janse to read the deposition that had been prepared at the request of the Swiss Chiropractic Association in relation to unqualified practitioners. This deposition was prepared under the instructions of Dr. Hendricks and Peterson and attached to the minutes of the previous mid-year meeting. The intent and contents of the deposition were unanimously approved of by the Council membership in attendance.

The next matter brought into discussion and consideration was the request submitted to the Council by Dr. Herman S. Schwartz, chairman of the Council on Chiropractic Psychotherapy, that support be afforded his new book "When Mental Illness Strikes Your Home." Following were some of the discussions and conclusions that ensued.

a. A study of the outline of the contents submitted by Dr. Schwartz to various of the school men revealed that the book was really not a textbook but more of a manual on home treatment in the management of the less formidable mental and emotional disorders. Hence it was finally concluded that the book could not be prescribed as a class room text but rather recommended as collateral reading and practice reference.

b. It was concluded that wherever possible texts and books written by members of the profession should experience greater support from the colleges either as prescribed texts or recommendation for collateral reading.

c. The value of texts and books written by competent members of the profession resided primarily in the fact that they portray the chiropractic concept.

d. The Director of Education advised that the various members of the accredited college faculties desirous of writing books and texts should be encouraged to refer to the clinical and chiropractic subjects rather than the basic sciences. The reason being that certainly in the average basic science there are already many fine texts available that probably could not be improved upon. On the other hand, there is an ever increasing need for texts in the various clinical phases of chiropractic.

e. It was also suggested that it might be of benefit to appoint a committee with the assigned responsibility of carefully reviewing and editing books written by doctors of chiropractic and to determine whether the NCA would be in a position to underwrite the expense of some of the better written texts if necessary. In this respect no further action was taken.

f. In a subsequent session Dr. Schwartz appeared before the Council and asked for assistance in assuring the distribution of his new book. Upon being asked as in what manner his needs would be best served he frankly acknowledged that he had no definite plan in mind and had hoped that probably the Council might make some recommendation to him. Further considerations led to the following conclusions:

(1) That various members of the Council carefully read the script of the book and conclude as to its merit and clinical value.

(2) That if the script proves to be as anticipated, the Council members make every sincere endeavor to incorporate its usage either as a prescribed text or a text for collateral reading in the accredited colleges.

(3) To recommend the book to the various professional groups encountered on the many appearances of the various Council members at state and national conventions.

(4) To encourage all the agencies of the NCA to lend themselves in similar support to the efforts and contributions of Dr. Schwartz.

The Council next carefully considered the ever increasing trend among basic science and composite medical boards toward the objective fill in, true and false, and multiple choice type of examinations.

a. Dr. Janse emphasized the importance of carefully estimating the effect of this trend upon chiropractic examinees and the methods of instruction in the various accredited colleges. He cited the instance of the Illinois Board which at the last two examinations resorted to the multiple choice questions in the basic sciences, and advised the Council that in this instance they were the same questions as used by the National Medical Board.

b. Dr. Nugent expressed the opinion that possibly once the technic of this type of examination be mastered they should not represent a hazard and might be less difficult to handle because in estimating chiropractic examinees one of their primary deficiencies is in the proper writing of discussion answers because of their incompetence in grammar.

c. Dr. Janse insisted that greater concern should be exercised in this respect. That it was fundamentally impossible to expect the average chiropractic student to fully parallel the academic capacities of medical students, because of the latter's pre-professional background and because the medical student in all instances represents a hand picked scholastic personality. The fact cannot be avoided that in many instances we are asking our chiropractic students to measure up to the talents of the medical student in every respect when neither his background or the depth of his education has privileged him to acquire these abilities.

d. Dr. Wolf, as a member of the South Dakota Basic Science Board, verified the statement of Dr. Janse maintaining that the average chiropractic examinee was not as well qualified for his examinations as the medical student.

e. The final conclusions after some further discussions were the following:

    (1) That a concentrated effort be made to obtain sample copies of the new types of examinations to be distributed to the accredited colleges.

    (2) That some competent member of one of the faculties be appointed to assemble and edit state board questions and possibly answers of all types. To properly catalog them and then to send them into the NCA offices for multigraphing. Drs. Hendricks and Janse were instructed to present this matter and request to the Executive Board for consideration.

    (3) That whenever possible the Council officers, the Director of Education as well as the various members of the Council should seek to mediate with the various basic science board and medical board members and draw their attention and consideration to the problem that confronts the chiropractic examinee and if possible seek to obtain some attitude of deference.

f. Dr. Hendricks then related the unfortunate happenings at the recent basic science board examinations in Florida, where some 70 chiropractic examinees of the P.S.C. sought to obtain certification by the board on the basis of the indiscretion of obtaining the questions by means of a "blind student plant" before the regular examination. This misconduct was apprehended and all 70 examinees denied the privilege of sitting for the examination by the office of the Governor directly.

The next matter for consideration related to the request by the Charles O. Puffer Public Relations Firm, under contract to the NCA, that all of the accredited colleges ready their facilities for the teaching of Civil Defense work.

a. Mr. Puffer contacted Dr. Janse and advised him that he had mediated with Mr. Val Peterson, National Director for Civil Defense, and advised him that he was certain the various NCA accredited colleges would be willing to cooperate with the various regional Civil Defense agencies and incorporate a course in Civil Defense (probably some 8 to 16 hours) in the regular first aid course of the curriculum. A regular Civil Defense instructor would come in to conduct the class during the period of specific instruction.

b. Dr. Janse had contacted all of the schools per letter and had received indications of readiness to participate if such an effort could be proven to be to the full interest of the country.

c. Dr. Weiant expressed the caution that the school men should only commit themselves to a participation if the entire program be kept away from any attempt to propagandize.

d. Dr. Haynes maintained that it should be left entirely up to the various colleges to determine whether they should or should not take part.

e. Dr. Nugent insisted that as citizens we should certainly be ready to do our part in the all important program of Civil Defense. He felt that not only the school but also the practitioners should seek to place their talents and facilities at the disposal of the regional agency. He agreed with Dr. Weiant that any participation should not be made the subject of a propaganda project.

f. Dr. Homewood stated that at the Canadian College a special course was being organized for the neighboring doctors of chiropractic.

g. Dr. DeRusha advised that in Minneapolis a local group of doctors of chiropractic had taken a course and upon their certificates no designation was made of their doctorate title or degree.

h. The final conclusion was that of having the various colleges establish their own programs of participation when requested and according to their own circumstances.

Dr. Hendricks then asked for further discussion of the matter that had been taken up in Toronto at the mid-year meeting in relation to encouraging the NCA to subsidize the accredited colleges in support of the recommended program to have certain members of the various faculties seek to return to college to do either graduate work, or work toward a baccalaureate degree in the progressive effort to more competently qualify our accredited college faculties for their work.

a. Dr. Nugent advised the Council that he had approached the Executive Board about the proposition and that consequently Dr. L.M. Rogers in his annual report to the House of Delegates had recommended that some $5,000 a year be set aside for this purpose. Dr. Nugent advised that he had recommended $10,000.

b. Dr. Janse asked for a rather broad interpretation of the prescribed privileges of participation. He cited the example of the fact that in all the accredited colleges there were permanent full time faculty members who had proven their capacities and value yet who did not possess a college degree although having had a number of years of pre-professional college training. It was felt that these men who had proven of such worth and who had contributed so much to the educational picture in the profession should certainly experience the privilege of participating in the program, permitting them to first obtain their baccalaureate and then eventually their graduate degree.

c. Dr. Nugent fully agreed with this recommendation acknowledging the fact that in all the accredited colleges were indispensable talented instructors who had never been privileged to obtain their collegiate degrees and certainly any program should include them within its privileges.

Dr. Nugent reiterated his difficulty in presenting a competent criterion of standards to any accrediting agency or group either of state or national government without having men with graduate degrees heading the various teaching departments, especially in the basic sciences.

d. Dr. Weiant agreed that sufficient latitude should be permitted in any evolved program to permit and encourage undergraduate work if necessary. Dr. Hendricks concurred with this premise as did all the other school heads.

e. Finally the following conclusions were reached:

(1)   That any program for advanced educational privileges for picked faculty members of the accredited colleges should be sufficiently broad to permit undergraduate work as well as graduate work so as to enable a larger percentage of the tried and proven faculty members of the various colleges to take advantage of the opportunity.

(2)   That each college in conjunction with the Director of Education seek to determine how the program might function most competently in relation to the individual needs of the various schools.

(3)   That the participating faculty member should be bound by certain stipulations to be set up and agreed upon by the Council. The reason for this being to avoid any tendency on the part of any participating faculty member to walk out on his obligations after the privilege of his background had been realized. In this respect the following suggestions were submitted for further consideration:

    (a)   That the participating faculty member sign a contract for 3 to 5 years tenure.

    (b)   That he not be employed by any of the other accredited colleges without the express permission of the administration of the college under whose auspices he obtained his extension education.

    (c)   That if he does decide to discontinue his affiliation with the college he reimburse the college and the NCA the amount spent on him by both organizations.

First session adjourned 5:30 p.m.

The second session of the Council was held Tuesday afternoon, July 3, with Dr. Hendricks presiding.

Dr. Hendricks, as chairman, advised that on Wednesday afternoon the Council had been invited to attend the special meeting to be held by the National Council of Chiropractic Examining Boards, at which Dr. John J. Nugent, Director of Education of the National Chiropractic Association, and Dr. C.A. Adams, Director of Education of the ICA had been invited to present the views and program of these respective associations on chiropractic education.

The chairman then asked for a discussion on the matter that had been brought up and considered in Toronto in relation to the possibility of all of the accredited colleges advertising collectively.

    a.   Dr. Hendricks advised the group that he had not gone through with the proposed ad for the special June convention issue of the New York Journal for the simple reason that all of the colleges had not answered his inquiry as to whether they desired to participate.

    b.   Dr. Haynes insisted that the accredited colleges should not be required to participate if they did not consider it advantageous because of regional limitations. Furthermore, that if the colleges advertise collectively in one journal they would out of common necessity have to advertise in all the journals and for that reason he felt that the colleges just should not advertise unless the ads are run as a help and courtesy to the colleges without charge.

    c.   Dr. Nugent maintained that the Chiropractic Editors Guild should be contacted and consulted, submitting the request that all state journals accept without charge a standard ad, listing all the accredited colleges and inviting those interested to contact the various registrars of the colleges.

    d.   Subsequent to the foregoing, Drs. Hendricks and Janse had occasion to talk with the editors of the Michigan and New York State Journals and the idea of granting the NCA accredited colleges the privilege of running without charge an ad in the journals with each publication might experience favorable consideration.

Dr. Hendricks then asked Dr. Janse to read a letter that he had received from Dr. D.R. McDowell, Secretary-Treasurer of the South Dakota Board of Chiropractic Examiners, and Chairman of the Committee on Standardization of State Board Examinations of the National Council of Chiropractic Examining Boards.

(Copy of Letter from South Dakota State Board of Chiropractic Examiners)
Sioux Falls, S. Dak., June 1, 1956
Dr. Jos. Janse, National College of Chiropractic, 20 N. Ashland Blvd., Chicago 7, Illinois
Dear Dr. Janse:

The National Council of Chiropractic Examining Boards meets in Chicago, July 3, 4 and 5. We have various committees such as Accrediting, Basic Science, Legislative and Standardization of State Board Examinations, of which I am Chairman. This committee is two years old and last year we made the following report to the Council:

"The basis of this report is examinations given in 26 states; namely, Arkansas, Arizona, California, Colorado, Connecticut, Delaware, Florida, Georgia, Idaho, Iowa, Kansas, Kentucky, Maine, Maryland, Michigan, Montana, Nebraska, Nevada, New Hampshire, North Carolina, North Dakota, South Dakota, Tennessee, Texas, West Virginia and Wisconsin.

Findings: - A total of 35 subjects are given in examinations. They are: Anatomy, Physiology, Pathology, Orthopedy, Symptomatology, Hygiene, or Public Health, Chemistry, Chiropractic Principles, Chiropractic Analysis, Jurisprudence, Chiropractic Philosophy, Chiropractic Adjusting, Bacteriology, Histology, Palpation, Nerve Tracing, Analysis of Spine, Toxicology, Neurology, Obstetrics, Gynecology, Physiotherapy, Urinalysis, Pediatrics, Diagnosis, Dietetics, Drugless Therapy, Sanitation and Public Health, Spinography, Embryology, Dermatology, Eye, Ear, Nose and Throat, Microscopy, Physical Diagnosis and Drugless Therapy.

Subjects examined vary from 6 to 18. Of these, Anatomy, Physiology, Pathology, Orthopedia, Symptomatology, Hygiene and Public Health, Chiropractic Principles and Bacteriology seem to predominate.

Other subjects appear in various exams in states from one to nine states using them. For example, two states give examinations in Obstetrics and nine states examine in nerve tracing.

Recommendations -

1. State Boards agree on subjects to examine applicants
2. Examine in subjects given by majority of states
3. Agree on definite number of subjects
4. Standardize terminology
5. Aim toward examination that is comprehensive
6. Decide whether to use multiple choice questions or true and false."

After reading the above, I am wondering if you could offer some suggestions on how we as examining boards could standardize our examinations for your students graduating and coming into those various states to appear before our boards.

Thanking you in advance for suggestions you can give us, I remain Sincerely, D.R. McDowell, D.C., Chairman, Standardization of Examinations Committee

Following is the letter that Dr. Janse as Secretary of the Council wrote Dr. McDowell.

June 6, 1956

Dear Doctor McDowell:

Your communication of the 1st relates to a matter of great importance to all of us school men. It is almost frightening to think that the heterogeneity of our chiropractic boards would compel us in the schools to ready our examinees for thirty-five different subjects. Correspondence will not permit a thorough explanation of this problem. Certainly, it has received extensive considerations from the members of the Council. In brief, the following would be some of our recommendations:

1. That all of the specialty subjects, such as orthopedy, chiropractic analysis, nerve tracing, etc., be included under one common designation, such as, chiropractic principles, mechanics and procedures.
2. That all of the phases of anatomy, such as embryology, microscopy and neurology be included under the general heading of anatomy.
3. That all the diagnostic divisions be included under physical and clinical diagnosis.
4. That all the specialty therapies, such as dietetics, physiotherapy, and drugless therapy be included under chiropractic practice.
5. That such clinical specialties as dermatology, E.E.N.T., etc., be lumped together under clinical practice.

Certainly, it would make it much easier for everyone concerned if such measures of correction could be contemplated. It would allow the school men to standardize their catalogues; it would avoid a great deal of obsolete terminology, and actually permit the state boards to do a better job at examining.

I hope that during the NCA Convention, this matter might experience a very careful and considerate deliberation.

With all good and bright wishes, I am Sincerely yours,   J. Janse, Secretary.

Consequent to the Council meetings Dr. Janse received the following statement from Dr. McDowell.

To: National Council of Chiropractic Examining Boards
Re: Standardization of State Board Examinations

At the 1955 meeting of the Council, the committee on standardization of examinations submitted a report taken from the studies of 26 state chiropractic laws.

They found that students upon graduation appearing before various state boards were confronted by 35 subjects given in the states, some of them now obsolete and not being taught in our accredited schools.

Using these 35 subjects as a basis, the committee this year contacted the accredited chiropractic colleges on the subjects now taught and we submit the following recommendations which should be taken home by the various state boards and bills introduced into the legislature to standardize our state board examinations.

1. That all of the specialty subjects such as orthopedy, chiropractic analysis, nerve tracing, etc., be included under one common designation such as, Chiropractic Principles, Mechanics and Procedures.
2. That all of the phases of anatomy such as embryology, microscopy and neurology be included under the general heading of Anatomy.
3. That all the diagnostic divisions be included, physical and clinical diagnosis.
4. That all the specialty therapies such as dietetics, physiotherapy and drugless therapy be included under Chiropractic Practice.
5. That such clinical specialties as dermatology, E.E.N.T., etc., be lumped together under Clinical Practice.

Further, we are of the opinion that 9 subjects should cover everything from an examination standpoint as follows:

1. Anatomy	4. Pathology	7. Diagnosis
2. Bacteriology	5. Physiology	8. Principles
3. Chemistry	6. Public Health & Hygiene	9. Method of Adjusting

Further, in states where doctors of chiropractic are permitted to practice obstetrics and gynecology, the subject should be optional.

Further, in states where it is impossible to change the wording of the laws they could break down the various subjects as follows and still have the graduates confronted with only 9 examinations.

Anatomy:-	Hygiene and Public Health:-
Histology	Sanitation and Public Health
Embryology	Bacteriology
Neurology	X-ray
Microscopy	Spinography
Physiology:-	Chiropractic Practice
Dietetics	Analysis
Pathology:-	Palpation
Microscopy	Nerve Tracing
Diagnosis:-	Orthopedy
Symptomatology	Adjusting
Physical Diagnosis	Obstetrics and Gynecology
Urinalysis	Drugless Therapy:-
Pediatrics	Physiotherapy
Dermatology	Dietetics
Eye, Ear, Nose and Throat	
Chemistry:-	
Toxicology	

Further, if a student has passed an examination under a basic science board that examines in either of the first five or six subjects, he should be excused from repeating them and be examined only in those subjects not covered by basic science. We feel that re-examining a student in the same subjects is a slap at the basic science boards and undue repetition for graduates. We also feel that examination questions should be to the point and of a comprehensive type and that true-false or multiple choice often times become a guessing game for the applicant.

Lastly, the terminology of questions should be on a par with those used in the accredited schools and state board members giving examinations should watch themselves as many have specialized in special fields and have a tendency in their examinations to over emphasize their particular specialty and require a higher level of knowledge than should be expected justifiably of the general practitioner.

Signed: Standardization Committee, Chairman, Dr. D.R. McDowell, South Dakota; Dr. Gruening, New Jersey; Dr. Smith, Maryland; Dr. Davidson, Indiana; Dr. Sierra, Puerto Rico

In concluding the discussions a unanimous motion was passed to have a committee formed for the purpose of making a careful study of the various state board subjects, to seek to classify and standardize the same, and then to submit recommendations to Dr. McDowell and his committee.

A brief discussion was next concluded in relation to possible teaching aids. Following were the major points brought out:

a.   The Ciba Pharmaceutical House, has prepared a series of kodachrome 35 millimeter slides on anatomy and gross pathology which are extraordinary. They can be procured at a relatively nominal price.

b.   It was recommended that every college obtain the catalog of the American Society of Bacteriologists. The same can be obtained by writing Dr. Henry E. Morton, Chairman of the American Society of Bacteriologists, University of Pennsylvania, School of Medicine, Philadelphia, Pennsylvania.

c.   Dr. Goldschmidt recommended that all the colleges write to the United Fruit Company and obtain their literature on the various food and vitamin values in fruits. He did commit himself to provide the library of each of the colleges with a packet of literature.

d.   Dr. Levine suggested that from time to time the various departments of the accredited colleges exchange examination questions to provide the various faculties with an idea as to what is going on in the other colleges from an examination standpoint. This would, he insisted, be especially helpful and interesting in the field of chiropractic principles and practice.

Dr. Hendricks next called for a report and discussion by the committee that was assigned in Toronto to investigate the matter of transfer students. Following was the report that Dr. John B. Wolfe, chairman of the committee submitted:

REPORT OF COMMITTEE ON TRANSFER STUDENTS
COMMITTEE MEMBERS: Drs. Haynes, Troilo, Wolfe.
RECOMMENDATIONS ON TRANSFER OF STUDENTS FROM ACCREDITED SCHOOLS TO ACCREDITED SCHOOLS.

1.   A system of uniform transcript form should be adopted.

2.   A system of standard titles to courses should be evolved in which the course content is similar among the various schools within limitations imposed by differences in school character.

3.   A minimum honor point rating should be established below which a transfer student should not be accepted except after a waiting period of approximately six months and then only by action of the work committee and under conditions of strict probation.

4.   Full credit should be given for all work done in accredited schools for completed courses even when the hours do not exactly

coincide except where state law demands specific hour requirements in listed subjects.
5. When a student requests a transcript it should be coded on it his rating such as:
           1. Undesirable   2. Desirable   3. Financial difficulties
Either the above system should be employed or the admittance committee should request a confidential letter of recommendation from the dean of the previous school to the dean of the admitting school.

RECOMMENDATIONS ON TRANSFER FROM NON-ACCREDITED CHIROPRACTIC SCHOOLS.

1. The council should adopt an evaluation standard for each non-accredited school on an individual basis. This standard should be based on past experience, recommendations of the director of education and other inspection agencies, the disposition of state boards, and the general agreement of the council. This action would discourage the continuous outcropping of inferior schools and stop the shopping of potential transfer students from the schools of convenience to ones of respectability for the best 'deal.'

RECOMMENDATIONS ON TRANSFERS FROM OTHER SCHOOLS OR COLLEGES.

1. Credits from accredited colleges offering a baccalaureate degree should be accepted as advance credit only in the pre-clinical level.
2. No credit should be granted from schools of physiotherapy, massage, machine-therapy, naprapathy, etc.
3. Where pre-professional requirements are required for admission to a chiropractic school credit should not be granted as both pre-professional and professional for the same course unit.

In the subsequent discussions the following major points were brought into observations:
a. Dr. Troilo drew careful attention to the final point three on the report maintaining that there is a rather common tendency on the part of some matriculants to expect to receive both pre-professional credit as well as professional credit from some of the their pre-professional college work. Certainly in instances where pre-professional education is required this doubling up should not be permitted.
b. Dr. Troilo passed out a Progress Report and Transcript sheet as used at the Texas College and advised the school men that this sheet was simply Photostatted and sent in to the various state boards.
c. Dr. Haynes maintained that a greater effort should be made to more thoroughly standardize the curricula of the various colleges. He further recommended that effort be made to standardize the freshman, sophomore, junior and senior years so that a student transferring would not have his progress too severely garbled or interrupted.
d. Dr. Janse insisted that although this does not constitute the ideal certainly it would be very difficult to attain primarily for the reason that some of the colleges included the teaching of physiotherapy in their curricula and others did not and hence in order to make room for this subject matter some restrictions had to be made elsewhere, or on the other hand fill-ins would have to be provided for in the curricula of schools not teaching physiotherapy.
Dr. Haynes suggested that all schools standardize their subject material to conform to the minimum of all state board requirements.
Dr. Wolfe expressed his keen interest in graduate and extension work. He insisted that sooner or later the various colleges would have to contemplate the organizing of courses along these lines. He requested that the Council seek to obtain as much information as possible from the Los Angeles College which has penetrated the subject extensively.
Dr. Weiant advised the Council members that at the Chiropractic Institute of New York graduate course effort had met with little success as comparatively few of the regional doctors had seemed sufficiently interested.
No further discussions were brought under consideration and hence the chairman called for a motion to have the report of the Committee adopted. The motion was seconded and unanimously passed.
The Council then received Dr. Gordon V. Pefley, Chairman of the Council on Chiropractic Physiotherapy. Dr. Pefley extended the appreciation of his Council to the Educational Council members for their support of the physiotherapy council's program. He advised the group that the Physiotherapy Council sought to submit the following unanimous recommendation: "That a course in physiotherapy be presented at all the accredited colleges if not a prescribed then at least on an elective basis."
Dr. Weiant next presented the suggestion that the various school heads on the Council set up a minimum standard for convention appearances of themselves and the various members of their faculty and clinic staffs as far as an honorarium is concerned. He maintained that in the past some of the school men had made convention appearances without charge and thus had established some embarrassment to those other school men who had stipulated an expense and an honorarium.
Dr. Wolfe strongly supported Dr. Weiant in this matter, both insisting that the minimum should include all expenses plus at least $25 a day honorarium. Dr. Levine added his support to this contention.
Drs. Hendricks and Janse expressed the opinion that this should remain an individual decision for the various schools; that the circumstances and reasons for convention appearances varied greatly from time to time and certainly each school man should be privileged to decide according to the personalized circumstances of his appearance.
It was further contended that if one lecturer charged less than the other it would result in competitive misunderstandings. Both Drs. Hendricks and Janse asserted that such had never been their experiences and that the issue about who gets how much had never been brought up.
Finally, after some further discussions a motion was presented that suggested that school men convention appearances, other than in

their home states, should be on the basis of all expenses paid plus an honorarium of not less than $25 a lecture day.

The recommendation was seconded and carried with a majority vote, Drs. Wolfe and Levine casting opposing votes, their objection being on the ground that first the motion merely suggested and second the charge of $25 was not enough.

The meeting was adjourned at 5:30 p.m.

The third and final meeting of the Council was held Thursday afternoon for the purpose of receiving the official report of the Committee on Chiropractic Educational Standards, with Dr. Hendricks presiding.

Dr. Janse advised the Council that his attention had been drawn to certain mistakes that had been made in reporting the minutes of the Toronto meeting and he assured that corrections would be made and that a copy of these corrections would be sent to every member of the Council.

Dr. Walter Wolf maintained that to date the Council minutes had never been voted on for approval and acceptance and certainly that should be done.

Dr. Nugent felt that the minutes were too voluminous and should be abbreviated and more carefully edited.

Following is the official report of the Committee on Educational Standards as read by Dr. Ralph J. Martin, Chairman of the Committee.

"Rumors that the Western States College will close are without foundation and will not be realized. With an enrollment of 75-76 they will graduate 26 this summer. However, they already have 30 signed up for enrollment in September and with new administrative heads which Dr. Higgins has secured, or is in the process of securing, he expects a total enrollment of between 80 and 100 or more. There has been many other unfortunate events at Western States since the death of Dr. Budden. In fact, there has been serious consideration by the Committee of recommending to the Council that the school be placed on a conditional approval basis. After extensive conference with the Board of Trustees of the college the Committee feels reasonably sure that the school will attain the standards required by the code of the Council at a very early date. In event plans do not materialize as expected it will be necessary to place the school on a provisionally approved basis."

"California's two-year pre-professional education requirement by the Board of Chiropractic Examiners has been delayed by superior court at Los Angeles pending further arguments which will be presented July 14th and 15th and which Dr. Nugent expects to go to California immediately to prepare for.

The trial in March, in the Superior Court in Los Angeles, resulted in the Judge awarding the Hollywood School a temporary injunction. By agreement between the Hollywood School and the Board of Examiners a decision was reached to take the case off the calendar for a period of 60 days for a possible out-of-court settlement. No settlement was reached, so work is directed toward placing the case back on the calendar. This work will be planned by Dr. Nugent and Mr. Von Herzen in July and is expected to go back to court for final settlement."

The extension courses of the Graduate School of the L.A.C.C. have been studied by the Committee appointed in Toronto by Dr. Hendricks with the following recommendations:

"The Graduate School commitment with the Michigan group is to be fulfilled. No further extension graduate classes outside California will be conducted without filing and consultation with the Council. Formulation of plans for post-graduate extension courses, correlated with all the faculties of the accredited colleges are being developed for submission to the Council as soon as possible for consideration."

"The Toronto agreement and commitments made by the National School have been delayed in fulfillment by several circumstances. We have kept closely in touch with the National School situation and with Dr. Janse and Mr. Miller since last February and have had several conferences with Mr. Otto J. Turek here in Chicago and with Dr. Janse and Mr. Miller. We are gratified to announce to the Council that Mr. Turek has promised to fulfill the stipulations agreed upon in Toronto of placing a chiropractor on the Board of Trustees of the National School and in all other ways will abide by the code and rules of this Council. A much better understanding exists now than has been enjoyed for the past couple of years and Mr. Turek has come to understand the purposes and objectives of the Council much more comprehensively than at any time in the past. Therefore, we feel that our problems with the National School have been definitely resolved at this meeting and the air has been cleared."

"The New York Institute has announced that Dr. Sol Goldschmidt has replaced Dr. John Nugent on the Board of Trustees."

"There are some significant changes in prospect in the Texas School which may be reported at the mid-winter meeting."

"All the accredited schools remain in about the same condition as at our last meeting but most of them are enjoying substantial enrollment increases."

Dr. Hendricks called for a motion to adjourn. This was made and seconded and approved by unanimous vote.

Minutes of the Mid-Year Meeting of the NATIONAL COUNCIL ON EDUCATION of the NATIONAL CHIROPRACTIC ASSOCIATION, Hotel Rowe, January 5, 6, 7, 8, 1957, Miami Beach, Florida

Dr. Arthur G. Hendricks, Chairman of the Council, presided at all of the meetings. In attendance were:

A. Administrative personnel of the accredited educational institutions of the National Chiropractic Association.

Dr. Arthur G. Hendricks, Chairman of the Council and President of the Lincoln Chiropractic College, Inc., 633 N. Pennsylvania Avenue, Indianapolis 3, Indiana

Dr. Joseph Janse, Secretary of the Council and President of the National College of Chiropractic, 20 N. Ashland Boulevard, Chicago 7, Illinois

Dr. Thure C. Peterson, President of the Chiropractic Institute of New York, 325 East 38th Street, New York 16, New York

Dr. George H. Haynes, Dean of the Los Angeles College of Chiropractic, 920 East Broadway, Glendale 5, California

Dr. Julius C. Troilo, Dean of the Texas Chiropractic College, San Pedro Park, San Antonio, Texas

Dr. John B. Wolfe, President of the Northwestern College of Chiropractic, 2222 Park Avenue, Minneapolis 3, Minnesota

Dr. Earl A. Homewood, Administrative Dean of the Canadian Memorial Chiropractic College, 252 Bloor Street West, Toronto 5, Ontario, Canada

Dr. Robert Elliot, President of the Western States Chiropractic College sent his excuses for being unable to attend.

B. Members of the National Committee on Educational Standards.

Dr. Norman E. Osborne, Chairman of the Committee, Longmeadows Extended R.D. 5, Hagerstown, Maryland

Dr. E.H. Gardner, Secretary of the Committee, 1655 N. Normandie, Los Angeles, California

Dr. Walter B. Wolf, 207 West Main Street, Eureka, South Dakota

Dr. Ralph J. Martin, 30 West Sierra Madre Boulevard, Sierra Madre, California

C. Special guests.

Dr. James N. Firth, President emeritus, Lincoln Chiropractic College.

Dr. Harry K. McIlroy, former executive director of the National Chiropractic Association.

Dr. Emmett J. Murphy, National representative of the National Chiropractic Association.

Dr. Frank G. Plodder, Vice-president of the National Chiropractic Association.

Dr. Hendricks as chairman of the Council had appointed an agenda committee and in the course of the morning the following matters were discussed and concluded.

Matter No. 1: Further discussion of the program that would provide for the continuing of the education of picked faculty members of the accredited schools, and which would seek financial support from the National Chiropractic Association, preliminary discussions had been conducted at Toronto and in Chicago.

Careful and deliberate discussions ensued which resulted in the unanimous passing of the following resolution:

"That any program for advanced educational privileges for picked faculty members of the accredited colleges should be sufficiently broad to permit undergraduate work as well as graduate work so as to enable a larger percentage of the tried and proven faculty members of the various colleges to take advantage of the opportunity.

"That each college in conjunction with the Director of Education seek to determine how the program might function most competently in relation to the individual needs of the various schools.

"That the participating faculty member shall be required, if he decides to discontinue his affiliation with the college, within three years after he has completed his training, to reimburse the college and the NCA prorate the amount spent on him by both organizations.

"The NCA shall retain all assigned funds in their possession and allocate them equally among all accredited institutions and to be disbursed by the NCA to the various colleges as each of their programs develops."

In a subsequent meeting with the Executive Board and Officers of the NCA, the resolution was submitted for their consideration.

Matter No. 2: Establishment of reduced membership fees in the NCA for faculty members of the accredited colleges.

It was the unanimous consensus of opinion that special rates for full participating membership in the National Chiropractic Association should be provided for the faculty members of the accredited colleges.

It was concluded that a request be made of the NCA Executive Board to consider the proposition of providing such faculty members with full membership privileges on a half-rate basis.

In the subsequent meeting with the Executive Board this proposition was presented and it was evident that it would enjoy full acceptance, with the general conclusion that it would create a definite interest in the National Association among all the faculty members of the accredited colleges and thus in turn extend this interest onto the student bodies.

Matter No. 3: Final settlement of the matter of advertising by the approved colleges.

It was fully agreed by everyone that the combined accredited group of NCA colleges should have more publicity. In a later meeting with the Executive Board this opinion was presented with the request that the NCA seek to effect some program that would give the accredited schools a greater extent of publicity and display, possibly at state and national conventions, at career day gatherings, as well as in high schools and junior colleges. The Executive Board indicated their readiness to consider the matter and report their conclusions to the Council at some later date.

It was further concluded that a definite effort be made to induce the editors of the various state publications to carry without charge a composite ad of the NCA accredited colleges as a service to the colleges and a compensation for the many services rendered the various state associations by the colleges.

Dr. Janse was instructed to contact Mrs. Arlene Raymond, public relations director of the Iowa Chiropractors Association and President of the Chiropractic Editors Guild, to determine whether at the next NCA convention, at which the Guild meets, this matter might be presented to the entire membership of the Guild.

Dr. Janse had the opportunity of contacting Mrs. Raymond before the printing of these minutes and he wishes to report that this appointment has been made.

It was further concluded that the individual schools should continue their contracts with the various state publications of the states in which they had their main constituents but wherever possible to refrain from extended commitments.

Matter No. 4: Coordination of curricula and a yardstick for evaluating transfer credits.

Dr. Haynes initiated the discussions by contending that there should be a much more thorough standardization of the curricula of the accredited colleges, insisting that it would reduce a lot of difficulty in evaluating the credits of transfer students and also provide a more standard criterion for state boards to work from.

After extended careful discussions a motion was unanimously passed "that all the accredited schools submit a run down on the contents of the basic science subjects to each of the other accredited colleges before the next meeting. This brief on each of the basic science departments was to be readied by the respective departmental directors and then submitted to the administrative dean or president who in turn would submit copies to the respective other accredited colleges."

Dr. Wolfe then brought the matter of transfer students into consideration. It was the general opinion that student transferring should be discouraged and controlled as competently as possible. It was acknowledged that possibly in some instances a student maladjusted at one school might find himself at another.

Finally after careful deliberations had been conducted the following resolution was unanimously passed:

"Any student transferring from one accredited college to another should be placed on probation until the registrar or administrative head of the college to which the student has transferred receives an official letter of release from the administrative officer of the school from which the student has transferred. Furthermore, if a student of an accredited college negotiates with the registrar's office of another accredited college and indicates his or her desire to transfer, the registrar or administrative officer of the college to which the student has written should contact the administrative officer of the school from which the student seeks to transfer and advise him of the same."

Further discussions led to the passing of another motion which reads as follows:
"If one of the accredited colleges dismisses a student for moral reasons or reasons of misconduct or total financial unreliability as well as academic incompetence his name, along with the stated reason, should be circulated among the accredited colleges."

Dr. Peterson then made the recommendation that if a student transfers into one of the accredited colleges from a non-accredited college, the tuition of which is much lower than that of the accredited college, this student be charged extra in tuition so that the total equals that of the regular students.

Matter No. 5: Discussion on the forthcoming book by Dr. Oetteking on the cranium.

Dr. Peterson advised the Council that Dr. Oetteking of the faculty of the Chiropractic Institute of New York would, within the next month or so, release a 200-page volume on the topographical and gross anatomy of the head. This book would represent a classic in this phase of anatomy because of Dr. Oetteking's extended knowledge and research in this field. The book was being printed in Germany and thus the price would be comparatively low. Each of the accredited colleges would receive a complimentary copy for review and it was hoped that the text might be recommended and used in the departments of anatomy of the approved schools.

Matter No. 6: The future economics of our accredited colleges and revaluation of tuition fees.

This subject commanded extended and penetrating discussions by all the members of the Council, including the Director of Education and the Committee on Educational Standards. Following were the major considerations and conclusions:

(1) Effort should be made by programs of public relations, advertising and personal contact to make the educational program of the NCA accredited colleges more attractive and thus possibly cut down on the number of students that are now matriculating in the non-accredited schools.

(2) An eventual approach will have to be made to the profession to subsidize the accredited colleges regularly with part of the operating expenses. It was agreed that the professional membership as a whole were not fully aware of the severe economic problems that confronted some of the accredited institutions.

(3) It was also agreed that sooner or later an effort would have to be made to seek contributions and endowments from foundations, industry and labor. The question being, however, how should this approach be made and by whom and whether it should be tried immediately or whether it would be wise to wait until all the accredited colleges had better facilities and greater faculty depth. It was the general feeling that although great care should be exercised and that possibly it was somewhat early to make the attempt, certain initial investigations should be made to determine just what attitudes and dispositions would be encountered.

(4) Attention was drawn to the fact that the country was entering a low available college students because of the low pre-war birth rate and that this low would extend over a number of years before the post-war increase in birth rate would make more candidates for college education available. Therefore, it was acknowledged that the next four or five years would provide but small enrollments and hence the economics of the accredited colleges would be under a compromise.

(5) By the majority it was deemed necessary to raise tuition and fees in general to help defray the current expenses of the institutions they represented.

(6) Dr. Nugent, Director of Education, submitted his dispositions on the subject which may be stated as follows:

    (a) Tuition should be raised and the Council should decide on a minimum tuition rate for all of the accredited colleges.

    (b) A vigorous campaign should be initiated to alert the profession to its responsibility of financially supporting the accredited colleges. This support should be in the form of a continuous endowment to help defray operating expenses.

    (c) If an approach is to be made to foundations, industry and labor it should be done by the Council rather than some other committee or body of the NCA for the simple reason that the welfare of the accredited colleges is most competently understood by the Council. He expressed the apprehension that if some other body would make the attempt it might result in frustration of intent. He further expressed the opinion that not sufficient progress had been made at the various schools to warrant the attempt, maintaining that until better facilities were realized by some of the schools and a greater depth in faculty personnel were accomplished along with a student body that possessed a higher prerequisite requirement, any attempt would be met with hesitancy and rejection on the part of the people in question. He insisted that first we must obtain from the profession the support necessary to enable the schools to raise themselves to that level of qualification that would make them acceptable to the stipulations of foundations, industry, labor as well as the government.

    (d) There should be a student procurement director in each of the accredited colleges. In other colleges throughout the country this has proven very successful and there is no reason why it would not be a successful plan for chiropractic schools.

(7) Dr. Nugent was then asked whether something might not be done toward getting the United States Government to recognize the accrediting agency of the National Chiropractic Association and thus possibly eventually obtain some government aid for the accredited colleges. In answer Dr. Nugent insisted that his original contact with the governmental agencies had been severely compromised by the counter efforts of the ICA representatives and the intrusions of the Dr. Norcross' efforts. He advised the Council that he was somewhat hesitant in making extended efforts because he felt that certain added improvements would have to be made at the accredited colleges before accreditation might be expected. When asked what these added features entailed he voiced the following:

    (a) Our schools will have to be accepted as institutional members of the American Educational Society.

    (b) Our schools must possess faculties that possess competent academic depth. This being the reason for his concern about the necessity of setting up a program that would permit chosen members of the faculties to continue their education on a leave of absence or part time basis.

    (c) All our schools must possess adequate laboratories and the technical talent to operate them.

    (d) Our schools must possess student bodies that possess adequate pre-requisite requirements and thus qualify the schools as institutions of higher education.

(8) Dr. Nugent did agree that a careful continued effort should be made to maintain contacts and an open door. He was encouraged by the entire Council membership to seek an appointment with the government officials in question and at least seek to determine whether or not they would recognize the Council as the only accrediting agency of the chiropractic profession. It was suggested by Dr. Peterson that when Dr. Nugent kept this anticipated appointment he seek to have with him officers and members of the Council as factual representatives of the Council and the accredited schools. This being acknowledged as a good recommendation.

(9) At this point the Council received Drs. Cecil Martin and Frank Plodder, members of the newly appointed NCA Committee on Endowments for the Accredited Colleges. Dr. Martin, as spokesman, asked the members of the Council for suggestions and recommendations. He advised the Council that he had made some precursory investigations especially in relation to industry and labor and he was of the opinion that some fruitful contacts might be established. The consequent discussions led to the following conclusions:

    (a) That Dr. Martin and his committee might continue to carefully investigate some of the possibilities of obtaining favorable connections with foundations, industry and labor.

    (b) That the present expansion and building programs of the various colleges should receive full encouragement and no efforts should be made to solicit the profession through the committee as such might possibly compromise these programs.

    (c) That probably the committee could function as the vehicle of prompting that might induce the Executive Board as well as the House of Delegates to prescribe a raise of the annual membership dues of the NCA members and assign the extra revenue pro rata to the maintenance of the accredited colleges.

(10) In conclusion of all the discussions it was agreed that every avenue of possibility should be penetrated and carefully evaluated. Certainly it will be necessary to alert the general professional membership to the need of lending financial support.

Matter No. 7: Consideration of the letter as directed to all of the accredited colleges by the Secretary of the Kansas State Medical Society in relation to our attitude toward basic science legislation.

The matter experienced careful study and it was concluded that although the Council could not necessarily condone the plans of this group to sponsor either a basic science law or a composite medical, osteopathic and chiropractic board, the Council should not alienate the group by an inordinate retort realizing that with the growth of the radius of chiropractic education, mediations with other professional groups would involuntarily crop up. The following letter was prepared and submitted to the Council. Unanimous approval was indicated and the Council secretary was instructed to send it.

Oliver E. Ebel, Executive Secretary, The Kansas Medical Society, 315 West 4th Street, Topeka, Kansas
Dear Mr. Ebel:

Your letters to the National Chiropractic Association and to the members of the National Council on Education were discussed at the semi-annual meeting of the Council, January 5, 6, 7 and 8. The following are the conclusions the Council reached:

1. Although no particular criticism of any composite board is intended, we are of the opinion that the best interests of the public and the members of our profession result under the guidance of independent professional boards composed of people of ability and integrity.
2. The National Chiropractic Association is concerned with the problem of protecting the people of Kansas and other states against inadequately trained practitioners, but we do not feel the solution you proposed will solve this problem in a practical manner.
3. Further study of this problem may provide a practical solution to the situation in Kansas.

We appreciate your consulting us in this matter. Sincerely yours, J. Janse, Secretary, National Council on Education of the NCA

Matter No. 8: A discussion on all pending chiropractic legislation and action throughout the country.

The following related matters and conclusions discussed and made:

(1) The unfortunate matter of the Maryland Homeopathic Board scandal was brought up. It seems that a member of the Homeopathic Board induced a number of chiropractors to take a special examination given by the Board after having obtained unauthentic documents of homeopathic training. That a number of homeopathic licenses had thus been issued with the promise that they could be further used to obtain reciprocity into other states and thus permit unrestricted medical practice. It was the unanimous opinion of the Council that a recommendation should be made to the NCA Executive Board that it be determined whether any of the involved chiropractors were NCA members and if they were they should be instructed to relinquish the thus obtained homeopathic diplomas and licenses or else be expelled from NCA membership. Drs. Haynes and Osborne were appointed as a committee of two to investigate the Maryland matter and to report their findings and recommendations to the Council and also the Executive Board of the NCA.
(2) Drs. Nugent and Haynes then reviewed the situation in California advising the Council that a decision was pending as to whether the proposed legislation of the California Chiropractic Association and supported by the Board of Chiropractic Examiners, requiring two years of pre-professional college education before entering an accredited college of chiropractic, was constitutional or not. If this decision would be in favor of such legislation and if the legislation went into effect, it would of course represent a distinct hazard to the low standards schools now competing with the Los Angeles College of Chiropractic.

Both doctors insisted that "Declaration of Policy" as prepared and published by the Council on the Council's attitude on the two-year pre-professional college requirement because of its "middle of the road" stand had been used by the opposition as well as statements out of context from some of the personal letters of Council members. For these reasons Dr. Haynes recommended the passing of the following resolution:

"We as a Council reaffirm our support in principle of the two year pre-professional requirement and we clearly, individually, and collectively present an attitude that cannot be assumed to directly or indirectly oppose the above statement." (The vote was unanimous.)

(3) Attention was drawn to the fact that the Wyoming Chiropractic Association this January was sponsoring legislation recommending two years of pre-professional college requirement. These two years would be required before entering chiropractic college, although no pre-chiropractic subjects were stipulated and was attended by the qualification that any student in full time attendance at one of the approved colleges at the time of the passage of the legislation would not be affected by the same. It was concluded that this legislation was rather severe and Dr. Troilo was instructed to contact Dr. Gordon Holmes, chairman of the Wyoming legislative committee and seek to induce him and his associates to alter the stipulations so as to permit an inclusion of the program of the Texas College of Chiropractic as it relates to its students procuring their college requirements at the San Antonio Junior College concurrent with their chiropractic education.
(4) The letter by Dr. Stanley Hayes, chairman of the legislative committee of the United Chiropractic Association of Arizona to all of the accredited colleges was read detailing the fact that the Association was intending to sponsor legislation that would require two years of college along with a four year chiropractic degree. The college work however could be obtained before, current to

and even after the chiropractic course.

(5) The Council membership was somewhat divided in opinion in relation to the two-year pre-professional issue. Some felt that the Council should declare itself for it without qualification and within the near future make it a requirement to matriculation. Others insisted that it should be left alone and permitted to evolve on the basis of individual state decision, the contention being that an immediate transition would so severely compromise the economics of the colleges that some of them would not be able to remain in existence. It was conceded that pre-professional college requirements were inevitable, yet the Council proper should not rush into any such stipulations because of the already existing hazards of reduced enrollments. Hence it was concluded to permit the matter to reside where it is and fully sustain the resolution submitted by Dr. Haynes.

Matter No. 9: Discussion of the possibility of readying state board questions by the NCA to be distributed at cost to the students of the accredited colleges.

(1) It was acknowledged that properly catalogued past state board questions especially in the basic sciences served as a distinct aid to students in readying themselves for state boards. Examples were cited to show that this practice was common in the medical and osteopathic professions as well.

(2) Dr. Janse advised the Council that in conformity with the instructions received at the previous meeting, members of the National College faculty as well as the senior class has proceeded to set up a catalogued set of basic science board questions for the last 10 years or so. That contributions had been made by Dr. Bierman of the Lincoln College and Dr. Haynes of the Los Angeles College.

(3) Dr. Janse was instructed to submit the set to the NCA as soon as possible so that they might be multigraphed and readied for use. In a subsequent meeting with the Executive Board, Dr. Rogers advised the Council that the Webster City office would seek to ready multigraphed sets as soon as possible.

(4) It was recommended by Dr. Peterson that the members of the National Council of Chiropractic Examining Boards be contacted at the time of the NCA convention and invited to consider the possibility of confining the practical examination in chiropractic to permitting the applicant to display the method of spinal examination and adjusting that he had been taught at the college attended and be evaluated on that basis rather than expecting him to display talent and knowledge of all the methods of spinal examination and adjusting that might be existent among the college and in the profession in general.

Matter No. 10: A discussion of the proposed roentgenological certification program of the National Council of Chiropractic Roentgenologists.

Dr. Hillary W. Pruitt, former secretary of the Roentgenological Council, had asked for the privilege of presenting the proposed program to the Council and resultantly he was in attendance at this discussion.

Dr. Pruitt advised the Council that the Council on Roentgenology sought the approval and sanction of the Educational Council for this program and desired to submit the program for study and consideration. At the request of the Council he read the terms and prescriptions of the program. Various corrections and suggestions were made by members of the Council. Dr. Pruitt asked for the opportunity to contact the officers of the Roentgenological Council to determine whether they would accept these recommendations. This courtesy was granted and in a subsequent session Dr. Pruitt advised the Council that his associates had agreed upon the suggestions and recommendations and that he was ready to submit the corrected outline of the program. The following submitted outline was unanimously approved and accepted by the Council:

NATIONAL COUNCIL OF CHIROPRACTIC ROENTGENOLOGISTS CERTIFICATION PROGRAM AS APPROVED BY THE NCA COUNCIL ON EDUCATION.

I. Purpose: To establish and maintain a certification program for the National Council of Chiropractic Roentgenologists.

II. Examining Board:

1. To consist of five men; including a president, vice-president, and secretary-treasurer.
2. The original Board of Examiners approved by the NCA Council on Education consists of:
    a. Waldo G. Poehner, D.C., Chicago, Illinois; b. Leo E. Wunsch, D.C., Denver, Colorado; c. Fred H. Baier, D.C., St. Louis, Missouri; d. M.A. Giammarino, D.C., Coatesville, Pennsylvania; e. Duane M. Smith, D.C., Huntington Park, California
3. Appointments to the Board shall be by the president of the N.C.C.R. from a list of ————— members submitted by the executive officers.
4. No member of the board may serve more than two consecutive terms.
5. Appointments to the initial board are to be made for one, two and three year terms respectively; thereafter, each appointment is to be for three years.
6. A temporary fund of $500 shall be deposited with the secretary-treasurer of the board, until such time as the fund is self-supporting.
7. Upon the death or resignation of any board member, it shall be the duty of the president to appoint a qualified member of the N.C.C.R. to serve the unexpired term.

III. Duties of the Examining Board:

1. To collect examination fees of $100 minimum.
2. To conduct an examination annually preceding or following the NCA annual convention or the N.C.C.R. symposium, or both, according to the discretion of the Board and other special examinations upon the approval of the N.C.C.R.
3. To issue a document of registration or fellowship to the applicant based on his or her qualification and examination results.
4. To issue a renewal certificate annually, contingent upon the certified attendance of the applicant at a two-day X-ray educational session, plus a renewal fee of $5.00.

IV. Board Member Expenses:
1. The secretary-treasurer is authorized to pay all expenses in connection with the examination, plus a $30 a day per diem, per member. All vouchers must be signed by the president and secretary-treasurer.
2. Secretary-Treasurer to be placed under an adequate bond.

V. Subjects for Examination:
1. X-ray physics and technic
2. Spinography
3. Chiropractic roentgenology

VI. Applicant requirements for those in the field at the inauguration of this program:
1. The applicant must be a graduate of a chiropractic college with a minimum of 5 years in X-ray practice in the field, and 3 years attendance at the N.C.C.R. symposia or its equivalent as determined by the Board of Examiners.
2. The applicant must be a licensed chiropractor.
3. The applicant must be a member in good standing of the National Chiropractic Association, National Council of Chiropractic Roentgenologists, and the state society within the state in which he or she practices.
4. There shall be paid to said board by each applicant a fee of not more than $100 to accompany the application.
5. Any applicant failing in any subjects may be re-examined in those subjects for a fee contingent upon the number of subjects.

VII. Applicant requirements after January 1, 1959.
1. The applicant must be a graduate of any NCA accredited college, plus 5 years of X-ray experience in the field, including 500 hours of continuing study in X-ray laboratories or colleges approved by the N.C.C.R.
2. The applicant must be a licensed chiropractor.
3. The applicant must be a member in good standing of the National Chiropractic Association, National Council of Chiropractic Roentgenologists, and the state society within the state in which he or she practices.
4. There shall be paid to said board by each applicant a fee of not more than $150 to accompany the application.
5. Any applicant failing in any subjects may be re-examined in those subjects for a fee contingent upon the number of subjects.

Matter No. 11: Revaluation of the Jr. NCA program in the accredited colleges.

The importance of attempting to have every student at the accredited colleges become a Jr. NCA member was emphasized. It was the general disposition that it should, however, still remain a volitional matter.

All the school men were encouraged to seek a 100% Jr. NCA enrollment on the $5 for the entire four-year program.

It was acknowledged that the entire program would experience stimulus if the program designed to enroll all the faculty members as NCA members could materialize.

Matter No. 12: Support for the research work of Dr. Illi.

Both Drs. Peterson and Janse had been contacted by Dr. Fred W. Illi of Geneva, Switzerland with the request that they submit to the Executive Board and the Council his request for substantial financial assistance in his plans for extended research work, especially as it relates to the taking of motion picture X-rays of the movements within the spine and pelvis.

Dr. Illi contemplated the purchase of a most expensive X-ray unit from the Phillips Co. in the Netherlands that would enable him to take X-rays of the spine and the pelvis with these structures in motion with commanding proficiency.

Dr. Peterson had received a short experimental film from Dr. Illi that had hurriedly been taken with this unit. This was shown to the Council and all agreed that it possessed definite promise.

In a previous conference with the Executive Board, Drs. Peterson and Janse had presented Illi's proposition to the Board and they had said that it would be brought under consideration.

Matter No. 13: Discussions pertaining to Dr. Herman Schwartz's request in relation to his recent new book.

The officers of the Council had received letters from Dr. Schwartz requesting that the school men of the Council consider the usage of his text, "Home Care For The Emotionally Ill," in the accredited colleges whenever possible.

It was the consensus of opinion that everything possible should be done by each school to augment the sale of the text, it being recognized that Dr. Schwartz had made a very definite and exceptionally worthy contribution to the profession.

Some of the school men went so far as to indicate that they would be willing to underwrite a hundred or more copies to be sold to the students and faculty.

Matter No. 14: Considerations of the request by Mr. Shelton, procurement director of the John Crerar Library, for chiropractic texts.

This library located in Chicago is considered one of the finest and largest research libraries in the world and Dr. Janse had contacted Dr. Illi with the request that he submit copies of all of his publications which Dr. Illi graciously complied with. In addition Dr. Janse presented the English edition of Illi's latest work, "The Vertebral Column," as well as the National College text.

It was recommended that the various schools make it a point to send into the library any of their school publications or texts which might be of value to the need of more competently portraying the principle and concept of the profession.

Matter No. 14: Discussions pertaining to extension, post-graduate and graduate courses.

The Council's attention was drawn to a recent communication received from certain elements of the profession in Rhode Island requesting the privilege of organizing an Internist group for the purpose of conducting extension courses. The Los Angeles College of Chiropractic had been requested to conduct the course.

The Council was advised by Dr. Nugent that this group in Rhode Island unfortunately wished to obtain instruction and conduct classes in clinical subjects that extended beyond the scope of chiropractic practice and hence their request should not receive compliance.

The Director of Education emphasized the need for exercising care in matters of this type insisting that no college should be too anxious to participate in programs of this type unless very careful and exacting arrangement can be agreed upon.

At this point Dr. Janse advised the Council that the Iowa Chiropractors Association, an NCA affiliated state association, had requested that the National College of Chiropractic conduct a series of 6 extension or post-graduate courses in Des Moines extending over Saturday and Sunday, the work being in chiropractic measures and X-ray as it relates to the spine and pelvis.

Dr. Haynes made the following motion, "That the Council give its consent to the National College to carry out its proposed extension class in Iowa under the conditions presented by Dr. Janse but without certification."

At this point it was considered advisable to have the Accrediting Committee to make its report because some of it related to this very question of extension and graduate courses.

Dr. Norman E. Osborne, as chairman of the committee, read the report and submitted a full copy to the Council secretary and which reads as follows:

"Report of the Accrediting Committee to the Council on Education"

"The first order of business of the Accrediting Committee was the reading of a letter from the National College of Chiropractic advising us of the appointment of Dr. Ralph C. King to the Board of Trustees. This addition of Dr. King to the Board of Trustees was well received by the full committee and meets the requirements set forth by the accepted code."

"A communication from Dr. Raymond S. Pierce, Providence, Rhode Island, was read in relation to the approval of an extension course desired in Rhode Island by a group of doctors. This course to be conducted by one of the approved colleges.

"This request then led to a long discussion on the subject of extension courses. From this discussion came the following suggestion for the regulation of the conducting of such extension courses:
   I.   The area which the courses encompass:
        (a)   Must remain within the scope of general chiropractic practice as described by the NCA code and or in accordance with the state laws and regulations.
        (b)   Instruction in the pre-clinical and clinical sciences — as taught by and in the approved schools.
   II. By whom shall this instruction be provided.
        (a)   Under the auspices of and by the approved schools
        (b)   Could and may be sponsored by state or national organizations
        (c)   Council shall be notified of the intentions to conduct such course and content of such course may be subject to review by the Council.
        (d)   The creation or organization of a post-graduate or extension course faculty from qualified men outside the regular faculty should the burden of such courses become too great and might in any way endanger the undergraduate school.
   III. Financial arrangements.
   (1)   The cost of conducting such courses shall be on a self-sustaining basis. At no time shall regular school funds be used for the conducting of such courses."

"Report on all the approved schools. No special recommendations of changes for any of the schools made and at the same time no changes of status of any of the schools were made.

"Full report on the California, Montana and Oregon situation was given by the Director of Education to the entire Council."

The report of the Accrediting Committee was unanimously approved and accepted.

Further discussion in relation to extension courses emphasized the fact that in California the extension courses conducted by the graduate school of the Los Angeles College of Chiropractic were definitely designed and set up for the purpose of offering credit and certification and any attempt on the part of the Council to alter this set-up in California proper would lead to a great deal of disturbance in California and a resistance that might prove severely hazardous.

Matter No. 15: Discussion of the position of the three schools that had been retained as institutions which subscribe to the program of the National Council on Education.

The Director of Education advised the Council that for the last several years no progress had been made at any one of these institutions, and that it was becoming increasingly more evident that they would not be able to comply with the standards of the Council; hence, they should no longer expect to be carried on the list of NCA approved or subscribing schools.

It was the final conclusion of the Council that the Council secretary should write a letter to the editor of the NCA Journal and advise him to delete the names of these institutions from the bottom of the page carrying the NCA approved schools, as subscribing institutions.

Matter No. 16: Brief discussion of the Student Loan Fund and the usage of the same by the students of the NCA schools.

The largest percentage of the students availing themselves of the Student Loan Fund have been students from the subscribing rather than the approved colleges.

It was deemed advisable to have the Webster City office advise the various school heads whenever a student or graduate failed to live up to the contract of the loan.

Following is the copy of the letter that the Council secretary directed to Dr. Rogers in relation to matters 15 and 16.

Dr. L.M. Rogers, Executive Secretary, National Chiropractic Association, National Building, Webster City, Iowa
Dear Doctor Rogers:

At the recent meetings of the National Council on Education, I was instructed by the membership of the Council to advise you of the following:

1. If from time to time your office notes that any of the students of the accredited colleges who have obtained assistance through the Student Loan Fund do not meet their obligations in relation to the contracts of the loan, your office advise the administrative heads of the colleges of this delinquency.
2. The Council unanimously recommends that from now on the page in the NCA Journal carrying the ad and listing of the accredited colleges, no longer at the bottom of the page carry the names of the Kansas State Chiropractic College, Missouri Chiropractic College and the University of Natural Healing Arts as schools which subscribe to the program of the National Council on Education. The reason being that none of these schools has been able to make any progress toward the fulfillment of the requirements of the Council.

With every good wish, I am Sincerely yours, J. Janse, Secretary

Matter No. 17: Mr. Harold Achenbach submitted to the secretary the following resolution as passed by the Executive Board in its meeting held concurrent with that of the Council.

"Motion by Dr. Wood, seconded by Dr. Martyn that a committee on research be established with authority to appoint a scientific editorial board as approved by the National Council on Education and publish research reports, when, as and if sufficient material is available." Motion was carried unanimously.

Matter No. 18: Discussions pertaining to the professional situation in Mexico.

The Council was advised by Drs. Peterson and Haynes that Dr. Luna, Chiropractor of Mexico City, is seeking to establish a college of chiropractic in Mexico. It seems that Dr. Luna has obtained from the Mexican Government the authority to be the certifying agent for chiropractic in that country. It appears to be the intention of the doctor to establish an understanding with one or more of the chiropractic colleges in the states and have them train students for chiropractic practice in Mexico but he would certify their credits and diplomas from his office in Mexico City.

To this end Dr. Luna has been in contact with several of the professional segments in the United States. It appears that some of these contacts are of an unfavorable disposition involving personalities that cannot be depended upon to maintain an integrity in behalf of the profession. For these reasons the Director of Education recommended that the Council seek to carefully investigate the matter and determine whether it, the Council, might not contact the Mexican Government as well as Dr. Luna and determine just what might be done constructively in relation to the matter of chiropractic in Mexico.

To accomplish this, two recommendations were concluded by the Council.

(1) That Drs. Weiant, Haynes and Troilo who have had the closest contact with the situation seek to probe it further and obtain as much information as possible, and probably before the next meeting one of the latter two, because of geographical advantage, make a trip into Mexico and seek to evaluate the matter.
(2) If possible the Council should seek to hold its next mid-year meeting in Mexico City, thus permitting the entire Council membership to get a first hand picture of the situation and also enable the Council representative to possibly have some conferences with the Mexican Government officials with the intent of getting them to recognize the Council and its directing position in the entire educational picture of the profession.

Matter No. 19: Election of Officers.

It was the unanimous decision of the Council members, other than those holding office who did not seek to cast a vote, that the present officers of the Council should be retained. Drs. Hendricks and Janse expressed their appreciation for the confidence shown and committed themselves to seek to continue to serve as competently as they could.

Extra Information.

On February 11, 1957 Dr. Joseph Janse, as secretary of the Council on Education, attended the annual meeting of the American Association of Basic Science Boards, held in Chicago, Illinois.

Dr. R.E. Medeck (chiropractor) and member of the South Dakota Board of Basic Science Examiners addressed the group on the subject entitled, "The Effect of Basic Science Laws on the Chiropractic Profession." Dr. Medeck did a commendable job and his comments were well received. He emphasized the fact that basic science legislation and the need for chiropractic students to take basic science boards augmented interest in and study of the basic sciences in the various chiropractic colleges, thus serving as an incentive toward a greater depth and breadth in the teaching of these subjects.

Dr. Janse was called on to say a few words in behalf of the Council on Education. He extended to the assembly of the Association its greetings and good wishes of the Council. He drew attention to the fact that the entire basic science issue in chiropractic education had come to enjoy a more generous and tolerant understanding, an that the entire basic science program was now looked upon with deference and determination. Dr. Janse did stress the fact that inasmuch as the doctor of chiropractic is a limited practitioner it is often a question and problem that confronts the educator in chiropractic as to how broad and wide the radius of education should be in any of the basic sciences, drawing attention to the fact that certain aspects of the basic sciences such as tropical microbiology, pharmaceutical experimental physiological and chemistry, as well as toxicological pathology, have very little relation to the clinical aspects of chiropractic. He contended that it is always difficult to teach any of the basic sciences or any aspect of the same without some eventual clinical reference or outlet.

It was evident throughout the subsequent discussions that as a whole a much more tolerant and respectful attitude was being sustained by the educators that constitute the members of most of the basic science boards toward chiropractic and its problems in education.

N.H. Serror, President of the Association of Basic Science Boards, instructed Dr. Janse to carry the good wishes of his association to the Council with the recognition of admiration for the diligent work that was being performed by the Council in its efforts to raise and supervise the educational program of the chiropractic profession.

Some of the pertinent points of information that might be of importance to the various accredited colleges are the following:

1. Rhode Island now sustains reciprocity by waiver or endorsement with the state of Colorado, and might within the near future also include Texas.
2. Minnesota has full reciprocity arrangement with the District of Columbia if one possesses two years of pre-professional college education.
3. Rhode Island has just defeated a bill that would have exempted medical candidates for licensure from basic science examination.
4. Most of the basic science boards that have tried the multiple choice question examinations as prepared by the Professional Examination Service have discontinued their usage. Attached was a brief submitted on that matter.

THE PRESENT STATUS OF OBJECTIVE BASIC SCIENCE EXAMINATIONS

The use of objective examinations in the basic sciences has been a question of interest to this Association for a number of years. The matter has been discussed at a number of the annual Association meetings. Several of the individual boards have conducted studies of their own and a number of them have used objective examinations under an established policy or experimentally. Representatives of the Professional Examination Service have addressed this group on several occasions and have urged the adoption of the PES exams by the several basic science boards. Two years ago at least one statement was made unofficially which indicated that the use of the PES examinations was being seriously considered by several boards.

Although opinion is by no means unanimous, the consensus of the board members attending Association meetings for the past few years has been that the use of the PES examinations is not desirable and that the disadvantages inherent therein far outweigh the possible advantages. The report presented today makes no pretense of studying this question nor does it undertake to review in any way the studies and discussions which have been presented before. This report merely summarizes the answers obtained by the Program Committee to a letter of inquiry which was directed to all basic science boards during the summer of 1956. This inquiry was meant merely to determine the current policy of the several boards with respect to the use of objective examinations, with particular reference to those furnished by the Professional examination service.

It is gratifying to report that all basic science boards, both members of the Association and non-members, replied to our letter of inquiry with the single exception of Alaska. Since this summary of information may be of interest to a number of individual board members, it is the recommendation of this Committee that these findings be made available to all basic science boards.

The following table summarizes briefly the information reported by the several Boards:

Numbered footnotes referring to the Boards noted above appear on the following page.

(1) The Colorado Board recently made an extensive study of the PES examinations and decided they were not comparable to the examinations given by that Board. A summary of these findings was presented to the Association in February of 1956. The Colorado Board has decided not to use the PES examinations and has refused reciprocity to several applicants whose certificates had been issued in another state on the basis of PES examinations.

(2) The District of Columbia reports that the question of the PES examinations was considered by the D of C Basic Science Board, the Professional Examining Boards, and the Commission on Licensure. All three groups voted against the adoption of objective type questions and they are continuing to use the essay type examinations which they feel have been very successful.

(3) The Michigan Board reports that it has never used these examinations although it has considered doing so. The Michigan Board has discussed the PES examinations with a representative of the Professional Examination Service. They feel that waiver and reciprocity between the several boards would be greatly facilitated if a majority of the basic science boards used these examinations.

(4) In 1953 the Bureau of Institutional Research at the University of Minnesota conducted a thorough survey of the status and use of examinations in the basic sciences in Minnesota. The findings of this report were subsequently reported to the Association and copies thereof were made available to the several basic science boards. Although the Minnesota Board used the PES examinations experimentally for a number of times, the Board decided against their continued use and has no further plans for the use of objective examinations in the future.

(5) Several years ago the New Mexico Board used the PES examinations in an experimental way. This Board, however, has discontinued the use of the PES examinations and apparently plans to use only essay type examinations in the future.

(6) The Oklahoma Board states that the matter of examination questions is left to the individual examiner. They consider multiple choice or completion type questions to be legitimate but feel that true and false questions are of no value. Although the practice in Oklahoma is not completely clear from the wording of their reply, it appears that objective examination questions may be used infrequently by individual examiners.

It is clear that all Boards have considered this matter of examination questions in some detail and that policy is rather definitely established in each case.

It is further clear that the preponderance of preference is in favor of the essay type examination over the objective. Nine boards report that they do not use the objective type examination at all. Four boards report that they use objective examinations infrequently or very seldom. Four more boards report that they use them in part but only in the case of South Dakota does their use extend to as much as 40%.

The consistent use of objective examinations is apparently restricted to the states of Connecticut, Florida and Wisconsin.

No basic science board currently employs the Professional Examination Service objective examinations. Apparently no board anticipates their use in the near future, with the possible exception of Michigan.

The objective examinations used by the Florida Basic Science Board are prepared by the individual examining members of that board. Information from the Florida Board makes it clear that they take pains to see that examination questions are not duplicated from one examination to the next. The questions used by the Connecticut and Wisconsin Boards are prepared by expert examiners who are faculty members of Universities within these states but who are not Board Members.

In all other cases, where the use of objective examinations is either infrequent or limited, the examination questions are prepared by the Board Members themselves.

Minutes of the Annual Meeting of the NATIONAL COUNCIL ON EDUCATION of the NATIONAL CHIROPRACTIC ASSOCIATION, Hotel Fountainebleau, June 15, 16, 17, 18, 1958, Miami Beach, Florida

The annual meeting of the Council on Education was held in conjunction with the annual convention of the National Chiropractic Association, June 15 through June 20, at the Hotel Fountainebleau, Miami Beach, Florida.

Dr. Arthur G. Hendricks, Chairman of the Council, presided at all the meetings. Those attending included:

A. Members of the Committee on Educational Standards.
   Dr. Norman E. Osborne, Chairman of the Committee, Long Meadows Extended #5, Hagerstown, Maryland
   Dr. Walter B. Wolf, 207 West Main Street, Eureka, South Dakota
   Dr. Ralph J. Martin, 478 N. Sierra Madre Boulevard, Sierra Madre, California
   Dr. John J. Nugent, Director of Education, 92 Norton Street, New Haven, Connecticut

B. Administrative personnel of the Accredited Educational Institutions of the National Chiropractic Association
   Dr. Arthur G. Hendricks, Chairman of the Council and President of the Lincoln Chiropractic College, Inc., 633 N. Pennsylvania Avenue, Indianapolis 3, Indiana
   Dr. Joseph Janse, Secretary of the Council and President of the National College of Chiropractic, 20 N. Ashland Blvd., Chicago 7, Illinois
   Dr. Thure C. Peterson, President, Chiropractic Institute of New York, 325 East 38th Street, New York 16, New York
   Dr. George H. Haynes, Dean, Los Angeles College of Chiropractic, 920 East Broadway, Glendale 5, California

Dr. Julius C. Troilo, Dean of the Texas Chiropractic College, 618 Myrtle Street, San Pedro Park, San Antonio, Texas

Dr. John B. Wolfe, President of the Northwestern College of Chiropractic, 2222 Park Avenue, Minneapolis, Minnesota.

Dr. Earl A. Homewood, Dean of the Canadian Memorial Chiropractic College, 252 Bloor Street, West, Toronto 5, Ontario, Canada.

Dr. Edward G. Hearn, President, of the Texas Chiropractic College, see above address.

Mr. Charles A. Miller, Vice-president, of the National College of Chiropractic, see above address.

Dr. Robert E. Elliot, President of the Western States College of Chiropractic, Portland, Oregon sent his regrets in not being able to attend.

The meetings extended over four days and following are the matters and topics brought forth in discussion.

Matter No. 1. Consideration of the report of the Committee on Economic Support of the NCA Accredited Colleges.

Dr. Peterson as chairman of this Committee assisted by the other members, Drs. Haynes and Wolfe had prepared and submitted to each member of the Council a handsomely prepared brief detailing reasons and needs for NCA support of the accredited colleges and setting forth a plan for the realization of the same. The substance of which included the creation of a National Fund for Chiropractic Education, a supervising Board of Trustees, a yearly assessment of each NCA member and the conditioned pro-rating of the monies accrued to the accredited colleges.

The discussions that ensued were as follows:

(1) Dr. Nugent advised the Council that the Board of Directors of the NCA had discussed the matter of school support extendedly and sustained rather concise attitudes.

    (a) All members of the Board of Directors acknowledged the need for school support.

    (b) Some felt that such support should be withheld until there was a consolidation of some of the accredited colleges. The attitude being that there are too many colleges to support.

    (c) Some doubt had been expressed as to the possible success of the building and expansion programs that all of the accredited colleges had initiated or were contemplating.

    (d) Both Dr. Rogers as Executive-Secretary of the NCA and Dr. Shafer as chairman of the Board of Directors in their annual report to the House of Delegates intended to make definite mention of the need for support of the accredited colleges.

    (e) The Board had been reminded of the marked academic advancements made by the various colleges and that extended benefit had been accrued by the NCA through the efforts of the accredited educational institutions.

    (d) Dr. Nugent had advised the Board that any thought of consolidation of any of the NCA accredited colleges would constitute a hazard and any such thought should be discouraged.

    (e) The Executive Board although aware of the need for support of the accredited colleges was definitely seeking a competent plan for the realization of the same.

(2) Dr. Hendricks expressed the conviction that any talk of the consolidation of accredited colleges represents a hazard and mitigating attitude.

(3) Dr. Janse advised that consolidation of accredited colleges would possibly drive some of the students involved in the process of amalgamation into ICA chiropractic schools.

(4) Dr. J. Wolfe expressed the feeling that advice should be given to Dr. Dewey Anderson as to the Council's interpretation of the need for consolidation, namely that effort along these lines should be directed toward measures that would absorb and consolidate those schools that resided outside the accrediting program of the Council.

(5) Dr. Wolfe further presented the argument that because of the increase in population there will be an increasing need for the NCA accredited colleges and it would be unwise and imprudent to encourage consolidation of any of the approved schools. Following being some pertinent statistical information that he submitted:

(blank space on two successive pages)

(6) It was unanimously concluded that in the joint session with the Executive Board the Council's unanimous attitude toward the consolidation concept should be definitely expressed. The basic reasons being:

    a. There is a definite need for regionally located accredited colleges.

    b. Consolidation of accredited colleges might give rise to the establishment of an ICA school in the area vacated by accredited college that was absorbed in the consolidation.

    c. It being questionable if all the students involved in the consolidation effort would seek to continue their education at the school of consolidation but probably some would seek matriculation at a non-accredited college of the region in question.

    d. With the increase in population there should definitely be an eventual increase in enrollment and if accredited schools were to be loaded to a near maximum by consolidation it would compromise their ability to handle any future increase in matriculants.

    e. There is an ever increasing need for doctors and the accredited colleges definitely play a role in the fulfillment of this need.

    f. The financial needs of a school should not constitute the sole criterion as to whether a school should be consolidated or not. The yard stick should be the professional and geographical need for the school.

(7) The report as submitted by the Peterson Committee was carefully gone over sentence for sentence. Certain changes and deletions were recommended and made. The following is the revised copy and the one submitted to the Executive Board and were the major revisions concluded after careful deliberation and consultation.

Pertaining to paragraph two on page three.

"This fund would be allocated evenly among the NCA accredited colleges and be dispersed as required to the individual accredited colleges according to demonstrated need, substantiated by proper investigation, and only after each school in question had demonstrated that it was operating without any wasteful expenditures, or inefficiency of administration. Should a school not use its allocation and permit the same to accumulate it may after some five years proceed to use the same for capital expenditure."

(8) Further discussions brought out the following points.

a. Every member of the Council would have to be most careful in his discussions with men in the field about school aid. The tendency to misinterpret, to overstate and to misrepresent the matter on the part of the general membership of the profession might negate the progress of the program.

b. There was some question about the Canadian Memorial Chiropractic College and just what position it might be asked to sustain in relation to the program. Unfortunately because of the strong central organization that was being created in Canada, Canadian membership in the NCA had declined noticeably and it represented a question whether the Americans would wish to assist a Canadian College under such circumstances.

(1) Dr. Homewood, Dean of the Canadian College acknowledged this issue and stated that some tenable understanding certainly could be reached.

c. It was concluded that the Peterson report was excellent and that a penetrating study had been made by the Committee.

Matter No. 2. Consideration of a special production by the Vitaminerals, Inc. and in the name of the National Council on Education with the intent of alerting the profession for the great need for support of the accredited colleges.

a. The production being in the form of a sound-slide visualization depicting the clinical progress of chiropractic yet the mitigating circumstances of the chiropractic colleges.

b. A special showing was held within the suite of the Vitaminerals people and it was the general consensus of opinion that it was a commendable effort and certainly the Vitaminerals Inc. should be complimented for their generous support of the accredited colleges in their efforts to maintain their standards.

Matter No. 3. Discussions relating to the evaluation of credits from non-accredited colleges.

1. The Director of Education advised the Council that in his many appearances throughout the country either in behalf of legislative efforts or in instance of court cases relating to chiropractic standards he often found his position compromised by the fact that the accredited colleges were granting credit for work done at non-accredited schools.

a. For these reasons he posed the question whether the Council was ready to make a decision to close the door against credits from unrecognized schools?

b. The consensus of opinion amongst the schoolmen of the Council was that at present such a conclusion would be impractical and probably could not be sustained.

c. The general disposition of the Council in relation to the matter was carefully reviewed and it was observed that the registrars' offices of the various accredited colleges had sustained a careful and particular decorum in relation to the matter.

d. In conclusion it was decided to establish regional evaluation committees whose duty it would be to evaluate the credits of all applicants to accredited colleges but who had done work at non-accredited schools. The purpose being to standardize this phase of credit evaluation and to reduce the tendency on the part of those students to shop amongst the accredited colleges for advantages and thus pit one against the other. Following are the primary prescriptions unanimously decided upon.

(1) That three regional evaluation teams be appointed, namely Western team consisting of Dr. Haynes and Martin, and servicing the Los Angeles, Texas and Western States Colleges. Midwestern team consisting of Drs. John Wolfe and Walter Wolf and servicing the National, Lincoln, Northwestern Colleges. Eastern team consisting of Drs. Peterson and Osborne and servicing the Chiropractic Institute of New York and the Canadian College.

(2) The registrars of each of the accredited colleges would have to be alerted as to this plan. They upon receipt of a transcript of credit obtained from a non-accredited college would make a tentative evaluation. This evaluation along with a copy of the transcript is to be sent as soon as possible to the regional evaluation team. They would proceed to conclude the evaluation, and immediately advise the other teams and schools of the conclusion. This conclusion as expediently as possible should be submitted to the registrar of the college in question and the student advised accordingly.

It was agreed that this program although somewhat involved would centralize the problem and avoid undue variation in the handling of an awkward issue.

It was further concluded that correspondence and conclusions should be conducted as quickly as time would permit.

The forgoing procedure was put in the form of a motion, it was seconded and unanimously passed by the Council.

Matter No. 4. Joint meeting with the Executive Board of the National Chiropractic Association.
    (1) At the invitation of the Executive Board the Council presented two major matters that had been considered in previous sessions.
        a. Dr. Hendricks as chairman of the Council advised the Board of the deliberations with reference to financial support of the accredited colleges and presented to the Board the concluded recommendations as readied by the Peterson committee.

The Board advised that definite considerations would be made and that Drs. Hendricks and Peterson would be advised of the decisions reached.

It was the overall opinion that plans and studies of the matter should proceed with care and that all deliberations were to be kept confidential so as to avoid any gossip or misrepresentation.
        b. Dr. Hendricks then advised the Board of the Council's conclusions with reference to the consolidation idea that appeared to be quite prevalent in the thinking of some of the NCA people.
            (1) Upon conclusion of Dr. Hendricks' presentation each school representative spoke briefly in support of the attitude sustained by the Council in this respect.
        c. The joint meeting with the Board was concluded with an attitude of satisfaction and mutual appreciation of both segments.

Matter No. 5. Miscellaneous matters that had been brought to the attentions of the Council.
      a.   Dr. Peterson advised the Council of the new book that was being presented by Drs. Weiant and Goldschmidt. This text is in the form of a detailed and catalogued reference to verifying statements and discussions about chiropractic and its principle in the literature of credited biologists, scientists and members of the medical profession, especially those in Germany.

Because of the fact that the text was being printed in Germany it would be made available to doctors and students at a comparatively very nominal price.

It was the conclusion that this text might serve as a handsome supplement to the course in principles and concept.
      b.   Dr. Janse drew the Council's attention to a small comprehensive text entitled "A Day in Court" as readied by Dr. Robt. T. Leiter of Macon, Georgia. It related to a competent catalog on actual cases as to how a doctor should conduct himself in court and what his responsibilities and privileges are.
      c.   The matter of the foreign student was brought into focus of discussion. Following were some of the major points referred to.
        (1) Too many of the foreign students were matriculating at non-accredited schools and efforts should be made by all the accredited colleges to interest the foreign students in the NCA educational program.
        (2) The large percentage of foreign chiropractors are graduates of the Palmer School hence the tendency to refer students to this school. Evidence was growing to indicate a steady turn to NCA concepts and this should be encouraged.
        (3) It is becoming increasingly more important to convey the idea of the NCA program into the chiropractic circles of foreign practitioners.
        (4) Dr. Troilo sought advice in relation to the tendency of some state boards to expect a defraying of expenses whenever an inspection of a college was made. Special reference was made to the Pennsylvania Chiropractic Board.

He was advised that others of the accredited colleges had been inspected by members of the Pennsylvania Board and that they had been paid for their expenses by the individual colleges. Dr. Peterson offered to investigate the matter inasmuch as a graduate of the New York school was on the Board and had demonstrated an understanding attitude toward matters of this type.
        (5) Dr. Janse submitted to the Council a letter received from Lester M. Wegner, Registrar of the Western States Chiropractic College requesting that something be done about the standardizing of transcript forms of the various accredited colleges especially those relating to those occasions when a chiropractic student sought to submit his chiropractic credits to a liberal arts college or university for evaluation and the granting of credit leading toward a baccalaureate degree.

The letter was attended by a suggested form, and a copy of which had been sent to the heads of all of the accredited colleges.

After some discussion it was concluded that the occasions where a chiropractic student sought to have his chiropractic credits evaluated by a college or university were actually quite infrequent and hence a readying of a special form for this purpose would be an expense beyond need.

It was however, concluded that effort should be made on the part of all the accredited schools to prepare a transcript form that would be in conformity with the general pattern of transcripts as used by various colleges and universities.
        (6) Dr. Hendricks then drew attention to a letter that had been received by the Webster City offices of the NCA and had been referred to the Council on Education. The communication had been written by Dr. Norman B. Bartlett of Rolla, Missouri and pertained to the ever existing question as to what is good scientific and clinical chiropractic and the responsibility of the school heads in establishing a competent yard stick of evaluation.

It was all agreed that a renovating of many of the ideas of chiropractic theory and concept should be conducted but it was also realized that there was always the problem of personnel, time and wherewith.

The secretary was instructed to write Dr. Bartlett and advise him of this problem that constantly confronts the chiropractic educators.
        (7) A similar communication had been received by Dr. Hendricks from a Dr. Larkins in Pennsylvania. Although the Council was fully sympathetic toward the disposition of the letter it was concluded as in instance of the Bartlett letter that at present all schools had their hands full without the assuming of the extended responsibility of attempting to standardize concept and technic.

Matter No. 6. Relating to the matriculating of blind students.

1.   Periodically certain organizations for the blind seek to put pressure on the accredited colleges to induce them to accept blind students.

2.   It was conceded that it constituted a touchy and hazardous subject especially with blind doctors of chiropractic in the field and whom neither the colleges nor the NCA wished to alienate.

3.   It was generally concluded that the schools should accept only those applicants who, by optometric test if necessary, could prove themselves qualified to do the classroom, laboratory and textbook work expected of the average student.

Matter No. 7. Discussion of the trend of thinking besetting segments of the National Council of Chiropractic Examining Boards, namely that the accrediting of chiropractic schools should be the function of an independent Committee set up by the Council of Examining Boards rather than the Council on Education.

1.   The Director of Education and other members of the Council voiced their concern about the inclination on part of certain elements in the Council of Examining Boards and also the NCA to sustain the promise that the accrediting of chiropractic schools should be the function of an independent Committee.

2.   It was acknowledged that the State Board of Examiners did constitute segments of assigned state authority, yet because of the varied and heterogeneous attitudes sustained amongst the various state board members any attempt on part of the Council of Examining Boards to assume the function of accreditation would result in confusion and indiscreet function.

3.   Any such action would give impetus and advantage to those schools that have withstood and flaunted opposition to the efforts of the Council on Education.

4.   It was realized that greater effort should be made to contact the various state board members and explain to them the exact function, and duties of the Council on Education and the need to leave the accrediting program in the hands of the Council.

5.   It was unanimously concluded that great detriment would be imposed upon the profession if the program of the Council were to be reduced in effectiveness by the mitigating influences of such a trend of thinking.

Matter No. 8. Pertaining to the request of the Internist Society of Rhode Island.

1.   Dr. Haynes submitted to the Council a letter that he had received from Dr. Daniel V. Nash encouraging the Council to grant official approval and accreditation of the course in various phases of diagnosis that had been conducted and completed by the Internist Society of Rhode Island.

2.   Dr. Pierce of Providence, Rhode Island had advised Dr. Nash, as

[PAGE 11 MISSING]

2.   Dr. Hendricks then proceeded to read the preliminary report and presented a copy to the chairman of the Executive Board. Upon the completion of the same he asked to be heard on a matter that concerned the entire membership of the Council, namely the issue of school consolidation and amalgamation. Dr. Hendricks advised the Board that the Council would urgently ask to dispel the idea of consolidation from the minds of the Executive Board as well as the entire membership of the NCA Following were the main points of reason for this stand by the Council.

a.   The Council on Education does not favor the consolidation of NCA schools but does definitely favor the inclusion of non-accredited schools.

b.   Any attempt at amalgamation of accredited schools would result in a loss of students to non-accredited schools.

c.   There is an ever growing need for accredited schools in strategic areas of the country.

d.   Amalgamation of accredited schools would encourage the establishment of unaccredited schools.

3.   The meeting was then opened for questions and answers and discussion.

a.   The question was asked of the Council whether there was a proposed plan for the raising of revenue and the administration of the same. Dr. Peterson as chairman of the Committee answered by stating the following points.

(1)   The entire membership of the NCA should support the schools by submitting to an increase in dues and that a Foundation with a Board of Trustees be created for the reception of these monies and the proper administration of the same.

(2)   That all the accredited colleges would have equal privilege and that the economically successful colleges would not be discriminated against but that arrangement would be made to permit them to use their share on capital improvements rather than on sustaining expenditures.

(3)   Dr. Peterson voiced the opinion that if the program could be evolved so that eventually the upkeep of the physical plant could be subsidized, student tuition should cover the academic program.

(4)   He cautioned against hurry in the entire matter acknowledging the need for educating the professional membership to the need of such a program.

b.   Dr. Murphy asked for the privilege of reading a letter he had received from Dr. Dewey Anderson, encouraging the consolidation of chiropractic schools and the establishment of a laymen's committee for the investigation of chiropractic colleges to determine their fitness to continue.

It was the general disposition that probably Dr. Anderson was not fully aware of the problem as defined by the Council and it was recommended that certain reliable elements of the Council seek to orient him as to the exact nature of the problem.

    c. Dr. John Wolfe emphasized the fact that all plans of the Executive Board and the Council should take the future into consideration. The ever increase in national population would demand more chiropractic doctors and as a result there will be an increasing need for all the accredited colleges.

He stressed the regional importance of the smaller accredited schools, and significantly drew attention to the possibility of alienating the loyalty of the alumni of the smaller schools if consolidation were to be effected and drive them into the ranks of the ICA

    d. Both Drs. Nugent and Peterson stressed the fact that professional colleges out of academic and clinical necessity cannot competently handle large student bodies.

    e. The question was asked as to whether by combining two or more of the accredited colleges the administrative costs would not be cut down accordingly? The answer was not proportionately.

    f. Drs. Haynes, Troilo and Janse then briefly spoke on the subject lending their support to the fact that there is a definite need for all of the present accredited colleges.

    g. Dr. Walter Wolf speaking in behalf of the Committee on Educational Standards voiced similar sustaining opinions and attitudes insisting that the ideal set up in professional education is the comparative small school.

    h. Dr. Peterson was then asked as to whether his Committee had considered any other plan for raising money other than increase in NCA membership dues? The doctor answered by saying that the Committee had but had come up with nothing of a substantial nature.

    i. The meeting terminated with mutual expression of awareness of the importance of the problem and a declaration of desire and intent to research the matter further until a competent solution was found.

Matter No. 10. Pertaining to the proposal of the Neurological Research Foundation, Inc. to have the clinical concept known as Autonomic Nerve Control introduced as undergraduate and graduate study into the accredited colleges.

1. Dr. Terrence J. Bennett the Founder of the Foundation and the originator of the clinical concept had submitted to all members of the Council a brief detailing the purpose of the Foundation, its financial status and the fundamentals underlying the clinical concept supported by the Foundation. This had been accompanied by an offer from him to submit the clinical concept to the accredited colleges for under graduate and graduate instruction.

    a. It was Dr. Bennett's original thought to have instructors from the Foundation periodically come to the accredited colleges and put on the course for the seniors of the undergraduate school and instruct them in the concept and technic of application. For this the college in question would charge an extra tuition of $75 to $95 out of which the expenses of the instructor from the Foundation would be paid.

Then at regular or special post-graduate sessions review, and refresher courses would be taught for which a nominal tuition of approximately $10 would be charged. These classes would also be conducted at the accredited colleges.

2. Careful discussion of Dr. Bennett's plan led to the conclusion that it would be impractical and rather impossible to attach another special course fee onto the undergraduate tuition. That it would be somewhat disturbing to the undergraduate student body to have such a special course taught by other than regular members of the chiropractic department teaching faculty. That the colleges would not, at the present time, care to assume the responsibility of organization, advertising and conducting "review" course in the work as handsome as it might be from a clinical standpoint.

3. Drs. Hendricks and Janse were instructed to contact Dr. Bennett and advise him of the same and to inquire as to whether some other arrangement might not be concluded.

4. Such was done and Dr. Bennett asked the Council submit to him and his associates a plan which might be compatible to the schoolmen. This invitation was responded to by the Council which submitted to Dr. Bennet the following proposal:

    a. That each accredited college appoint a faculty member to attend a special class of instruction for this purpose only. This class would be held in a centrally located city to which all of the appointed faculty members from the accredited colleges would come to take the course.

        (1) It was suggested by Dr. Ralph Martin, who knows the work thoroughly, that the teaching of the course be divided into two sections as seeking to absorb it entirely in one teaching might be difficult.

        (2) It was also concluded that it would be a matter of individual volition as far as the schools were concerned. No college would be made to participate if its administration did not see fit to do so.

    b. That upon the completion of this special instruction period the faculty members would return to their respective colleges and carefully seek to introduce it into the undergraduate course, as a special class in the senior year.

    c. The Foundation would be paid by each college the regular tuition fee for the course as taken by the assigned faculty member. The traveling expenses of the faculty members from the various colleges would be prorated.

    d. If deemed necessary a review course might be conducted for the faculty group that was participating in the program.

e.   The schoolmen felt that they did not want to assume the responsibility of having their respective institutions advertise, organize or conduct any review courses for the graduate doctors and sought to encourage the Foundation to conduct these at their own discretion and disposition.

f.   As an alternative it was suggested that if it were not possible to have a special class for the faculty group it might then be possible for each college to send a faculty member to one of the regular classes that would be regionally held in the vicinity of the college.

4.   Dr. Bennet was again contacted by Drs. Hendricks and Janse and he indicated his acceptance of the above recommendations. He suggested that if such were done that the undergraduate class simply be called "Reflexology" rather than Autonomic Nerve Control and thus avoiding any pin-pointing of the concept.

5.   Further discussion by the Council resulted in the conclusion that the matter might be worked out satisfactory to everyone and that further study of the possibilities should definitely be conducted.

Drs. Haynes and Martin were instructed to mediate further with Dr. Bennett and his associates. They were asked to especially determine whether anyone of the colleges wishing to include it in their graduate or post-graduate schools might do so without financial obligation to the Foundation.

Matter No. 11 - Council received Mrs. Walter B. Rich, President of the National Chiropractic Auxiliary.

1.   Mrs. Rich advised the Council that the Auxiliary's stationery project for purpose of raising funds for their scholarship program had bogged down and asked that the colleges support the project by carrying a small announcement of the same in their college journals.

2.   She informed the Council that the first $300 scholarship had been consummated and that the first year recipient the Northwestern College had cooperated in a most handsome manner in the presentation of the same.

3.   It might be mentioned that Dr. Janse as secretary of the Council during the convention week addressed the auxiliary and spoke on the subject of the Future of Chiropractic Education. Consequent to his address the Auxiliary went on record of initiating a program entitled "Dollars for Chiropractic Education."

Matter No. 12. Council received Dr. M.A. Giammarino, Executive-Secretary of the National Examining Board of Chiropractic Roentgenologists.

1.   Dr. Giammarino sought to advise the Council that the program creating a specialization, namely Chiropractic Roentgenologists, devised by the Council on Chiropractic Roentgenology, and approved of by the Council on Education, had been successfully brought into being.

a.   The first examination had been held in Omaha in conjunction with the annual x-ray symposium as sponsored by the Council on Roentgenology. Some 20 applicants had taken the examination and three had successfully passed the same, others having failed in one or more subjects and who had been invited to repeat.

b.   That in May in conjunction with the annual convention of the Illinois Chiropractic Society, the second examination had been held at which five new applicants and three repeaters had participated. At this time one of the new applicants passed all the examinations and one of the repeaters was successful in obtaining his certification.

c.   Dr. Janse who had taken the Omaha examination advised the Council of the competence and quality with which the examinations had been conducted and verified to the general attitude of respect that all examinees held in regard to the examination.

d.   Dr. Haynes advised the Council that Dr. Smith the California member of the National Board was very pleased with the conduct of the Board and the caliber of examination given.

e.   Dr. Giammarino advised that to date there were then 5 who had been certified by examination as Chiropractic Roentgenologists, as well as the three men from California who qualified by waiver privileges on strength of the qualifying program that had been conducted by the California Roentgenological Society, and then of course the three original members of the Board, namely Drs. Wunsch, Giammarino and Smith.

d.   Dr. Giammarino did seek to advise the schoolmen that the following major deficiencies were noted in the majority of the examinees:

1. Radiological anatomy
2. Correlative diagnosis
3. Poor incompetent clinical terminology
4. Vague and protopathic concept of basic spinography
5. Weakness in interpretation of lumbosacral mechanical pathologies.

e.   The following list of registered chiropractic roentgenologists was submitted:

(1)   Those having passed the Board: Dr. L.P. Rehberger, Dr. Earl Rich, Dr. Leonard Richie, Dr. Ronald Watkins, Dr. Joseph Janse.

(2)   Those having received certification by waiver: Dr. Clifford B. Eacrett, Dr. Chas. A. Moran, Dr. James O. Empringham

      (3)   Those constituting the original Board: Dr. Leo E. Wunsch Sr., Dr. Duane Smith, Dr. M.A. Giammarino

    f. Dr. Giammarino mentioned that the Council on Roentgenology had contemplated appointing at present just one person to replace Drs. Poehner and Baer both of whom had passed away. At a subsequent meeting of the X-ray Council Dr. L.P. Rehberger was appointed as the new member of the National Examining Board in Chiropractic Roentgenology.

Matter No. 13. Relating to the request of Dr. Joseph Samskey, the Director of the Chiropractic Section of the Healing Arts Board of Kansas to determine what might be done with those students of those schools which the Kansas Board could not approve.

    1. Dr. Nugent advised the Council that in counsel with Dr. Samskey he had been informed that the Healing Arts Board had denied approval or recognition of the following two chiropractic colleges in Kansas, namely the Kansas State Chiropractic College and the Harris College of Chiropractic, and that he Dr. Samskey had been instructed by the Department of Education to advise the administrative officers of these institutions to terminate their efforts.

    2. The concern that now confronted Dr. Samskey was what to do with the comparative few students who are now being trained at these colleges.

    3. Dr. Nugent advised the Council that in conversation with Dr. Nash the Executive Secretary of the Healing Arts Board in Kansas the opinion was expressed that some deference and consideration should be extended these students, because they were confronted by a compromise of economics and time.

    4. Dr. Janse recommended that Dr. Samskey be encouraged to advise these students to make application for transfer to any one of the accredited colleges of choice, and that the registrar's office of that college seek to process the evaluation of their credits as prescribed by the previous conclusions of the Council in relation to credits from non-accredited colleges.

    5. It was concluded that this should be done and the secretary of the Council was instructed to write Dr. Samskey accordingly. Following being a copy of the letter so directed.

Dr. Joseph M. Samskey, Member, Healing Arts Board of Kansas, 500 North 4th. Street, Kansas City 1, Kansas.
Dear Doctor Samskey:

    In response to your request that the Council on Education determine what considerations might be afforded by the accredited colleges to those students of the schools which have been rejected by the Kansas Board, may we submit the following:

    1. That these students be encouraged to make application for transference to the accredited college of their choice.

    2. To send a complete transcript of their credits to this college as soon as possible.

    3. The registrars' offices will make a tentative evaluation which is to be sent to the Committee of Evaluation of Credits of the Council. This Committee will come to a definite conclusion. The student in turn will be advised by the registrar of the college to which application has been made.

    4. The Council has decided upon this procedure so as to mitigate any tendency for a student to "shop" amongst the accredited colleges to determine where he or she might be able to obtain the best "deal."

    5. It is the concurrence of the Council membership that these students should be assisted as competently and substantially as possible.

    We of the Council at this time wish to express our sincerest admiration for you and your associates on the manner in which you have handled a most difficult and compromising problem. If at any time we can be of further help please do not hesitate to let us know.

    With every good wish I seek to remain, Most sincerely yours, J. Janse, Secretary.

Matter No. 14. Relating to the possible consolidation of the Carver College with the Texas College.

    1. Dr. Osborne as chairman of the committee on educational standards advised the Council that the Committee, the Director of Education had been in conference with Drs. Troilo and Hearn, Dean and President of the Texas Chiropractic College, respectively and consulted with them about the possible merger of the Carver College with the Texas College.

    2. It was the general consensus of opinion that this would indeed be a fine thing and represent a benefit to the entire profession in the Southwest.

    3. Dr. Osborne then read the following recommendations of the Committee to the Council, which were unanimously approved.

        a. That the officers of the Texas College be privileged to proceed to negotiate with the Carver College and effect a merger if possible.

        b. That in instance of Carver students having but a semester or two left at the Carver College be permitted to go to the Texas College to finish that amount of time at the same and then receive their degree as issued in the name of the Carver College.

        c. Those students having more than one or two semesters left are to go to the Texas College and to simply continue their training under the program of the Texas College and upon completion of the same receive their degree as issued by the Texas College of Chiropractic.

    The secretary of the Council was instructed to write Dr. Troilo a letter and advise him to this effect. Following is a copy of the same.

Dr. Julius C. Troilo, Dean, Texas Chiropractic College, 618 West Myrtle Street, San Pedro Park, San Antonio, Texas.
Dear Doctor Troilo:

This is to officially advise you that the Council on Education at its recent mid-year meeting in Miami Beach, Florida reviewed the possibility of a merger between the Texas College and the Carver Chiropractic College. In such a merger the Council sees marked benefit to the profession especially throughout the southwest and the Council seeks to encourage you and your associates to bring this about.

The Council also agrees to the recommendations of the Committee on Educational Standards in relation to the processing of Carver students if the merger is effected.

1. In instance of Carver students having but one or two semesters left in their training program be permitted to go to the Texas College and finish that amount of time at the same and then receive their degree as issued in the name of the Carver College of Chiropractic.
2. Those students having more than one or two semesters left are to go to the Texas College and to simply continue their training under the program of the Texas College and upon completion of the same receive their degree as issued by the Texas College of Chiropractic.

May we hope that you and your associates will be able to bring about this merger and we wish to extend every good wish in this effort. If the Council can be of any further service please do not hesitate to seek the same.

Sincerely yours, J. Janse, Secretary.

4. Dr. Peterson asked that the students at Carver be privileged to seek transfer to any of the other accredited colleges if they desired. He cited the example of the fact that inasmuch as the Chiropractic Institute had always emphasized the Carver concept and was really the product of amalgamation between a Carver conceived school in the East with others, some students had inquired about the possibility of transferring to New York. It was acknowledged that in the final summation students could not be assigned colleges to go to.

Matter No. 14. Relating to the issue as to whether a schoolman should attend the inspection of a chiropractic college.

1. The Director of Education brought the Council's attention to the fact that he had been asked to accompany Dr. Samskey and two medical members of the Healing Arts Board of Kansas in an inspection of the Cleveland College resident in Kansas City, Missouri.
2. Inasmuch as the National College had been included in the literature of the Bill creating the Healing Arts Board as the school of standard he had deemed it advisable to contact Dr. Janse and request that he accompany Dr. Nugent in the inspection of the Cleveland College of Chiropractic.
3. Dr. Janse after deliberation and consultation with members of the Committee on Educational Standards, and the Chairman of the Council proper had declined the request on the grounds that decision of the Council of some three years ago had stipulated that no school man should be asked to inspect another school.
4. The question now is should this conclusion be maintained or should a schoolman under certain special circumstances be asked to attend a school inspection. The general conclusion being that with the circumstances as they are in the profession it would represent somewhat of a compromise of any schoolman to inspect another school and such a requirement should be avoided whenever possible.
5. It was maintained that such a function pertained to the Committee on Educational Standards and should be contained and retained within the same.

Matter No. 15. Relating to the teaching of hypnosis at the accredited colleges.

1. Dr. Herman S. Schwartz, Chairman of the Council on Psychotherapy appeared before the Council and asked that the Council voice a definite attitude against the teaching of hypnotic procedures to the undergraduates in any of the accredited colleges.
2. Following resolution was unanimously passed by the Council in this respect. "The Council on Education of the National Chiropractic Association strongly recommends that the principle and technic of hypnosis be excluded from undergraduate instruction in any of the accredited colleges. The Council feels that the teaching of this subject to the undergraduate student would be wrought with hazard and indiscriminate attempts at clinical application."
3. Dr. Schwartz also drew attention to the fact that the National Association For Mental Health had made an unwarranted attack on chiropractic and he felt that something should be done about it. Inasmuch as this organization was going to hold a meeting soon in New York, Dr. Peterson said that he and Dr. Weiant would look into the matter.

Matter No. 16. Relating to a joint meeting of the Council on Education and Council of Chiropractic Examining Boards.

1. At the invitation of Dr. Melvin Klette, Chairman of the Council of Examining Boards the Council met in joint session with all the attending state board examiners.
2. After statements of deference and welcome from both chairmen the meeting was opened for general discussion.
3. Dr. Peterson asked for the privilege of recommending to the Council of Examining Boards that if possible all the chiropractic colleges be reacquainted with the rulings on reciprocity and exemption by waiver that were now being sustained by the various Boards. He advised that it was exceedingly difficult for the registrars' offices of the colleges to maintain an up to date file on these matters and advice as to the current situation from each Board would be most helpful.

4. Dr. Guy Smith then asked about the Council's on Education attitude toward the two year college program preceding or attending the professional course. Drs. Peterson, Nugent and Janse fully detailed to the assembly the Council's stand on the matter and referred all in attendance to the published policy of the Council on the matter.
5. The Council on Examining Boards were encouraged to seek methods whereby subjects and questions on state board might become somewhat more standardized

[missing page(s)]

6. Six years from now the U.S. population is estimated will be 200,000,000. Applying the same figures as above the chiropractic population in 1964 should be 200,000,000 divided by 6600 or 30,350 to maintain existing ratio. The loss per year in 1964 should be 30,350 x 0.0316 or 958. Additional new graduates required in 1964 to accommodate a population growth of 3,000,000 for that year is 3,000,000 divided by 6,600 or 456. Total graduates needed in 1964 to maintain chiropractic strength at present level in relation to population 958 plus 456 equals 1414.
7. Chiropractic population (student) necessary in 1963 to graduate 1414 students.

    Freshman 1414 x 100/75   1886
    Sophomores 1414 x 80/75   1510
    Juniors   1414
    Seniors   1414
    Total   6224

Total school population required in 1964 to maintain present chiropractic population in relation to general population is 6224. If it is assumed that the accredited colleges will contain only 50% of the students in chiropractic the figures will be 3112 students or many hundreds of students beyond the present maximum capacity of all the accredited schools (2500)

8. If this figure appears high it is because total chiropractic population has possibly been exaggerated by reporting agencies over the years. If the figure of present chiropractic population is arbitrarily reduced to introduce realism or conservatism and the same calculations are repeated.
9. Estimated present chiropractic strength — 25,000, conservative estimate.
10. Ratio of chiropractors to population, 1/7250
11. Chiropractic strength estimated in 1964 is 200,000,000 divided by 7250 or 27,600
12. New loss per year in 1964 is 27,600x 0.0316 or 874
13. Yearly increment of increase in chiropractic graduates to accommodate 3,000,000 yearly population increase is 3,000,000 divided by 7250 or 413.
14. Total yearly graduates necessary in 1964 to maintain existing ratio 874 plus 413 equals 1287.
15. Total students necessary in 1964 to produce 1287 graduates

    Freshman 1287 x 100/75 =   1722
    Sophomores 1287 x 80/75 = 1377
    Juniors   1287
    Seniors   1287
    Total   5673

16. Using the conservative estimate of 25,000 chiropractors total today, in 1964 the present accredited schools would have to accommodate 2836 students to maintain the existing ratio of 1/7250. This is more than the maximum capacity of the present schools.
17. Conclusions.

The above set of figures is intentionally ultra-conservative, still they prove the contention that our present schools are needed for the future. These figures do not allow for chiropractic growth in relation to population.

Minutes of the Mid-Year Meeting of the NATIONAL COUNCIL ON EDUCATION of the NATIONAL CHIROPRACTIC ASSOCIATION, Baker Hotel, January 3, 4, 5, and 6, 1959, Dallas, Texas
Dr. Arthur G. Hendricks, Chairman of the Council, presided at all of the sessions.

In attendance were:
A. Administrative personnel of the accredited educational institutions of the National Chiropractic Association.
   Dr. Arthur G. Hendricks, Chairman of the council, and President of the Lincoln Chiropractic College, Inc., 633 N. Pennsylvania Avenue, Indianapolis 3, Indiana
   Dr. Joseph Janse, Secretary of the Council, and President of the National College of Chiropractic, 20 N. Ashland

Blvd., Chicago 7, Illinois

Dr. Thure C. Peterson, President of the Chiropractic Institute of New York, 325 East 38th. Street, New York 16, New York.

Dr. George H. Haynes, Dean of the Los Angeles College of Chiropractic, 920 East Broadway, Glendale 5, California.

Dr. John B. Wolfe, President of the Northwestern College of Chiropractic, 2222 Park Avenue, Minneapolis 3, Minnesota.

Dr. Julius C. Troilo, Dean of the Texas Chiropractic College, 618 West Myrtle Street, San Antonio, Texas.

Dr. Edw. B. Hearn, President of the Texas Chiropractic College, 220 N. Zangs, Dallas, Texas.

Dr. A. Earl Homewood, Dean of the Canadian Memorial Chiropractic College, 252 Bloor Street West, Toronto 5, Ontario, Canada.

Dr. Robert Elliot, President of the Western States College of Chiropractic, sent his excuses for being unable to attend.

B. Members of the National Committee on Educational Standards.

Dr. John J. Nugent, Director of Education, National Chiropractic Association, 92 Norton Street, New Haven, Connecticut

Dr. Walter B. Wolf, Chairman of the Committee, 207 West Main Street, Eureka, South Dakota

Dr. Norman E. Osborne, Secretary of the Committee, Longmeadows Extended R. D. 5, Hagerstown, Maryland.

Dr. Ralph J. Martin, 478 N. Sierra Madre Blvd., Sierra Madre, California.

The Council was advised that the President of the NCA with the approval of the Executive Board had appointed Dr. F.C. Etheridge, Jr., 106 Howard Street, Rossville, Georgia, to fill the vacancy left by the retirement of Dr. E.H. Gardner.

Dr. Hendricks as chairman of the Council had appointed an agenda committee and in the course of the meetings the following matters were discussed and concluded.

Matter No. 1. A study of the professional situation in Louisiana and an evaluation of the pending federal court case as it relates to the Louisiana situation.

a. The deliberations extended over several sessions and involved the participation first of the Council members, then with representatives of the Louisiana Chiropractic Association, the Executive Board of the NCA, the legal counsel of the NCA and finally with the counsel for the Louisiana group. The discussions were extended and involved and following are the pertinent points and conclusions:

(1) That although the Louisiana Medical Practice Act provided for the practice of chiropractic it certainly did not clearly define the privileges or restrictions, nor the qualifying requirements.

(2) That various amendments to the Medical Practice Act completely prohibited any possibility for the chiropractic profession to seek function under the act.

(3) That the medical board of examiners assigned the responsibility of administering the Act had been capricious and unfair in their relation to the chiropractic profession for the following reasons:

(a) Had openly derogated chiropractic and announced the determination to exclude doctors of chiropractic from obtaining licensure under the Act.

(b) Had refused to inspect or accredit any of the existing chiropractic schools.

(c) Had insisted that any examinee who would seek to take the Board would have to pass examinations in materia medica and surgery.

(4) That as the result of this situation and because within recent years the practicing doctors of chiropractic in Louisiana had been constantly harassed and subject to arrest, the Legal Action Committee of the Louisiana State Chiropractic Association had employed counsel and taken action to mitigate the problem. This action to date had resolved in the following:

(a) The decision to carry the issue into the Federal Courts on the basis and argument that the conduct of the Medical Board being capricious and unfair had infringed upon the constitutional right of the Louisiana practitioners and hence it became a matter of federal court deliberation.

(b) At first the district federal court rejected this appeal but later rescinded its decision and by majority vote submitted the conclusion that "they the chiropractors should have their day in court, to prove the merit and clinical value of their practice".

(c) In consequence the chiropractors in Louisiana and their counsel proceeded to conclude that they were going to accept this privilege and seek to ready their case of "proof and evidence". All this being attended by the following surmises:

(1) That if they win their case it would force the State of Louisiana to instruct the Legislature to enact a chiropractic law and it would set a precedence, because of Federal Court involvement, that might be referred in the support of chiropractic legislation elsewhere.

(d) However, the need for financial and documentary help became increasingly more pressing. Appeal had been made to various groups and segments of the profession. At first the ICA had hesitated in its willingness of support. Subsequently, probably on the anticipation that a favorable decision would provide a wedge for other legal actions against medical boards, readiness for support was indicated.

(e) Questioning of the Louisiana representatives and counsel revealed that it had been their intent to submit their case on the basis of the typical limited ICA definition and interpretation of diagnostic and practice scope. It also became obvious that these people had been misinformed about the status of chiropractic practice under the medical acts of such states as Illinois, New Jersey, and Indiana.

(f) This of course provoked concern and caution in the minds of the Council Members and the counsel of the NCA as well as the Executive Board. In fact the following points of hazard were brought up for study and observation and exactingly detailed to the Louisiana representatives and their counsel.

    (1) That federal courts in the past had not been too favorable in their attitudes toward chiropractic.

    (2) That a favorable decision by the federal court of that area yet on the basis of a limited definition and interpretation of practice would have harmful extending effect in states where the practice of chiropractic enjoyed comparative broad interpretation and practice.

    (3) That an unfavorable decision by the federal court would provide the opposition with a precedence which they might well employ against chiropractic all over the country.

(g) The Louisiana representatives and their counsel at first mitigated the significance of these apprehensions but progressively sensed their importance and granted deference. However, they expressed their determination to go ahead with their case.

(h) Further deliberations of the Council with the NCA counsel and executive officers led to certain conclusions which were submitted to the Council by the Executive Secretary of the NCA and which was distributed to each Council member as a confidential directive by the chairman of the Council. Essentially these conclusions provided both financial aid and documentary assistance to the Louisiana group under the stipulation of certain reservations.

Matter No. 2. Discussion of the professional and legal situation in some

(a) The NCA counsel advised the Council group of the recent events in Wisconsin as relating to the Grayson case, namely that the decision of the court prohibited the use of instrumentalities of therapy but did grant the continuance of the use of instrumentalities of diagnosis and analysis.

(b) The Director of Education advised that in Montana the situation had resolved itself in the Court ordering the Examining Board to permit the two P.S.C. applicants to sit for the examination. That to this extent the P.S.C. had been recognized in Montana. That the Court had not instructed the Board to extend the P.S.C. unqualified accreditation. That it was hoped that the state legislature might be prevailed upon to amend the chiropractic act and empower the Examining Board to uphold its conclusions on what schools of chiropractic it would or would not recognize.

(c) The Council was advised that in Illinois the NCA affiliated State Society had been working with the state's attorney's office in conducting suits against unlicensed practitioners and that this effort was beginning to take effect. Furthermore, that the chairman and the secretary of the Council had been asked by the State Society to appear at a hearing before the Illinois Medical Commission at which the Society submitted to the Commission a printed brief on the Society's position relative to the efforts, conduct, intrusions of the unlicensed practitioners as well as the attitude of the licensed group toward the present mechanism of licensure under the Medical Act. A copy of this report to the commission might be obtained from the Secretary of the Illinois Chiropractic Society, Dr. L.E. Fay, 694.5 W. Grand Ave., Chicago, Ill.

Matter No. 3. Review of the effectiveness and accomplishments of the regional NCA seminars.

(a) Although of no great pertinence the opinion was expressed that probably the timing of the seminars might be studied a little more carefully as well as consultation with local personnel in obtaining hotel arrangements would possibly enable reduction in expense and inconvenience.

Matter No. 4. Conclusion of the matter of business pertaining to the National Board of Certified Chiropractic Roentgenologists.

(a) The secretary of the Council submitted a letter as directed to the Council by the secretary of the National Board in relation to a matter that had come up and on which the Board sought the advice of the Council. It was about the fact that several Canadian doctors of chiropractic had indicated their desire to write the National Board, but they did not sustain membership in NCA nor the National Council of Chiropractic Roentgenologists, and they had requested that the National Board consider special dispensation of their case.

(b) The discussions which included the opinion and advice of the dean of the Canadian school eventuated into the following conclusions which the secretary of the Council submitted to the secretary of the National Board.

    (1) That those Canadians desirous of becoming Certified Chiropractic Roentgenologists through examination by the Board in question should definitely hold membership in the NCA

    (2) That the National Board should be privileged to honor their membership in the Canadian National Council of Chiropractic

Roentgenologists in lieu of membership in the National Council of Chiropractic Roentgenologists.

(3) That the National Board could certainly recognize the necessary qualifying credits as provided by programs of training accredited by the Canadian Roentgenological council.

(4) The National Board might be encouraged to eventually include a qualified Canadian as a member on the Board.

Matter No. 5. Study of the effectiveness in function of the regional evaluating committees that had been created at the previous mid-year meeting.

(a) It was acknowledged that at times the function of the committees had been a little cumbersome and possibly responses somewhat delayed but in over all a competent purpose had been accomplished.

(b) Several additional ideas were suggested but finally it was concluded to recommend that the committees and the personnel of the same continue to function as were.

(c) The following conclusions and instruction were unanimously decided upon:

(1) Upon receipt for advanced standing on the basis of having obtained work at an non-accredited college the school in question should have the registrar's office send to the elected regional committee the name of the applicant, the date of application and the non-accredited school at which the work was obtained.

(2) The above should be attended by a suggested evaluation.

(3) The evaluation committee in question should establish an official conclusion, advise the school in question of the same and also the other evaluating committees, and thus avoid the possibility of the applicant making two applications to two different schools and have his work evaluated by two different committees.

Matter No. 6. Complete review of the fund for chiropractic education and a study of the plan effected by the Executive Board and referred to as FACE

(a) This matter represented the major matter for discussion and concern within the Council. It involved extended deliberations which resulted in a joint meeting with the Executive Board and other officers of the NCA The primary elements of attitude, conclusion and decision are presented as follows:

(1) There was a general attitude of disappointment and disfavor among the Council members in relation to the action of the Executive Board with the establishment of FACE

(2) It was the feeling that the original recommendations of the Council through its authorized committee had been side-stepped and a rather ineffective substitute effected.

(3) That FACE and the monies contained under its prescription represented more of a "figures on paper" proposition, rather than actual tangible aids to accredited schools.

(4) That a substitute for an actual assessment of the membership would represent little promise and contain but small potential.

(5) That some of the Executive Board members proper were dissatisfied with the program of FACE and expressed the opinion that it would result in but minimal benefit.

(6) Finally the related Council Committee consisting of Drs. Peterson, Wolfe, and Haynes were instructed to draw up a set of exact recommendations to the Executive Board and which were to be presented to the same by the Council chairman and the committee members in a full formal joint meeting of the Council with the Board and the NCA officers. Following are the stipulations that were drawn up, unanimously decided upon and submitted accordingly:

I. Opening remarks - Expression of thanks to the NCA Executive Board. Recapitulation of the history of the Council's request for economic aid.

(1) Expression of regret for the lack of consultation with the Council and its committee in the formulation of the program. Reminding the Board of the Council request in Miami for further consultation and the surprise of the Council membership to be made aware of the nature of the program not through private consultation with the Council, but rather through a public announcement.

II. Inadequacy of their present program.

(1) Gifts from foundations will not come to Funds controlled by a service organization. The present corporate status of FACE would place it in the order of a service organization controlled fund.

(2) The yearly revenue from the $50,000 endowment fund of FACE would be so small as to hardly make a splash in the field of research. Furthermore research grants are not to be considered as an economic aid to a college, for the equipment and expense of a research program generally exceeds the monetary value of the grant. Even if the $50,000 is many times increased, the revenue would not be adequate to underwrite major research programs. The accredited colleges were forced to request the NCA to withdraw their offer of $1000 per college for research purpose as we felt unable to carry on such a project to completion on such a budget.

(3) The operating fund could be of great assistance to the profession. However, under the present conditions there are no provisions made to assure the availability of adequate operation assistance to the colleges year after year. The only assured fact is that this

year the accredited colleges could obtain up to $43,200; but what about 1960, 1961 and 1962 and years thereafter. We all know that monetary assistance predicated upon the possibility of future donations from members of our profession is, to say the least, wishful thinking. To prove it just look at the history of the C.R.F.

It is you gentlemen, year after year, who have contributed to the welfare of the profession. It is now time that all members of the profession take over the load. Are you not tired of being the bankers of the profession? How many more dedicated men like you will continue to give and give?

III- Changes requested.

(1) It is our recommendation that the control of this fund be vested in a board of trustees embracing prominent laymen to induce the flow of non-professional donated funds.

(2) We suggest a Board consisting of: 1. The Director of Education; 2. A representative of the accredited colleges; 3. Three prominent laymen who have had experience in the business world in administrative capacities; 4. A representative of the Executive Board.

(3) Methods of raising money.

    (a)   As it has been clearly demonstrated, the only dependable and equitable method of supporting the growth and progress of a profession is by the raising of membership dues. We, therefore, feel that it is necessary to increase the NCA dues and such an increase to be earmarked for the educational fund. We request the equivalent of seven cents per day from every NCA member for this fund.

    (b)   A suitable percent of the public relations appropriation should be transferred to the operational fund of FACE to be used as intended by the colleges as outlined in a later section.

    (c)   Continue the solicitation of funds from the profession as encompassed in the present plan.

    (d)   Set into motion the solicitation of funds from non-professional sources.

IV. How the funds received are to be used by the colleges.

(1) The colleges need funds for an active procurement program. This involves the hiring of a representative who will make personal calls on high schools and colleges. He would place literature and speak to students in these schools. This is a public relations program that cannot be equaled as it involves personal contact.

(2) The colleges are in need of adequate funds to increase faculty salaries to retain and attract men of great ability. Living costs have increased but faculty salaries have not changed.

(3) A great deal of equipment becomes obsolete each year and there are no adequate funds from which to replace said equipment.

V. Conclusion.

(1) We, therefore, request $5000 for each college to set into motion the student procurement program. We further request the allocation of the equivalent free printing credit of $1000 (retail value) of promotional material for each college.

(2) Though the premature announcement of the FACE program might have produced an unfavorable atmosphere for the request of funds from the profession, we feel that by added collective work we will be able to obtain general cooperation for this program.

(3) The thought of a bankroll of $92,000 does decrease the willingness to donate or contribute to such a fund, as the assumption would be that such an amount is sufficient to meet all demands. Only your Board and we of the Council know better.

(4) If you gentlemen of the Board feel reticent to carry this matter through the House of Delegates we are ready to stand with you before the State representatives and help you get it through.

(7) It is to be noted that the foregoing is a verbatim copy of the recommendations made to the Executive Board and Officers of the NCA in a joint meeting with the full membership of the Council.

(8) It was at this joint meeting that the Executive Secretary of the NCA expressed his surprise at the dissatisfaction displayed by the Council with the organizing of FACE insisting that it represented the conscientious effort on the part of the NCA to provide the accredited colleges with rather immediate and tangible assistance.

(9) It was further expressed by the chairman of the Executive Board that the reason why an increase in membership for support of the accredited schools had not been considered advisable was contained within the fact that the California Chiropractic Association had disaffiliated itself from the NCA and this had represented quite a loss in membership.

(10) The Executive Board and Officers of the NCA were encouraged to consider the recommendations as submitted by the Council and drawn up by the Council Committee on Financial Aid for the Accredited Colleges.

(11) Consequent to the Dallas meetings directives had been received from the Secretary-Treasurer of the NCA detailing the conclusions and decisions of the Executive Board in relation to the recommendations of the Council in relation to FACE and the problem of financial aid for the schools.

    (a)   These directives have been submitted in confidence to all members of the Council.

Matter No. 7. As pertaining to the credentials of qualification as well as advanced standing for foreign students, especially those from France.

    (a)   NCA accredited colleges were increasingly being investigated by European students as possible institutions for chiropractic education. Some of these students sustain backgrounds of training in medical physical therapy, or massage and medical gymnastics.

The former course in such countries as France, Germany and Sweden entails from 3 to 4 years of education with a pre-professional requirement equivalent to approximately one year of college work, and the latter some two years of training with a pre-professional requirement of work equivalent to high school.

(b) It was acknowledged that the training in these courses in Europe entailed more study in both the basic sciences and clinical aspects than probably here in the United States and that any graduate of the same should experience the privilege of some advanced standing.

(c) After a careful analysis of the matter it was finally concluded that any person of any one of these European countries who could evidence having had training as a medical physical therapist might receive some two semesters (8 months) of advanced standing, and that any applicant being able to evidence having had training in medical message and gymnastics might be granted one semester (4 months) of advanced standing.

(d) Any school granting these privileges to foreign students should advise the regional evaluating committee of this action along with submitting the name of the student or students.

Matter No. 8. Pertaining to the teaching of audiometry in the accredited colleges.

(a) The chairman and secretary of the Council respectively had been contacted by the distributors of a national brand of "hearing-aid" unit to determine whether the colleges would be interested in instituting a course in audiometry.

(b) Finally it was concluded unanimously that the teaching of audiometry might be encouraged and arranged for if the manufacturers and sales organizations are willing to install the necessary equipment solely on the basis of a diagnostic study and service and without any obligations on the part of the schools.

Matter No. 9. As pertaining to the directive received from the Secretary of the California Board of Chiropractic Examiners.

(a) The dean of the Los Angeles College of Chiropractic advised the Council that the directive from the Secretary of the California Board was actually the consequence to an inquiry that he made to the Board for a clarification of what the Board would advise as to what the course in First Aid and Minor Surgery should include.

(b) The secretary of the Council advised that he had received a phone call from the secretary of the California Board advising that it was not the intent of the Board to prescribe the course completely but simply to advise the various schools what the Board thought the course should include and what the Board will examine in.

(c) It was concluded that each school would seek to evaluate the course in question. Determine what depth and extent the course might experience at the school in conformity with the tradition geographical and legal stipulations that surround it.

Matter No. 10. Relating to the recommendation as made by Dr. Mellon of Michigan suggesting that the colleges proceed to conduct aptitude tests amongst high school and college students to determine their inherent qualifications to take up chiropractic.

(a) It was conceded that the idea was worthy, yet at present somewhat impractical inasmuch as yet the student bodies of high schools and colleges were not accessible to representatives of chiropractic colleges, and as yet the volume of high school and college students interested in chiropractic was as yet too minimal to warrant such a venture.

(b) It was, however, concluded that it would be advisable for all the colleges to investigate the possibility of providing all new matriculants with the privilege of an aptitude and orientation test.

Matter No. 11. Relating to the letters distributed by the ICA over the signature of the counsel and secretary of the ICA and relating to another appeal for "unity" on certain professional aspects.

(a) Both letters mentioned certain resolutions that had been passed by the Board of Control of the ICA and pertained to the recommendation that a United Front Committee be formed consisting of representatives of C.C.A., ICA, NCA, North American Association of Chiropractic Schools, and the National Council on Education, for the purpose of determining a basis for "unity."

(b) Careful deliberations by the Council resulted in the conclusion that these letters should be answered in the form of a general public statement from the Council. Drs. Haynes, Nugent and Janse were appointed as a committee to draw up this statement which was to appear in the NCA Journal.

Matter No. 12. Consideration of the letter written by the chairman of the National Council on Chiropractic Physiotherapy recommending that all the accredited colleges institute a department of physiotherapy.

(a) It was the unanimous opinion that no college should be instructed to teach physiotherapy unless it was so disposed.

(b) Several of the schoolmen indicated that they were contemplating the possibility of such an action at some advantageous time in the future.

(c) The secretary of the Council was instructed to direct a letter to the chairman of the Council on Physiotherapy and advise him of these attitudes and conclusions.

Matter No. 13. Discussions relating to the request for accreditation of a course in orthopedics and certifications of the participants as submitted by the Florida Board of Orthopedic Review.

(a) Most of the schoolmen had received a number of communications from this Floridian group requesting that they participate in a graduate course in orthopedics, at the completion of which the participants would be certified as chiropractic orthopedists.

(b) It was the unanimous opinion of the Council that certainly any certification of any group of chiropractors as specialists in chiropractic orthopedics would be premature, and represent a compromise of clinical integrity.

(c) The observation was made that the popular trend toward "chiropractic specialties" constituted a hazard in that so often those participating advertised themselves as being a great deal more than they were, and were capable of representing.

(d) It was the consensus of opinion that the entire matter should experience careful control and judicious supervision. As a result when the representative of the Floridian group appeared before the Council he was advised of the following conclusions of the Council:

    (1) The Council on Education of the National Chiropractic Association requests letters from the Board of Chiropractic Examiners, and the Florida Chiropractic Association that the term "specialist" will not be used by those to receive training in chiropractic orthopedics.

    (2) That the Council on Education is willing to suggest to the House of Delegates of the National Chiropractic Association that the first steps to be taken to establish a Council on Chiropractic Orthopedics, which is the establishment of a Committee on chiropractic orthopedics. After this committee has been in existence for a set period of time and has acquired a certain membership, application for Council status may be made.

    (3) When and if a Council on Chiropractic Orthopedics is established it is agreed that no member of this Council will use the designation of "orthopedic specialist" in any of his listings, but may use the term "member of the National Council of Chiropractic Orthopedics."

    (4) If the foregoing stipulations are acceptable to those concerned and such is officially indicated the Council on Education would be willing to designate a course in which its accredited colleges will be permitted to participate at invitation.

        (e) The Council secretary was instructed to officially mediate these conclusions to the chairman of Florida Board of Orthopedic Review, the secretary of the Florida Board of Chiropractic Examiners, and the President of the Florida Chiropractic Association.

        (f) Subsequent to the above communications have been received from these three agencies indicating acceptance and approval of the Council recommendations.

Matter No. 14. Miscellaneous and concluding transactions.

    (a) The Council was advised that the Michigan Basic Science Board had evaluated the examinations in the basic science subjects as given by the California Board of Chiropractic Examiners and had indicated its readiness to recognize them as equivalent to their examinations and grant reciprocal certification accordingly. Three such privileges had already been granted.

    (b) The Council was also advised that the Internists Program once contemplated by a group in Rhode Island had evidenced no further activity.

    (c) The Utah situation came in for a brief discussion. Comment being made that sooner or later NCA representation would have to seek to establish contact with the agencies concerned. At present the Utah Board of Chiropractic Examiners would not accept the applications of graduates from schools teaching physiotherapy.

    (d) Mention was made of members of the National Board of Roentgenological Examiners participating in an educational program of a non-accredited college. It was encouraged of all schoolmen not to lend themselves in any way to the educational endeavors of any non-accredited school or group.

    (e) All schools were encouraged to augment the activities of their Jr. NCA programs, seeking to institute mechanisms that would make every student a Jr. NCA member.

    (f) Comment was made about the request by certain elements in the profession to have a meeting of representatives of the Council on Education, the North American Committee of Chiropractic Schools and the National Council of Chiropractic Examining Boards. It was concluded that the Council would in no way participate in any attempt to establish a schoolmen's organization outside the confines of the National Chiropractic Association and would not dignify any such effort by any degree of participation.

    (g) In a final discussion in relation to the matter of financial aid for the accredited colleges the following decisions were concluded: A committee consisting of Drs. Hendricks, Haynes and Nugent was assigned to meet with the Executive Board and the officers of the NCA on the afternoon following the Council meetings and detail to them the conclusions and recommendations of the Council in relation to FACE and the entire matter of raising funds for the support of the accredited colleges.

It was also agreed in general by the Council that unless some changes were made in the working mechanism of FACE the Council would not take advantage of the grants of funds at this time.

    (h) The election of officers for the coming year resulted in the resignation of Dr. Arthur G. Hendricks as Chairman and Dr. Joseph Janse as Secretary and the unanimous election of Dr. Joseph Janse as Chairman, and Dr. John B. Wolfe as Secretary.

Respectfully submitted, Dr. Joseph Janse, Secretary

Minutes of the Regular Convention Meeting of the COUNCIL ON EDUCATION, NCA, at the Leamington Hotel, Minneapolis, Minnesota - July 3 through July 7, 1960.

The meeting was called to order on Sunday, July 3, 1960 at 10:30 A.M. by Dr. George Haynes, president.
Members in attendance:
Presiding: Dr. George H. Haynes, Dean, Los Angeles College of Chiropractic.
    Dr. Jos. Janse, President, National College of Chiropractic.
    Mr. Charles A. Miller, Vice President, National College of Chiropractic.
    Dr. Thure C. Peterson, President, Chiropractic Institute of New York.
    Dr. Arthur G. Hendricks, President, Lincoln Chiropractic College.
    Dr. J.G. Anderson, Dean, Graduate School of L.A. College of Chiropractic.
    Dr. Julius C. Troilo, Dean, Texas Chiropractic College.
    Dr. Edward B. Hearn, President, Texas Chiropractic College.
    Dr. Robert E. Elliot, President, Western States College of Chiropractic.
    Dr. Earl A. Homewood, Dean, Canadian Memorial Chiropractic College.
    Dr. John B. Wolfe, President, Northwestern College of Chiropractic, recording secretary of the council.

    Accrediting Committee:
    Dr. John J. Nugent, Director of Education.
    Dr. Walter B. Wolf, Chairman.
    Dr. Norman E. Osborne.
    Dr. Ralph J. Martin.
    Dr. F.C. Etheridge.

The order of business was as follows:

Letter from Dr. Illi regarding qualifications of European students. No action was taken because the Council on Education has previously indicated to the chiropractors of Europe that it is cooperating in properly screening students from European countries.

Report by FACE Liaison Committee by Dr. Thure C. Peterson.
Dr. Peterson reported that the liaison committee had met with the Executive Board on Saturday, July 2, at 2:00 P.M. At this meeting Dr. Peterson presented the Council's mortgage purchase plan as a funds distribution program and discussed its merits. It was reported that there remains a difference in the opinion of the Executive Board and the Council on the basic elements of the plan as well as the steps to be followed in gaining accreditation for the schools. In the discussion the Executive Board asked the Council for recommendations with respect to Western States College and the Canadian Memorial College.
    A general discussion of alternate plans for distribution of FACE funds and the essential steps for gaining accreditation followed. As a conclusion to the above discussion Dr. Troilo proposed and Dr. Wolf seconded the following resolution which was then unanimously adopted:

Resolved: That the Council on Education reaffirm its previous position that the Council on Education be the sole accrediting agency for the NCA and that Dr. Nugent shall be instructed by the Council to proceed with the program of gaining approval of the Council on Education as an accrediting agency from the Department of Education in Washington.

Badger Report.
After discussing the apparent uses to which the Badger report was put by the Executive Board and the need for the Council to know the information contained therein, the following resolution was proposed by Dr. Peterson, seconded by Dr. Hendricks and unanimously adopted.

Resolved:
That the Council on Education through its president request a copy of the secret Badger report as a matter pertaining to education at the earliest practical time.

MEETING with Dewey Anderson.
The good that might come from having an informal meeting with Dr. Anderson was discussed. It was agreed by consent that the president should invite Dr. Anderson to meet with the Council later today.

Council on Examining Boards.

The problems of exchanging mutually beneficial information with the Council on Examining Boards was next introduced by the president. The subject was concluded when the following resolution was made, seconded and unanimously adopted:

Resolved: That a committee consisting of the president, a member from the accrediting committee, and a member from among the school-men be appointed by the president whose purpose shall be to meet with a similar committee constituted from among the members of the Council on Examining Boards at mutually convenient times during the National Chiropractic Conventions to establish liaison; and that the secretary be instructed to invite the Council on Examining Boards to take similar action.

Meeting recessed until 4:00 P.M. to allow members to attend House of Delegates to hear reports.
MEETING CALLED:
    4:20 P.M. Sunday, July 3, Dr. Haynes presiding.

Dr. Dewey Anderson was present and related for the Council his experiences in inspecting the three schools, Lincoln, National and Los Angeles. He discussed at length the Anderson report which was submitted to the Executive Board as a result of his examination of the schools. In addition to reaffirming the conclusions reached in his report he stated that the Council on Education was the logical agency to seek approval as an accrediting agency for our profession. He concluded by recommending that the Council seriously consider possible compromise in the differences existing between itself and the Executive Board in matters pertaining to accreditation and FACE funds allocation in order that the whole program could be launched without further delay.

Further discussion of the same points was held after Dr. Anderson's departure.

Meeting recessed at 5:30 P.M.
MEETING CALLED at 7:30 P.M. - July 3, 1960 by Dr. Haynes.

FACE Liaison committee report.
Dr. Haynes called upon Dr. Peterson to present the committee's proposals on tentative compromise measures to be suggested to the Executive Board. Dr. Peterson reported the following committee recommendations:
    A. That the mortgage purchase proposal made by the Council earlier be withdrawn.
    B. That the Council reaffirm its recommendation that funds be requested by each school at the beginning of each school year on a proposed budget for specific purposes of upgrading and that the schools understand that either the money is to be used for these purposes, within approximately 10%, or an amended budget proposal is to be submitted to the Executive Board for approval. Further, that the schools are to submit exact reports of expenditures at the end of each school year.
    C. That accreditation be left solely in the hands of the Council on Education.
    D. That the application for approval of the Council on Education which is pending in the Department of Health be pursued until its conclusion or until recommendations from that department suggest a different course.
    E. That Dr. Nugent be retained as Director of Education until the present phase of gaining accreditation is accomplished.
    F. That the individual schools will continue self examination by a local committee based on the Los Angeles pattern.
After discussing each proposed point the following resolution was made, seconded and unanimously adopted.

Resolved: That the Council on Education adopt the recommendations of the liaison committee in their entirety and authorize the FACE Liaison Committee to convey these new proposals to the Executive Board.

Meeting recessed at 10:20 P.M.
MEETING CALLED at 2:10 P.M. Monday, July 4, 1960, Dr. Haynes presiding.

Montana.
Dr. Getchell reported results of supreme court decision relative to PSC and asked for a review of the circumstances by the Council and advice. He was referred to the Director of Education and his committee and NCA Legal Counsel.

Inspection of Northwestern College of Chiropractic.
The president, with the consent of the members, set 9:00 A.M. Wednesday, July 6, as the hour when the full council with the accrediting committee would inspect Northwestern.

FACE Liaison committee report.
Dr. Peterson reported that the FACE funds and accreditation proposals had been conveyed to the Executive Board verbally at a 10:00 A.M. meeting Monday. He related that there seemed to be general acceptance of the points presented and that each of the members of the Executive Board indicated that they were confident that agreement could be reached within the frame work of the proposals. Since our

proposals did not include recommendations concerning the exact distribution of FACE funds on a percentage basis, the Executive Board suggested that the Council recommend such a formula as early as possible.

Canadian Memorial Grant.

The president then took up the subject of student procurement grant request which was made by the Canadian Memorial College with the support of the entire Council. After reviewing the facts relative to omission of the Canadian School from the list of recipients the council unanimously adopted the following resolution:

Resolved: That in the interests of Canadian Memorial Chiropractic College and of the relationship of the NCA to Canadian chiropractors it is moved that the Council on Education reaffirm its request that the Canadian school be given a student procurement grant of $4800 similar to the other accredited schools.

Western States Chiropractic College.

General discussion about the Western States school followed. It was disclosed that:

   A.   Western States is in the process of negotiating a cooperative agreement with Columbia Christian College, Church of Christ, through which basic sciences subjects may be taught in the Columbia plant using Columbia's facilities.

   B.   It has modified its entrance requirements to conform to those of surrounding states and thus expects to increase enrollments.

These changes and others justify a further study of Western States. No action. The committee will submit its recommendations later.

Approval of Minutes.

Dr. Martin moved, Osborne seconded, and the following resolution was unanimously adopted:

Resolved: That the minutes of the Midyear Meeting at Los Angeles in 1960 be amended by deleting the portion of the paragraph on page 13 entitled Report of Accrediting Committee which reads, "After that date the accreditation is to be removed. This action is based upon the economic conditions of the college," and substitute therefore "or otherwise securing adequate financial resources and a dynamic program for improving their small enrollment and laboratory deficiencies."

   The following resolution was then moved, seconded and unanimously adopted.

Resolved:That the minutes of the Midyear Meeting of the Council on Education held in Los Angeles in January 1960 be accepted as amended.

Allocation of FACE funds.

By consent the FACE Liaison committee was requested by the president to draw up a recommendation for funds allocation among the accredited schools on a percentage basis.

Meeting recessed until 8:00 P.M.

MEETING CALLED AT 8:00 P.M. July 4, 1960 by President Haynes.

FACE funds allocation.

Dr. Peterson reported for the FACE Liaison Committee. He recommended the adoption of the following formula for funds allocation among the accredited schools. These figures are based to a large extent upon the percentage allocation derived from the mortgage purchase needs submitted by the various schools:

   Los Angeles 18%   Northwestern   14%
   National   18%   Texas   14%
   New York   18%   Lincoln   18%

This proposal was discussed at length. The president then polled the members for comments and finally the following resolution was moved, seconded and unanimously adopted:

Resolved: That the Council on Education adopt the proposal for funds allocation as submitted by the committee and embody it in their recommendations to the Executive Board. By consent the FACE Liaison Committee was then instructed by the president to prepare a memorandum to the Executive Board containing the points of tentative agreement as well as the funds allocation proposal.

Western States

After Report by Chairman of Accrediting Committee (Dr. Wolf) and a discussion of position of Western States it was agreed by consent that Western States College of Chiropractic would be omitted from the above proposals but that the Council would support Western States in a special appeal to the Executive Board based on its altered circumstances.

Meeting recessed at 10:20 P.M.

MEETING CALLED AT 10:30 A.M. Tuesday, July 5, by President Haynes

Report on schools approved by Examining Boards of various states. Dr. Janse reported that there is no positive findings as yet from his committee. His committee is preparing the questionnaire to circulate to the various boards.

X-Ray Course Approval.
Dr. Ulrich of Florida requests approval of Course in X-Ray to be conducted under the sponsorship of Lincoln school by Dr. Rich. No action necessary inasmuch as course is sponsored by Lincoln.

Ratification of Memorandum to Executive Board by Council on Education dated July 5, 1960
Dr. Peterson, as chairman of the FACE Liaison committee, read the entire memorandum draft. After every point was discussed and accepted by the Council the following resolutions were moved, seconded, and unanimously adopted:

Resolved:That the memorandum as read be adopted in its entirety by the Council on Education and that the FACE Liaison Committee be authorized to convey it to the Executive Board.
Resolved:That paragraph 8 be added to the memorandum reading as follows: "And further the Council on Education reaffirms its unanimous recommendation that the Canadian Memorial Chiropractic College be given a $4800 student procurement grant - similar to the student procurement grants previously awarded the other accredited schools."

Meeting recessed.
ASSEMBLY 9:00 A.M. Wednesday.
The Council on Education with the Accrediting Committee and four members of the Council on Examining Boards inspected the Northwestern College of Chiropractic in Minneapolis. The group examined the classrooms, laboratories, library, teaching aids, clinic, and records of the school. Interviews were conducted with students and faculty.

MEETING CALLED AT 11:30 A.M. Wednesday, July 6, 1960 by President Haynes.
FACE Liaison Committee Report.
Dr. Haynes reported for the liaison committee on its meeting with the Executive Board for the purpose of conveying the Memorandum containing the Council's funds allocations recommendations and restating the previous areas of tentative agreement. He reported that the Executive Board accepted the memorandum for consideration with the following conditions:
1. Delete reference to $10,000 in Paragraph 2A
2. Modify wording through memorandum to change the sense from understanding or agreement to request or recommendation.
3. Delete the references to Dr. Nugent contained in the balance of the Paragraph 5 following the phrase "be continued to its conclusion."
Dr. Haynes reported that the Executive Board suggested these changes because if the Council's request was found to be acceptable it would be laid before the FACE Trustees and the employment of Dr. Nugent was not rightly a matter which should be considered by that body. The Liaison Committee reported accepting the suggestions pending approval by the Council on Education.

Action of the FACE Liaison Committee was approved by appropriate resolution, moved, seconded and unanimously adopted. The president then asked the FACE Liaison Committee to draw up a memorandum containing the Council's recommendations regarding the Director of Education, Dr. Nugent, to be presented to the Executive Board.

Council on Orthopedics.
Dr. Ploudre requested the Council on Education to consider the problems facing the California and Florida groups of orthopedists and to help in setting up minimum standards for certification. He was assured the Council was working toward that end in its cooperation with the Council on Orthopedics.

Appointments:
The following appointments were fixed for Wednesday afternoon. Dr. Pressor, 2:30 P.M.; Dr. Pruitt, 2:45 P.M.; Dr. Fay, 2:50 P.M.; Dr. Higley, 3:00 P.M.; Dr. Schwartz, 3:45 P.M.

Meeting recessed.
MEETING CALLED at 2:00 P.M. Wednesday July 6 by President Haynes.

Accreditation and Dr. Nugent's role.
 The president requested the individual school heads and members of the accrediting committee to express their personal thoughts as to the work done by Dr. Nugent and as to the value of Dr. Nugent's continuation or his substitution in his work particularly in the preparation of

the material requested by the Dept. of Health, Education and Welfare and in the approval of the Council on Education of the NCA by the above department. Each of the school heads and Dr. Wolfe as speaker for the committee expressed their position on the above points in a very clear, firm and positive manner. They did so, not basing themselves on personal likes or dislikes, but upon the welfare of their schools, chiropractic education and the progress of the profession. Based on this the FACE Liaison Committee was instructed to prepare the July 6 memorandum to the Executive Board.

The following resolution was then moved, seconded and unanimously adopted.

Resolved:That the MEMORANDUM FROM THE COUNCIL ON EDUCATION, NCA, TO THE EXECUTIVE BOARD dated July 6, 1960 be adopted as read and that the FACE Liaison Committee be instructed to convey it to the Executive Board.

Council on Orthopedics.
Dr. Prosser asks the Council's recommendations and suggestions concerning the Council on Orthopedics' proposed constitution and bylaws.

Research Council, NCA.
Dr. Higley reported the results of publication of Section I of "The Intervertebral Disc Syndrome" and plans to complete Section D which will be a clinical research study conducted through the facilities of the clinics of the accredited schools in accordance with the published Protocol.

Dr. Herman Schwartz accompanied by Dr. Tom Lawrence reported the book, "Home Care for the Emotionally Ill" had been approved by the Department of Medicine and Surgery of the VA after deletion of reference to chiropractic. Dr. Schwartz then recommended that psychotherapy be introduced in school clinics and that it be taught in extension courses sponsored by the schools.

Meeting recessed at 4:00 P.M. to allow FACE Liaison committee to meet again with the Executive Board.
MEETING CALLED AT 9:00 A.M. Thursday by President Haynes.

FACE Liaison Committee report.
Dr. Peterson reported that the Memorandum of July 6th pertaining to Dr. Nugent had been transmitted to the Executive Board at 4:00 P.M. Wednesday. No decisions were announced by the Executive Board.

Field Representatives
The subject of field representatives for accredited schools was reintroduced for action. The question: whether to approve faculty representatives residing in distant states who were not actively teaching. The following resolution was made by Dr. Peterson, seconded by Dr. Wolf, and unanimously adopted.

Resolved: That the Council on Education does not approve at this time the appointment of field faculty men by the member schools whose function would be to conduct or supervise extension courses.

The following resolution was then moved, seconded and unanimously adopted:

Resolved: That any consideration of the qualifications to be used as standards for selecting faculty for extension courses is to be referred for study to the Committee on Accreditation.

Council on Orthopedics.
At the request of the Council on Orthopedics the following recommended changes in the proposed bylaws of the Council on Orthopedics were moved, seconded and unanimously approved:

Article V, Sec. 1, line 1 change to read:
"The Council on Education of NCA shall sponsor, etc."
Article VI, Sec. 1, paragraph 2, line 1 change word "elected" to "nominated" and delete the balance of the paragraph following the phrase "in these bylaws." Substitute following for deleted portion "These nominees shall then be submitted to the Council on Education of the National Chiropractic Association for approval." The nominees shall present such evidence of educational background and experience as shall be requested by the Council on Education."
Article VI, Sec. 2, line 2, delete phrase "one of whom is to be elected by the National Council on Education".
    Line 5, delete sentence "Mechanics for selecting the first Examining Board shall be agreed upon later," and substitute "The members of the first Examining Board shall be nominated by the Society of Orthopedists from among the members of the Society who meet the

qualifications for Fellow as contained in Article V, Section 2 above." These nominees shall then be submitted to the Council on Education of the National Chiropractic Association for approval. The nominees shall present such evidence of education and experience as the Council may request.

Entrance Examination for Enrollees.
The Entrance Examination Committee, Dr. Troilo, chairman, presented the proposed entrance examination evolved by his committee. By appropriate action it was laid over until the January meeting.

Agenda: The following points on the Agenda were laid over to the January meeting.
    8. Action on report of the Fund for Chiropractic Education Committee, Dr. Hearn, chairman.
    13. Efforts to improve caliber of enrolling students.
    15. Degrees from accredited schools after previous graduation.
    16. Uniform policy for accepting students who have failed in another school.

Report on Vitaminerals Scholarship.
Dr. Haynes reported the Activity of the Council on Education in promoting publicity for the Vitaminerals Scholarship and urged each member of the Council to do his utmost to assist in making the program successful.

Louisiana Brief, as Text.
Dr. Etheridge recommended the employment of the Louisiana Brief as a text. Discussion disclosed that most schools used it in connection with jurisprudence classes.

Chiropractic a Career pamphlet.
By consent the president referred the request of Dr. Pruitt for revision of the pamphlet, "Chiropractic a Career" to the Director of Education, Dr. Nugent, with the request that he revise the booklet.

Approval of Extension Courses.
By appropriate resolution unanimously adopted the following extension courses were approved.
Lincoln's Florida X-ray course.
National's Kansas diagnosis course.

Dr. Etheridge's service on Illinois committee.
No action necessary because the council members had individually previously agreed to his participation.

Hood Color.
Dr. Wolfe reported no progress in getting hood color, forest green, registered because registration depends upon accreditation.

Veteran's Care, Dr. Pefley.
Dr. Pefley requested information through the schools about the amount of pre-professional college training individual practicing chiropractors possess. This information to be used to establish qualifications for possible eligibility to care for veterans. It was agreed by consent that the secretary would write to Dr. Pefley asking for further information and suggesting a central registration center through which to gather this information.

Report to NCA.
Dr. Haynes called attention to the report of the Council on Education's activities for the year which was submitted to the Executive Board. It was ordered filed.

Unsponsored lectures by faculty members of the accredited schools were disapproved by appropriate resolution.

Site of midyear meeting was left to be determined at a later date through a mail ballot.

Minutes of the Meeting of the COUNCIL ON EDUCATION of the NCA, Las Vegas, Nevada - June 11-17, 1961

In attendance
>   Dr. George H. Haynes, Dean of the Los Angeles College of Chiropractic, President of the Council
>   Dr. Robert E. Elliot, President of the Western States Chiropractic College
>   Dr. Arthur G. Hendricks, President of the Lincoln Chiropractic College
>   Dr. A. Earl Homewood, President of the Canadian Memorial Chiropractic College
>   Dr. R.N. Thompson, New President of Canadian Memorial Chiropractic College
>   Dr. Joseph Janse, President of the National College of Chiropractic
>   Dr. Thure Peterson, President of the Chiropractic Institute of New York
>   Dr. Russell, President of the Texas Chiropractic College
>   Dr. Julius Troilo, Dean of Texas Chiropractic College
>   Dr. John Wolfe, President of Northwestern College of Chiropractic, Secretary of the Council
>   Dr. Walter Wolf, Chairman, Accrediting Committee
>   Dr. Francis C. Etheridge, Jr.
>   Dr. John Nugent, Director of Education
>   Dr. Norman Osborne

The meeting was called to order at 9:00 a.m. Monday, June 12th. The order of business was as follows:

Item 1. Council of State Chiropractic Examining Boards
The invitation of the Council of State Chiropractic Examining Boards extended to our Council was read. The matter was discussed and it was decided that the Council on Education of the NCA, in the interest of maintaining good relations with the Council of Examining Boards, would accept their invitation to present the education criteria of our Council and the history and procedure for Federal Accreditation and to participate in a panel discussion with the ICA representatives.

The following presentation in an outlined form, prepared by the president, was unanimously approved, and Dr. Haynes was authorized to present it before the Examining Boards.
1.   General statement of appreciation for the work of the Council of Examining Boards
2.   Qualifications of the speaker
3.   Outline of the educational problem

I. Meaning of national accreditation
II. Benefits of accreditation as related to our profession:
>   A. Tangible
>>   1. to the schools - negligible Government assistance - proof-list of all educational assistance laws and where they can be obtained.
>>   2. to the individual D.C. - Health insurance participation and Health assistance laws
>   B. Intangible - prestige to the schools and the profession at large
III. Procedure
>   A. Department of Health, Education and Welfare. Ref. - criteria to met by agency.
>>   1. Scope of operation
>>   2. Need for such an agency
>>   3. Freedom of judgment
Compare NCA and ICA Councils on Education and reference to B report obtained by the ICA
>>   4. Public knowledge of its operation
>>>   a. Criteria - NCA - 1939 to 1947, ICA - 1955
>>>   b. Reports - NCA-continued
>>>   c. list of schools, NCA 1st.
>>   5. Adequate organization and effectiveness of agency to:
>>>   a. obtain quantitative and qualitative information regarding the schools
>>>>   1). Accrediting committee - ICA?
>>>>   2). Director of Education - Adams
>>>>   3). Outside education (NCA evidence) - ICA?
>>>>   4). Self-evaluation - ICA?
>>>   b. Periodical re-evaluation of the schools
>>>   c. Financial stability of agency

               NCA, ICA - new agency? how?
      6. Accredits only schools that meet or approaches standards
      NCA - (evidence)
      ICA - Ref. - B report of ICA, page 70 #2
      7. Length of life of agency
      NCA-1939 on, ICA-1955, new agency - delay
      8. General recognition of agency
      NCA - all schools but one, State Boards (chart), etc.
      9. Economic independence
      NCA - ICA - new agency?
IV. Present chiropractic accrediting agencies
    NCA - Ref. - Kersey report, probably Badger report
    ICA - Ref. - ICA - B report
    evidence actual NCA criteria, ICA criteria?
V. Need to raise standards need of one standard only based on academic concepts and not politics.

The chair appointed Drs. Troilo, Peterson, and W. Wolf as the committee to appear with him before the Council of State Chiropractic Examining Boards.

Item 2 - Report on Accreditation
    Dr. Nugent was called upon to give his report on the status of accreditation. He reported that in his opinion our request for approval as an accrediting agency for the chiropractic profession was sympathetically received. He indicated that it appeared that on the basis of the long history of effort and the most recent achievements of the NCA our request would be the only one seriously considered. The letter of non-acceptance from the Department of Education was presented and discussion was had as to its effects upon our program. Based upon Dr. Nugent's talk with Dr. Coronet and Dr. Haynes; talks with the Western College Association, the Arts & Science local accrediting agency, it appeared that often the first and second applications by agencies were rejected and that the rejection apparently did not harm the progress of the agency towards recognition.
    The balance of the morning and afternoon sessions of the Council were dedicated to the discussion of each of the points enumerated in the letter setting forth the current deficiencies of the Council on Education and its schools. The conclusion was that with concentrated effort and sufficient funds these deficiencies could be eliminated in a reasonable time and that the NCA Council on Education then had a good chance for recognition.

    Motion - It was unanimously approved that Dr. Nugent's work be accepted.
    The secretary was then instructed to request from the Executive Board of the NCA an appointment to present Dr. Nugent's report.

Meeting recessed.
Meeting called to order at 10:35 a.m. Tuesday morning.

    Dr. Haynes reported that beginning at 9:00 a.m. the committee met with the Council of State Examining Boards and that he gave his report substantial as it had been approved and that it was well received.

Item 3 - House of Delegates.
    A committee appointed by the House of Delegates for exchange of information between the House and the Council on Education was received. Dr. Gordon Pefley of Oregon outlined its general purposes. The Committee consisted of:
    Dr. Gordon Pefley - Oregon, Chairman; Dr. Jack Sample - Kansas; Dr. M.E. Calhoun - Arkansas; Dr. C.S. White - Connecticut; Dr. Truman Walters - Kentucky

    Their questions as to the activities of the Council were answered. To their inquiry as to how they could assist the Council it was generally suggested that a closer relationship between the Delegates, Executive Board and the Council would greatly benefit the accreditation program.

Item 4 - Dr. Nugent's services.
    It was agreed by consent that since the process of accreditation had reached a critical stage, and since it appeared possible that the Council on Education of the NCA could gain approval as the accrediting agency for the chiropractic profession with stepped-up, sustained action, Dr. Nugent's uninterrupted services were therefore more important than ever.
    By agreement the president appointed a committee to draft a request to the Executive Board regarding the position of the Council as it affects Dr. Nugent. The Committee follows: Dr. Joseph Janse, Chairman; Dr. Norman Osborne; Dr. Arthur Hendricks; Dr. Robert

Elliot; Dr. John Wolfe

Meeting recessed at 12:05 p.m.
Meeting called at 2:05 p.m.

Council on Examining Boards
The committee reported on its participation with the Council on State Examining Boards and ICA Committee beginning at 1 p.m. Report of the Committee was satisfactory.

Dr. Nugent's Services
The proposed memorandum (attached as appendix I) to the Executive Board was read by Dr. Janse on behalf of the committee. The following resolution was then adopted without any dissent.

Motion - That the memorandum be approved as read and be transmitted to the Executive Board by the Committee at the earliest practical time.

Meeting adjourned at 5:00 p.m.
Meeting called at 9:00 a.m. Wednesday

Accreditation
A further discussion of the general needs of the schools to qualify for accreditation occupied the morning.

Meeting called at 2:00 p.m.

Item 5 - Clinical neurology
Dr. Ralph Martin's proposals for eventual formation of a council on clinical neurology as a means of evaluating technic methods were given informal approval by the Council on Education.

Item 6 - The alumni luncheon
It was made clear by the president that he or the Council were not responsible for the luncheon or its program. Furthermore, Dr. Haynes stated that he had not been asked or consulted as to his participation as presiding officer at the luncheon nor given any outline of the program to be expected. His first knowledge as to his part in the luncheon was obtained from the printed program.

Item 7 - Mr. Christian E. Burckel
Mr. Burckel presented to the Council his views on the course of action which should be pursued by the NCA in order to obtain school accreditation along with his ideas on how to raise the necessary funds to achieve these purposes.
Mr. Burckel was informed of the supposed charge of collusion with Council members regarding his remarks during his talks. He stated his talk was based on his opinion only. He was also informed as to an apparent difference in facts relating to our dealings with the Department of Education. Mr. Burckel stated that he would not argue against ghosts but that he requested an opportunity to discuss the facts face to face with Dr. D. Anderson and anyone else who was supposed to have personal and direct information from the Department of Education and who claimed Mr. Buckel's statements to be incorrect.
Various members of the Council voiced their opinions. The general conclusion was that the apparent shadow-boxing was extremely detrimental to the well being of the accrediting program and to the profession and that it was creating a picture of disagreement and antagonisms between the Executive Board and the Council on Education that had not existed and should not exist. It was the general opinion that a meeting be brought about between Dr. J. Nugent, Dr. Dewey Anderson and Mr. C. Burckel, all of whom claimed direct contact and knowledge from the Department of Education, for them to discuss the matter and determine the truth. The members of the Executive Board and members of the Council, who do not claim direct knowledge and contact with the Department of Education, to act as non-participating members of the meeting, and therefore as judges of the veracity of the information presented. This opinion of the Council members was made known to the chairman of the Executive Board by Dr. Wolf, Chairman of the Accrediting Committee, and the president of the Council.

Meeting recessed.
Meeting called to order at 9:00 a.m. by Dr. Haynes.

Item 8 - Research committee report
Dr. Haynes called upon Dr. Henry Higley who discussed the progress report of the research on "The Intervertebral Disc Syndrome". Copy of the report is on file with the secretary.

Item 9 - Uniform college accounting

The uniform chart of accounts procedures contained in the report "Suggested chart of accounts following the recommended form of the Department of Health, Education and Welfare," prepared at the LACC were presented by Dr. Higley and discussed by the Council. The forms were distributed to all council schools as a guide to setting up the uniform accounting procedures as adopted by the Council's January 1961 meeting.

Meeting interrupted and recessed at 10:50 to attend Dr. D. Anderson's and House of Delegates' discussion of our accreditation program.

Meeting called at 12:30 p.m. by Dr. Haynes to prepare the recommendations of the Council on Education as requested for presentation to the House of Delegates at 2:00 p.m. as per resolution recessing the delegates meeting for luncheon.

The following recommendations were adopted after due discussion:

1. The Council on Education is to continue its attempts to meet the criteria for accreditation and particularly on the points found wanting as per the Department of Education letter of May 22, 1961, namely points 5a, b, c, d, and 6, 8 and 9.

2. In order to promote a better liaison between the Executive Board, House of Delegates and the Council on Education a committee from each body be appointed to discuss the progress and planning of the accreditation program, and that all information and reports relative to the welfare of the program be freely interchanged.

The Council on Education is to continue to report to the Executive Board and House of Delegates as in the past.

3. That Dr. Nugent, with the title of Director of Education, is to continue the efforts towards accreditation because of his background of experience and contacts with the Department of Education.

To assure the continuation of the accrediting program that a man be trained immediately to ultimately take over the full position of Director of Education.

4. A much larger proportion of FACE funds be released as soon as possible so that the program can proceed at a faster pace, and the House of Delegates devise ways and means of raising additional funds with the knowledge that the greater amount of funds that are made available will increase the rate of our progress and assure our ultimate success.

Dr. Dewey Anderson was invited to participate in the discussion. Dr. Anderson stated he had no objection to any part of our proposed recommendations to the House of Delegates.

Meeting recessed at 2:05 p.m. to appear before the House of Delegates.

Meeting called on Friday at 9:00 a.m. by Dr. Haynes.

Item 10 - Entrance screening.

Entrance examination as adopted at the January 1961 meeting (S.A.T.) was discussed again. Drs. Hendricks, Peterson and Janse presented some of the difficulties encountered by the application of this requirement.

Various points of view presented were finally reconciled resulting in the following motion to modify the previous action which was passed unanimously:

Motion Resolved - That the previous motion requiring the S.A.T. entrance examination for all entering students beginning September 1961 be amended to exclude the following specific applicants for admission:

a) Those who have satisfactorily completed 14.5 units of college education.

b) Foreign students.

c) Special cases which are admitted for cause by the school admission committee. These cases shall be subject to review on demand by the Council on Education.

Item 11 - Agenda subjects

Points on proposed agenda for the June 11-17, 1961, meeting and not considered as yet were laid over to a future meeting by consent.

Questions regarding the actual present duties, responsibilities and jurisdiction of the Council on Education and its position as the result of this motion adopted by the House of Delegates could not be answered. Nor the question regarding the effect of this motion on point 3 of the criteria for accrediting agencies of the Department of Education.

The time and place of the next meeting was left open and to be discussed by mail.

Dr. Haynes requested the election of a new president as he had already served a year and one half. His request was denied and the Council re-elected the present set of officers.

The meeting adjourned to allow the committee to meet with the Executive Board.

APPENDIX I
TO THE EXECUTIVE BOARD OF THE NCA

To the full membership of the National Council on Education it is evident that significant progress has been made toward federal accreditation through the efforts of Dr. John J. Nugent as Director of Education of the National Chiropractic Association.

Recent conferences and events in Washington support these facts. We are all, therefor, charged with the responsibility of continuing this program to completion.

It is apparent that a break-through has been accomplished. It is the responsibility of all of us to exploit this break-through.

The members of the Council who over many years have sought with concern and diligence to gain this accreditation, are apprehensive about any change which may weaken our efforts to accomplish this end.

It is evident that the entire NCA membership is vitally concerned about this matter. Expressions by general members, as well as members of the House of Delegates give indication that they demand the maximum of effort which will insure success.

Thus the Council members unanimously and urgently recommend that the services of Dr. Nugent as Director of Education be continued.

Minutes of the COUNCIL ON EDUCATION Mid-Year Meeting, FEBRUARY 19, 1962, BILTMORE HOTEL, LOS ANGELES, CALIFORNIA

Those in attendance:
George H. Haynes, President, LACC
John Wolfe, Secretary, NWCC
Joseph Janse, NCC
Thure Peterson, CINY
Arthur Hendricks, LCC
Julius Troilo, TCC
Robert E. Elliot, WSCC
Donald McMillan, CMCC
Accrediting Committee: Walter Wolf, Chairman, Asa J. Brown, Orval Hidde,
Edward Poulsen - not present

Monday, 10:00 a.m.
The meeting was called to order by president, Dr. George Haynes.
MINUTES - The minutes of the Council on Education meeting at Las Vegas, 1961, were unanimously approved as published.

ACCREDITING COMMITTEE - Report of the Accrediting Committee of the Council on Education as given at the Las Vegas meeting was approved and ordered filed.

AGENDA - The following agenda was formed and approved.
1. Scholarships for academically superior students.
2. Committee of the Profession on Education. Past meeting and coming meeting on textbooks. National Examining Boards in Chiropractic and Basic Science Boards.
3. Status of accredited schools with regard to approval by State Boards of Examiners.
4. Changes in Criteria for Accreditation, Council on Education.
5. Distribution of FACE funds.
6. Insurance for clinic, malpractice.
7. Orthopedic Council.

REPORT - COMMITTEE OF PROFESSION ON EDUCATION
Dr. Haynes reported the action of the C.P.O.E. in approving jointly the basic division of the curriculum as contained in the final report. He indicated it differed slightly from the Council on Education's current criteria and should therefore require Council action to modify the criteria. He recommended approval of the curriculum division as adopted by the C.P.O.E.
MOTION: A resolution to adopt the foregoing report of the C.P.O.E. was unanimously passed.

The president then requested the secretary to inform the Executive Board of Directors that the above action had been taken and that the action would be effective after similar action had been taken both by the Board of Control of the ICA and the Council of State Examining Boards.

TEXTBOOKS
Dr. Haynes then discussed the report on textbooks he had compiled and his recommendation on textbook selection which he proposed to

take to the next C.P.O.E. meeting in Detroit.

MOTION: By unanimous action Dr. Haynes' report was approved and the committee ??????? present it to the C.P.O.E.

DEWEY ANDERSON

MOTION: It was unanimously adopted that a letter requesting ??????? Dewey Anderson meeting with the Council on Education be transmitted to the Executive Board of Directors.

MOTION: A motion was adopted to extend to Mr. Bellevue an invitation to appear before the Council at the Detroit meeting.

MOTION: A motion was unanimously adopted to ask the Executive Board to again consider the problems of Teacher Retirement and Malpractice Insurance.

MEETING ADJOURNED

TUESDAY DAY

The individual school representatives met with the inspection committee of the Committee on Chiropractic Standards of the NCA during the day.

The following actions were presented for the consideration of the full Council by the Committee on Educational Standards of the NCA:

1. Our inspection indicates the need to bring the Educational Standards for Chiropractic Schools, 1955 Edition up to date through revision to meet developments that have taken place during the past seven years. In doing so, it is suggested that a committee work closely and directly with the U.S. Office of Education, which is the final authority in listing accredited schools.

2. Pending revision of the Standards and the development of any other plans for reorganization or improvement in our educational system, all colleges be continued as "Provisionally accredited" by the NCA.

3. A regional plan of education should be adopted. This should take into account possible amalgamations, establishment of new schools, individual school surveys and plans, raised standards and adequate financial support.

4. The national wide alumni should be organized through the NCA, with appropriate participation and leadership being ???? by the individual schools. Its programs should include an active recruitment, fund raising and distribution effort, as well as an awakening and development of membership and public interest in chiropractic education.

5. FACE should be encouraged and strengthened to become a major effort of the NCA, and the vehicle through which alumni and other contributions can be channeled for educational support. A new program of financing the schools should be developed in which FACE should participate. This could include a substantially increased membership contribution.

6. A qualified and experienced educator should be appointed to the NCA staff to act as its expert, and to cooperate with the membership, schools and government authorities in developing the educational program.

7. A national plan of records and reports should be developed to insure minimum standards and proper uniformity among approved schools. For this purpose a cooperative committee of the Board and council should be established.

8. Every encouragement should be given the Council on Education by the NCA through its Executive Board of Directors. To this end, and appropriately as to time, place and circumstance, the Board should acquaint the Council of its deliberations and seek close cooperation in working out whatever plans and programs may be developed as a result of this inspection and report.

Point #1 was modified to read:

1. That a revision of the Educational Standards for Chiropractic Schools, 1955 Edition, be made to meet developments that have taken place during the past seven years. In doing so, it is suggested that a committee work closely and directly with the U.S. Office of Education, which is the final authority in listing accredited schools. The NCA Executive Board of Directors to appoint a three-man committee composed of one member from the accrediting committee, one of the school administrators and one member selected by the Board. Also that in the meantime, if a Director of Education is appointed he should have a part in this.

The change was unanimously approved.

Point #2 was not acted upon but left open for further discussion to determine the possibility of finding an acceptable modification.

Point #3 was not acted upon because it dealt with a matter not within the real of authority of the school representatives. It was informally agreed that the individual schools would submit point #3 to their respective Boards for their consideration.

Point #4 was unanimously passed in the following modified manner:

4. The NCA should encourage the organization and correlation of the alumni of each accredited school with appropriate participation and leadership being exercised by the individual schools. The program should include an active recruitment, fund-raising and distribution effort, as well as an awakening and development of membership and public interest in chiropractic education.

Point #5 was unanimously passed in the following modified manner:

5. FACE should be encouraged and strengthened to become a major effort of the NCA and a vehicle through which alumni and other contributions can be channeled for educational support to augment direct gifts to the schools. A new program of financing the schools should be developed in which FACE should participate. This could include a substantially increased membership contribution and the continuity of its support maintained in accordance with policies established by the Trustees of FACE.

Point #6 was unanimously adopted as proposed.

Point #7 was unanimously adopted in the following modified form.

7.   A national plan of records and reports (financial, student, accounting, bulletins) should develop minimum standards and proper uniformity among approved schools. For this purpose, a cooperative committee of the Board and the Council on Education should be established.

Point #8 was unanimously adopted as proposed.

MEETING ADJOURNED.

TUESDAY EVENING

Joint meeting of the Accrediting Committee and the Council on Education at which the Accrediting Committee's report, FACING THE FUTURE, was discussed.

MEETING ADJOURNED.

WEDNESDAY

After consultation with the NCA Executive Board, points #2 and #3 were acted upon.

Motion was made and unanimously approved to accept the following wording for point #2:

2.   Pending revision of the educational standards, all colleges will receive a bill of particulars covering the points that need to be brought up to date to meet the present criteria of the Council. The classification (certification) of the individual schools made under these criteria will be determined within the academic year - Sept. 1962 to June 1963 - to be based on the extent of compliance with the corrections requested under the revised standards. During this period, colleges are to be continued under the house definition of accreditation, functioning under the provisions of the NCA Executive Board and the Council on Education. The house definition of "accredited" for internal use only is that it is clearly understood as it applies to all colleges will be considered as provisional, subject to further inspection under the revised criteria. The accredited rating of colleges shall remain undisturbed for public purposes during this temporary period of pending the outcome of the procedure outlined above.

The following form of point #3 was approved. Each of the school administrators will present to his respective Board of Trustees for their consideration and decision the following recommendation of the Committee on Educational Standards of the NCA - "a regional plan of education should be adopted. This should take into account possible amalgamations, establishment of new schools, individual school surveys and plans, raised standards and adequate financial support."

The following changes in the criteria for accreditation were officially adopted by unanimous vote of the Council on Education:

Page 9 - Add to paragraph #3:

No trustee shall serve in an administrative or instructional capacity in the institution of which he is a trustee.

Page 9 - Change paragraph #4 to read:

The chief administrative officer of the school may be appointed by the Board of Trustees and his power shall be initiatory and executory and shall be directly responsible to the Board. He shall select, appoint or employ all other employees of the school, however, the appointment or employment of administrative personnel is subject to approval of the Board. All powers and duties delegated to the chief administrative officer are to be executed in accordance with the policies adopted by the Board. All other officers of the school shall be responsible to the chief administrative officer.

Page 10 - Financial management - delete paragraphs #4, #5, #6, etc. until page 11 - Records - For it substitute the following:

As far as it is possible. the financial accounting and reporting system should follow that suggested by the National Committee on Standard Reports for Institutions of Higher Education.

The basic principles of college and university accounting is made clear by the following material from their manual:

"Colleges and universities are nonprofit institutions. It is essential, therefore, that they set up their budgets, maintain their accounts, and present their financial reports in accordance with generally accepted accounting principles appropriate to nonprofit enterprises."

"Since service rather than profit is the primary objective of education institutions, the accounting procedures differ from those of commercial enterprises. In commercial activities there is usually a direct relationship between revenue and expenditures; in colleges and universities income, for the most part, is obtained independently of expenditures. In commercial accounting emphasis is given to the determination of net profit and net worth; in accounting for nonprofit organizations no such objective exists."

The accounts should be classified in balanced fund groups and so followed in the books of accounts and financial reports.

The financial transactions should be reported by fund groups without intermingling of detailed items.

The following fund groups are recommended:

1.   Current Funds - which includes funds available for general operating and for current restricted purposes.

2.   Loan Funds - Includes only funds which can be loaned to students, faculty and staff.

3. Endowment and other non-expendable funds - Includes only funds which are non-expendable at the date of reporting.
4. Annuity Funds - Includes funds designated or expended for the acquisition of physical property used for institutional purposes.
5. Agency Funds - Includes funds in the custody of the institution, but not belonging to it.

The completed form RSS-041 of the Department of Health, Education and Welfare, Office of Education shall be forwarded to the Chairman of the Council on Education.

Page 13 - Student-Faculty ratio - delete last sentence of paragraph #1 and substitute the following:

With the growth of the student body the number of teachers should be correspondingly increased so as to maintain a faculty-student ratio of one to fifteen.

Page 14 - Conditions of service - Third paragraph - add:

They should be encouraged and assisted to pursue a program of post-graduate studies in their own and related fields.

(add to paragraph #6)

...and a plan for faculty retirement should be adopted.

Page 15 - Admission - Change first sentence to read:

The number of students admitted shall be limited to the facilities of the college as determined by the Council on Education through inspection.

(add just before "age")

An entrance examination should be required, preferably one compiled and administered by recognized testing agencies.

Page 15 - Pre-professional education - Change section "A" of first paragraph to read:

a) Completed 16 units of work with at least a C average in an accredited high school.

(Delete fifth paragraph and specific course outline and substitute the following)

Liberal arts education has, since the history of the professions, been considered a basic foundation for fundamental culture required of all those who deal with the sensitive mental, physical, social, and spiritual development of the people. Liberal arts training is the essence of cultural foundation.

The prospective student should have such a cultural foundation, as well as an adequate background in chemistry and the biological sciences.

Page 16-17 - Orientation of new students - Add after last paragraph:

A well organized program of student counseling should be established which will encourage and assist every member of the student body to realize and accept the importance of multi-degree attainment.

Page 23 - (Library) Change paragraph #3 to read:

The Library holdings should number at least 3,000 volumes, of which at least 1,000 volumes should be current, i.e., less than 10 years of age. Mere numbers etc.

MEETING ADJOURNED

THURSDAY

The status of the NCA schools with regards to their approval by State Boards of Examiners was discussed. The final recapitulation of the answers received from the State Boards were presented by the president. Copy is hereby attached.

The election of officers for the next year was then considered. Dr. George H. Haynes was elected president and Dr. John Wolfe was elected secretary by unanimous vote.

The president was requested to codify the minutes of the Council and to bring up to date the by-laws and constitution of the Council.

MEETING ADJOURNED.

Minutes of the Annual Meeting of NATIONAL COUNCIL ON EDUCATION, June - 1962

Those in attendance:
> Dr. George Haynes, LACC, presiding
> Dr. John Wolfe, NWCC, secretary
> Dr. L.F. Bierman, Dean, LCC
> Dr. Frank G. Ploudre, President, LCC
> Dr. James Russell, President TCC
> Dr. Thure Peterson, President, CINY
> Dr. Joseph Janse, President, NCC
> Dr. Robert E. Elliot, Dean, WSCC
> Dr. D.W. McMillan, Dean, CMCC
> Dr. R.N. Thompson, President, CMCC

Members of Committee on Standards:
Dr. Walter B. Wolf, Chairman
Dr. Asa Brown
Dr. O.L. Hidde
Dr. Dewey Anderson

Meeting of Council on Education without Committee on Standards met at 10:00 AM Monday, Dr. Haynes presiding.

Minutes
Minutes of the midwinter meeting were reviewed and approved by unanimously adopted motion.
Agenda:
An agenda was discussed and tentatively laid out to cover the week. It was agreed to begin with reports of college heads on their status and attitudes of their boards with respect to the regional school proposals.
College Reports:
The reports of the school heads were given over the balance of Monday.
Tuesday
MEETINGS
Canceled during the day to allow all school representatives to appear before the Executive Board and the Board of Directors of FACE individually to give their reports to the boards. These reports were the same as those reviewed on Monday by the Council.
Tuesday PM
A meeting was held of the full council at which Dr. Dewey Anderson distributed his reports and summary reports covering the school inspections and the conclusions and recommendations formulated by the Committee on Standards.
Wednesday:
Meeting called by the chairman, Dr. Haynes, at 9:00 AM.

RESEARCH
Dr. Henry Higley distributed copies of his report on research on the Disc Syndrome and elaborated upon it and commented upon it. He asked for more cooperation from the school administrators and clinic directors in insuring the increased flow of data to the research project. He then described certain of the methodology employed in the period.

Next Dr. Higley tentatively outlined his itinerary to visit the clinics of each school to discuss the research project further.

VOCATIONAL GUIDANCE
Mr. Belleau, author of Chiropractic as a Career, as well as a guidance film on chiropractic, described the effectiveness of the items and requested assistance of the Council in having them adopted by the NCA as official guidance material.

Dr. Haynes' material on vocational guidance, prepared at LACC, was studied. His monograph outline was elaborately prepared.

Resolution: It was resolved that Dr. George Haynes should appear before the Executive Board and indicate to them our general approval of Dr. Belleau's guidance book and discuss with them their possible use.

BOOKKEEPING POLICY
Previous discussions concerning approved methods of bookkeeping according to HEW standards were recalled. It was the consensus that all schools would start their fiscal years concurrently with the beginning of the fall term and set up their books in accordance with COLLEGE AND UNIVERSITY BUSINESS ADMINISTRATION, Volume 2, if they had not already done so.

CONSTITUTION AND BY-LAWS
The proposed constitution and by-laws for the Council as prepared by Dr. Haynes from extracts of previous official action of the Council was studied in detail by the Council. The substance was accepted by consensus with several minor changes recommended and with the stipulation that it be referred to a committee for changes and expansion to fill our needs. The chairman then appointed the following committee to complete this work: Dr. Bittner - CINY; Dr. O. Hidde - Committee on Accreditation.

"FULL TIME" FACULTY MEMBER
After discussion by consensus it was agreed that a full time faculty member is one who devotes the major portion of his time to college work.

The Council was entertained and edified by pre-luncheon cocktails and a skillful presentation of current research at CMCC on measurements of spinal deviations, static and dynamic. The members were: Dr. R. Bartlow, V.P. CCA;   Dr. D. Sutherland, Research Director; Dr. L. Johnston

The Council reconvened after lunch.

NATIONAL COUNCIL OF CHIROPRACTIC ROENTGENOLOGY

Dr. Ronald J. Watkins addressed the Council concerning the advisability of undertaking to standardize terminology describing normal and abnormal spinal mechanics.

RESOLUTION: It is moved that the Council on Education endorse the plan of the NCCR to standardize terminology in spinal mechanics and recommends that the NCCR exercise the initiative and leadership in accomplishing the task; that the schools are urged to assist when called upon.

COUNCIL ON ORTHOPEDICS

Dr. William O. Watkinson, president of the Council, appeared before the Council on Education. He requested cooperation of the CE and the school administrators in keeping the Council on Orthopedics in closer touch and in better control of the orthopedic courses conducted by the schools. He made the following requests:

    a.   That outlines and syllabi of all courses be submitted early to CO.

    b.   That specially trained orthopedic instructors from the council be included with every course whenever feasible.

    c.   That faculty and student lists of all courses be submitted to CO.

    d.   The school should closely supervise the hours of attendance at these courses as well as the records of examinations. That a certificate at completion implies that the man has satisfactorily met both requirements.

    e.   That copies of certificates be sent to CO.

Resolution: It was moved that the Council on Education expresses its agreement with the above requests and that the member schools are urged to cooperate accordingly.

Thursday

Thursday was spent in informal discussion and in individual conferences with the FACE Board.

July 11, 1962

Dr. L.M. Rogers, Secretary, National Chiropractic Association, National Building, Webster City, Iowa

Dear Dr. Rogers:

The General Committee of the Profession on Education met in Detroit on Sunday, June 24, 1962. Dr. Janse did not arrive until the following day so I had Dr. Peterson join Dr. Wolfe and myself to complete our panel.

The first item of business was consideration of a suggested uniform certification of credits for all State Boards of Examiners. The form I presented was modified as shown in the attached sheet. This certification to be accompanied by the explanatory sheet as enclosed. Unanimous agreement was reached on this point.

The second matter on the agenda was the survey of the entrance requirements based on the answers received to my questionnaire.

In general the entrance procedures were acceptable to all with the following comments:

Age limit - agreed that students must be over 21 to graduate.

Grade average - The ICA schools will consider the "C" grade requirement for entrance.

Entrance test - The ICA will consider the institution of a college entrance test, conducted and graded by an outside agency.

Finger prints - was recommended for use by all schools - action pending.

College of Arts & Science - on a limited basis of subject per subject.

D.O. or M.D. school - limited as above and only applicable to basic science subjects.

The entrance requirement proposals will be considered by the individual schools.

The chair requested that Dr. Coggins and I should appear before the Council on State Boards. Dr. Coggins and I accepted the invitation.

Discussion was had as to the sequence to be followed in our future meetings. No decision was reached. I did present the idea of a sort of code of ethics to govern student procurement, using as an example for the need of code of ethics was the fact that friends of an ICA school had approached three of the LACC students and finally one of the students agreed to sign a scholarship application to that college. Whereby the college in question granted this student a $900 scholarship even though they were aware that this student was completing the second semester at the LACC. In general all agreed that the above procedure was not proper.

At our appearance before the Council of Examining Boards, that body voted to approve the general curriculum and list of textbooks as presented by us.

Dr. Holman will prepare the minutes and notify us of the agenda for the meeting to be held in the future.

Each member of the Council has a copy of the "Entrance Requirements" form but possibly they would want a copy of the other items.

Sincerely yours, George H. Haynes, D.C., President

Enclosures

COUNCIL ON EDUCATION, NATIONAL CHIROPRACTIC ASSOCIATION
Mid-Year Meeting at Los Angeles Chapman Park Hotel
January 19 through January 24, 1963

Meeting called to order by president, George Haynes at 10:00 A.M. on January 19th.

Those in attendance:

Dr. George Haynes, dean, LACC, president
Dr. John Wolfe, pres. NWCC, secretary
Dr. Robert Elliot, dean, WSCC
Dr. Julius Troilo, dean, TCC
Dr. James Russell, pres., TCC
Dr. Joseph Janse, pres. NCC
Dr. L.F. Bierman, dean, LCC
Dr. Frank G. Ploudre, pres. LCC
Dr. Thure C. Peterson, pres., CINY
Dr. Herbert M. Whims, dean, CMCC
Dr. W.F. Trelford, chairman, CMCC

Committee on Accreditation:

Dr. Walter Wolf, Chairman
Dr. Dewey Anderson
Dr. Asa Brown
Dr. O.L. Hidde

RESOLUTION: Minutes of Detroit Convention meeting of June 1962 were approved as published.

AGENDA: The following agenda was adopted by consensus.
1. Meeting Wednesday at 10:00 A.M. with representative of Vitaminerals regarding reactivation of the Vitaminerals scholarship program.
2. Student procurement.
3. School interim reports and plans.
4. Foreign students.
5. Restriction of FACE funds.
6. Printing allotment.
7. USAC
8. Summer sessions.
9. College contact page.
10. Licensure conditions - Canada - U.S.
11. Curriculum - allotment of hours.
12. Constitution and By-laws.
13. Psychiatry hours.
14. Criteria revisions.
15. Inspection rating forms.
16. Executive Board Liaison.

It was agreed that the preceding items of the agenda would be acted upon in the order decided upon by the president.

LICENSURE CONDITIONS - CANADA - U.S.

Dr. Himes and Dr. Trelford gave their report on qualifications for licensure in the provinces of Canada and suggested that each school catalog show exact educational requirements for licensure.

Utah - It was brought out that the Utah Board was not consistent in its stand on physiotherapy and therefore was open to attack on that basis.

LICENSURE CONDITIONS - CANADA - U.S.
Dr. Himes and Dr. Trelford gave their report on qualifications for licensure in the provinces of Canada and suggested that each school catalog show exact educational requirements for licensure.
Utah - It was brought out that the Utah Board was not consistent in its stand on physiotherapy and therefore was open to attack on that basis.
Hawaii, Minnesota, Wisconsin, and California have endorsed the application for licensure forms suggested by the Committee on Education for the profession.

USAC
After a report on the last meeting of the USAC by Dr. Himes and a general discussion of its objectives, constitution, and by-laws - the following action was approved:

RESOLVED: That while the goals and objectives of USAC are considered to be commendable the nature of its organization indicates that it cannot be given approval by school administrations or access to school funds.
Sunday, January 20, no meeting was called in order that Council members could attend the business sessions of the NCA - California Seminar.

Monday, January 21, meeting called by president Haynes at 9:30 A.M.
PSYCHOTHERAPY
Dr. Herman Schwartz's recommendations concerning hours and methods of teaching were discussed - the following hours were reported:

Table Appendix B-1. Entrance Requirements.

Hawaii, Minnesota, Wisconsin, and California have endorsed the application for licensure forms suggested by the Committee on Education for the profession.

USAC

After a report on the last meeting of the USAC by Dr. Himes and a general discussion of its objectives, constitution, and by-laws - the following action was approved:

RESOLVED: That while the goals and objectives of USAC are considered to be commendable the nature of its organization indicates that it cannot be given approval by school administrations or access to school funds.

Sunday, January 20, no meeting was called in order that Council members could attend the business sessions of the NCA - California Seminar.

Monday, January 21, meeting called by president Haynes at 9:30 A.M.

PSYCHOTHERAPY

Dr. Herman Schwartz's recommendations concerning hours and methods of teaching were discussed - the following hours were reported:

	From	To	
National		96	115
CMCC		108	108
CINY		120	130
TCC	135	135	
LACC		72	108
LCC	80	160	
NWCC		240	180
WSCC		72	72

It was concluded that no specific action could be taken until Dr. Schwartz's recommendations were clarified.

COLLEGE CONTACT PAGE

Following a general discussion of the purpose of the page it was concluded that it should contain articles which would convey the general education problems to the profession. Each council member therefore agreed to submit a subject to be written up by Tuesday morning.

The following resolution was adopted unanimously:

RESOLVED: That the Council on Education of the National Chiropractic Association herewith conveys to Mrs. Arthur Hendricks its sympathy upon the recent death of her husband, Dr. Hendricks.

The council and Dr. Hendricks are inseparably tied together in the history and development of chiropractic education. His determination, patience, strength, humor and integrity were the qualities upon which the council leaned heavily to make possible the success of its labors.

In addition, his warmth and friendship made the council's work pleasant. The body of work he helped to create and the affection felt for him by his colleagues will keep his memory alive.

The secretary was instructed to convey the foregoing resolution to Mrs. Hendricks.

CURRICULUM - CREDIT HOURS

A general discussion of credit hours based on the different term lengths ensued. No conclusion was reached.

MONDAY A.M.   Dr. Haynes presiding.
EDUCATIONAL CRITERIA

The revised criteria were taken up paragraph by paragraph.
MONDAY P.M.   Dr. Wolfe presiding.
STUDENT RECRUITMENT

Dr. Russell outlined what Texas College was doing. Spot radio and T.V. short announcements and releases were obtained free, as public service information. One minute statements stressing doctor shortage. Listeners wrote to stations who forwarded names to Texas College. Two Dallas, three or four Houston, and other smaller stations co-operated - also were given highway poster space but had to pay for paper and labor.

Dr. Elliot has similar arrangements as public service, emphasizing their clinic and child health program.

Drs. Peterson and Troilo both lauded the direct mail approach.

Dr. Himes advocated using available personnel principally alumni - provided folder costing $1.45 to alumni members.

The PR firm of J.P. Stewart wrote releases for Texas. It was suggested that NCA PR firm could do the same for schools.
FOREIGN STUDENTS

General discussion of enrollment of foreign students ensued. The great success of PSC in this field was noted, and Dr. Himes stated that they received no special considerations while he was at PSC. However PSC did give hundreds of scholarships some of which went to foreign students. It was concluded that the best approach to obtain such students was through alumni in such countries.

It was moved by Dr. Brown, seconded by Dr. Troilo that the executive board be requested to adopt a uniform scholarship program for all NCA schools. Passes.
PRINTING ALLOTMENT

Dr. Wolfe pointed out that there was a lack of information, and as a result he lost out on use of allotment. It was moved by Dr. Russell and seconded by Dr. Elliot that the executive board be urged to allot the funds again this year and to give each school a specific listing of what printing comes under the allotment. Passes.
DR. HERMAN SCHWARTZ AND PSYCHIATRY COURSES

The request of Dr. Schwartz for more emphasis upon his approach in the teaching of Psychiatry was discussed and in the absence of the letter to Dr. Walter Wolf this matter was discussed in general and then laid over to the next day.

TUESDAY

Deliberations were resumed on the criteria.
WEDNESDAY

Continuation of criteria discussion. The following resolution adopted unanimously:
RESOLVED: While in full agreement that the authority and responsibility for accreditation approval or disapproval of any college ultimately rests with the profession through its House of Delegates and executive board of the National Chiropractic Association, there is a divergence of view within the council as to the composition of the accrediting agency. There is no divergence of view respecting the objective sought, namely the approval and maintenance of colleges, which in all essentials are professional institutions of high standards. It is the means of reaching this level of attainment which underlies the divergence that exists.

The institutional members of the council maintain that this can be done through a structure of equal voting power within the accrediting agency which structure has been satisfactorily functioning for approximately twenty years. The Committee on Accreditation feels that until such time as fully accredited colleges are in existence, this can be achieved better and sooner with the full responsibility residing in its hands. The expectation is that possibly within the future one or more schools will qualify as accredited by NCA, and the section on structure and function will then be amended by recommendation of the council and approval of the NCA Executive Board in the light of the facts then prevailing.

Therefore, while not concurring in the view of the Committee on Accreditation concerning this section on "Structure and Function," and in order to expedite the important business of establishing a revised Educational Standards for use of the NCA in its forthcoming re-inspection, for guidance of the colleges in their work, and of the Foundation for Accreditation of Chiropractic Education in its deliberations, the institutional members of the council will accept the decision of the NCA Executive Board respecting this matter.

VITAMINERALS SCHOLARSHIP

The new scholarships offered to the accredited schools were described by Mr. Vogel. The council expressed its approval and its willingness to cooperate in the conduct of the selection.

CRITERIA

The following resolution was unanimously adopted:

RESOLVED: That the chair appoint a three man committee to draw up an outline of specific procedures necessary to implement the Education Standards for Chiropractic Colleges adopted by the Council - one man from an institution, one from the accrediting committee and Dr. Dewey Anderson. The chair then appointed with the approval of the council: Dr. D. Anderson, Dr. W. Wolf, Dr. G. Haynes.

ELECTION OF OFFICERS

The present officers were re-elected by acclamation -

President, George Haynes

Secretary, John Wolfe

There being no further business - the meeting was adjourned until the national convention in Chicago.

Annual Convention Meeting, COUNCIL ON EDUCATION, NCA - 1963
Monday, June 24th, 1963, 10:00 A.M., Sheraton Chicago Hotel, Chicago

Meeting was called to order by the president, Dr. George Haynes

Those attending:

    Dr. George Haynes, dean, LACC, president

    Dr. John Wolfe, president, NWCC, secretary

    Dr. James Russell, president, TCC

    Dr. Julius Troilo, dean, TCC

    Dr. Thure Peterson, president, CINY

    Dr. Frank Ploudre, chairman, LCC

    Dr. L.F. Bierman, president, LCC

    Dr. Robert Elliot, president, WSCC

    Dr. Joseph Janse, president, NCC

    Dr. Herbert Himes, dean, CMCC

Accrediting Committee

    Dr. Walter Wolf, chairman

    Dr. Dewey Anderson, consultant

    Dr. Asa Brown

    Dr. O.L. Hidde

    Dr. Edward Poulsen

MINUTES

By appropriate resolution the minutes of the midyear meeting of January 19-24, 1963 at Los Angeles were approved as published

AGENDA

Drs. LaRoche and Gravelle from Quebec, Canada are scheduled to meet with the Council on Wednesday at 3:00 P.M.

NCA JOURNAL PAGE

Dr. Haynes urges the schools to complete the articles for publication in the Journal which were assigned to them by agreement and by his memo as soon as possible.

CHIROPRACTIC AS A CAREER

A discussion of the pamphlet disclosed that there was agreement that it was obsolete and therefore no longer used by majority of schools. Only two use it. It was agreed therefore that the chairman would again bring this fact to the attention of the executive board and request that it be revised.

GRADUATE STUDY

Discussion centered about the lack of supervision and organization of some graduate study being conducted by individuals for various councils of the NCA. The conclusion was reached that all graduate study involving academic credit must flow from the schools exclusively. Therefore the following resolutions were unanimously adopted.

RESOLVED: That the Council on Education will recognize and approve the granting of credit only for courses conducted under the administrative control of schools approved by the council.
RECESS

Monday afternoon session called by Dr. Haynes. The previous discussion of graduate study was resumed.
RESOLVED: All academic requirements adopted by the present or future councils of the NCA toward membership or certification must be based upon credits officially earned and certified by a college approved by the Council on Education. Motion made by Dr. W. Wolf, seconded by Dr. R. Elliot.

RESOLVED: That a college in the council can only certify academic credits presented under its own administrative control.
Dr. Haynes then pointed out that the adoption of the foregoing motions placed a great deal of responsibility on the schools to formulate and develop uniform courses of study to provide qualifications for persons seeking to acquire certification in the various specialty councils such as orthopedics, X-ray, physiotherapy, and psychotherapy.
Faculty salaries for these courses are recommended to be $10 to $15 per hour. Total cost of course should allow for moderate return to the school above costs of approximately 15%.
Dr. Haynes suggested the invitation of heads of X-ray, orthopedics, physiotherapy, and psychotherapy councils to meet with Council on Education to discuss the foregoing problem. Time was set at 2:30 P.M. on Tuesday.

COMMITTEE ON EDUCATION REPORT
Results of meeting on Sunday, June 23rd with representatives of Board of Examiners and ICA.
1. It is recommended that a search be made by all schools and a compilation of all books written for the profession be completed - as found in their libraries.
2. The committee will undertake to obtain from the state boards of examiners the following information:
    a. Students passing and failing in each subject and school which they represent.
    b. List of new licenses issued by state annually.
    c. Number of licenses lost from all causes.
    d. Total licenses existing in state with increase or decrease during past year.
3. Schools requested to formulate questions which can be used by National Board of Chiropractic Examiners - questions to be of nature that can be answered by yes or no - or multiple choice. The examinations are to be held at various schools under the supervision of the national examiners. All schools agreed to propose questions.
RECESS - Meeting to resume at 10:00 A.M. Tuesday

TUESDAY
Meeting called by Dr. Haynes, president, at 10:00 A.M.
CHIROPRACTIC EDUCATION - OUTLINE OF A STANDARD COURSE
Rules and procedures for implementing the criteria is the subject for discussion.
Dr. W. Wolf suggested that the following particular aspects be discussed:
    a. Definition of financial stability
    b. Definition of full time faculty member
General discussion of the rules followed. It was suggested by Dr. Thure Peterson that a revision on page 7 be made specifying that a school can be accredited by only one chiropractic professional agency.

Page 7: it was further suggested that in the subject matter on page 7 the provision should be stated that the accrediting committee should be required to state specifically the particular aspects in which a school fails to meet the criteria in its reports to the school
Page 8: should include the provision that a school must have a federal tax exemption.
Page 12: it was recommended that on page 12 some provision should be made to retain instructors in basic sciences who have been long in the service to the school but who are not academically qualified.
Page 13: it was suggested that a full time instructor should be defined as one who spends a minimum of 25 hours weekly on the school premises.
It was recommended that the section dealing with pre-professional training of 60 units should not mention the course or subject material to be included.
Page 18: provision should be made prohibiting the duplicate use of pre-professional credit units as advance credit.
RECESS until 2:30 P.M.

The meeting was called by Dr. Haynes with the following council heads sitting in:

Dr. W.A. Watkinson, president, Council on Orthopedics

Dr. A.L. Hancock, secretary, Council on Orthopedics

Dr. Ed Kropf, president, Council on Roentgenologists

Dr. Ralph A. Power, president, Council on Physiotherapy

Dr. H.S. Schwartz, president, Council on Psychotherapy

Dr. Haynes gave a general presentation of the Council on Education's position regarding graduate study requirements as outlined in the resolutions adopted Monday afternoon. The councils on psychotherapy and physiotherapy have no graduate study requirements currently. Dr. Watkinson and Kropf expressed agreement in principle with the resolutions. Dr. Watkinson then stated the general objectives of the orthopedics council in graduate study:

a. That special graduate study be made available to as large a portion of the profession as possible.

b. That the presentation be taken to all geographical areas so that field doctors need travel only short distances.

c. That it be provided at a reasonable cost - such as $1.50 per hour provided there are sufficient enrollees.

RECESS until Wednesday at 2:30 P.M.

Dr. Haynes called the meeting to order at 2:30 P.M. The morning having been spent in individual school interviews with the executive board directors.

Dr. Haynes introduced Drs. LaRoche and Gravelle from Quebec, who described formation of the Royal Commission on chiropractic conducted by the honorable judge Gerard LaCroix of the Quebec Superior Court. He stated that the judge intended to visit CINY, LCC and WCC in the relatively near future and that the judge would make known his plans in advance. He then described the activities of the Quebec chiropractors in support of legislation and outlined what the schools could do to assist in providing documentary proof of the merit of the profession. The council assured the doctors of Quebec they would help in every way possible.

CHIROPRACTIC RESEARCH

Dr. Higley then presented his fifth report on the activities of the Research Department. A discussion followed on ways and means to improve the volume of patient reports from the schools. Dr. Wolfe suggested that a monthly reminder be sent to the school heads. Dr. Peterson indicated that cooperating with the research project cost CINY considerable money annually and suggested that some form of remuneration to the clinic director responsible for the examination and reports be devised.

FACE FUNDS

It was suggested by Dr. Troilo that the FACE matching fund raised by the school be freed from restrictions as to use. Agreement was expressed by the school heads. Dr. Wolf indicated he would discuss the matter with FACE as a member of the accrediting committee.

POLICY OF NCA ON PRINCIPLES

A discussion followed on Mr. James Bunker's communications to members of C of E. Dr. Janse suggested the formation of a committee of faculty members to establish principles which could then be discussed by the council.

FACE POLICY

It was suggested by Dr. Haynes and concurred in by other member schools that Dr. W. Wolf recommend that FACE establish a regular policy of grants to schools so that the pressures of uncertainty are relieved and so that budgets can be worked out some time in advance. Schools should present requests and budgets in January at mid-year meeting so that final action can be completed at least by June. A regional director of NCA should sit with the school heads during preparation of reports and budgets to obtain advice and assistance.

RESOLUTION: The preceding suggestions was put in the form of a resolution by Dr. Elliot, seconded by Dr. Bierman and unanimously adopted.

DIGEST OF CHIROPRACTIC ECONOMICS

After discussing recent developments the following motion was made by Dr. Peterson, seconded by Dr. Elliot and adopted, CMCC not voting.

RESOLVED: Hereafter the accredited schools of the NCA will not provide articles to the Digest of Chiropractic Economics.

It was agreed that Dr. Homewood would be requested by Dr. Haynes to convey to Mr. Wm. Luckey the reasons for the council's action and that Dr. Janse who was absent should be sent letter explaining action.

CHIROPRACTIC AS A CAREER

Mr. Belleau reported to the council that he would agree to print monograph for NCA schools exclusively provided council would guarantee purchase of 6000 at $350 per 1000.

A motion to guarantee purchase of 6000 monographs by members of the council did not carry. The following alternate motion was unanimously adopted:

RESOLVED: That Mr. Belleau be requested to print the NCA version of "Chiropractic as a Career" and all schools will purchase as many as they can.

MIDYEAR MEETING
Time and place selection to await developments.

ADJOURNMENT
5:30 P.M.

Minutes of the Mid-Year Meeting of the COUNCIL ON EDUCATION of the ACA, JANUARY 12, 1964, HOTEL RIVIERA, PALM SPRINGS, CALIFORNIA

The Council on Education was called to order at 9:00 A.M. January 12, 1964 by President George H. Haynes. The following is a list of the attendees:

> Dr. George H. Haynes, President
> Dr. John Wolfe, Secretary
> Dr. Dewey Anderson, Director of Education of the ACA
> Dr. O.D. Adams, Assistant to the Director of Education
> Dr. Walter Wolf, Chairman of the Accrediting Committee
> Dr. Asa Brown, Member of Accrediting Committee
> Dr. Orval Hidde, Member of Accrediting Committee
> Dr. J.R. Quigley, Member of Accrediting Committee
> Dr. Herbert M. Himes, Dean, Canadian Memorial Chiropractic College
> Dr. Thure Peterson, President, Chiropractic Institute of New York
> Dr. Sol Goldschmidt, Regent, Chiropractic Institute of New York
> Dr. Helmut Bittner, Dean, Chiropractic Institute of New York
> Dr. L.F. Bierman, President, Lincoln Chiropractic College
> Dr. Frank Ploudre, Trustee, Lincoln Chiropractic College
> Dr. John L. Prosser, Trustee, Lincoln Chiropractic College
> Dr. Vierling Kersey, President, Los Angeles College of Chiropractic
> Dr. Joseph Janse, President, National College of Chiropractic
> Dr. John B. Wolfe, President, Northwestern College of Chiropractic
> Dr. Julius Troilo, President, Texas Chiropractic College
> Dr. James M. Russell, Regent, Texas Chiropractic College
> Dr. Robert Elliot, President, Western States Chiropractic College
> Dr. Devere Biser, President, Council of State Examining Boards
> Dr. Robert Runnells, Vice-President, Council of State Examining Boards
> Dr. Gordon Holman, Secretary, Council of State Examining Boards

Visitors:

> Dr. William N. Coggins, President, Logan Chiropractic College (who on 1-14-64 became a full member of the council)
> Dr. Ernest G. Napolitano, President, Columbia Institute of Chiropractic

After having called the meeting to order, President Haynes welcomed the guests and read the agenda. Dr. Haynes then turned the next portion of the meeting over to Dr. Anderson and Dr. Wolf for the reading and interpretation of the "Educational Standards for Chiropractic Colleges."

Dr. Wolf informed the Council that the Logan College of Chiropractic had applied for accreditation to the Accreditation Committee of the ACA. Dr. Wolf further stated that the school had been inspected and was in the process of being rated.

Dr. Wolf next informed the Council that the Columbia Institute of Chiropractic had applied for accreditation to the Committee and that their status was now being considered in the Committee's meetings.

Dr. Anderson reviewed and clarified his interpretation of the different points comprised in the booklet "Educational Standards for Chiropractic Colleges."

A one hour general discussion followed Dr. Anderson's presentation.

It was brought out that the Council must be considered in the ACA as a direct continuation of that one under the NCA and not as a new or modified council. H.E.W. requires a ten year life of an accrediting agency before it can be recognized by its department of education.

Dr. Peterson stated that he felt that faculty seminars and faculty retirement insurance should not be the plan of an individual school, but an action of the Council.

Dr. Anderson stated that he was in full accord with this thought and suggested the Council propose such an action to the ACA Board. Dr. Wolf was in agreement with this.

Dr. Bittner advised not to mix scope of practice with scope of instruction.

Afternoon Session:

The full Council reconvened at 1:30 P.M. and the proposed "Outline of Standards" was read and discussed.

On the matter of procedure Dr. Hidde objected to the statement referring to the sections requiring the Committee on Accreditation to consult with the full Council before they made their decisions on accreditation.

Dr. Haynes expressed his feelings that the full Council should have the privilege of knowing who is being considered for accreditation, and of expressing their views. He further pointed out that the Committee still has full power of accreditation after listening to the views of the schoolmen.

Dr. Holman expressed the feeling that the whole Council should be made aware of the actions of the Accrediting Committee.

Dr. Wolf questioned the accrediting Committee's need for haste in its decisions.

Dr. Haynes stated that the Council members only asked for discussion before a decision was made by the Accrediting Committee.

No questions were raised regarding the section on revocation.

Dr. Adams questioned the non-profit provision. After general discussion the President asked for a vote on this matter. The vote was unanimous for retaining the non-profit status requirement.

No objections were raised to the sections on Financial Stability and Internal Organization.

On the matter of educational requirements of faculty, Dr. Hidde expressed his feelings that instructors in the clinical science subjects should have A.B. or higher scholastic degrees.

Dr. Faye pointed out that in the clinical sciences experience is the most important factor.

Dr. Anderson stated that the schools should try for a B.S. degree in the clinical sciences faculty.

Dr. Quigley noted that the degree did not insure quality.

Dr. Haynes brought out the fact that in medicine the instructors in the clinical sciences had no additional degree requirement.

Dr. Anderson agreed that the M.D. has an academic background.

Dr. Haynes pointed out that an M.D. degree is a professional degree and is no higher or better than a D.C. for the respective field.

Dr. Wolfe stated that provisions should be for specialization of the faculty in specific areas of the basic sciences. It met with general approval.

No comment was had on "Faculty-Student Ratio" or "Teaching Load." It was pointed out that the faculty salaries are still too low.

Dr. Anderson stressed the need for a strong counseling program.

Under the section on Students, Dr. Hidde expressed the feeling that something should be developed in regard to pre-professional training.

Dr. Haynes said the credits should be transferable and leading towards a B.S. degree.

Dr. Holman stated that the requirement of pre-professional training should be held up until there is a surplus of students.

Dr. Hidde expressed his feelings that the requirement of pre-professional education will not ruin the schools.

Dr. Holman stated that the state board level should not be where the pre-professional requirement originates, that it should come from the profession as a whole and that it should be realistic.

The matters of curriculum, attendance, advance standing, clinical training and physical plant were considered.

January 13, 1964 - 9:00 A.M.

Meeting was called to order by the President.

"Quantitative Questionnaire" was discussed.

Dr. Bierman asked if part time instructors should be included in Student-Faculty ratio; and if the 16 hours per week to compute the full-time faculty equivalent referred to clock or semester hours.

Dr. Haynes explained that part-time teachers are to be converted into full-time faculty equivalents on the basis of 16 semester hours.

Dr. Himes asked if guest lecturers should be listed as faculty, Dr. Haynes answered that they should.

Dr. Wolf stated that if a man taught 1 or 2 hours per semester that he was listed as a guest lecturer, but if he taught 1 class per semester, he should be classified as a part-time instructor.

Dr. Coggins asked for a definition of semester hours. Dr. Haynes answered that one hour per week of lecture for one semester, 16 to 18 weeks equals 1 credit or semester hour. 2 or 3 laboratory hours per week for one semester constitutes one semester hour.

Dr. Bierman asked if technic was a lab. Dr. Haynes answered that in his concept it was a lab.

Dr. Peterson asked what credits should be given for clinic. Dr. Haynes answered that clock hours should be given but not credits.

Dr. Adams asked if clinic hours are considered as lab. Dr. Haynes answered no.

Dr. Peterson noted that a total number of credits has never been set. Dr. Haynes stated that it could not be uniform.

The "Qualitative questionnaire" was then considered.

Dr. Haynes stressed the need for the institution to state its objectives which in turn should be included in the statement of policy of the school. Dr. Troilo stated that the statement of policy should be included in the catalogue.

Dr. Haynes stated that H.E.W. will judge the objectives of the accrediting agency not that of the schools. The accrediting agency is to take into account the objectives of the schools, which should be more or less uniform but leaving it up to the individual school as to how they carry out their objective.

The manual of instruction for the preparation of self-evaluation report of the college and that for the preparation of the inspection by the inspecting team.

Dr. Wolf stated that after a second inspection the institutions could expect a visit from the Director of Education at any time without prior notice.

Dr. Haynes asked if anything should be deleted or added to the rating sheets.

Dr. Wolf answered that the student follow up should be deleted. He asked if the State Boards would assist in this area.

Dr. Holman answered that the individual State Boards are hesitant to give out any information.

Dr. Haynes stated that determining whether or not a graduate became a success in practice was not the duty of the schools because it is not an academic procedure, but should be the duty of the State Boards or profession. He went on to state that it would be up to the schools to maintain records after they are given the information, but they have no way of collecting it directly.

Dr. Haynes stated that information from State Boards as to the results of examinations and the individual subjects that their students passed and failed would be of value to the schools in determining academic procedures.

Dr. Holman displayed the forms used by the Council of State Examining Boards to show the break down of licenses granted, revoked, lost through death etc.

Dr. Haynes suggested a questionnaire be sent out with the license renewal form requesting information as to practice status. He went on to say that this would give the position of the profession in each state.

Dr. Holman stated that the matter will be presented at the next meeting of the Council of State Examining Boards.

The Council reconvened at 1:30 P.M.

(This was a closed meeting with only the full members of the Council in attendance.)

President Haynes asked Dr. Wolf to present the activities and actions of the Accrediting Committee.

Dr. Wolf began the discussion by stating that the Logan Chiropractic College had been reinstated to a provisionally accredited status as enjoyed by all other ACA schools and thus eligible for full membership in the Council. He said that the first inspection of Logan had disclosed findings similar to those obtained on the first inspection of the other ACA Colleges.

Dr. Wolf state that Logan had been removed from the list of provisionally accredited schools because of the following reasons:

1. At that time Logan was attending meetings of the NCA as well as ICA
2. Logan was asking their students to keep confidential the contents of some of their technic courses.
3. There existed an incompatibility between Dr. Logan and Dr. Nugent.
4. Dr. Logan refused inspection.

(Introduce attached matter.)

Dr. Wolf stated that a self-evaluation had been submitted by the Missouri Chiropractic College, by Dr. Otto Reinert. After a preliminary inspection by Dr. Anderson the Accrediting Committee adopted a resolution based upon Dr. Anderson's recommendation that the Missouri Chiropractic College is not eligible for a full inspection.

Dr. Wolf stated that the Columbia Institute of Chiropractic had made a request for inspection. The self-evaluation form had been completed and will be appraised at the meetings of the Accrediting Committee. Dr. Anderson feels after a preliminary inspection that the school is worthy of a full inspection.

Dr. Wolf stated that some conferences had been held between Atlantic States Chiropractic College and Dr. Anderson.

Dr. Wolf's presentation covered the following points:

1. Western States College of Chiropractic
   a) Notice has been given to Western States College of Chiropractic on January 12, 1964 that they had failed to correct their deficiencies.
   b) The Accrediting Committee has revoked the status of provisionally accredited. The school is now on a conditionally approved status.

The Western States College of Chiropractic has been informed that unless they improve their deficiencies in six months, their status of conditionally approved would be revoked.

2. Texas Chiropractic College

The Accrediting Committee noted that the Texas Chiropractic College program was good and that if a building site could be bought by June and that an architectural design and feasibility of a new school could be shown that the school would retain their provisionally accredited status.

3. A similar statement was made regarding the Northwestern College of Chiropractic.
4. Chiropractic Institute of New York

The Accrediting Committee stated that the Chiropractic Institute of New York has a good plan, action on the June resolution has been deferred pending determination of the feasibility of the building plan. The Chiropractic Institute of New York retains their status of provisionally accredited.

5.   Los Angeles College of Chiropractic, Lincoln College of Chiropractic, and National College of Chiropractic.
The Accrediting Committee stated that these schools are making good progress and will retain their status of provisionally accredited.

With the Accrediting Committee's presentation completed, a question and answer period followed.

Dr. Elliot requested a hearing of appeal of the Western States College of Chiropractic to the Accrediting Committee and to be conducted in the presence of the full Council.

It was decided by the two involved parties that the appeal hearing would be held Wednesday, January 14, 1964 and asked Dr. Haynes to preside. The chair accepted after general agreement that he would have the power to stop any direct exchange or argument between individuals and confine the floor to members of the Accrediting Committee and Western States College of Chiropractic representatives. The chair warned that all parties concerned should be fully prepared.

The efforts and progress made by the Accrediting Committee towards application for approval from H.E.W. was then discussed.

Dr. Haynes reiterated that it will be the Accrediting Agency that will be approved by H.E.W. rather than the individual schools.

Dr. Anderson related his unofficial talks with Dr. Cornet of H.E.W. held on December 24, 1963.

Dr. Anderson stated that approval had been denied the 5-22-61 application because of failure to comply with the H.E.W. criteria set in 1952.

Dr. Haynes asked if the information in 5a of the H.E.W. criteria had been collected and Dr. Anderson answered that it had not.

Dr. Anderson stated that he could work informally with Dr. Cornet until the Accrediting Committee is ready to go to H.E.W. with their formal request for approval.

The Council reconvened on January 14, 1964 to attend the Western States College of Chiropractic appeal hearing before the Accrediting Committee.

ORDER ON REINSTATEMENT OF ACCREDITED STATUS

Re: Logan College of Chiropractic
WHEREAS, the accredited status of the Logan College of Chiropractic was revoked by the Council on Education of the National Chiropractic Association during the annual meeting held in Los Angeles, California in July 1953, and

WHEREAS, the reasons for revocation were stated to be:

1.   Refusal by Dr. Vinton Logan to permit inspection of the Logan College by the Director of Education
2.   Participation in the accrediting organization known as North American Association of Chiropractic Schools and Colleges.
3.   Continued separatism in the actions of Dr. Vinton Logan. (Details set forth in the minutes of the Council.)
4.   Failure of Dr. Logan to attend meetings of the National Council on Education, and

WHEREAS, the Logan College of Chiropractic requested a re-inspection of the college and reinstatement of accredited status on the basis of an expressed intent to comply with the criteria and standards of the Council on Education of the National Chiropractic, and
WHEREAS, an intensive inspection of the Logan College of Chiropractic by an Accrediting Committee on October 3-4, 1963 revealed that the objectionable items causing the 1953 revocation of accredited status had been removed and substantial progress had been made toward meeting the criteria for chiropractic colleges.
NOW THEREFORE, BE IT RESOLVED, that the Committee on Accreditation of the American Chiropractic Association does hereby order the reinstatement of the "Accredited Provisionally" status for the Logan College of Chiropractic.

W.B. Wolf, Chairman, Committee on Accreditation, January 12, 1964

The Full Council meeting was called to order by the Secretary John Wolfe in the absence of President Haynes.

Dr. Wolf called for comment on post-graduate classes and their relation to the other Councils of the ACA.

It was generally agreed that certification is a job of the profession and not that of the schools.

Dr. Janse stated that Dr. Wunsch, President of the Board on Certified Roentgenologists, feels certification should come from the Board. They feel they have the right to present this work themselves but will recognize credits given by teachers holding their certification. They will put on classes independently of schools and Council on Education.

Dr. Adams stated that they have no legal grounds to do this and that in effect they are chartering themselves as a school.

Dr. Hidde expressed his feeling that this would be a step backward.

Dr. Janse stated that the certified men know their work and in some cases they might be more qualified to teach than the men teaching in our schools, but that every man who was certified was not qualified to teach.

At this time Dr. Haynes took back the chair and welcomed Dr. Coggins as a full member of the Council due to the formal action taken by the Accrediting Committee the previous afternoon.

Dr. Anderson stated that the schools are competent to teach X-ray and orthopedics and that this principle must be recognized by the profession to protect the schools. He warned against letting the specialty boards make the decision for it would be detrimental to accreditation.

Dr. Haynes stated that a school could not grant credits for work not conducted under their direction and control.

Dr. Haynes stated that at the Los Angeles College of Chiropractic in the teaching of post-graduate classes in a specialty they had met with a tendency on the part of the specialty to dictate to the school who could teach and what to teach. Dr. Haynes stated this had been the case in minor surgery and obstetrics which had resulted in an unfavorable reputation for the entire college, which took him years to rectify.

Dr. Haynes stated that the Council on Roentgenology and the Council on Orthopedics have done an excellent job and the Council on Education would assist them in every way possible.

The matter of "course peddling" was then discussed.

Dr. Haynes brought up the matter of the publication, "Chiropractic Economics" and the fact that according to the action of the last meeting of the Council, Dr. Homewood had contacted the editor. He had informed Mr. Luckey to publish news of the schools but not as reports from the schools because of the undesirable advertising appearing in the magazine.

Dr. Hidde pointed out that the ACA Journal now had some of the same advertising.

Dr. Janse said he believed that the schools reports were not to be given to Mr. Luckey. Dr. Haynes stated that reports were not being given but that the pictures of the school heads were still on articles that were being printed.

Dr. Coggins offered to talk to Mr. Luckey to persuade him to stop the articles. The chair accepted the offer.

Dr. Haynes suggested that a Council policy statement should be prepared for action by the Council. Dr. Faye and Dr. Brown were appointed to prepare such a resolution.

Dr. Anderson stated that if a technic is valuable it should be taught through the schools and not through an outside channel. Dr. Himes and others pointed out the need for policy on this matter. It was also pointed out that there are a number of committees in the ACA whose work appears to be related to technics and procedures now being peddled to the profession.

Dr. Anderson asked why these committees existed and if they give out a bill of particulars in the realm of their functions. It was suggested that the ACA Committees be disbanded after 2 years if they do not render a service.

The matter of the Jr. ACA was brought up and the matter of increased dues was discussed.

Dr. Pruitt appeared before the Council to clarify the changes. He stated that dues of $5.00 per year is not too high.

He stated that it should be voluntary on the part of the student to be a member of the Jr. ACA. The Board feels it is better to create an interest in the student. The Board wants an active organization, a junior organization that will serve the same purpose as the senior organization. Dr. Pruitt further stated that a Jr. ACA member is entitled to the first year of senior membership at a lower rate.

Dr. Haynes pointed out that since 1948 Jr. NCA membership was mandatory at the Los Angeles College of Chiropractic and the NCA fee (now ACA) was made a part of the student body fee. Dr. Janse pointed out their recent change to this ACA dues inclusion in the student body fee. A discontinuance of this system will cause a decrease in membership.

Most schools are meeting resistance from the students to the increase in dues.

SCHOLARSHIP

Dr. Anderson asked how the scholarship plan is implemented.

Dr. Pruitt explained that a mailing had been sent to all Jr. Colleges explaining the program. He further stated that another mailing will be made and the program will be publicized in the journal.

Dr. Anderson stated that each school has their own program.

Dr. Hidde asked what became of a student who did not win an award.

Dr. Pruitt said that their names would be turned over to the proper school.

Dr. Prosser asked why the school had to pay half of the scholarship when even the full tuition was not paying the cost of education.

Dr. Pruitt answered that the ACA paid the public relations cost and that there was no help from FACE on this project.

The meeting of the Full Council was called to order by President George Haynes on 1-14-64 at 1:30 P.M.

Dr. Haynes stated that a report would be presented by Dr. Henry G. Higley, Director of Research of the ACA and turned the meeting over to Dr. Higley.

Dr. Higley began by stating that the Dept. of Research had been created in 1959 for the purpose of conducting organized research to back up the claims made by the profession. He went on to say that the Intervertebral Disc Syndrome had been the first project and that the Low Back Syndrome had been next. The results had been published and have been accepted favorably within the profession and without. Dr. Higley stated that these reports had been examined by many agencies, two of which were the Department of Labor and H.E.W. and that the responses had been good. Dr. Higley added that he had received a request for information from the United States Air Force.

Dr. Higley stated that the research had been started with a search of literature dealing with the spine. He stated that 980 documents had been researched, from which 3,000 abstracts have been obtained. Dr. Higley stated that the Chiropractic research had been accepted on the same level as other research by men of science.

Dr. Higley stated that the data coming from school research must be accurate and valid and that each school is given proper credit.

Regarding the Low Back Syndrome Dr. Higley stated that he was not receiving enough cases and that the re-checks were not coming in as they should. Dr. Higley stated that the four following points are necessary in the research projects if they are to be successful.

1. Send in all applicable cases. (Only those cases satisfactory will be accepted.)
2. The re-checks are vital.
3. The correct dates are very important.
4. The reports should not come in all at once, rather that the information should be sent in immediately.

Dr. Higley stated that he had been requested by the Executive Board to ascertain the average number of hours per week the research staff of each school devoted to the preparation of these reports. He cited for an example that the Los Angeles College of Chiropractic spent 8 hours per week in the preparation of these reports and that this amount of time is inadequate.

Dr. Higley then asked for any questions.

Question: What if patient is well before 4 weeks?
Answer: Consult the Manual
Question: How do you get the patient back if he is well before 4 weeks?
Answer: Call them

Dr. Hidde suggested that the patient should be informed that he is part of a research program.

Dr. Adams stated that if this (L.B.S.) became a fact, it could be sold to the compensation insurance companies.

Dr. Anderson asked when the project started.
Answer: 1959 - First set of reports in 1962.

Dr. Higley stated that there had been an improvement in the results between the first and second years and that the school's participation in the project had been noted by FACE.

Dr. Elliot stated that Dr. Higley's personal visit and his chart had been very helpful.

Dr. Haynes stated that he felt the research had started slowly because the clinicians and externs were very busy but that it will now proceed faster.

Dr. Higley stated that three articles have been published in the ACA Journal and more will be published.

Dr. Higley stated that every full time profession should devote a certain amount of time to research. Dr. Higley stated that the research should be prepared in proper form, the final form being done by a technical writer. He further said that the faculty should be stimulated to do simple research and that several books are available on the subject, etc. Unusual cases in private practices should also be reported.

Dr. Anderson stated that an understanding of research required the ability to read and understand literature and suggested the teaching of scientific methodology.

Dr. Haynes stated that the Department of Research in the school should use the students to search the literature. He cited several research projects completed and published by members of the Los Angeles College of Chiropractic faculty.

1. Nilsson and Carlson - Cranial Resistance to Mechanical Force.
2. Vampa - Examination of Cervical Area Before and After Adjustment
3. Nilsson - Study of Nerve Root
4. Nilsson - Head of Rib - Relation to Intervertebral Disc.

Dr. Haynes stated that this research was not opinion but statement of fact.

Dr. Ploudre stated that the offer of a cash grant would be of value.

Dr. Higley said that this had been done and only 2 papers were submitted. Dr. Higley said that the papers must be of scientific merit.

Dr. Anderson stated that research submitted should be a factor considered in the grading in obtaining an additional degree.

Dr. Holman suggested research on technic peddling.

Dr. Anderson pointed out that the Haynes Report had been paid research done by Stanford.

Dr. Quigley pointed out that the practitioner is more reluctant to open his records for research than are the schools.

Dr. Bittner outlined a proposed Scientific Journal. He stated that the President of each school should submit once every three months one article authored by a member of his faculty after he had judged the article worthy of being published. The article would then be evaluated by an editorial committee. Reference texts on thesis writing were suggested. It was hoped to have the Journal ready for distribution by the June Convention.

I.   The Research Director will submit twice a year or on request to the FACE Board of Governors of the American Chiropractic Association, Director of Education and the Accrediting Committee an evaluation of the research activities of each institution. The evaluation will be based on the degree of adherence to the "Protocol" and Manual of Procedure in each case.

II.   The Research Director will submit twice a year at the regular meeting a written and an oral report of the Department of Research and Statistics to the Board of Governors of the ACA and to FACE.

III.   Research proposals
    Institutions desiring to submit a research proposal to the ACA will do so by submitting such proposals to the Research Director.

The proposal must consist of the following information.
1. Objectives
2. Brief history
3. Relationship and value in relation to the general aim of the ACA.
4. Qualification and experience of principle investigation.
5. Methodology to be used.
6. Bibliography of pertinent and relative work including published work of investigation.
7. Budget

    The Research Director is to study and analyze such proposals. Considering each one of the seven points listed above, and also the degree of duplication with other projects submitted or in process.
    Value of the proposed research in accelerating, aiding, clarifying or in any other way helping in the over-all research program of the ACA.
    The Director of Research will prepare and submit to FACE his recommendation with a copy of the proposal for action and disposition by the Board of Directors of FACE.

    Wednesday, January 15, 1964
    Meeting called to order by President Haynes to consider resolutions and motions.
    It was moved by Dr. Wolf that the "rules of Procedure" (outline of standards) be referred back to Committee. Motion was adopted.
    It was moved by Dr. Peterson, and seconded, that the following motion be adopted:
    The Council on Education supports the action of Dr. Dewey Anderson in respect to the steps taken and to be taken in line with the application to H.E.W. to obtain approval for the Accrediting Agency of the ACA.
    It was recommended and requested by Dr. Anderson that the colleges re-prepare their financial analysis as discussed at the meeting. This material to be sent to Dr. Haynes for integration and tabulation.
    A motion was made to bring to the attention of the Board of the ACA the matter of "course peddling" and its reflection on the profession with the view of setting a program to correct this condition. Motion was adopted.
    Motion was made to commend the Roentgenological Council and Certifying Board of their fine work and for the excellent symposium that they sponsor.
    Motion was adopted.

    The following recommendation was presented. It is recommended that after functioning for two years, each Council established within the American Chiropractic Association be required to submit evidence to the House of Delegates that it is serving a useful and constructive purpose. If such evidence is not demonstrated, said Council shall not be permitted to continue to function.
    The recommendation was adopted.

    A motion was made that a committee of three members of the Council on Education be appointed by its chairman to act as liaison with the various councils appointed by the Executive Board and whose activities are related to chiropractic education and in which we, as a Council are vitally interested.
    Motion was adopted.

    Dr. Holman presented the aim and work carried on by the Examining Boards. This materials is attached to these minutes.
    The Chair declared the floor open to nomination for Council on Education officers.
    Dr. Janse nominated Dr. Haynes for chairman. Dr. Haynes requested his name be removed from nomination and that a new chairman be selected.
    Dr. W. Wolf moved that Dr. Haynes and Dr. J. Wolfe be retained in their present posts, seconded by Dr. ??? and Dr. Holman. Dr. Wolfe asked for the vote and the motion carried.
    Meeting was adjourned.

AREA OF RESPONSIBILITY OF STATE BOARDS COMMITTEE

    To obtain, correlate and make available information relative to individual State Boards of Examiners to the Council of Education of the ACA.
    At the suggestion of the General Committee of the Profession and at the direction of the membership of the Council of Examining

Boards necessary forms and procedures have been prepared. The forms were first mailed out December 1963. Some 20 states have responded as of January 9th, with their 1963 reports. It is expected that a small percentage of State Boards will not respond with all the information requested. In these cases we will proceed to gather all information legally available. Sample forms are enclosed.

The Council of Examiners is also active in other areas, namely:

Standard Basic Curriculum

Certification of Credits, forms.

List of accepted text books, phase I

Library list of Chiropractic text books and related subjects - in process

List of teaching text books - in process - 80% complete

National Board of Chiropractic Examiners was formed in April 1963 and incorporated in June 1963. First examination in phase * - Target date January 1965.

Council of Examining Boards is active in several other fields such as:

Radiation Control

Definition of clinics

Reciprocity between states

Policing powers of State Boards

December 15, 1963, Lincoln Chiropractic College, Indianapolis

Dear Sirs,

This letter is written to you on account of a special group of Swedish chiropractors. Those who are not graduated from any chiropractic school in the U.S.A.

They are people who have been active chiropractors for many years. Between 10-30 years. Their chiropractic education is of different origin and length, some very brief, perhaps, to start with but surely accumulating through the years.

This group and some graduated chiropractors did form the first Swedish Chiropractic Association of which I now am the chairman.

In Sweden, there is no special law about chiropractic, there is just one law stating what an M.D. is supposed to do and his associates as nurses, physical therapists and so on. Then there is another law for "laymen, " that is - all the rest in the healing profession.

However, we do feel the impact of the Swedish government upon "laymen" doctors and would very much like to raise the chiropractic education amongst our members. We have been discussing this issue and found that the interest for a course at a Chiropractic School is great but that the amount of prospective students hardly amounts to more than ten (a variation possible both up and down). The length of time should be three or four months. The subjects of special interest:

1. Chiropractic philosophy.
2. Physical examination, all aspects.
3. Chiropractic analysis, all different types (those who are built on X-ray findings only very short as we are not allowed to use X-ray here in Sweden).
4. Chiropractic listings.
5. Chiropractic adjusting techniques, all different types.
6. Office procedures.
7. X-ray film reading-interpretation.

We welcome suggestions on other subjects and so on.

This group of people consists of no great linguists, but the members do understand clearly and slowly spoken English.

The writer of this letter is a graduate of the P.S.C. in 1950, and visited your country for chiropractic studies three years 1947-1950, and two months in 1962, and is willing to take part in this course both for re-education and as an interpreter for the group, if necessary.

Now gentlemen to the questions:

A. Is it possible for you to arrange such a course and if so preferably during the time May - October?
B. What would be the estimated cost?
C. We understand that such a course, perhaps could not give a diploma of the usual type but nevertheless there has to be some kind of a written certificate. Could that be issued?

D. I am sure there are questions not mentioned here that have to be discussed before any decision can be made on either side but this is just a preliminary letter and I am very interested to get your reaction and will be very happy to hear from you and get all the information you may care to send.

Sincerely yours, Kurt Malmberg, D.C.

Minutes of the Meeting of the COUNCIL ON EDUCATION of the ACA
January 16 to 21, 1965, Des Moines, Iowa

The Council on Education was called to order at 9:00 AM on January 17, 1965, by President George Haynes. The following were present:

Dr. George H. Haynes, (L.A.C.C.) Council President
Dr. Jack Wolfe, (Northwestern C.C.) Council Secretary
Dr. John Fisher, Director of Education
Dr. Walter Wolfe, Chairman of the Accrediting Committee
Dr. Herbert Hinton, Member of the Accrediting Committee
Dr. Edward Poulsen, Member of the Accrediting Committee
Dr. J.R. Quigley, Member of the Accrediting Committee
Dr. Herbert M Himes, Dean of the Canadian Memorial Chiropractic College
Dr. Thure Peterson, President, Chiropractic Institute of New York
Dr. Ernest Napolitano, President, Columbia Institute of Chiropractic
Dr. Lewis Bierman, President, Lincoln Chiropractic College
Dr. William Coggins, President, Logan College of Chiropractic
Dr. Joseph Janse, President, National College of Chiropractic
Dr. Julius Troilo, President, Texas Chiropractic College
Dr. Robert Elliot, President, Western States College of Chiropractic
Dr. Gordon Holman, Secretary of the Council of State Boards of Chiropractic Examiners
Dr. Helmut Bittner, Dean, Chiropractic Institute of New York
Dr. Leonard Fay, Assistant to the President, National College of Chiropractic
Dr. Henry G. Higley, Research Director, Los Angeles College of Chiropractic
Dr. Frank Ploudre, Trustee, Lincoln Chiropractic College
Dr. E.M. Saunders, President of the National Board of Chiropractic Examiners.

Dr. Orval Hidde, Member of the Accrediting Committee, was unable to be present and sent his regrets.

Notice was made of the meeting of the individual colleges administrators with the Accrediting Committee which were held on Saturday, January 16, 1965.

The agenda was adopted by the Council as presented.

The minutes of the last meeting were approved as read with the correction of an omission, so that on page 4 of the minutes, the first paragraph dealing with the report of the Accrediting Committee should read: "4-Logan, Lincoln, National, Los Angeles, and Chiropractic Institute retain their status of provisionally accredited".

The Chair welcomed Dr. Schierholz and the members of the Board of FACE who were invited guests of the Council.

The Chair also welcomed Dr. Hinton, newly appointed member of the Committee on Accreditation of the ACA.

Dr. Fisher was introduced by the Chair and invited to address the Council. Dr. Fisher stressed the need for planning for the future in conformity with the changing times. He presented a set of charts based on surveys made by the government and discussed the following points:
1) Population changes outlook
2) Trends in jobs and job training
3) Trends in educational enrollments
4) Economic outlook and increased cost of education
5) The meaning of the above points to chiropractic education

Like all other colleges and universities we must consider the demand for better education; both in breadth and depth. This raises a number of questions to which we must prepare the answers.
1) What is the estimated chiropractic enrollment for the next ten years?
    a)   What is the optimum capacity of our schools?

  b)   Is the betterment of student quality dependent on pre-educational requirements? If so:
    1)   How are we to get the quantity of students needed and how long will it take to do so?
    2)   How good a quality are we to demand?
 2)   On what rests the quality of our faculty?
  a)   Degrees?
  b)   Scholastic Attainments?
  c)   Faculty salary scale?
 3)   What will the effect of the changing times be on the operational budget? How high will it go? The present level is $1,600,000 for our nine schools. What about capital expenses?
 4)   Where is this money coming from?
  a)   From students?
  b)   From endowments?
  c)   From gifts and grants?
  d)   From other sources?
 5)   What is the plan that answers these questions?
  a)   To whom must we sell our program? Who is to sell it? The schools? The Council? FACE? The ACA?

He cautioned the Council to remember that a prospective donor wants to see a ten year projected plan and budget before he will become an actual donor.

Dr. Fisher was then asked to report on the present status of our presentation before H.E.W.

Dr. Fisher reported that no further material has been presented before H.E.W. and that our application has not been re-opened. During an official discussion with Dr. Coronet of H.E.W.'s Department of Education, Dr. Fisher gathered the impression that the departments consider that we need at least two and a half years before being ready for approval, and that at least two of our schools must be fully accredited before the case is re-opened in Washington.

General discussion followed; there was a general agreement on the following points:
1)   The need to introduce the two year pre-professional requirement.
2)   The need to increase the number of chiropractic students.
3)   The need to increase the security of opportunity to establish a successful practice.
4)   The need to increase the stature and prestige of our profession before the public.

Dr. Schierholz extended a welcome to the members of the Council and informed us of the progress of the ACA program. He explained the difficulties and enormous work entailed in the moving of the ACA headquarters and his assumption of the new duties as Executive Director of the ACA.

Dr. Schierholz was commended by the Council for the praiseworthy manner in which he had handled the difficult task.

Dr. Schierholz and the Board of FACE excused themselves and left to resume the meeting of their Board.

Dr. Walter Wolf then presented the problem of grading the inspection findings through a point system. Discussion was held and at the expressed wish of the Council, the Chair appointed a committee to work out the point system.

The Chair appointed to this committee all the members of the Accrediting Committee, Drs. Fisher, Fay, Coggins, Bittner and Haynes.

Dr. Fay presented the report of the meeting of the Clinic Directors held at the National College on October 31 and November 1, 1964. The report was received, and a vote of appreciation was extended to Dr. Fay. The next Clinical Director's meeting will be held at the Logan College.

Dr. Ploudre announced that the International College of Chiropractic intends to make a presentation to each college possibly in September.

Dr. Fisher presented a plan for uniform financial reporting by all the colleges. After much discussion the plan was adopted after making a few modifications. Dr. Fisher was asked to send copies of the approved chart of accounts to each one of the colleges.

The report from the National Board of Chiropractic Examiners, presented by its president, Dr. E.M. Saunders was received. The first examination will be held on March 4, 5, 6, and 7, 1965, at four locations: Los Angeles, California, Davenport, Iowa, Indianapolis, Indiana and New York City, New York. At present ten State Boards will accept these examinations towards licensure.

The report from the Council of State Boards of Chiropractic Examiners, presented by its secretary, Dr. Gordon Holman, covering the analysis of 41 State Board statistics was received.

Dr. Holman was thanked for his report and praise was given for the publishing of their directory. It was requested that Dr. Holman check if the agreed upon certification form is actually accepted by the Boards that have voted it. He was also requested to continue to gather the licensing statistics from the different states.

Means of improving the efficiency of the Junior ACA program was discussed. The Chair appointed a committee consisting of Dr. Bierman as Chairman, and Drs. Napolitano, Higley and Fay to prepare recommendations on the above matter for presentation to the ACA The report is made part of these minutes.

Dr. Wolf reported the recommendations from the committee on grading the inspection findings through a point system, copy of which is attached to these minutes. Final action on this report was left for the next meeting of the Council in June 1965.

Dr. Rich appeared before the Council to present his program with regards to the post-graduate program in the field of Roentgenology as agreed upon with a section of the Certifying Board.

It was with regrets that the Council was forced to reject the suggestions as to size and dates of classes, tuition and other charges, organization and control of classes, splitting of tuition income with the Certifying Board and pay for instructors as all of these items are part of the duty and power of the individual colleges. Acceptance of the proposed terms would place the chances for accreditation in jeopardy.

The proposed outline for the course could not be acted upon at this meeting as it arrived too late to allow the Roentgenology Departments of our colleges to pass upon its merits.

The Accrediting Committee reported the following actions:

1) The Los Angeles College of Chiropractic, the National College of Chiropractic and Texas College of Chiropractic retain their present status as provisionally accredited.
2) The Lincoln and Logan Colleges retain their status as provisionally accredited with the understanding that an internal reorganization is to take place so that the full power of administration shall rest on the college's executive officer.
3) The New York Institute and Columbia Institute retain their status as provisionally accredited and were given six months to find a solution to their problems.
4) The Northwestern College remains on the provisionally approval list for six months, pending a report from Dr. Fisher.
5) The Western States College was given notice of revocation of their provisional approval status.
6) The committee has accepted the official request from the Canadian College for inspection.

Dr. Higley, Director of Research of the ACA gave his report. He has received from our clinics reports covering over 500 cases of low back involvement for tabulation. Each college was to report the cost of their clinical research program on the low-back syndrome.

His department has been commissioned by FACE to prepare 20 research proposals. Dr. Higley asked the Council for assistance for this program.

1) Moved that the point system of grading the inspection findings be printed and acted upon at the Florida meeting, Passed.
2) Moved that the clinic report be accepted and an expression of thanks be extended to Dr. Fay. Passed.

Dr. Ploudre announced that FACE has allocated funds for the transportation of the clinic directors to the next meeting, to be held at the Logan College.

3) Moved that Dr. Fisher proceed to print copies of the approved chart of accounts and financial reporting form to be distributed to all the approved colleges, Passed.
4) Moved that a vote of thanks and appreciation be extended to Dr. Saunders for his excellent work on the National Board of Chiropractic Examiners. Passed.
5) Moved that a vote of thanks be extended to Dr. Holman for his excellent work in the Council of State Boards of Chiropractic Examiners. Passed.
6) Moved that a vote of thanks be extended to Dr. Haynes and Dr. Higley for the analysis of the State Board statistics. Passed.
7) Moved that the colleges in the area of test sites for the National Board Examination require their Junior and Senior students to take the examination. Failed
8) Moved that the colleges in the area of test sites for the National Board Examination will strongly recommend their Junior and Senior students to take the examination. Passed.
9) Dr. Coggins as chairman of the committee, appointed to consider the problems raised by the institution of pre-professional requirements presented his report.

Moved that the report presented by Dr. Coggins be received and a vote of thanks be extended to Dr. Coggins and his committee. Passed.

The Chair appointed the following committees:

10) Moved that we approve in principle the phasing of the two year pre-professional requirement for matriculation to be instituted on September 30, 1968 by institution, if possible, a one year pre-professional requirement by September 30, 1967 or before.

Moved that the Council go on record as approving President Johnson's proposals for federal support of general education and health education. Passed.

Moved that the Council go on record as approving the proposals of granting income tax exception to those pursuing their education. Passed.

Moved that Dr. G.H. Haynes and Dr. H.G. Higley be commended for their action concerning the San Diego State College class on Health Education Quackery. Passed.

Move that the Council proceed with the formation of a speakers bureau to represent chiropractic at all health education and allied classes presented through colleges all over the United States. Passed.

Moved that the ACA approved colleges accept the request received from the European Chiropractic Union. Passed. Letter is attached to the minutes.

Dr. Bittner made an appeal for cooperation from the colleges in publishing of a quarterly scientific journal.
Meeting adjourned.
Respectfully submitted, Jack Wolfe, Secretary

Minutes of the Meeting of the COUNCIL ON EDUCATION of the ACA
Hollywood, Florida, June 19 through June 25, 1965

The meeting of the Council on Education of the ACA was called to order by the President, Dr. George H. Haynes, at 9:00 A.M., Monday, June 21, 1965, at the Diplomat Hotel, Hollywood by the Sea, Florida.
Council President, Dr. George H. Haynes, Los Angeles College of Chiropractic, Present
Council Secretary, Dr. John Wolfe, Northwestern College of Chiropractic, Present
Director of Education, ACA, Dr. John A. Fisher, Present
Accrediting Committee, Dr. Walter Wolf, Present, (Chairman)
Accrediting Committee, Dr. Orval Hidde, Present
Accrediting Committee, Dr. Herbert Hinton, Present
Accrediting Committee, Dr. Edward Poulsen, Present
Accrediting Committee, Dr. J.R. Quigley, Present
Chiropractic Institute of New York, Dr. Thure Peterson, Present (President)
Columbia Institute of Chiropractic, Dr. Ernest Napolitano, Present (President) from June 23 on
Lincoln College of Chiropractic, Dr. Earl Rich, Present, (President)
Logan College of Chiropractic, Dr. William Coggins, Present, (President) from June 23 on
National College of Chiropractic, Dr. Joseph Janse, Present (President)
Texas College of Chiropractic, Dr. W.D. Harper, Present, (Dean)
Council of State Chiropractic Examining Boards, Dr. Robert Runnels, Present
Council of State Chiropractic Examining Boards, Dr. Gordon Holman, Present

Also present:
Canadian Memorial College of Chiropractic, Dr. Herbert Himes, (Dean)
Western States College of Chiropractic, Dr. Robert Elliot, (President)
Chiropractic Institute of New York, Dr. Helmut Bittner, (Dean)
Lincoln College of Chiropractic, Dr. Chester Stowell, (Dean)
Los Angeles College of Chiropractic, Dr. Henry Higley
National College of Chiropractic, Dr. Leonard Fay, (Vice-President)
Texas College of Chiropractic, Dr. James Russell, (President, Board of Regents)
National Board of Chiropractic Examiners, Dr. E.M. Saunders, (President)

The minutes of the mid-year meeting held at Des Moines, Iowa, were approved as read.

COMMUNICATIONS:
Letter to President Johnson and reply relative to the Council's endorsement of his national program of financial assistance for higher education.
Letter from the Wyoming Department of Education forwarded by Dr. Napolitano relative to the Columbia Institute of Chiropractic's attitude towards blind students. The Council President's reply was approved as representing the policy of the Council and it is to be introduced as part of these minutes.
ELECTION OF OFFICERS:
The chair reminded the Council that the election of officers should have taken place at the mid-year meeting and suggested that the Council should proceed to remedy this oversight.
Dr. Peterson, seconded by Dr. Janse nominated Dr. Haynes to the Presidency. Dr. Walter Wolf nominated Dr. John Wolfe for

Secretary. Dr. Harper called for a vote and Dr. Wolfe was re-elected Secretary.

Their term of office will expire at the time of the mid-year meeting of the Council in early 1966.

DR. JOHN A FISHER, DIRECTOR OF EDUCATION:

Indicated there had been no further contact with H.E.W. and briefly discussed the ACA Scholarship Program.

DR. E.M. SAUNDERS, PRESIDENT OF THE NATIONAL BOARD OF CHIROPRACTIC EXAMINERS:

Presented his report on the Board's activity for the past year. A discussion on the results of the last examination. Dr. Saunders was highly commended for his work. Dr. Saunder's written report is attached.

DR. GORDON HOLMAN, SECRETARY OF THE COUNCIL OF STATE CHIROPRACTIC EXAMINING BOARDS:

Presented his report. The directory published by the Council of State Boards was praised by those present. Dr. Holman's written report is attached.

DR. LEONARD FAY, CHAIRMAN OF THE CLINIC DIRECTORS SEMINAR:

Presented his report. Discussion was had on the progress of the seminar and of the Committee on Standardization of Clinic Forms. The written reports are attached.

DR. HENRY HIGLEY, DIRECTOR OF RESEARCH FOR THE ACA;

Presented his report and recommendations. The importance of departmental research in all the colleges was stressed. Written report is attached.

DR. EDWARD POULSEN, CHAIRMAN OF THE COMMITTEE ON LEGISLATIVE DIRECTION OF THE COUNCIL;

Presented his report.

DR. O.L. HIDDE, CHAIRMAN OF THE PROFESSIONAL AWARENESS COMMITTEE OF THE COUNCIL;

Presented his report.

DR. WILLIAM COGGINS, CHAIRMAN OF THE COMMITTEE ON STUDENT ADMISSIONS AND COUNSELING OF THE COUNCIL;

Presented his report.

Dr. Lee Arnold, President of the Florida Chiropractic Association and Dr. Herman Ulrich, Chairman of the Scholarship Committee appeared before the Council. Dr. Arnold presented the student admissions and counseling program of the Florida Association followed by a general discussion on the subject. Dr. Arnold and the Florida Association were commended for their program and the Council tendered their full support.

Dr. Ulrich discussed the Scholarship Program. His written report is attached.

Mr. Simone and Dr. Adams of Louisiana were invited to speak on the present status of the England Case and discuss the implications of this court action on the chiropractic profession. A general discussion followed. Mr. Simone expressed the need of a strict scientific approach to the practice of our profession the avoidance of the concept of one cause for all disease and urge the approach of considering the M.D. profession as a branch of Medicine, namely as the allopathic branch. Mr. Simone was extended the Council's appreciation for the valuable information and advise that he presented to the group.

Dr. Haynes presented his report on the Speaker's Bureau. He emphasized the need for this program and mentioned that the Los Angeles College of Chiropractic had been once more called to represent Chiropractic, this time at the San Francisco State College, written report is attached.

Note was made that Junior ACA membership is now mandatory at the following colleges: Texas Chiropractic College, Lincoln Chiropractic College, National College of Chiropractic, Northwestern College of Chiropractic, Chiropractic Institute of New York, Los Angeles College of Chiropractic and Western States College of Chiropractic.

Dr. Ulrich and Dr. Howard appeared on behalf of the Council on Roentgenology to present the nominations for the Certifying Board of Examiners and educational provisions of their constitution. The Council on Education promised its prompt consideration of their request for approval.

Dr. Janse presented the report of the Committee on Standardization of Chiropractic Principles. A copy of the written report "Chiropractic of Today" was distributed and superficially discussed. Dr. Janse and his committee were commended for their untiring work on behalf of the profession.

Discussion was had on the subjects of NCIC Malpractice Insurance Plan for the college clinics and the matter of faculty pension and retirement plans.

The Council went into executive session to receive the report from the Accrediting Committee.

Dr. Wolf, the chairman, reported as follows:

1. Lincoln, Los Angeles, National and the Texas College retain their present status as provisionally accredited.
2. The Logan College retains its provisional accreditation subject to the second inspection.
3. The New York Institute and Columbia Institute retain their provisional accredited status subject to certain conditions made known to said colleges.
4. Northwestern College retains its conditional approval status subject to certain conditions made known to said college.
5. The Western States College lost is conditional approval.

Dr. Wolf also announced that the schools will be inspected during the coming year. The inspection team will include two outside educators, experts in the Basic Sciences, two members of the profession, and the ACA Director of Education. The Chiropractic doctors will not be assigned to inspect their alma mater.

The rating procedure will follow the point system as adopted at the last meeting including the 20 points on student body.

Each school is to file a progress report before the winter meeting. It should follow the criteria outline.

Dr. Wolf also asked that each school supply the committee the available statistics of their students, regarding the National Board Examinations.

The Council took the following actions:

1. A vote of thanks was extended Dr. Saunders and the National Board for their excellent work.
2. Dr. Holman and the Council of State Boards were commended for their work and particularly for the excellent directory that they published.
3. Adopted policy, motion by Dr. Bittner, seconded by Dr. Rich and passed unanimously.

The clinic Directors Seminar shall be conducted under the Council on Education through a chairman appointed by the Council and assisted by the host Clinic Director. The chairman shall be directly responsible to the Council.

The next seminar will be held at the Logan College probably on October 30 and 31, 1965.

4. All chairmen and members of the following committees were re-appointed and commended for their work.
   a. Legislative Direction Committee
   b. Professional Awareness Committee
   c. Student Counseling and Admission Committee
5. The Professional Awareness Committee was instructed to implement recommendation #3 of their report. Recommendations #1 and #2 were accepted. (unanimous vote)
6. The Legislative Direction Committee was instructed to implement recommendation #1 of their report. (unanimous vote)
7. Roentgenology, motion by Dr. Fay, seconded by Dr. Russell and passed unanimously.

"The Council on Education approves, in principle, the X-Ray post graduate course outline presented by the Council on Roentgenology."

Moved by Dr. Russell, seconded by Dr. Peterson and passed unanimously.

"The Council on Education approves the educational provision of the constitution and by-laws of the American Council of Chiropractic Roentgenologist regarding the preparation of X-Ray papers by senior students in our colleges."

Moved by Dr. Peterson, seconded by Dr. Janse and passed unanimously.

The Council on Education approves the appointment to the American Board of Chiropractic Roentgenologists of the following: President - Leo E. Wunch, D.C., Vice-President - Duane M. Smith, D.C., Secretary-Treasurer - Michail A. Giammarino, D.C.

The Council on Education feels that Donald Hariman, D.C., and James J. McCarthy, D.C. are no doubt qualified to serve on this Board but must withhold approval until receipt of documentary evidence of their educational qualifications similar to those now on file for the approved members."

8. England Case

Moved by Dr. W. Wolf, seconded by Dr. Peterson and unanimously approved.

"The Council on Education requests the Board of Governors of the ACA to extend all possible support to Dr. Adams and Mr. Simone in the conduct of the England Case. The council petitions the Board of Governors to obtain a copy of the transcript of the court proceedings of the England Case that includes Drs. Janse's and Harper's testimony and make a copy available to each member of the Council on Education."

9. "Chiropractic of Today" presented by Dr. Janse. Motion by Dr. Rich, seconded by Dr. Harper and passed unanimously.

The Council on Education expresses its full confidence and support of the work done by the Committee on Standardization of Chiropractic Principles. The Council endorses in principle the paper prepared by Dr. Joseph Janse, as Chairman, Dr. Helmut Bittner, Dr. William Harper, Dr. Earl Homewood and Dr. Clarence Weiant as members of this committee.

A careful analysis and bibliography must be prepared to see that no part of this paper can be misinterpreted or be claimed to be without adequate written authoritative background.

The Council recommends that each of its members carefully review the material presented and supply to Dr. Janse by October 15, 1965, a written report and bibliography references for the Committee's consideration.

The Council also recommends that after receipt and collation of the material from the Council members, the Committee meet prior to the mid-year Council meeting to prepare and assemble work for final discussion.

10. Oklahoma School

Motion by Dr. Wolf, seconded by Dr. Janse and passed unanimously.

"The Council on Education expresses a desire to cooperate in any way necessary in the matter of the establishment of a Chiropractic College at the Bethel Baptist University of Oklahoma."

11. Faculty and pension and retirement plan.

The Council appointed Dr. Fay and Dr. Bittner to investigate, consult and prepare a report relative to faculty pensions and retirement plans for possible use by the ACA colleges.

12. Accrediting Committee's Report - National Board.

It was generally agreed that the colleges did not have adequate records of the results of the National Board of Examiners to supply the statistics requested. It was agreed that the Committee could request this information directly from the National Board as it would relate to the ACA colleges.

13. NCIC Clinic Coverage

It was generally agreed that the proposed NCIC clinic malpractice insurance places a very heavy load on the schools, particularly when a number of faculty members do assist the regular clinicians.

14. School Classification

Moved by Dr. Wolf, seconded by Dr. Hinton and passed unanimously.

"The Council creates a chiropractic college classification of 'Affiliate of the Council on Education of the ACA' This classification is hereby defined as follows: A school that subscribes to the policies and regulations of the Council on Education of the ACA but does not yet meet the accreditation standards."

15. Western States College of Chiropractic and Canadian Memorial College of Chiropractic.

Motion by Dr. Wolf, seconded by Dr. Poulsen and passed unanimously.

The Western States Chiropractic College and the Canadian Memorial Chiropractic College are granted the classification of "affiliate of the Council on Education of the ACA."

16. Blind Students

The Council on Education adopted the following statement as part of its policy:

The general consensus of the Council is that a person visually handicapped should be treated no different than any other student. He should not be denied admittance, nor should higher scholastic requirements be demanded of him nor should he be granted special scholastic or other types of privileges because of his visual handicap.

They, like all other students, must carry out laboratory assignments, including microscopic work and X-Ray Interpretation. If they can do this work, pass oral, written and practical examinations and meet all the requirements of the college, they can graduate.

Meeting adjourned June 25, 1965.

Respectfully submitted, John Wolfe, D.C., Secretary

The following reports are on file with the Secretary. These reports were placed in the hands of members of the Council as presented.

1. Report on Analysis of National Board of Chiropractic Examination, 1965. Prepared by Dr. Harrison C. Godfrey, presented by Dr. Edward M. Saunders.
2. Report of Council of State Chiropractic Examining Board. Presented by Dr. Gordon L. Holman.
3. Report of Clinic Directors Seminar. Presented by Dr. Leonard Fay.
4. Report of Committee on Standardization of Clinic Forms. Prepared by Dr. Glenn C. Olson, presented by Dr. Leonard E. Fay.
5. Outline of report of Department of Research and Statistics. Presented by Dr. Henry G. Higley.
6. Report of Committee on Legislative Direction. Presented by Dr. Edward C. Poulsen.
7. Report of Professional Awareness Committee. Presented by Dr. Orval L. Hidde.
8. Report of Committee on Student Admissions and Counseling. Presented by Dr. William N. Coggins.
9. Report of ACA Scholarship Committee. Presented by Dr. Herman O. Ulrich.
10. Report on Visiting Lectureship Program. Presented by Dr. George H. Haynes.
11. Report on Speakers Bureau. Presented by Dr. George H. Haynes.
12. Report on ACA Council on Chiropractic Roentgenology. Presented by Dr. Herman O. Ulrich.

Minutes of the Meeting of the COUNCIL ON EDUCATION of the ACA
Des Moines, Iowa, January 18 through January 22, 1966

The mid-year meeting of the Council on Education of the ACA was called to order by the President, Dr. George H. Haynes, at 9:10 A.M., Tuesday, January 18, 1966, at Johnny and Kay's Motel, Des Moines, Iowa.

Roll call:

Council President, Dr. George H. Haynes, Los Angeles College of Chiropractic, Present
Council Secretary, Dr. John Wolfe, Northwestern College of Chiropractic, Present
Director of Education, ACA, Dr. John A. Fisher, Present
Accrediting Committee Chairman, Dr. Walter Wolf, Present
Accrediting Committee, Dr. Orval Hidde, Present
Accrediting Committee, Dr. Herbert Hinton, Present
Accrediting Committee, Dr. Edward Poulsen, Absent
Accrediting Committee, Dr. J.R. Quigley, Present
Columbia Institute of Chiropractic, Dr. Ernest Napolitano, Present
Chiropractic Institute of New York, Dr. Thure Peterson, Present
Lincoln Chiropractic College, Dr. Earl Rich, Present
Logan College of Chiropractic, Dr. William Coggins, Present
National College of Chiropractic, Dr. Joseph Janse, Present
Council of State Chiropractic Examining Boards, Dr. Robert Runnells, Present from January 21 on.
Council of State Chiropractic Examining Boards, Dr. Gordon Holman, Present
Council of State Chiropractic Examining Boards, Dr. Howard Fenton, Absent

Also present:

Canadian Memorial College of Chiropractic, Dr. Herbert Himes, (Dean)
Western States College of Chiropractic, Dr. Robert Elliot, (President)
Chiropractic Institute of New York, Dr. Helmut Bittner (Dean)
Los Angeles College of Chiropractic, Dr. Henry G. Higley
National college of Chiropractic, Dr. Leonard Fay, (Vice-President)
National Board of Chiropractic Examiners, Dr. E.M. Saunders, (President)

The minutes of the June Meeting of the Council on Education held in Hollywood, Florida were read and approved.

The letter of invitation to Drs. Palmer, Cleveland, Jr. and Cleveland, Sr. were read. No reply from either of the Doctors Cleveland was received. The tardy reply from Doctor Palmer was read.

It was decided to allow Dr. McAndrews, Assistant Dean at Palmer College of Chiropractic, to sit in at the meetings of the Council on Wednesday, January 19, 1966.

The request from the Japanese organization asking for support for their proposed school was considered. It was agreed that the colleges may extend aid but not sponsorship to their program.

The request to invite Dr. Roney of the Stanford Research Institute was approved. An invitation to the Board of Governors of the ACA to attend the meeting with Dr. Roney was approved.

COUNCIL MEETINGS AT THE CONVENTION:

It was agreed that the Council's meeting at the convention would begin on the evening of June 23. The convention dates are June 19 to 25, 1966 at the Biltmore Hotel, Los Angeles, California.

The Chairman was instructed to request the ACA and FACE to consider the dates of their mid-year meetings with a view to avoid conflicts with the beginning of semester dates of our member schools.

THE FLORIDA STATE CHIROPRACTIC ASSOCIATION'S REQUEST REGARDING PRE-CHIROPRACTIC STUDY PROGRAM was discussed. Dr. Fisher's letter to them for use by the Florida Department of Education and Public Instruction was approved. This may allow the inclusion of our colleges in the list of college recommendations published by the Department.

The qualitative and quantitative pre-professional requirements were discussed.

DRS. SCHIERHOLZ AND GEARHART APPEARED BEFORE THE COUNCIL.

Dr. Schierholz extended an invitation to meet with the Board of Governors to hear Mr. Simone and other attorneys on the England case. The meeting to be held Thursday morning.

He also requested that the colleges consider the offering of post-graduate seminars to replace the itinerant type of lectures. Further, he requested the information regarding college seminars be supplied to the ACA for publication, without charge, in the association's journal.

Dr. Gearhart urged the colleges to assist in the growth of the Junior ACA chapters and to assist the journal in its quest for new articles.

ON WEDNESDAY MORNING, DR. MCANDREWS OF THE PALMER COLLEGE was welcomed to attend the council meeting as an observer.

The matter of a uniform Hood color for all the colleges was discussed. The council had adopted the Hunter's Green as the official color.

COLLEGE YEAR, UNIT SYSTEM AND GRADE POINTS:

The following survey was completed.

CLINIC SEMINAR

Dr. Fay presented his written report and recommendations.

THE CHIROPRACTIC OATH

The desirability for a uniform Chiropractic Oath was discussed.

LECTURING PROGRAMS

The matter of minimum honorarium for faculty while lecturing at conventions and seminars was discussed.

CHIROPRACTIC FRATERNITIES

The advisability of administration control of the fraternities and their campus activities was discussed. It was determined that all colleges do exercise proper control.

INSTRUMENTATION

Dr. Himes supplemented his written report by an extensive oral presentation of the aims and problems faced by the Canadian Memorial College of Chiropractic in the development and use of their instrument, Synchrotherme. He indicated the value of this instrument to the profession and the need for support. CMCC is willing to weigh any recommendation the Council will make. Dr. Himes did indicate the probable conflict with the F.D.A. Considerable discussion was had as to the promotional program in operation, the validity of the interpretation of the temperature findings and of the lease program offered.

CHIROPRACTIC QUARTERLY

Dr. Bittner requested the cooperation of the Council in starting the publication of the Quarterly.

FACULTY PENSIONS

Dr. Fay and Dr. Bittner presented a written report together with copies of insurance plans.

CURRICULUM

It was decided that this matter should be discussed at a future meeting.

NATIONAL BOARD

Dr. Saunders presented his report and stated that out of 433 non-candidate applicants to the first Board examinations, 400 had converted and obtained their grades.

It was the unanimous opinion of the colleges present that the National Board should not send copies of past examinations to any one other than to official governmental Boards or departments.

COUNCIL OF STATE BOARDS.

Dr. Holman reported the activities of his council. Copies of the questionnaire sent to all State Boards were distributed.

Dr. Holman indicated that the next meeting of the General Committee for the Profession on Education would probably be held in August of this year in Davenport.

CHIROPRACTIC OF TODAY

The prepared manuscript, "Chiropractic of Today" was carefully considered. The discussion brought out an appreciation for the value of the work done by Doctors Bittner, Weiant, Homewood and Harper under the able chairmanship of Dr. Janse.

UNIFICATION COMMITTEE

The report of the unification committee appointed by the ACA was read and discussed.

RESEARCH

Dr. Higley presented his written report on the progress of the Low Back Syndrome research.

Dr. Higley also elaborated on the need for the faculties of the colleges to participate in educational and scientific societies.

The Stanford Research Institute's proposed study of Chiropractic Education and related facts was discussed.

REPORT OF THE ACCREDITING COMMITTEE

The Lincoln College, National College and Los Angeles College have applied for full accreditation and have been supplied with self-evaluation forms.

The Lincoln College has completed its self-evaluation and this report will be studied by the accrediting committee and the college will probably be inspected in March of this year.

Action on the Columbia Institute of Chiropractic and the Chiropractic Institute of New York has been deferred awaiting developments. The two schools will be visited by the committee.

The Texas and Logan Colleges will be asked to file a new self-evaluation report.

The Northwestern College was complimented for the progress that the school has accomplished in the past few months. It will retain its present classification.

The Committee suggested changes in the "Foreword" of the criteria. The matter was discussed.

MOTIONS AND RESOLUTIONS ADOPTED.

1. Moved by Dr. Fay, seconded by Dr. Quigley and passed: "That the special meeting with Drs. Palmer and Cleveland Jr. and Sr. be canceled because of lack of cooperation."
2. It is the Council's recommendation that the ACA assist in the development of new speakers by using younger members of the faculty of the ACA colleges as speakers at the convention and assist them financially to make possible their participation in the convention program.
3. Moved by Dr. Rich, seconded by Dr. Coggins and passed: "The Council feels that specific credit requirements in the sciences and humanities are not to be included in pre-professional enactments, but rather be provided for on a broad flexible basis by the colleges. College catalogues should suggest from 12 to 30 semester hours in the sciences with the emphasis in biology and chemistry. From 30 to 48 semester hours should be divided somewhat evenly between the humanities and the social studies including communications and history."
4. Moved by Dr. Quigley, seconded by Dr. Harper and passed;
    a) Credits to meet the pre-professional requirements will be accepted from institutions listed in "Educational Director, Part 3, Higher Education", United States Office of Education under "Classifications" I and II, and all under "Type of Program" excepting "a" group.
    b) Applicants must have been graduates from, or be eligible to return to the last institution attended from which credits are acceptable or transferable to meet the pre-professional requirement.
5. Moved by Dr. Coggins, seconded by Dr. Peterson and passed:
    The council recommends support of the England case but suggests that the ACA does not enter the case as a friend of the court.
7. Moved by Dr. Harper, seconded by Dr. Napolitano and passed;
    The following unit system is hereby adopted by the Council on Education for use by its member colleges:
    Semester unit equals 16 to 18 hours of didactic work or 32 to 36 hours of laboratory or related work.
    Quarter unit represents 12 hours of didactic work or 24 hours of laboratory or related work and is equal to two-thirds of a semester unit.
8. Moved by Dr. Quigley, seconded by Dr. Rich and passed;
    The Council adopts the alphabetical grading system and following unit grade point system for the use of its member colleges:
    One unit of A grade equals 4 grade points
    One unit of B grade equals 3 grade points
    One unit of C grade equals 2 grade points
    One unit of D grade equals 1 grade points
    One unit of F grade equals 0 grade points

College	System	Unit	No. of Weeks per Term
Chiropractic Institute of New York	Trimester	S.U.=16 hrs.	16
Logan College of Chiropractic	Trimester	S.U.=16 hrs.	16
Columbia Institute of Chiropractic	Trimester	S.U.=16 hrs.	16
Canadian Memorial College of Chiropractic	Semester	S.U.=16 hrs.	18
National College of Chiropractic	Trimester	S.U.=16 hrs.	16
Lincoln College of Chiropractic	Trimester	S.U.=16 hrs.	16
Los Angeles College of Chiropractic	Semester	S.U.=16 hrs.	18
Northwestern College of Chiropractic	Quarter	Q.U.=12 hrs.	12
Texas College of Chiropractic	Semester	S.U.=16 hrs.	18
Western States College of Chiropractic	Semester	S.U.=16 hrs.	18
Palmer College of Chiropractic	Quarter		12

9.   On motion made by Dr. W. Wolf and seconded by Dr. Napolitano, the following action was adopted by the Council:

Approved the continuation of the Clinic Directors' Seminar. Suggested the consideration of palpation methods and regulations for patient handling. Approved the Los Angeles College of Chiropractic as the next site for the meeting. Dr. Fay asked to continue as the Council's representative.

10. The President appointed a committee to prepare a short chiropractic oath for use by all the member colleges. The committee consists of Drs. Fisher, Janse, and Napolitano.

11. The Council once more approved the following as the minimum fee schedule for faculty members lecturing at conventions and other professional gatherings: $100 per day of lecture and full coverage of travel, food, and lodging expenses.

12. The President appointed Dr. Hinton to survey the existing Honorary Fraternities of the Chiropractic Colleges with the view of the formation of a national honorary fraternity.

13. Moved by Dr. Fay, seconded by Dr. Hinton and passed:

Hypnotherapy has been and should be taught as part of the course in psychology. The principles of hypnosis, preparation of the patient, limitations inherent in hypnosis as a therapeutic tool, its analgesic implications, and its use as a supplemental device in psychotherapy should be presented.

14. Moved by Dr. Bittner, amended by Dr. Rich, seconded by Dr. Holman and passed;

The Council on Education views with great concern the promotion of the vasomotor monitoring instrumentation program by the Canadian Memorial College of Chiropractic. It recommends its discontinuance until sufficient evidence justifying the suggested clinical interpretation of the Synchrotherme readings has been obtained. This evidence should be obtained through recognized formal research procedures. The Council does not endorse nor support the above instrumentation program.

15. Moved by Dr. W. Wolf, seconded by Dr. Holman and passed;

The Council on Education of the ACA formally notify the Canadian Memorial Chiropractic College of their violation of the rules of the Council by conducting extension seminars outside their area of residence without prior approval from the council.

16. The following recommendations from Dr. Fay and Dr. Bittner were adopted:

That the Faculty Pension Plans presented by the Committee be refereed to the ACA with a request for their professional study, evaluation and advice.
The CMCC is to be notified that it must adhere to all the rules of this council and must immediately cease to violate them.

17. The Council on Education took the following action regarding the prepared manuscript, "Chiropractic of Today":

a)   It is a valuable paper representing the combined work of fine men of great ability and high reputation.

b)   It should not be published as the work of an official committee of the ACA nor a part of the policy of the association, but as the work of fine outstanding individuals.

c)   The Council and each individual member offers all support and assistance that the fine authors may desire.

d)   The Council congratulates them for their outstanding efforts and dedication to the profession.

18. Moved by Dr. Janse, seconded by Dr. Wolf and passed;

That the Council on Education cannot accept the proposed definition or scope of practice proposed by the Unification Committee of the ACA.
Moved by Dr. Napolitano, seconded by Dr. Quigley and passed;
That Dr. Haynes' letter of December 7, 1965 be considered as also representing the feeling of the Council is strongly opposed to any attempt to define chiropractic.

19. Motion by Dr. Fay, seconded by Dr. Runnells and passed;
The Council on Education and its member schools will cooperate with the Stanford Research Institute in their survey on Chiropractic education.
The following recommendations were adopted:

1)   That copies of all reports of research dealing with the healing arts and conducted by the Stanford Research Institute be made available to all members of the Council.

2)   That there be an extensive interchange of ideas, contacts and information regarding this survey.

3)   That there be only one official channel of communication with the Stanford Research Institute.

4)   That these recommendations be implemented through Dr. Fisher, the Director of Education of the ACA.

20. The following extension courses were approved:
Western States College - Seminar in Washington
National College - Seminars in Kansas and Florida
Lincoln College - Seminar in Alabama

21. Moved by Dr. Wolf, seconded by Dr. Bittner and passed;
That the "Foreword" in the booklet, "Educational Standards for Chiropractic Colleges" be amended to read:
"A Doctor of Chiropractic is a physician concerned with the health needs of the public. He gives particular attention to the relationships of the structural and neurological aspects of the body in health and disease. He is educated in anatomy, biochemistry, microbiology, pathology, physiology, public health, clinical disciplines and related health sciences.

The purpose of his professional education is to prepare the doctor of chiropractic to diagnose, treat or refer to other physicians. The colleges approved by the American Chiropractic Association are dedicated to the purpose of producing a competent practitioner.

The Council on Education and the Committee on Accreditation of the American Chiropractic Association have validated the Educational Standards for Chiropractic Colleges operating on approval of the association. In doing so they are aware of the importance of these professional colleges to the profession and to the public which it serves. These standards indicate the training received in the approved colleges by Doctors of Chiropractic.

The qualities of a college are vested in the character of its students, the ability of its teachers, the soundness of its instruction and the adequacy of its equipment. This booklet sets forth the educational standards of the profession."

Motion by Dr. Bittner, seconded by Dr. Quigley and passed;
That Dr. Fisher be authorized to reward the section headed "Principles and Criteria".

ELECTION OF OFFICERS
Dr. Janse moved, seconded by Dr. Bittner, that Dr. Haynes be re-elected President and that Dr. John Wolfe be re-elected Secretary. Moved by Dr. Holman, seconded by Dr. Rich that the nominations be closed. Dr. George Haynes and Dr. John Wolfe were elected as President and Secretary for the forthcoming year.
The president was authorized to appoint new committees on Legislative Direction, Professional Awareness and Student Admission and Counseling.
Meeting adjourned, January 22, 1966
Respectfully submitted, John Wolfe, D.C., Secretary

Minutes of the Meeting of the COUNCIL ON EDUCATION of the ACA
Los Angeles, California, June 22 through June 25, 1966

The meeting of the Council on Education of the ACA was called to order by the President, Dr. George H. Haynes at 1:00 P.M., Wednesday, June 22, 1966 at the Biltmore Hotel, Los Angeles, California
ROLL CALL
Council President - Dr. George H. Haynes, Los Angeles College of Chiropractic, Present
Council Secretary - Dr. John Wolfe, Northwestern College of Chiropractic, absent on Wednesday, June 22, but present the rest of the meeting.
Director of Education - Dr. John A. Fisher, Present
Accrediting Committee Chairman - Dr. Walter Wolfe, Present
Accrediting Committee - Dr. Orval Hidde, Present
Accrediting Committee - Dr. Herbert Hinton, Present
Accrediting Committee - Dr. J.R. Quigley, Present
Accrediting Committee - one vacancy
Columbia Institute of Chiropractic - Dr. Ernest Napolitano, absent Wednesday, June 22, present the rest of the meetings.
Chiropractic Institute of New York - Dr. Helmut Bittner, Present
Lincoln Chiropractic College - Dr. Earl Rich, Present
Logan College of Chiropractic - Dr. William Coggins, Present
National College of Chiropractic - Dr. Joseph Janse, Present
Texas College of Chiropractic - Dr. William Harper, Present
Council of State Chiropractic Examining Boards - Dr. Howard Fenton, Present
Council of State Chiropractic Examining Boards - Dr. Gordon Holman, Present
ALSO PRESENT:
Canadian Memorial College of Chiropractic - Dr. Ronald J. Watkins
Western States College of Chiropractic - Dr. Mel Higgins, present on Wednesday, June 22, absent rest of the meetings.
National Board of Chiropractic Examiners - Dr. E.M. Saunders
Chiropractic Institute of New York - Dr. Thure Peterson
Lincoln College of Chiropractic - Dr. Chester Stowell

Los Angeles College of Chiropractic - Dr. Henry Higley and Dr. Earl Homewood
National College of Chiropractic - Dr. Leonard Fay

The minutes of the Council meeting of January 22, 1966 were corrected to show the Texas College of Chiropractic, represented by Dr. William Harper, on the roll call as present. The minutes were then approved.

Discussion was held on the date for the mid-year meeting of the Council. The reports from the schools indicated that the beginning of the Spring school term would rule out the month of January as a mid-year meeting time.

The Director of Education gave a brief summary of his activities during the past year.

The matter of the Stanford Research Institute proposed survey was discussed.

COMMITTEE ON ACCREDITATION

The matter of the progress made by the Committee on Accreditation, which is the accrediting agency for the ACA, in meeting the H.E.W. criteria was opened by Dr. Haynes by reviewing its back history as follows:

"In order for any school of Chiropractic to be listed by H.E.W. as an institution of higher learning, it is necessary that an agency in the field of chiropractic be recognized by the Federal Department of Education.

Our ACA agency formally applied to H.E.W. in January, 1961, and the application was denied on May 22, 1961, with words of commendation and a suggestion to re-apply at a later date.

In July of 1961, I made certain suggestions for the continuation of our program with a view to meet the objections raised by the H.E.W. No action followed and the NCA suggested a wait-and-see policy program. Soon after the Council on Education was replaced by the Accrediting Committee as the accrediting agency.

Dr. D. Anderson, the Director of Education, received an informal, unofficial letter from Dr. Coronet of the Department of Education, dated June 26, 1964, pointing out some of the sections of the H.E.W. criteria that needed to be met by our agency.

Since then, we have not had any report of activity in relation to work done to qualify the agency under H.E.W. except in the area of up-grading the schools.

The up-grading of our schools will be the basis for the agency to qualify under sections 1, 2, 3, 4, 5-b, c, d and 7, 8 and 9 on the basis of their activity and progress in areas external to the schools.

Acceptance of the agency depends upon the presentation of documentary evidence to satisfactorily prove to H.E.W. the agency's compliance with all of the nine sections of the federal criteria.

This evidence must be documented and must be, in many instances, initiated by the agency and must cover an adequate expanse of time.

The colleges have been working diligently to merit the status of institutions of higher learning and have gone to the field to raise funds by dangling the silver lining of the accreditation goal. We are now heavily questioned as to the time table to reach our goal, and we must have an answer to give.

Based on my study of the criteria, H.E.W. letters and conversations, I present the following questions with regards to the agency's preparation to qualify under the federal criteria.

Federal Register - Criteria

The agency or association:
1. Is regional or national in the scope of its operations. (Regional as here used means several states):
    A.   What evidence has been developed and gathered to prove it is a national agency? From:
        a) Schools of chiropractic?
        b) Practicing profession?
        c) Accrediting bodies of other health professions?
        d) Other accrediting agencies - national and regional?
        e) Non-chiropractic schools?
        f) State Department of Education?
        g) Federal agencies?
    B.   What period of time is covered by this evidence?
2. Serves a definite need for accreditation in the field in which it operates:
    What evidence has been developed and gathered to prove the need for this agency?
    A.   Chiropractic profession
        a) What is the evidence that it is a science and not a cult?
        b) What evidence has been developed and gathered that the public employs the profession?
            1) Areas where it functions?
            2) Numbers that use it?
            3) Insurance companies recognizing it?
            4) States licensing it?

       c)   What evidence has been developed and gathered to prove the size of this profession?
            1)   From licensing bodies?
            2)   State government publications?
            3)   Federal publications?
            4)   Private publications?

B.   Public Welfare
    a)   What evidence has been developed and gathered to show that public welfare demands a classification of chiropractic schools?
         1)   Are there chiropractic colleges of varying quality of educational programs?
              a)   Schools curriculum?
              b)   Inspection reports?
              c)   Licensing Boards?
              d)   State publications?
              e)   Private publications?
         2)   Is there a difference in the services rendered by the graduates of the different schools?
              a)   In examination procedures, diagnosis and prognosis?
              b)   In quality of treatment?
              c)   In scope of referral and consultation?
              d)   And thus in the protection of the patient treated?
    b)   What evidence has been developed and gathered to show that this agency has helped to improve the quality of at least some of the graduates of our profession?

C.   Need for a new agency
    a)   What evidence has been developed and gathered to show there is no other agency able to do this?
         1)   Have other established national or regional agencies been contacted? Could any of them pass upon the chiropractic schools?
    b)   What evidence has been developed and gathered as to the ACA and non-ACA schools?
    c)   What evidence has been developed and gathered to show the educational services rendered by this agency? to:
         1)   Chiropractic colleges?
         2)   Profession?
         3)   General public?

3. Performs no functions that might prejudice its independent judgment of the quality of an educational program:
What evidence has been developed and gathered to show that the agency
    a)   Allows academic freedom?
    b)   Sees that the college administration accords academic freedom?
    c)   Is not subject to political considerations in its operations?

4. Makes available to the public current information covering: (a) criteria or standards for accreditation, (b) reports of its operations, (c) a list of accredited institutions, courses or educational programs:
    a)   What evidence has been developed and gathered to prove the agency has distributed it? And where?
        Library of Congress? Educational bodies? State Departments of Education? Educational institutions?
    b)   Is it workable?
    c)   Is it stable and endowed with permanency?

5. Has an adequate organization and effective procedures to maintain its operations on a professional basis. Among the factors to be considered in this connection are that the agency or association:
    a)   Secures sufficient and pertinent data concerning the qualitative and quantitative aspects of the work of an institution, including data on such items as the educational objectives, educational programs, admission practices, training and experience of teachers, financial stability, laboratory and library resources.
         1.   Where is this information found?
         2.   Are adequate records kept?
         3.   Uses justifiable procedures?
         4.   Reflects a pattern of relationship to colleges?
         5.   Reflects a pattern of relationship to public welfare?
    b)   Uses qualified examiners to visit institutions and inspect courses, programs and facilities and who prepare written reports and recommendations for the use of the reviewing body — and causes such examination to be conducted under conditions that assure an impartial and objective judgment.
         1)   Are the reports and recommendations on record?
         2)   Are they of a professional type and form?
    c)   Re-evaluates at reasonable intervals the accredited institutions, programs and courses of study.

        1)   Are there adequate records to prove it?

        2)   Are the publications dated?

   d)   Has financial resources as shown by its current financial statements, necessary to maintain accrediting operations in accordance with published policies and procedures.

        1)   Thus the agency uses a budget of record?

        2)   Is there recorded evidence of ACA financial status and support of the agency for the past and future?

6.   Accredits only institutions which are found upon such examination to meet specific standards for accreditation, established in advance in terms that include the factors above described:

(Must distinguish between schools)

   1.   Are the "specific standards" established in advance?

   2.   Is there permanency to these standards?

   3.   Do they cover the necessary points?

7.   Has had not less than two years' experience as an accrediting agency, or in the alternative demonstrates to the satisfaction of the Commissioner that it has been organized under conditions that reasonably assure stability and permanence and that it has gained the acceptance required under 8 below during such shorter period:

   a)   ACA new or a continuation of NCA?

   b)   What evidence has been gathered to prove this point?

8.   Has gained acceptance of its criteria, methods of evaluation, and decisions, by educational institutions, practitioners, licensing bodies and employers throughout the United States:

Who has accepted this agency?

   a)   The chiropractic colleges? How many? To what extent? What is the evidence?

   b)   The profession? ACA? ICA? State organization? What evidence has been gathered?

   c)   Licensing Bodies? Chiropractic Boards? Mixed Boards? Council of State Boards? National Board? Basic Science Boards? What evidence has been gathered?

   d)   Department of Education? Federal? State? Which States? Veterans' Administration? Immigration Department? What evidence has been gathered?

   e)   Accrediting Agencies? National in the field of healing? Other national agencies? Regional? Which? What has been done in this direction? What is the evidence?

   f)   Other Educational Institutions? Which? What has been done in this direction? What evidence has been gathered?

9.   Assurance is given that accreditation for the purpose of the act will not be conditioned on the payment of any sums of money: Provided, however, that a reasonable charge may be made by the agency or association for its services hereunder not exceeding the actual cost of the accreditation."

Discussion was had upon the above material. Documentation for many of the above points were found wanting and it was generally agreed that all members of the Council will assist the Committee and Director of Education in developing and completing this documentation.

COUNCIL ON ROENTGENOLOGY

    Dr. Ulrich, accompanied by Drs. Howard, Duane Smith and others from the Council on Roentgenology, appeared to present a resolution on ACCR education requirements for our Council's consideration.

CLINIC DIRECTORS SEMINAR

    Dr. Leonard Fay presented a written report on the Clinic Directors' Seminar.

CANADIAN MEMORIAL CHIROPRACTIC COLLEGE

    Dr. Watkins made a presentation regarding the CMCC's instrumentation program. The full implication of the resolutions passed by the Council on Education at the January 1966 meeting was made clear to him. Dr. Watkins was requested to contact his college Board with a view of obtaining an official answer to the Council's resolutions regarding CMCC's instrumentation program. Dr. Watkins announced the cancellation of their Los Angeles seminar and of a forthcoming official answer to the Council's letter.

RESEARCH DEPARTMENT

    Dr. Henry Higley, ACA Director of Research, filed a written report and spoke on the procedures to be followed in filing and reporting on all research projects. All research request reports are to be directed to his office as per recommendation from FACE on a quarterly basis.

COUNCIL OF CHIROPRACTIC EXAMINING BOARD

    Dr. Saunders presented a written report on the activities of the National Chiropractic Examining Board. Extensive discussion was had on the results of the last two national examinations.

INTER-RELATIONSHIP BETWEEN ACA APPROVED COLLEGES

    General agreement was reached on the following points:

1. Transfer of students among the member schools of the Council are not to be sought. Transfer students will not be accepted without a letter of recommendation from the Dean of the school from which they are transferring. This does not apply to drop-outs.
2. Dismissed or suspended students from any of our schools will not be accepted for enrollment without consultation with the school prescribing the penalty.
3. None of our schools will grant a Doctor of Chiropractic degree to anyone already having such a degree from another school unless the person retakes the full prescribed course without the grant of advanced standing.
4. The school members of the Council will refrain, with full allowance for the special geographical conditions pertaining to the four Midwestern schools, from mass solicitation for funds and students in each other's state of residence. This agreement shall in no way interfere with the normal rights of the college in soliciting from their respective alumni.

SCHOLARSHIPS

Scholarship offerings were discussed and some pointed out the advisability of refraining from offering large numbers of scholarships that are not backed by hard money less they be considered as discounts of tuition.

LINCOLN BULLETIN MAILING

Dr. Rich explained the reasons and the program proposed in their mailings. General discussion followed.

ROENTGENOLOGY RESIDENT PROGRAM

Dr. Wolfe presented a proposed Roentgenology resident program to be conducted at the Northwestern College of Chiropractic. It was generally agreed that this was an internal program of the Northwestern College, not subject to nor requiring Council action.

REPORT OF ACCREDITING COMMITTEE

The Committee reported as follows:
1. The Lincoln and National Colleges, after inspection, have been granted an accredited status.
2. There is no change in the ratings of the other colleges.
3. The LACC and Logan Colleges have submitted their self-evaluation reports. The Logan College has been asked for certain additional information.
4. The two New York schools are still considering amalgamation. Each will submit their self-evaluation report.
5. The Texas and Northwestern Colleges are preparing their self-evaluation reports.
6. The affiliated schools remain in that status, but there is grave concern regarding the activities of the Canadian Memorial Chiropractic College.

MOTIONS AND RESOLUTIONS

1. Dr. W. Wolf made the motion, seconded by Dr. Fay, that the Accrediting Committee's report be accepted. Passed.
2. Motion by Dr. Bittner, seconded by Dr. Harper that all the colleges send a copy of the National Board grades to Dr. Fisher for the use of the Committee on Accreditation. Passed.
3. Motion was made and passed that the Council recommend a February date for the mid-year meeting.
4. Motion was made, seconded and passed that all members of the Council assist in the collection of the necessary documentation needed for our H.E.W. application and that all evidence or information should be mailed to Dr. Fisher.
5. Motion was made, seconded and passed approving the request from the Council of Roentgenology in the following manner: post graduate courses on Roentgenology presented by our schools after June 1967, shall cover 300 hours of study. The Council on Education of the ACA fully approves paragraphs #2 and 3 of the Council on Roentgenology, dealing with the hour requirement, but not for the reason as listed in paragraph #1 of the resolution.

The Council on Education feels that there should be a very low percentage of the applicants qualified to meet the high requirements to become a diplomate of the American Board of Chiropractic Roentgenologists.

6. Motion was made, seconded and passed that each school is to conduct a careful comparison between school grades and national scores, and so bring such comparisons to the mid-year meeting for discussion with the National Board and their grade analyst.
7. Motion was made, seconded and passed that the Council prepare a program for presentation at the mid-year meeting dealing with continuing education. The Council President was empowered, at his discretion, to appoint a committee to assist him in this program preparation.
8. Motion was made, seconded and passed to request from the ACA a $25/month support for the operation of the office of the President of the Council on Education.
9. Motion was made, seconded and passed that approval be given for the meeting of the Clinic Directors Seminar to be held at the Los Angeles College of Chiropractic on October 29 and 30, 1966 and thanks be extended to the International College of Chiropractic, to Dr. Ploudre and to the Foundation for Accredited Chiropractic Education for this support of the program.
10. Motion made by Dr. Janse, seconded by Dr. Harper and passed: This Council considers that the Committee on Accreditation of the NCA provided for the continuation of its program of accreditation regardless of any change of the parent organization.

FINAL MEETING

On Saturday, June 25, a meeting was held with the Board of Governors of the ACA and the California Board of Chiropractic Examiners.

Dr. Hastings, President of the Board of Examiners, presented a report of the findings of a survey conducted by the Board during the last two examinations. The survey dealt with the practical clinical experience of the applicants for licensure. General discussion followed.

Meeting of the Council adjourned June 25, 1966.
Respectfully submitted, John Wolfe, D.C., Secretary

Minutes of the Meeting of the COUNCIL ON EDUCATION of the ACA
Atlanta, Georgia, February 7 through February 10, 1967

The meeting of the Council on Education of the ACA was called to order by the President, Dr. George H. Haynes at 2:30 P.M., Tuesday, February 7, 1967 at the Biltmore Hotel, Atlanta, Georgia.

ROLL CALL

Council President - Dr. George H. Haynes, Los Angeles College of Chiropractic, (PA) Present
Council Secretary - Dr. John Wolfe, Northwestern College of Chiropractic, (AC) Present
Director of Education - Dr. John A. Fisher, Present
Accrediting Committee Chairman - Dr. Walter Wolf, Present
Accrediting Committee Secretary - Dr. Orval Hidde, Absent
Accrediting Committee - Dr. Herbert Hinton, Present
Accrediting Committee - Dr. J.R. Quigley, Present
Accrediting Committee - Dr. Anthony Bazzano, Present
Columbia Institute of Chiropractic - (PA) Dr. Ernest Napolitano, Present
Chiropractic Institute of New York - (PA) Dr. Helmut Bittner, Present
Lincoln Chiropractic College - (A) Dr. Chester Stowell, Present
Logan College of Chiropractic - (PA) Dr. William Coggins, Present
National College of Chiropractic - (A) Dr. Joseph Janse, Present February 7 & 8, absent the rest of the meeting
Texas College of Chiropractic - (PA) Dr. William Harper, Present
Council of State Chiropractic Examining Boards - Dr. Howard Fenton, Present on Feb. 7 & 8, absent rest of the time
Council of State Chiropractic Examining Boards - Dr. Rex Wright, Absent
Council of State Chiropractic Examining Boards - Dr. Gordon Holman, Present

ALSO PRESENT:

Canadian Memorial College of Chiropractic - (affiliate of the Council) Dr. Earl Homewood
National Board of Chiropractic Examiners - Dr. E.M. Saunders
National College of Chiropractic - Dr. Leonard Fay
Lincoln College of Chiropractic - Dr. Elmer A. Berner
Los Angeles College of Chiropractic - Dr. Henry Higley

On motion of Dr. Janse and seconded by Dr. W. Wolf the minutes of the Council meeting of June 22-25, 1966 were approved.
The following points were discussed:

1. CHIROPRACTIC EDUCATIONAL FOUNDATION

The background information was presented by Dr. Haynes and Dr. Fisher. The statement in the letter as to H.E.W. approval of the C.E.F. formation was discussed and dismissed as an erroneous interpretation of H.E.W. policy of hands-off on the nature of a criteria prepared by an proposed accrediting agency as proved by H.E.W. letters in the files of Dr. Haynes and Dr. Fisher.

Dr. Rutherford's apparent claim of H.E.W. approval of the C.E.F. agency were denied by H.E.W., Dr. Fisher reported.

The futility of the political approach to H.E.W. was brought out as well as the wasted effort and TIME in attempting to develop a new accrediting agency. The C.E.F. appears to present a criteria more suited to secondary schools than colleges of higher learning.

It was made clear that any participation in any other chiropractic accrediting agency by this council will wreck any chances of attaining H.E.W. recognition of our agency. It was also clarified that our agency cannot be subjected to political pressure or be involved in professional politics if it hoped to be accepted by H.E.W. as the accrediting agency for chiropractic colleges.

2. NATIONAL HONORARY SOCIETY

Following a brief discussion it was agreed that the formation of a National Honorary Society would be advantageous.

3. CONTINUING EDUCATION

Dr. Haynes presented the report on Continuing Education and his recommendations, considerable discussion followed.

The status designations used by the profession in relation to Orthopedics and Roentgenology were considered.

4.   RESEARCH

Dr. Higley presented his written report and elaborated on the progress of the Low-Back Research. He brought out that the National College has reported the largest number of rechecks and that the Chiropractic Institute of New York was second in the number of rechecks done. The Council extends their appreciation to Dr. Higley for his work.

5.   CLINIC DIRECTORS SEMINAR

Dr. Fay, Chairman of the Clinic Directors Seminar, presented his printed report which was then discussed. The Council extended their appreciation to Dr. Fay for his work. Clinic patient load and extern training was reviewed.

6.   GENERAL COMMITTEE OF THE PROFESSION ON EDUCATION

Dr. Haynes made an oral report on the Kansas City meeting of February 5, 1967 to supplement his written report on the August 1966 meeting of this committee.

7.   COUNCIL OF STATE CHIROPRACTIC EXAMINING BOARDS

Dr. Holman presented a written report supplemented by an oral elaboration. It was thought advisable to use the credit hour instead of the clock hour in evaluating chiropractic education.

8.   FOREIGN CHIROPRACTIC ASSOCIATIONS AND THEIR EDUCATIONAL REQUIREMENTS

Dr. Haynes presented a resume of the educational requirements of foreign associations. Extensive discussion followed dealing with our relationship with the various nations.

9.   WESTERN STATE COLLEGE (Affiliate of the Council)

Dr. Elliot's letter explaining the reasons for his absence from the meeting was read.

10.   CHIROPRACTIC OATH

Dr. Fisher requested that this matter be left for the June meeting.

11.   STUDENT COUNSELING

In the absence of Mr. Collins, Dr. Fisher reported. Mr. Collins has been visiting the different colleges and has spoken before several alumni groups. Dr. Haynes inquired if Mr. Collins had developed a set student counseling program. Drs. Wolfe, Stowell and Janse felt he had.

12.   NATIONAL BOARD OF EXAMINERS

Dr. Saunders presented a written report, which was then discussed. The Board will request from the schools additional set of questions for the area of diagnosis, chiropractic principles, jurisprudence, X-ray and physiotherapy.

Through the testing consultant of the Board, guides to the mechanics of the multiple choice question and accompanying bibliography will be made available to the colleges.

13.   REPORT BY DR. FISHER

A written report summarizing the H.E.W. Criteria was presented. Extensive discussion was had regarding our application to the H.E.W. It was the consensus of opinion that no further delay can be allowed and that the approval of the agency by H.E.W. shall be pursued with vigor and speed until accomplished.

14.   SCIENTIFIC QUARTERLY

Dr. Bittner once more made his plea for scientific articles from the colleges for the publication of the Scientific Quarterly. He reminded the colleges of the previous approval of the program by the Council and of the format for the articles which was distributed to all the colleges.

15.   REPORT OF THE ACCREDITING COMMITTEE

Dr. W. Wolf reported the completion of the inspection of Los Angeles College of Chiropractic, Chiropractic Institute of New York, and Columbia Institute of Chiropractic. He informed the Council of the receipt of the self-evaluation form from the Northwestern College of Chiropractic.

Dr. Wolf announced the change of status for Los Angeles College of Chiropractic from provisionally accredited to accredited. There is no change in the ratings of the other colleges.

The Easton College of Ohio has requested information and consideration from the Accrediting Committee of the ACA

MOTIONS AND RESOLUTIONS

National Honorary Society

moved by Dr. Fay, seconded by Dr. Napolitano and passed - that Dr. Hinton be instructed to present a plan for the formation of a National Honorary Society.

Continuing Education

moved by Dr. W. Wolf, seconded by Dr. Bittner and passed - that paragraphs #1, 2, 3, 5 of the recommendations presented by Dr. Haynes on 'continuing education' be adopted.

1.   The Council considers that the program of post-graduate study conducted by its member colleges in the field of specialties is adequate. It should be strongly promoted by the ACA
2.   The Council recommends that the Councils on Psychotherapy and Physiotherapy (and any new councils that may be formed) be encouraged to set yearly academic requirements for membership.
3.   The Council recommends to our colleges an increase in the presentation of short seminars for the average practitioner.

5. The Council recommends that each ACA delegate be requested to interest the ACA members of his area in continuing education and to have them petition the council for post-graduate classes.

moved by Dr. Fay, seconded by Dr. Quigley and passed - that paragraph #4 of the recommendations be changed to read:

The Council recommends that the program utilizing the ACA Bureau of Investigation in the presentation of communications media conferences in various cities be approved. If it is determined there is need, or it is advisable, that an educational session be presented concurrently with the Bureau's program, arrangements shall be made with the local sponsoring ACA college.

moved by Dr. Coggins, seconded by Dr. W. Wolf and passed - that the chairman be instructed to contact the Roentgenology and Orthopedic Councils with a request for a copy of their present constitution and rules and regulations, particularly those related to the standing or classification of their members in the specialty, terms used to designate and requirements to attain such standing.
Clinic Directors Seminar
moved by Dr. Stowell, seconded by Dr. Harper and passed - that the Council authorizes a meeting of the Clinic Directors for 1967 to be held at the Texas College and that future meetings be held at a different ACA school and that not until all the colleges have been so visited would a non-college site be considered.

moved by Dr. Fay, seconded by Dr. Coggins and passed - that the Council approves the request for the presence of Dr. Higley at future Clinic Directors Seminars.

moved by Dr. Napolitano, seconded by Dr. Stowell and passed - that the Council authorizes the use of a letter-head "ACA College Clinic Director" under the Council on Education and that its use be cleared through Dr. Fay and Dr. Fisher and that the last two named shall formulate the restrictions for the use of such letterhead.
General Committee of the Profession on Education
moved by Dr. J. Wolfe, seconded by Dr. Bittner and passed - that a letter of thanks be forwarded to Drs. Fenton, Wright and Holman.
Foreign Chiropractic Associations
moved by Dr. Stowell, seconded by Dr. Harper and passed - that 1) the chairman be instructed to compile an accurate list of the individual educational requirements of the foreign chiropractic associations, 2) request their compliance with our entrance requirements, 3) the Council colleges to have all foreign transcripts evaluated by a proper educational agency, 4) that the Council colleges may grant advance standing to foreign educated students only on a course by course consideration and based on the above mentioned proper educational agency evaluation.
Student Counseling
moved by Dr. Bittner, seconded by Dr. Harper and passed - that Mr. Collins admission counseling work as directed by a special committee of this council consisting of Dr. Haynes, Dr. Fisher and Dr. Fay.

moved by Dr. Napolitano, seconded by Dr. Quigley and passed - that the Council, with the assistance of the ACA mail a white paper to the profession at large stressing the need for more students and monetary contributions. This mailing to include a return post card for names of prospective students.

moved by Dr. Harper, seconded by Dr. Fay and passed - that the individual college follow the above mailing in three weeks with a similar mailing to its alumni and friends.

moved by Dr. Fay, seconded by Dr. Bittner and passed - that the counseling department prepare two brochures - one describing the one-year and the other the two-year pre-chiropractic requirements with due consideration to local New York and Texas conditions.

motion by Dr. Fay, seconded by Dr. Napolitano and passed - that the Council and ACA prepare and send to each member of the House of Delegates a white paper explaining the conditions facing the chiropractic educational institutions and the profession with the advent of the pre-professional requirements, request for H.E.W. approval, and economic changes to motivate them to work for membership, fund raising, student search and support, and existence of the profession through preservation of its birthplace - the schools.

The Council is to stress to the Board of Governors and House of Delegates the importance of the "status" of the profession the "economic remuneration" of the practitioner, and the "scope of privileges" of the practitioner in the demanding of longer and tougher education to be levied on the students of chiropractic.

moved by Dr. Napolitano, seconded by Dr. Bittner and passed - that a chiropractic college register be published, including information on scholarship offerings not specifically directed to a given college.

moved by Dr. Bittner, seconded by Dr. Napolitano and passed - that a set of color projection slides featuring all Council schools be prepared for use at state and national conventions and other meetings.

moved by Dr. Bittner and seconded by Dr. Fay and passed - that each school is to submit to Dr. Fisher by April 15, 1967 a list of speakers. The format for the speakers' qualifications and topics will be furnished by Dr. Fisher. From the information a roster of speakers will be compiled and made available to all Chiropractic groups.

moved by Dr. Napolitano, seconded by Dr. Bittner and passed - that Dr. Fisher prepare and send articles to all state publications relative to the Council on Education.

H.E.W. Application

moved by Dr. Coggins, seconded by Dr. W. Wolf and passed that the following time table be adopted:

1. The committees assigned to collect the evidence to prove compliance with H.E.W. criteria points 1, 2, 3, 4, 5, 6, 7, and 9 are to complete their work by May 1, 1967.
2. The committee assigned to cover criteria #8 is to complete the work by June 1, 1967.
3. Dr. Fisher and the special committee assigned are to complete the preparation and integration of the evidence collected for presentation to H.E.W. by September 1, 1967. Allowance to be made for the growth in membership of the ACA to meet H.E.W. criteria #1.
4. The council authorized the formation of a committee to assist in the direction of the application presentation consisting of Drs. Fisher, W. Wolf and Haynes.

Procedure Rules

The accrediting committees recommendation that the accredited colleges are to be re-inspected and re-evaluated every three years or as indicated and all other schools every two years or as indicated was unanimously adopted.

motion by Dr. Napolitano, seconded by Dr. Coggins and approved - that credits from chiropractic colleges not in the list published by the accrediting agency of the ACA may be accepted but only on a provisional basis subject to internal rules of the college. A copy of these rules are to be filed with the Director of Education of the ACA

moved by Dr. Harper, seconded by Dr. J. Wolfe and approved - that each semester, starting a month before enrollment, the schools supply Dr. Fisher with the names of students refused admission and with the reasons for said refusal. Dr. Fisher is to make this list available to all other colleges.

moved by Dr. Coggins, seconded by Dr. J. Wolfe and passed - that the council authorizes the chairman to act on the request of the Texas College to present a neuro-physiology class in the State of Washington upon receipt of basic outline and written request from the college.

moved by Dr. Fay, seconded by Dr. Wolf and passed - that the school forward to Dr. Fisher a copy of their list of books requested by the faculty for library holdings. Dr. Fisher is to compile the lists and make them available to all the schools.

Election of officers

moved by Dr. Fay, seconded by Dr. Napolitano that the present officers of the council be re-elected. Motion by Dr. Coggins, seconded by Dr. Bittner that the secretary cast a unanimous ballot for the re-election of Dr. Haynes as president and of Dr. J. Wolfe as secretary. Motions approved.

The Council received Dr. David Palmer, Dr. O.D. Adams and Dr. Jerry McAndrews for an informal conference. Dr. Palmer stated that we were all in agreement to the need for accreditation under H.E.W. and extended his apology for Dr. Rutherford's statement at the last Parker Seminar that appeared to mean that C.E.F. had been approved by H.E.W. as an accrediting agency, which was not true.

General discussion followed and the meeting ended with mutual agreement of the need for further conferences.

Respectfully submitted, Dr. John Wolfe, Secretary of the Council

Minutes of the Meeting of the COUNCIL ON EDUCATION of the ACA
St. Louis, Missouri, June 28 through July 1, 1967

The meeting of the Council on Education of the ACA was called to order by the President, Dr. George H. Haynes at 9:00 a.m. Wednesday, June 28, 1967 at the Chase-Park Plaza Hotel, St. Louis, Missouri.

ROLL CALL

Council President - Dr. George H. Haynes, Los Angeles College of Chiropractic, (A) Present
Council Secretary - Dr. John Wolfe, Northwestern College of Chiropractic, (A.C.) Present
Director of Education - Dr. John A. Fisher, Present

Accrediting Committee Chairman - Dr. Walter Wolf, Present
Accrediting Committee Secretary - Dr. Orval Hidde, Present
Accrediting Committee -   Dr. Herbert Hinton, Present
Dr. J.R. Quigley, Present
Dr. Anthony Bazzano, Present
Columbia Institute of Chiropractic - (P.A.), Dr. Ernest Napolitano, Present
Chiropractic Institute of New York - (P.A.), Dr. Helmut Bittner, Present
Lincoln Chiropractic College (A) - Dr. Chester Stowell, Present
Logan College of Chiropractic (P.A.) - Dr. William Coggins, Present
National College of Chiropractic (A) - Dr. Joseph Janse, Present
Texas College of Chiropractic (P.A.) - Dr. William Harper, Present
Council of State Chiropractic Examining Boards -
Dr. Howard Fenton, Absent
Dr. Rex Wright, Absent
Dr. Gordon Holman, Absent

The three above members were present only to report on the National Board and Council activities.
ALSO PRESENT
Affiliated Colleges - Canadian Memorial College of Chiropractic, Dr. Earl Homewood
And - Western States College of Chiropractic, Dr. Robert Elliot
Lincoln College of Chiropractic - Dr. Elmer Berner
Los Angeles College of Chiropractic - Dr. Henry Higley
National College of Chiropractic - Dr. Leonard Fay

On motion of Dr. Walter Wolf and seconded by Dr. Janse, the minutes of the meeting of February 7 through 10, 1967 were approved. After the reading of the correspondence received, the following points were discussed:

1.   HONORARY CHIROPRACTIC SOCIETY FOR THE COLLEGES
Dr. Hinton reported progress. Will continue preparing the format and requested suggestions from the members of the Council.

2.   UNIFORM CHIROPRACTIC OATH
Dr. Fisher reported inability of the committee to meet. He will try to have a report ready for the mid-year meeting.

3.   NON-AMERICAN CHIROPRACTIC PRE-PROFESSIONAL REQUIREMENTS
Dr. Haynes submitted a written report which was made a part of these minutes.

4.   PRACTICE DESIGNATIONS UNDER THE ACA COUNCILS
Dr. Haynes presented a written report which is a part of these minutes.

5.   EXTENSION CLASSES
Reports of the extension classes presented during the year were given by Los Angeles College of Chiropractic, Northwestern College, Lincoln College, Logan College, National College, Chiropractic Institute of New York, and Texas College of Chiropractic. The other colleges promised to send their reports.

6.   CLINIC DIRECTORS' SEMINARS
Dr. Fay presented a written report which is part of these minutes. The uniform clinic forms are being prepared by both the Columbia Institute of New York and by Los Angeles College.

7.   COUNCIL OF CHIROPRACTIC EXAMINING BOARDS
Dr. Fenton presented the report including a suggestion of having the chiropractic accrediting agency sponsored by both National Associations. He also presented a copy of the chiropractic definition adopted by the Council.

8.   NATIONAL BOARD
Dr. Saunders presented a written report which is a part of these minutes. Dr. Holman suggested that the colleges require all students to take Part I and Part II.

9.   STUDENT COUNSELING PROGRAM
Dr. Haynes presented a written report regarding the program requested by the member colleges and agreed upon at the Chicago meeting of the appointed committee and Mr. Collins. Because of time difficulties the program is not yet in operation.

Mr. Collins presented his report and brought out the inability of one man to accomplish the work without the full cooperation of the colleges. Up to now only three council schools have appointed a school admissions director to work with Mr. Collins.

Most schools feel that Mr. Collins' efforts have increased the number of applicants for enrollment. Dr. Walter Wolf suggested the distribution of admission efforts in a better geographical manner.

10.   IMPACT
Through the courtesy of the Logan College the Council was informed by a delegation from Impact - a student political action group - of their activities. The group originated at the Logan College in order to assist the State Association and the profession in the area of political action. The group was commended for their excellent organization and accomplishments.

11. RESEARCH

Dr. Higley presented a written report which is a part of these minutes. He reported on his recent visit to Washington, D.C. and on his meetings with the different Federal agencies dealing with research. He will be meeting with them again in the spring of 1968.

The Federal agencies are primarily concerned with the basic science facilities and staff of our colleges. There is a good possibility that our schools could obtain Federal research contracts. The colleges are to prepare individual proposals and submit them to Dr. Higley.

12. SYNCHROTHERM

Dr. Homewood discussed the present status of the Synchrotherm. It was generally agreed that all the colleges would be willing to assist in the collection of data on the use of this instrument under a program prepared by the Research Department.

13. JOURNAL OF CLINICAL CHIROPRACTIC

It was agreed that we should encourage the publication of scientific chiropractic journals. It was further agreed that participation in the Journal of Clinical Chiropractic shall be considered the prerogative of each college.

14. CLINICAL REQUIREMENTS FOR GRADUATION

This matter was discussed and general agreement was reached.

15. SCIENTIFIC QUARTERLY

Dr. Bittner's program for the publication of a scientific quarterly was once more discussed. The need for a careful editing was stressed.

16. RELEASE OF CONFIDENTIAL INFORMATION

The release of confidential college information by the accrediting committee was discussed.

17. FACULTY LECTURES

The role of itinerant chiropractic lecturers in approved colleges as well as the role of extension faculty in itinerant lecturing was considered. The freedom of faculty members to accept lecturing invitations was discussed.

It was agreed that the president would be allowed to investigate the above matter and report at the next meeting.

18. Ph.C. DEGREE

It was brought out that the Council, several years ago, decided that none of its college members would issue the Ph.C. degree.

19. FULL TIME FACULTY

The matter of a more efficient utilization of the full time instructor was discussed and will be reconsidered at our next meeting.

20. BASIC MEDICAL WRITING COURSE

Dr. Hidde presented the advisability to train the chiropractic students in the area of basic medical writing. He suggested contacting the editor of the Journal of the American Osteopathic Association for their booklet on this matter.

21. ROENTGENOLOGICAL COUNCIL

Dr. Howe presented the names of Drs. Moran, Ray and Swallen for appointment to the Roentgenological Board of Examiners. The request was accompanied by the written qualifications of the candidates.

22. ORTHOPEDIC COUNCIL

This Council presented its modified by-laws for approval of the educational provisions. Action was postponed pending further study.

23. APPLICATION TO H.E.W.

The program of preparing the application to H.E.W. for the acceptance of our accrediting agency was discussed. The progress made was considered satisfactory. Further work on this program was assigned. Dr. Fisher is to prepare a list of material obtained to meet the nine points of the H.E.W. criteria in preparation for a meeting of Drs. Fisher, Wolf and Haynes to consider the form of the application.

24. OTHER ACCREDITING PROBLEMS

The discussions with the Palmer College were reported by the committee of the Council. It was decided that further meetings are desirous. The committee was given guidelines to follow at the next meeting with the Palmer Colleges. It was agreed that our application to H.E.W. cannot be retarded because of these talks.

25. REPORT OF THE ACCREDITING COMMITTEE

The Chairman of the Committee opened a Council discussion on the proposed demotion of the two New York institutions. It was pointed out that a bill of particulars had been presented to the Chiropractic Institute of New York in 1963 and to the Columbia Institute of Chiropractic in 1964 followed by extension of time for compliance up to the present date. Dr. Wolf pointed out that the action of the agency was not based upon the recent inspection except as related to the original bill of particulars.

Dr. Haynes, as Chairman of the Council, rechecked the procedures stated by the accrediting committee to determine compliance with the rules of procedure. There being no further discussion, the accrediting committee presented the following report:

The Chiropractic Institute of New York and the Columbia Institute of Chiropractic have been demoted from the provisionally accredited status to that of approved conditionally.

The Northwestern College of Chiropractic has been raised to the provisionally accredited status from that of approved conditionally.

The present status of the Colleges is as follows:

(A) Accredited - Lincoln College of Chiropractic, Los Angeles College of Chiropractic, National College of Chiropractic

(PA) Provisionally Accredited - Logan Chiropractic College, Northwestern College of Chiropractic, Texas College of Chiropractic

(AC) Approved Conditionally - Chiropractic Institute of New York, Columbia Institute of Chiropractic

The report was received. Dr. Napolitano requested an official notice from the accrediting committee.

MOTIONS PASSED BY THE COUNCIL

Non-American Pre-professional Requirements
Moved by Dr. Bittner, seconded by Dr. Stowell and passed that the report of the committee on non-American pre-professional require-ments, after approval from Dr. Grillo of the European Chiropractic Union, be published in a pamphlet form as a guide for the colleges of the Council and for use by the non-American Chiropractic Associations as part of a student counseling programs.
Practice Designations
Moved by Dr. Coggins, seconded by Dr. Harper and passed that the Council on Education recommend that the use of the terms "Roentgenologist", "Orthopedist", "Orthopod", "Specialist", or similar terms applied to a practitioner in a chiropractic specialty field be discouraged and eliminated. The use of the term "Diplomate" and terms designating the field of practice concentration, but not the indi-vidual himself, be considered acceptable if the practitioner meets the requirements set by the corresponding councils of the ACA.

Moved by Dr. Wolf, seconded by Dr. Hidde and passed that the other Councils of the ACA be contacted and requested to adopt a similar stand as the above and that this information be conveyed to all boards governing the licensure of doctors of chiropractic.
Extension Classes
Moved by Dr. Bittner, seconded by Dr. Stowell and passed that the members of the accrediting committee be notified of the extension classes presented by the colleges that are members of the Council and that an invitation be extended to them to attend and evaluate such classes.
Clinic Directors' Seminar
Moved by Dr. Stowell, seconded by Dr. Wolf and passed that a vote of thanks be extended to Dr. Fay for his excellent work as the Council's representative to the Clinic Directors' Seminar.
Council of State Chiropractic Examining Boards
Moved by Dr. Harper, seconded by Dr. Wolfe and passed that a vote of thanks be extended to the council of State Chiropractic Examining Boards for their outstanding work as reflected in their 1967 "Official Directory" and for their suggestion to solve the matter of a common accrediting agency for the profession.
National Board of Chiropractic Examiners
Moved by Dr. Wolfe, seconded by Dr. Quigley that a vote of commendation be extended to the National Board of Chiropractic Examiners for their accomplishments on behalf of public health and the chiropractic profession.
Department of Research
Moved by Dr. Janse, seconded by Dr. Wolf and passed that Dr. Higley be commended for the progress made by the Department of Research under his direction.
Scientific Quarterly
Moved by Dr. Napolitano, seconded by Dr. Stowell and passed that the Council on Education once more endorse Dr. Bittner's proposal for the publication of a "Scientific Quarterly" and that the colleges that are members of the Council supply at least one article to Dr. Bittner by December 1, 1967. The Council requests that the Council secretary and Dr. Fisher contact each college once each month on this matter until their articles are received.
Impact
Moved by Dr. Napolitano, seconded by Dr. Janse that the Council on Education extend its thanks and appreciation to "Impact" for their visit to the Council and for their excellent work.
Student Counseling Program
Moved by Dr. W. Wolf, seconded by Dr. Bittner and passed to accept the reports of the Admission Counseling Committee and Mr. Collins and to express to Mr. Collins the willingness of the colleges to assist him in the execution of his program.

Moved by Dr. W. Wolf, seconded by Dr. Fay and passed that Mr. Collins be asked to report to the Council at each of its meetings.
Release of Information by Accrediting Agency
Moved by Dr. Hidde, seconded by Dr. J. Wolfe and passed that the Accrediting Agency of the ACA may release confidential material dealing with the colleges to other qualified accrediting agencies when requested and considered useful.
Appointments to the Board of Roentgenology
Moved by Dr. Janse, seconded by Dr. J. Wolfe and passed that the Council on Education approves the nominees of the Council on Roentgenology for the appointment to the Board of Roentgenology. The nominees approved are Dr. Anthony Moran, Dr. Douglas Ray and Dr. Earl W. Swallen.
Clinic Graduation Requirements
Moved by Dr. Coggins, seconded by Dr. Hidde and passed that the clinic graduation requirements starting with the students entering the clinic for the year 1967-1968, shall include: (1) 25 physical examinations of which at least 10 will involve outside patients; (2) the study

of at least 30 are x-rays; (3) laboratory work to include 25 urinalyses, 25 CBC's and 10 blood chemistries; (4) a minimum of 250 patient visits when treatment is rendered.

Respectfully submitted, John Wolfe, D.C., Secretary of the Council

Minutes of the Meeting of the COUNCIL ON EDUCATION of the ACA
Las Vegas, Nevada, February 1, 2, 3, 4, 1968

The Meeting of the Council on Education of the ACA was called to order by the President, Dr. George H. Haynes, at 9:15 a.m. Thursday, February 1, 1968, at Caesar's Palace Hotel, Las Vegas, Nevada

ROLL CALL

Council President - Dr. George H. Haynes, Los Angeles College of Chiropractic, (A) Present

Council Secretary - Dr. John Wolfe, Northwestern College of Chiropractic, (P.A.) Present

Director of Education - Dr. John A. Fisher, Present

Accrediting Committee Chairman - Dr. Walter Wolf, Present

Accrediting Committee Secretary - Dr. Orval Hidde, Present

Accrediting Committee -   Dr. Herbert Hinton, Present

Dr. J.R. Quigley, Present

Dr. Anthony Bazzano, Present

Columbia Institute of Chiropractic - (A.C.) Dr. Ernest Napolitano, Present

Chiropractic Institute of New York - (A.C.) Dr. Thure Peterson, Present

Lincoln Chiropractic College (A) Dr. Chapel, Present

Logan College of Chiropractic (P.A.) Dr. William Coggins, Present

National College of Chiropractic (A) Dr. Joseph Janse, Present

Texas College of Chiropractic (P.A.) Dr. William Harper, Present

Council of State Chiropractic Examining Boards

Dr. Howard Fenton, Present

Dr. Rex Wright, Present

Dr. Gordon Holman, Present

ALSO PRESENT

Affiliated Colleges - Canadian Memorial College of Chiropractic - Dr. Earl Homewood

And - Western States College of Chiropractic, Dr. Robert Elliot

Columbia Institute of New York - Dr. Allen

Lincoln College of Chiropractic - Dr. Elmer Berner

Los Angeles College of Chiropractic - Dr. Henry G. Higley

National College of Chiropractic - Dr. Leonard Fay

Texas College of Chiropractic - Dr. Howard Pierce??

The Minutes of the Council Meeting of June 28 through July 1, 1967 were adopted after correcting line 10 & 11 on page 6 to read:

"The report was received. Dr. Napolitano requested an exact copy of the statement made by the Accrediting Committee to the Council on Education when they, the Accrediting Committee, reported the change of status of the C.I.C. He not only requested what was printed in the publication on standards, but what was read to the Council by Dr. Hidde that was handwritten on a yellow sheet of paper."

After reading of the correspondence, the following points were discussed:

1.   The request from FACE to meet with the Council was approved.

2.   The correspondence between Dr. Haynes and Dr. D. Palmer was considered.

Willingness to discuss the Accreditation of Chiropractic Colleges with Dr. Palmer was expressed, provided that there would be no political matters involved. Dr. Fisher reported his talks with Dr. McCarrel, who finally has agreed to a meeting without a set agenda, to discuss the Accreditation of Chiropractic Colleges. The Council to select from two possible March dates.

3.   PROPOSED MEETING OF REGISTRARS

Dr. Homewood's suggestion was considered as very valuable, but the present economic condition does not allow such a meeting in the near future.

4.   VOCATIONAL GUIDANCE

Members of the Council bought, through Dr. Peterson, a copy of "Chiropractic Career" booklet, published by the Vocational Guidance Manuals of New York for examination. The booklet will sell for $1.65 unless better arrangements can be made through the ACA.

5.   CONVENTION SPEAKERS - LETTER FROM ACA BOARD

It was made clear that the Council on Education has never had any official part in selecting the speakers.

Full desire to assist the ACA Board of Governors was expressed. It was considered that those attending the Convention, desire speakers that will give them something they can use in their practice. They are interested in the areas of Adjustive Technics and Practice Building.

The lack of adequate financial recompense deters many of the speakers or potential speakers from undertaking the long hours and days of preparation of their talks needed to bring out new factors into their lectures. The presentation should be at a graduate level and not at the undergraduate one.

6.   CHIROPRACTIC "BASIC PRINCIPLES" - LETTER FROM ACA BOARD

Due to the fact that the different members of the Council on Education voiced a wide variety of interpretations to the wording of the resolution passed by the Board of Governors on this matter, the Council requested Dr. Hightower and Dr. Kimmel to explain the purpose of the resolution.

The Council extends its thanks to both Dr. Hightower and Dr. Kimmel for accepting our request.

Dr. Kimmel summarized the purpose behind the resolution as referring to the concept of the subluxation and its possible effect upon the function of the nervous system, as being the property of the Chiropractic profession. The Council was in full agreement with Dr. Kimmel.

7.   LETTER FROM "PSYCHIATRIC NEWS"

Dr. Kimmel explained to the Council the background of this letter, and was assured of the full cooperation from our colleges.

8.   HONORARY CHIROPRACTIC SOCIETY

Dr. Hinton reported a lack of progress. Will continue working on it.

9.   UNIFORM CHIROPRACTIC OATH

Dr. Fisher reported a lack of progress due to failure of Committee meeting.

10.   MEMBERSHIP

Dr. Schmidt requested the Council to assist the membership drive by including a preferential financial arrangement for ACA members in relation to non-members in seminar and courses presented under the approval of the Council and member colleges.

11.   CLINIC DIRECTORS' SEMINAR

Dr. Fay presented a written report and elaborated on it. The Council commended Dr. Fay for his excellent work.

12.   DEPARTMENT OF RESEARCH

Dr. Higley presented a written report and elaborated on it. He stressed the need to obtain Federal grants for research and reported that two proposals have been filed.

13.   PENSION PLAN

Dr. Howard Pierce?? presented a pension and retirement plan for the consideration of the Colleges. This plan allows for the selection of its own insurance company by each College. A written brochure was made available to each member of the Council.

14.   GENERAL PATTERN FOR PRE-PROFESSIONAL REQUIREMENTS

Dr. Hidde brought out the need to outline the general areas of study covering the 60 unit requirement for enrollment. It was agreed that the Chairman of the Council was to appoint a Committee to prepare such a program for the consideration of the Council.

15.   CRITERIA REVISION

Dr. Hidde suggested that the Chairman appoint a Committee to examine the criteria adopted by the Council to determine if there is a need for modifications, particularly in the wording dealing with appeals. The Council approved his request.

16.   REPORT OF COUNCIL OF STATE CHIROPRACTIC EXAMINING BOARDS

Dr. Holman presented the report assisted by Dr. Fenton and Dr. Wright.

The standard basic curriculum was discussed. Further action on this item will be considered after Dr. Haynes completes his research project on curricula

It was agreed that the textbook list should be reviewed. It was further agreed that the Review Committee on Books and Publications should remain dormant.

The Council was informed that a file of updated Chiropractic laws with amendments, board rulings and attorney general interpretations, and court cases involving law, will be kept in the Council on Examiners' offices.

The possibility of a meeting of all Chiropractic College heads under the auspices of the Council of Examiners was discussed.

17.   NATIONAL BOARD OF CHIROPRACTIC EXAMINERS

Dr. Saunders reported on the activities of the National Board and presented the brochure that they have prepared, which will sell for $2.50. He discussed the idea of making the National Board Examination a pre-requisite to graduation, and the Illinois examination.

18.   ADMISSIONS DIRECTOR

Mr. Mel Collins reported on the activities of his department. It was brought out, the possibility that a college may include a pre-chiropractic course in their curriculum which would be promoted by their eleven counselors that now cover the area from the Rockies east.

19.   OFFICE MANAGEMENT COURSE

The possibility of having successful alumni present seminars for the new graduates was presented. It was agreed that all colleges would supply Dr. Homewood with the outline of the present undergraduate courses in office management.

20.   EXTENSION COURSES

The time table for request of approval for extension courses was discussed.

It was stressed that the presentation of seminars or courses by the member colleges within their state or province of residency do not require approval of the Council but only of those conducted out of state.

All member schools agreed that, at each meeting, they will submit to the Council Chairman, a list of all seminars or courses presented in the previous six months. This list to include in-state and out-of-state presentations.

21.   ORTHOPEDIC OUTLINE

The Council on Orthopedics' suggested outline of the post-graduate course to be used as the minimal coverage of the course was presented.

22.   The Board of FACE was received by the Council.

Dr. Schierholz presented a program that will allow the individual Jr. ACA Chapter to take over the sale of the seals. The Chapters will be allowed to retain 20% of the sales for local use.

He stressed the need for a more active participation in the ACA Scholarship program and again requested the report on grants and donations received by the colleges since 1959.

23.   SELECTIVE SERVICE

The directives of the Selective Service and their effect upon the draft deferment of our students was discussed. The need for active ACA representation before the bodies concerned with the draft was brought out. The help received from Mrs. E. Murphy and the late Dr. E. Murphy was recalled.

Mr. Rosenfeld appeared before the Council and assured us of his full support and assistance.

24.   REPORT OF THE ACCREDITING COMMITTEE

Dr. Walter Wolf reported that an appeal hearing on the demotion of the status of the Columbia Institute had been held and that the transcript of this hearing will be made available to the institutional members of the Council for their comment.

The Committee reported that there had been no change in the status of the member colleges from that reported at the last meeting.

MOTIONS PASSED BY THE COUNCIL

1.   Motion by Dr. Janse and Seconded by Dr. Harper:

The Council on Education to appoint an advisory committee to suggest topics and speakers for the ACA Convention and regional seminars. This committee to include representatives from the colleges of the area where the convention is to take place, and the committee's suggestions are to be reviewed by the full Council before presentation to the ACA Carried.

2.   Motion by Dr. Janse and Seconded by Dr. Napolitano:

The Council on Education will extend its full cooperation to the intent of the resolution passed by the Board of Governors relating to the "Basic Principles" of Chiropractic as clarified by Dr. Kimmel. Carried

3.   The Chairman was instructed to inform the ACA that the Council will cooperate with the request regarding the Life Foundation.

4.   Motion by Dr. Janse and Seconded by Dr. Napolitano:

That the Council direct the Chairman of the Clinic Directors' Seminar to advise the Council on Chiropractic Roentgenology that the x-ray residency program as presented has been tabled. Carried.

Motion by Dr. Janse and Seconded by Dr. Napolitano:

That the Chairman of the Council on Education communicate to Dr. Fay, the suggestions of the members of the Council as they relate to the proposed x-ray residency and that the Clinic Directors re-discuss this matter, and their conclusions be submitted to the Council on Education for decision. Carried.

5.   Motion by Dr. R. Wright, Seconded by Dr. W. Wolf:

The Council recommends that the National Board Examination should be a requirement for graduation. Carried.

6.   Motion by Dr. Fenton, Seconded by Dr. Wright:

That the Council on Education appoint two members to attend a meeting to be held in Chicago on March 15, 16, 1968, to discuss accreditation of Chiropractic Colleges if such a meeting is held. Carried.

7.   Motion by Dr. Janse, Seconded by Dr. Harper:

The Council on Education approves the attendance of the official representatives of the Institutional Members and Representation of the Council of State Examining Boards at a meeting at Chicago on March 6 and 7, 1968, as being arranged by Dr. Fisher and Dr. McCarrel to discuss the accreditation of Chiropractic Colleges if such a meeting takes place. Carried.

8.   Motion by Dr. Hinton and Seconded by Dr. Hidde:

The request for approval of extension classes must be submitted to the President of the Council at least 30 days prior to the beginning date of such a class. Carried.

9.   Motion by Dr. Janse and Seconded by Dr. Harper:

The Council approves the outline of Orthopedics presented by the Council on Orthopedics as the minimal educational standard for this post-graduate course. Carried.

10.   Motion by Dr. Hinton, Seconded by Dr. W. Wolf:

On the basis that the Ph.C. degree is not listed as legitimate and considered as a spurious one, the Council on Education goes on record as not recognizing the Ph.C. degree and opposing its use. Carried.

11. Motion by Dr. Napolitano, Seconded by Dr. W. Wolf:

    The Council on Education removes the mandatory program requiring the A.C.T. or S.A.T. test for enrollment and recommends that efforts be made to find a suitable Chiropractic aptitude test. Carried.

12. Motion by Dr. Napolitano, Seconded by Dr. J. Wolfe:

    That a letter of thanks and appreciation be sent to Dr. L. Fay, National Board, Council of State Boards, Dr. Higley, and Mr. Rosenfield. Carried.

13. Moved by Dr. J. Wolfe, Seconded by Dr. Hinton:

    The Council on Education recommends to the ACA and FACE the continuation of the scholarship program. Carried.

14. There was unanimous agreement on the following points:

    A. To supply FACE with the information requested regarding grants and donations received since 1959.

    B. More active participation in the ACA Scholarship Program.

    C. All colleges to send to the Chairman of the Council, the number and percentage of their students subject to draft. This information to be given to Mr. Rosenfeld.

    D. All colleges to re-evaluate tuition rates. Dr. Fisher to survey and report the tuition rates without reference to the individual colleges.

    The yearly election of Council Officers took place. Dr. Janse moved that the Council unanimously re-elect Dr. G. Haynes as President and Dr. J. Wolfe as Secretary. It was seconded by Dr. Napolitano. Dr. W. Wolf called for the question and the motion carried.

    Meeting adjourned at 1:35 p.m., February 4, 1968.

Respectfully submitted, John Wolfe, D.C., Secretary of the Council

Minutes of the Meeting of the COUNCIL ON EDUCATION of the ACA
New York, N.Y., June 30, July 1, 2, 3, 4, 5, 1968

The Meeting of the Council on Education of the ACA was called to order by the President, Dr. George H. Haynes, at 10:00 a.m. on Sunday, June 30, 1968, at the Americana Hotel, New York City, New York.

ROLL CALL

    Council President - Dr. George H. Haynes, Los Angeles College of Chiropractic, (A) Present

    Council Secretary - Dr. John Wolfe, Northwestern College of Chiropractic, (P.A.) Present

    Director of Education - Dr. John A. Fisher, Present

    Accrediting Committee Chairman - Dr. Walter Wolf, Present

    Accrediting Committee Secretary - Dr. Orval Hidde, Present

    Accrediting Committee -   Dr. Herbert Hinton, Present

    Dr. J.R. Quigley, Present

    Dr. Anthony Bazzano, Present

    Columbia Institute of Chiropractic - (A.C.) Dr. Ernest Napolitano, Present

    Chiropractic Institute of New York - (A.C.) Dr. Thure Peterson, Present

    Lincoln Chiropractic College (A) Dr. John Pierce, Present

    Logan College of Chiropractic (P.A.) Dr. William Coggins, Present

    National College of Chiropractic (A) Dr. Joseph Janse, Present

    Texas College of Chiropractic (P.A.) Dr. William Harper, Present

    Council of State Chiropractic Examining Boards:

    Dr. Howard Fenton, Absent

    Dr. Rex Wright, Present

    Dr. Gordon Holman, Present

ALSO PRESENT:

    Affiliated Colleges - Canadian Memorial College of Chiropractic - Dr. Earl Homewood

    And - Western States College of Chiropractic, Dr. Robert Elliot

OTHERS:

    Drs. Leonard Fay, Henry Higley, Charles Crosner, Anton Latham, McCarran, Chester Stowell, D.P. Casey.

The Minutes of the Council Meeting of February 1, 2, 3, 4, 1968, were adopted by motion made by Dr. Harper and seconded by Dr. Elliot.

The following points were discussed:

1.   A uniform Chiropractic Oath - Dr. Harper presented the oath used at the Columbia Institute of Chiropractic, for future consideration.
2.   APPOINTMENT TO THE ROENTGENOLOGICAL EXAMINING BOARD
     The American Council on Chiropractic Roentgenology submitted the name of Dr. Joseph Howe to fill the vacancy in the American Board of ???...

     Dr. Holman presented the Report of this Council covering their activities for the past six months. It was announced that their Directory will be published every other year with a supplement being published in the alternate year. He strongly recommended the establishment of better liaison with the other branches of the healing arts. [page missing]
5.   NATIONAL BOARD OF EXAMINERS
     Dr. Saunders presented the Report of the activities of this Board. 1478 applicants have passed this Board to date, and about 500 State Licenses have been granted on the basis of the National Boards' Certificates.
6.   VITAMINERALS SCHOLARSHIP PROGRAM
     Mr. Robert Swan, Vice President of Vitaminerals Inc., presented to the Council, a modified scholarship program. In the future, the scholarship grant will be based on a set figure for the four year period. One school at $2500, two schools at $3000, and seven schools at $3600 for the four year scholarship. Other provisions of the scholarship program remain unchanged.
7.   DRAFT PROBLEMS
     The discriminatory application of the Selective Service Act was discussed. A Committee under the Chairmanship of Dr. Fisher was appointed to prepare a brief for presentation to the ACA, with a request for vigorous efforts to place the draft status of chiropractic students and practitioners on the same basis as those of the other two major health fields, osteopathy and medicine. (M.D.)
     Mr. Rosenfeld, ACA's Washington representative joined in this discussion.
8.   AMERICAN COUNCIL ON CHIROPRACTIC ORTHOPEDICS
     The Orthopedic Council requested an opportunity to give a preliminary evaluation of future courses on Orthopedics so that they could submit their suggestions before the Council on Education acts on the approval of such courses.
     The Council on Education approved the request.
9.   PRE-PROFESSIONAL REQUIREMENTS AND ACCREDITATION PROCEDURES
     Lengthy discussion was held on the matter of the pre-professional requirements as found in the Council's Criteria and their effect upon the present colleges of chiropractic.
     Drs. Wright and Holman evaluated their Washington, D.C. investigation of the need for the pre-professional requirements and summarized their findings. The pre-professional educational requirements are not demanded in writing for the recognition of an accrediting agency for a profession, but is generally understood that such recognition could not be expected without such pre-professional requirements. This expression agrees with the individual findings and conclusions expressed in the past by Dr. Fisher, Dr. Walter Wolf and Dr. George Haynes.
     The Chair clearly stated that no action by the Council on Education was needed for the implementation of the 2 year, 60 unit pre-professional entrance requirement to go into effect as the governing rule for all graded Chiropractic Colleges within the Council on September 30, 1968. However, an action by the Council on Education is necessary in order to modify this rule or to prevent its implementation on September 30, 1968.
     No motion was offered on this matter.
     The Accrediting Committee's procedures, particularly as they relate to the Texas Chiropractic College, was discussed before the full Council by mutual consent of the two parties involved. It appeared that a satisfactory classification of this problem was reached.
     The Chair broached the subject of modification of the composition of the Accrediting Agency, moved by Dr. Harper and seconded by Dr. Fay, that this matter be tabled.
     Motion passed.
10. ROENTGENOLOGY
     Dr. Joseph Howe presented Mr. Jerome I. Levine, Health Physicist of the National Center for Radiological Health, who spoke on the educational program dealing with radiation.
11. FOUNDATION FOR CHIROPRACTIC EDUCATION AND RESEARCH
     A valuable and informative discussion was held between the trustees of F.C.E.R. and members of the Council, on the economic problems facing the further progress of chiropractic education.
     The Council extended its thanks and appreciation to Dr. Wunch, Dr. Schierholz, and to the other members of the Board of Trustees of F.C.E.R. for their informative presentation and their excellent cooperation and assistance.
12. COUNCIL OF DELEGATES
     The Council on Education and Trustees of F.C.E.R. appeared before the Council of Delegates of the ACA and fully acquainted them with the program on accreditation and the problems, economic and otherwise, facing chiropractic education because of this program.
     The Council on Education expressed its thanks and appreciation to the Council of Delegates and its presiding officer, Dr. Brassard, for patience in listening to us, and for their wholehearted support as evidenced by their accomplished and attempted actions to relieve the economic difficulties facing our Council's activities.
13. The following points were approved:

A) Students who present pre-professional college records of 26 to 29 semester hours or its equivalent in quarter units under the 1 year, 30 unit enrollment requirement, and those that present 52 to 58 semester hours, or its equivalent in quarter hours under the 2 year, 60 unit requirement with a grade point average of at least 2.25 (on a 4.00 scale), and who meet all other admissions requirements, may be admitted on a provisional basis for a period of one calendar year during which the deficiency must be corrected.

Motion by Dr. Stowell and Dr. Janse.

B) Students who present a minimum of 30 semester hours under the 1 year, 30 unit requirement or 60 semester hours under the 2 year, 60 unit requirement with a grade point average of 1.75 to 1.99 (on a 4.00 scale), and who meet all other admissions requirements, may be admitted on a provisional basis for a period of one calendar year during which a grade point average of 2.00 (on a 4.00 scale) must be earned.

Motion by Dr. Fay and Dr. Stowell.

C) Only 10% of the admitted class may be admitted under each of the above rules.

Motion by Dr. Fay and Dr. J. Wolfe

D) By motion of Dr. Stowell, seconded by Dr. Fay, and passed, a committee was appointed to deal with the matter of mature applicants and ex-servicemen who apply for admission and do not meet the present pre-chiropractic college requirements.

The committee appointed consists of: Drs. Coggins, Harper, Fay, Wolfe, and Bazzano, under the chairmanship of Dr. Fisher.

E) On motion from Dr. Fay, seconded by Dr. Quigley, the Council approved in principle, the awarding of scholarships to the underprivileged.

A committee consisting of Dr. Fay, Chairman, Drs. Hinton, Quigley, and Kavaler, was appointed to study the above matter.

F) The Chair was instructed to send a letter to Dr. MacDonald explaining the impossibility to approve his request that chiropractic colleges issue a four year Doctor of Chiropractic Diploma to those holding 18 month diplomas after a certain number of credits are earned at extension courses.

Motion by Dr. Stowell, seconded by Dr. Peterson.

G) APPROVAL OF EXTENSION COURSES

    1.   New York Institute of Chiropractic
            Course in Orthopedics - Approved.

    2.   National College of Chiropractic
          1)   Roentgenology 850, North Dakota (25 Sessions)
          2)   Roentgenology of the Spine & Pelvis - Kansas (7 Sessions)
          3)   Roentgenology of the Spine & Pelvis - Pennsylvania (7 Sessions)
          4)   Orthopedics 830, Ohio (20 Sessions)
          5)   Orthopedics 830, On Campus (20 Sessions)
          6)   Special Orthopedic and Adjustive Technic - Arkansas (10 Sessions)
          7)   Clinical Neurology - Pennsylvania (3 Sessions)
          8)   Athletic Injuries - Missouri (4 Sessions)

All of the mentioned requests were approved.

REPORT OF THE ACCREDITING COMMITTEE

Dr. W. Wolf reported that there had been no changes in the status of the Member Colleges since last Meeting.

    The Meeting adjourned at 12 m, July 4, 1968.

Respectfully submitted, John Wolfe, D.C., Secretary of the Council

Los Angeles College of Chiropractic

920 East Broadway * Glendale, California 91205

George H. Haynes, D.C., Administrative Dean

October 28, 1969

TO ALL MEMBERS OF THE COUNCIL:

    I'd like to acquaint all members of The Council on Chiropractic Education of the proceedings at a recent meeting of Chiropractic College Presidents as it relates to chiropractic education.

    May I make it clear that I attended such a meeting not in the capacity of member or president of The Council on Chiropractic Education but simply as the executive officer of the Los Angeles College of Chiropractic. To my understanding all the other college representatives were likewise only representing their respective schools.

    In early September, Dr. Jack Fisher informed me of a probable October meeting of all chiropractic college presidents. I received a letter from Dr. W.D. Harper, dated September 8, 1969 that opened as follows: "A single room has been reserved in your name at the Royal Coach Inn, 7000 Southwest Freeway, Houston, Texas for arrival on Tuesday, October 21, 1969, for the meeting of all college presidents, called by Dr. McCarrell and Dr. Fisher to review and establish a working basis for criteria that would be acceptable to all."

Naturally with the possibility of finding an avenue for a unified criteria I was eager to attend. Such a move followed right along with the action of The Council on Chiropractic Education last June, inviting the Palmer College to attend the next meeting of The Council as a means of developing better communications and searching for a way of presenting a unified chiropractic college front.

The meeting of the presidents was held October 21st and 22nd, 1969, as scheduled, with all eleven U.S. chiropractic colleges represented by their respective administrator.

All the college presidents agreed on the following points:
1. Need for a unified college group.
2. The Chiropractic Accrediting Agency should be autonomous and not politically dominated.
3. A desire for a HEW approved Accrediting Agency for chiropractic education.

I moved to approve, in principle, the following reorganization plan with the statement that the name, number of respective representatives, and even the addition of groups to be represented was open for modification.
1. Name - "The Council on Chiropractic Education."
2. Composition - Institutional members composed of one official representative on the administration level of each member College.

Accrediting Commission composed of representatives from the Chiropractic Colleges, Council of State Chiropractic Examining Boards, International Chiropractic Association and American Chiropractic Association.

3. Purpose - The Council on Chiropractic Education is an autonomous national organization advocating high standards of quality in chiropractic education, establishing criteria of institutional excellence, evaluating and accrediting colleges through its Accrediting Commission, and publishing lists of those institutions which conform to its standards and policies.

The Council on Chiropractic Education is sponsored and supported but not governed by the American Chiropractic Association, the International Chiropractic Association and the Council of State Chiropractic Examining Boards.

Vote on Accreditation - The Accrediting Commission would decide by vote accreditation status. Decisions of the Accrediting Commission on accreditation status may be appealed to The Council on Chiropractic Education.

My motion and proposed plan was based on the following reasons:

1. The information that I gathered through discussions with Mrs. Theresa Wilkins while connected with HEW Department of Education and the June and July, 1969 meetings in Washington with Mr. Profett and Mr. Pugsley of the same department.
2. Joint professional and school representation appears to be prevalent in the composition of those HEW approved and recognized agencies to grant specialized accreditation to professional schools such as, medicine, dentistry, optometry, etc.
3. My belief that the profession is vitally concerned and affected by the federal recognition of an agency for the accreditation of the Chiropractic colleges, and therefore has the right and responsibility to participate in the accrediting program.

Some of the college presidents expressed the opinion that the members of the practicing profession and representatives from non-chiropractic academic world were not knowledgeable of the problems of chiropractic education and would tend to demand or impose educational demands that our colleges could not accept. Two of the college presidents expressed strong opposition to professional members on a chiropractic Accrediting Agency.

Action - Six negative votes were cast constituting a majority. My proposal was not adopted.

Dr. Harper presented a prepared set of Articles of Incorporation and a set of by-laws for the formation of an Accrediting Agency composed of the eleven U.S. chiropractic colleges.

It embodied the following:

1. Name - "The Association of Chiropractic Colleges."
2. Composition - "The association is and shall be comprised of the presidents, or their chief executive officer or their designated representatives of each of the member Chiropractic Colleges in the United States." (To be called Trustees.)
3. Purpose - "...Specifically and without limitation of the generality of the foregoing, to inspect from time to time all duly recognized chiropractic educational institutes, to set standards, rules and regulations for the administration and conduct thereof, to issue certificates of recognition to withhold or withdraw such certificates and to do all things and have such other powers necessary in order to carry out a complete program of accreditation of chiropractic educational colleges and..."
4. Vote on Accreditation - "A majority vote of all Trustees either in person or by proxy shall be required to accredit a college or, to remove a college from the accredited list."

Dr. David Palmer moved the adoption of the Articles of Incorporation and by-laws presented by Dr. Harper.

Some of the college presidents expressed doubt that an accrediting agency composed of only the eleven chiropractic colleges would be acceptable to the Federal Department of Education. The following telegram sent to all eleven college presidents was brought out.

Royal Coach Inn   7000 Southwest Frwy Houston
Dear Doctor Haynes:

Tried to contact Dr. Dicky this date. He was not in the city and not expected back until wed. Talked to Jerry Miller, Associate Director to Dr. Dicky. He stated he did not believe that a group of Education people of our colleges could be acceptable as the sole members of an Accreditation Committee. He further stated that we must have a group of people of a wide variety. He suggested that four categories be presented. 1. Institutional member, 2. Examining Board members, 3. Members of and from both national groups, and 4. Lay people (an additional feature that to date has not been included by any faction in the profession). In forming any program we should always have a wide range of views to be able to meet any prospective problems. I offer you this information not to champion anyone, but hoping that you will give this your very personal attention in the present meeting on Accreditation.
Rex A. Wright, D.C., President of the Council of State Chiropractic Examining Boards.

I moved that the motion be tabled until all eleven college presidents would meet as a unit with Dr. Dicky of the National Commission on Accreditation and representatives of the Federal Department of Education to clarify the acceptability of an accrediting agency composed of only chiropractic college representatives.

Action - My motion was defeated by the casting of six negative votes.

I made it clear that I should not be placed in a position to vote on Dr. Palmer's motion endorsing such a program when there was a clear doubt of the acceptability of the composition of such an accrediting agency. Dr. Janse recommended that a plain association of our eleven colleges could be formed. Dr. Simon proposed the deletion of the accrediting provision of the proposed articles of incorporation or modification of the composition of the proposed association.

However, the question was moved for the proposed articles of Incorporation and by-laws. Six votes were cast in favor. Five colleges could not accept the proposal.
Sincerely, George H. Haynes, D.C

Appendix C

REPORT OF AN EXAMINATION OF THE CLEVELAND CHIROPRACTIC COLLEGE, KANSAS CITY, MISSOURI, FOR THE ASSOCIATION OF CHIROPRACTIC COLLEGES, OCTOBER 13-15, 1971

The Cleveland Chiropractic College was founded in 1922 by Dr. C.S. Cleveland, Sr. and has been in continuous operation since. Dr. C.S. Cleveland, Sr. was President until 1967, and was succeeded by the current incumbent Dr. C.S. Cleveland, Jr. The College is a privately supported college chartered under the laws of the State of Missouri, as a non-profit educational institution. The college is located at 3700 Troost Avenue, Kansas City, Mo. The College has adequate land for its purposes and for expansion.

The enrollment for the current quarter consisted of 192 students, with 110 of them being enrolled in the day division and 82 in the evening division. Ninety of the students were enrolled in the lower division and 102 in the upper division.

PURPOSE

The purpose of the college as stated in the self study are well defined and clearly stated. The committee felt that the program was organized to fulfill the stated purposes and was being revised as the administration and faculty changed or modified their goals. The self study was well done in general, but the committee felt that some of the material presented reflected goals and not actualities. The college has not had an adequate catalog to this date, but an examination of the proofs for a new publication indicated that the new edition will be adequate and accurate.

ADMINISTRATIVE ORGANIZATION

The governing board of the college, the Board of Trustees, operates under an adequate set of by laws. It is believed the Board concerns itself with policy and not with administrative matters and has properly delegated the responsibility for the administration of the college to the President. The Committee recognizes the need for an active Board for the Alumni Association, but felt that in the case of the Cleveland College many policy matters were referred to the Alumni Board and their recommendations were given equal weight with those of the Board of Trustees. It is suggested that this relationship be clarified and that the policy decisions of the Trustees be the final decision.

The financial report of the college for the fiscal year ending Dec. 31, 1970 had not been audited and it is the strong recommendation of the committee that an outside auditor be employed to make an annual audit. The small balance of $5,241 of income over expenses for this fiscal year was an evidence of prudent and careful management on the part of the administration. It is also recommended by the committee that a more complete accounting system developed for the American Council on Education and used by the vast majority of colleges and universities.

The College does not have tax exempt status with Internal Revenue and this must be applied for as soon as possible. We found no evidence of any reason why this should not be granted upon application.

The budget of the college was adequate and supports the programs of the college very well within the funds that are available. It is evident that the areas of purchasing, plant management, plant utilization, and general administrative matters were well handled. In the area of support it is the strong recommendation of the committee that the fees charged students be increased to a minimum of $250 per quarter. This recommended increase will be comparable with similar colleges and will provide much needed revenue to strengthen several of the educational programs. It is also the strong recommendation of the committee that entering classes be accepted only two times a year. This point is made to reduce the duplication of instruction that is inevitable with a small faculty and with four entering groups each year.

While the committee recognizes the problems students have financially and is aware of the fact that for almost fifty years the college has operated separate day and evening programs it is the strong suggestion that the college devote serious study to the idea of operating only one program for all of its students.

FACULTY

The faculty is adequately qualified by training and by experience. The staff is recruited from graduates of the college and an attempt should be made to add members who have had their training in other institutions. The actual teaching faculty at the time of our visit was much smaller than the faculty section in the self study would indicate. We found no evidence of any tenure provisions and the scale of salaries was quite low. The college provides no fringe benefits other than social security. Most of the faculty maintain private practices and yet carry a rather heavy load at the college partially because of the two separate divisions and the necessity to teach in both. In spite of these facts the faculty is experienced and their length of service to the college is above average.

The faculty committees that are listed provide an adequate means for the faculty to influence educational policy and the morale of the faculty is at least average. Because of the scheduling problems the faculty is not available for student consultations, for research work and writing, and for communication with each other as much as would be desirable. Academic freedom does not appear to be an issue with the current staff, but the committee urges that increased emphasis be placed on more faculty involvement with educational planning. The general level of class room instruction that we observed was quite acceptable. We felt that there should be more faculty syllabi and more instructional aids. It is because of these factors the recommendation was made for a fee increase so that more full time faculty members could be added and the loads reduced for the reasons stated above. It was the general feeling of the committee that the college was providing its students with good basic training in the basic subjects offered and in the clinical work that makes up a necessary part of the training of a qualified chiropractor.

The teaching staff does not have private offices and consultations with students are thus difficult to arrange. In spite of these difficulties the rapport between faculty and students was quite good.

EDUCATIONAL PROGRAM

The college operates on the quarter system. The admissions procedures seemed quite adequate except for the lack of any standardized examinations. The college does not have a formalized orientation program of any length and the college is aware of the need for a more detailed, functional program. The number of foreign students is small and thus a formal program for them is not essential.

The curriculum is a standard one for chiropractic colleges and is changed infrequently. Examination procedures are determined by the instructors and seem quite good. While the committee recognizes the necessity of the basic course work required in the training of chiropractors it is believed that with classes entering four times a year students at Cleveland College are subjected to an above average amount of duplication.

The clinic facilities were superior and were well maintained. The new record system is superior and the clinic load of patients was good. The clinic procedures were good and were designed for maximum supervision of the student doctors and for complete protection of the patients. The student clinic operated quite successfully and with less close supervision by the clinic director. It is recommended that the student doctors in their final year be given more freedom in the handling of their patients so the transition from college to private practice will be less abrupt. It was felt that the clinic hours should be increased as soon as practicable and that effort should be exerted to increase the number of clinic patients. Some additional small items of equipment must be procured. The teaching function of a practicing clinic can not be over-emphasized in the training of chiropractors and it was believed that an above average job was being done at the Cleveland College in Kansas City.

LIBRARY

The greatest weakness of the educational program at the college was the library. The College must employ an adequately trained librarian and must keep the facility open for student and faculty use for a reasonable number of hours for both divisions. The library has a small, basic collection of books, a less than adequate collection of periodicals and must become a more functional part of the teaching function of the college. We believe the administration and faculty of the college are aware of this deficiency and that every effort will be made soon to correct it.

STUDENT PERSONNEL SERVICES

The committee felt that the admissions program was acceptable. The college has the facilities for a larger student body and as soon as practicable steps should be taken to increase enrollments. The financial aids program for students was minimal and as soon as practicable should be financed more adequately. Health provisions for students were acceptable. The range of extra curricular activities was quite small and should be expanded when possible.

The committee was made aware of the plans for a remodeling project to provide an adequate student lounge. We consider this item to have a top priority and urge that every effort be made to provide a well equipped lounge for students and faculty. This need is of prime importance.

The alumni program seemed to be adequate. As soon as possible the college should employ at least a part time alumni director who could devote a major part of his time and attention to securing increased alumni support in several areas.

The procedures used in registration seemed to work quite well and the student records that were kept are quite acceptable. It is believed however, that immediate attention should be devoted to increasing the security of the records as they are not at present adequately protected against either fire damage or alteration by unauthorized people. As a minimum they should be kept in a fire resistant, locked file or cabinet.

PHYSICAL PLANT

The physical plant and the site of the college are in general quite good. The buildings are kept in good condition and the college is aware of its needs in this area. Space is very well utilized in the main building and the plans for future construction seem to be soundly conceived. Hopefully the college in due time will be able to finance and build some student housing. As resources permit the campus should be landscaped and the parking facilities should be surfaced and marked for more orderly parking.

SUMMARY

Cleveland College of Chiropractic in Kansas City, Missouri has many strengths, including a sound basic program, a loyal and interested faculty, a functional physical plant and a student body that believes it is receiving a fine educational training. In the opinion of the committee the college is graduating competent chiropractors. The main areas of concern are with the library facilities, the lack of a student lounge, the relatively small size of the student body, the small faculty, and the need for more responsibility being given the students in the clinic before they are graduated. While the committee agrees that the choice of technique to be taught is a matter for the college to decide, we do agree with some student opinion to the effect that before graduation they should be given the chance to learn several other technique approaches that have wide acceptance in chiropractic.

We feel strongly that only two, and at most three, entering classes should be accepted each year. We can not accept the duplication of instruction that students receive because of the small faculty and the four admission per year policy. We also believe that the advantages of a single session per day would far outweigh the dubious claim that many students could not attend unless separate day and evening colleges are maintained.

The committee does feel that the administration and faculty of the college have complete awareness of the areas of the program that must be strengthened.

EXAMINING COMMITTEE

H. Ronald Frogley	Executive Vice-President, Palmer College of Chiropractic, Davenport, Iowa (College Repr.)
William W. Kalas	Glendale, Arizona (Practicing Chiropractor and State Board of Chiropractic Repr.)
Joseph P. Mazzarelli	Pennsauken, New Jersey (Practicing Chiropractor)
Ted McCarrel	Education Consultant, Sun City, Arizona (Generalist)

Appendix D

CHRONOLOGY OF EVENTS AND ACTIVITIES RELATED TO THE APPLICATION FOR CORRESPONDENT STATUS OF THE SHERMAN COLLEGE OF CHIROPRACTIC

This appendix chronicles the events during the application for Correspondent Status by Sherman College of Chiropractic (SCC) (now named Sherman College of Straight Chiropractic - SCSC) to the Commission on Accreditation (COA) of the Council on Chiropractic Education (CCE). (CCE Archives, file #14-06-1983)

1. 8 January 1974. Letter from the President of the CCE, Dr. Orval Hidde, to Dr. T.A. Gelardi, President of SCC, inviting Dr. Gelardi and other SCC representatives of the institution to attend any or all of the CCE meetings scheduled for February 1974, and also to meet with representatives of the COA.

2. 7-10 February 1974. Drs. T.A. Gelardi and Marvin Buncher, representatives of SCC, meet with the CCE and the COA. The accreditation process is discussed.

3. 4 July 1974. Drs. Gelardi and Buncher meet with the COA in formal session. Progress of the college and the accreditation process are discussed.

4. 5-7 July 1974. Drs. Gelardi and Buncher participate in the CCE meetings.

5. February-August 1974. The CCE President, COA Chairman, and CCE Executive Secretary respond to numerous telephone and written requests from SCC representatives for information on the accreditation process.

6. August 1974. Draft of the SCC Institutional Analysis Report is submitted to the CCE Executive Offices. CCE staff requests additional materials.

7. 13 December 1974. The revised SCC Institutional Analysis Report is submitted to the COA (dated 27 November 1974) under cover letter from SCC Dean JoAnn F. Eastes.

8. 13 February 1975. Dr. Gelardi meets with the COA to discuss the report. The Commission decides to send a three-person Evaluation Team to visit the institution.

9. 20-22 May 1975. Evaluation Team conducts an on-site visit. The team is accompanied by an observer, appointed by the United States Office of Education (USOE), Dr. George W. Villafranca, Professor of Biology, Smith College.

10. 22 May 1975. Findings of the Evaluation Team are discussed with Dr. Gelardi and SCC legal counsel during the exit interview.

11. Period between 22 May 1975 and 23 July 1975:
    A. Initial draft composite of the Evaluation Team report is submitted to Dr. Gelardi for review and correction (if appropriate) of factual errors.
    B. Final composite Evaluation Team report is submitted to Dr. Gelardi with opportunity to provide written comment.

12. 23 July 1975. The COA conducts a hearing on the application. Present were: SCC President, Dr. Gelardi; all three members of the Evaluation Team; and, Mr. Larry Freidrich, staff representative of the Division of Eligibility and Agency Evaluation of the

USOE.

13. 24 July 1975. The COA adopts a resolution denying the application of the SCC for Correspondent status. The resolution is read to Dr. Gelardi before the full Commission and questions concerning the resolution are answered. The resolution encourages the institution to address its deficiencies and reapply.
14. 1 October 1975. The SCC files and appeal memorandum with the CCE.

15. 25 November 1975. The CCE files its response to the appeal.

16. 16 December 1975. A three member Appeal Panel is appointed.

17. Period between 16 December 1975 and 29-30 January 1976:
    A.   The Appeal Panel selects its own Chairman and Secretary.
    B.   The Appeal Panel receives written material from both appellant and the appellee.

18. 29-30 January 1976. The Appeal Hearing is conducted in Atlanta, Georgia. An observer appointed by the USOE is Dr. John Barrows, Director of Institutional Studies, University of Kentucky.

19. 31 January 1976. The Appeal Panel distributes its report. The decision of the Appeal Panel is to unanimously sustain the decision of the COA to deny the application of the SCC for Correspondent Status.

20. 27-29 January 1977. The COA votes unanimously to invoke the waiver of confidentiality clause in the Educational Standards for Chiropractic Colleges, in response to an action of the SCC in disclosing a part of the confidential accreditation process to the Board of Medical Examiners of the State of New Jersey.

21. Period following 31 January 1976:
    A.   The SCC does not reapply for status with the CCE;
    B.   The SCC changes its name to the SCSC.

REFERENCES

ACA has new librarian. ACA Journal of Chiropractic 1970 (Nov); 7(11): 18

ACA Journal of Chiropractic 1964a (Sept); 1(9): 15

ACA Journal of Chiropractic 1964b (Nov); 1(11): 24

ACC/American College of Chiropractors. Medical education versus chiropractic education. Pamphlet, "National Publicity Series No.3." New York NY: the College, 1927

ACC accredited colleges represent more than 71% of chiropractic students. Association of Chiropractic Colleges, news release, July 18, 1974 (CCE Archives)

Accreditation opposed. American Medical News, April 30, 1973a, p. 9

Accreditation committee meets, unpublished, November 10-11, 1973b (CCE Archives)

Achenbach HF. A comprehensive report of the most outstanding convention in history. Journal of the National Chiropractic Association 1961 (Aug); 31(8): 9-22, 56, 58, 60, 62, 64, 66, 68

ACEI/Allied Chiropractic Educational Institutions. In the matter of the preservation of chiropractic: an address. Issued July 20, 1940 (Ratledge papers, Cleveland Chiropractic College of Kansas City)

ACEI/Allied Chiropractic Educational Institutions. Minutes of special meeting, March 15, 1941, Oklahoma City (Ratledge papers, Cleveland Chiropractic College of Kansas City)

Acquaviva JA. Standardization of curricula is our greatest need. The Chiropractic Journal (NCA) 1934 (Oct); 3(10): 8, 30, 32

Adams AA. Basic science data: the first compilation of pertinent basic science information. ICA International Review of Chiropractic 1957 (May); 11(11): 14-6

Adams PJ. Report on the England case. Journal of the National Chiropractic Association 1961 (Jan); 31(1): 22

Adams PJ. Trial of the England case. ACA Journal of Chiropractic 1965 (May); 2(5): 13, 44

Advertisement for the National College of Chiropractic. Bulletin of the American Chiropractic Association 1927 (Mar); 4(2): rear cover

Advertisement for Cale Chiropractic Naturopathic College. The California Chiropractor 1928a (Dec); 1(6): 29

Advertisement for sale of physiotherapy equipment by Hugh B. Logan. The California Chiropractor 1928b (Aug); 1(2): 28

Advertisement for "Logan and Logan." The California Chiropractor 1928c (Dec); 1(6): 29

Advertisement for the Affiliated Universities of Natural Healing. The Chiropractic Journal (NCA) 1935 (Dec); 4(12): 41

Advertisement for the Cleveland Chiropractic College. The Chiropractic Journal (NCA); 1936 (Feb); 5(2): 40

Advertisement. National Chiropractic Journal 1948 (Nov); 18(11): 70

Ambrose ES. Letter to Leonard W. Rutherford, D.C., 3 July 1974 (CCE Archives)

American Association of Colleges of Osteopathic Medicine. The education of osteopathic physicians, 1979-80. Washington DC: AACOM, 1979

American Chiropractic Association: the ICA position. Digest of Chiropractic Economics 1963; June, p. 8

American Chiropractic Association. Chiropractic: state of the art, 1991-1992. Arlington VA: the Association, 1991

Anderson D. My impressions after a first reading of the report, "Chiropractic in California." Journal of the National Chiropractic Association 1960 (Oct); 30(10): 9-11, 73-5

Anderson D. Chiropractic in California - and the nation. Webster City IA: National Chiropractic Association, 1961

Anderson JG. Letter to J.C. Keating, 10 January 1992

Anderson JG. Interview with J.C. Keating, 20 November 1995

Anderson JG, Dishman RW. Interview with J.C. Keating, M. Oliva and R.B. Phillips, 14 February 1992

Anderson RT. Letter to J.C. Keating, 21 November 1995

Announcing - post-graduate classes in advanced technique, Bio-Mechanics=Bio-Engineering, free to all NCA members! The Chiropractic Journal (NCA) 1938 (Feb); 7(2): 4

Announcing the Graduate School Program of the Chiropractic Institute of New York; brochure, 1954 (CCE Archive)

Annual convention of the International Chiropractic Research Foundation. The Chiropractic Journal (NCA) 1934 (Oct); 3(10): 18

Application to the Committee on Educational Standards for the National Chiropractic Association from the American School of Chiropractic, Inc., 1941 (CCE Archives)

Application to the Committee on Educational Standards for the National Chiropractic Association from the Metropolitan College of Chiropractic; 24 June 1941b (CCE Archives, file #35-18-1941)

Aquarian-Age Healing (advertisement). The Chiropractic Journal (NCA) 1933 (July); 1(7): 25

Armstrong KS, Moore L, Wise LM. A report on chiropractic politics and education. Atlanta GA: Chiropractic Foundation of America, Inc., 1979

Articles of incorporation for The Chiropractic College, April 16, 1913 (Special Collections of the Library of the Texas Chiropractic College)

Articles of incorporation of the Los Angeles College of Chiropractic. October 18, 1911, Office of the Secretary of State, Sacramento CA

Articles of incorporation for the North American Association of Chiropractic Schools and Colleges (NAACSC), March 1, 1952 (Cleveland papers, Cleveland Chiropractic College of Kansas City)

Articles of incorporation of the Association of American Chiropractic Colleges. (CCE Archives, #31-02-1968)

Articles of incorporation for the Association of Chiropractic Colleges. November 3, 1969, Scott County, Iowa, Book 21 of Incorporations, Page 181 (CCE Archives)

Articles of incorporation of the International Chiropractic College of Neurovertebrology. Sacramento CA: Office of the Secretary of State, January 31, 1973

Ashworth SL. Letter to A.W. Schweitert, D.C., 16 October 1928 (Ashworth papers, Cleveland Chiropractic College of Kansas City)

Ashworth SL. Letter to Ruth Cleveland, D.C., 30 August 1944 (Ashworth papers, Cleveland Chiropractic College of Kansas City)

Association notes: Ernest J. Smith: the oldest practicing D.C.? Chiropractic History 1988 (Dec); 8(2): 6

Association of Chiropractic Colleges: a Digest report to the profession. Digest of Chiropractic Economics 1971; May/June: Supplement B-C

Association of Chiropractic Colleges. Report to the CCE. January 1984

Association of Chiropractic Colleges. Report to the CCE. January 1988.

Association of Chiropractic College Presidents. Report to the CCE. 26 January 1984.

A tribute. ICA International Review of Chiropractic 1951 (Sept); 6(3):8

Baer HA. Practice-building seminars in chiropractic: a petit bourgeois response to biomedical domination. Medical Anthropology Quarterly 1996; 10(1): 29-44

Barad AD. Pre-chiropractic - a future necessity! National Chiropractic Journal 1948 (Jan); 18(1): 27-8, 54

Bargain day in California. Fountain Head News 1917 [A.C. 22] (May 26); 6(37): 6

Basic science mess. ICA International Review of Chiropractic 1948 (Nov); 3(5): 13

Bauer JM. Letter to C.S. Cleveland, D.C., 29 March 1937 (Cleveland papers, Cleveland Chiropractic College of Kansas City)

Beatty HG. Strengthening the foundation of chiropractic. The Journal (NCA) 1931a (Mar); 1(3): 14-5

Beatty HG. Letter to Stanley Hayes, D.C., 30 March 1931b (Collected papers of Stanley Hayes)

Beatty HG. Basic science effects on chiropractic schools. The Chiropractic Journal (NCA) 1935b (Mar); 4(3):8

Beatty HG. NCA schools council. The Chiropractic Journal (NCA) 1935c (June); 4(6):16

Beatty HG. Basic science laws: shall we use them to our benefit or detriment? National Chiropractic Journal 1940 (Aug); 9(8): 27

Beaumont IDE. The making of a chiropractor [a biography of M.B. DeJarnette, D.O., D.C.]. Unpublished manuscript (Archives of Palmer College of Chiropractic/West)

Bebout ER. John J. Nugent -oo-oo-oo! Bebout College of Chiropractic Newsletter 1951a; December: 4-5 (CCE Archives, #35-25-1951)

Bebout ER. Selfish expediency. Bebout College of Chiropractic Newsletter 1951b; December: 4-5 (CCE Archives, #35-25-1951)

Bebout ER. Letter to B.J. Palmer, D.C., 17 December 1952 (CCE Archives, file #35-25-1951)

Beck BL. Magnetic healing, spiritualism and chiropractic: Palmer's union of methodologies, 1886-1895. Chiropractic History 1991 (Dec); 11(2): 10-6

Becker CU, Secretary of State. Letter to C.S. Cleveland, D.C., 22 August 1922 (Cleveland papers, Cleveland Chiropractic College of Kansas City)

Beginning - the twenties. Cleveland Chiropractic College Alumni News 1987 (Fall); 10(3): 3-5

Beideman RP. 65th anniversary of National College of Chiropractic. ACA Journal of Chiropractic 1971 (Sept); 8(9): 14-6

Beideman RP. Seeking the rational alternative: the National College of Chiropractic from 1906 to 1982. Chiropractic History 1983; 3: 16-22

Beideman RP. Oakley Smith's schism of 1908: the rise and decline of naprapathy. Chiropractic History 1994 (Dec); 14(2): 44-50

Beideman RP. In the making of a profession: the National College of Chiropractic, 1906-1981. Lombard IL: National College of Chiropractic, 1995

Bell TH. Letter to Orval L. Hidde, D.C., J.D., 26 August 1974 (CCE Archives)

Bell TH. Letter to Orval L. Hidde, D.C., J.D., 11 December 1975 (CCE Archives, #37179)

Berch FL. Legislation: a national problem. ICA International Review of Chiropractic 1949 (May); 3(11): 25-6

Bethea VC. Correspondence schools a menace to chiropractic. Bulletin of the American Chiropractic Association 1927 (Nov); 4(6): 5-7

Bierman LF. Library information committee needs your help. ACA Journal of Chiropractic 1969 (Dec); 6(12): 23

Bierring WL. An analysis of basic science laws. Journal of the American Medical Association 1948 (May 1); 137(1): 111-2

Biggs L. "Hands off chiropractic": Organized medicine's attempts to restrict chiropractic in Ontario, 1900-1925. Chiropractic History 1985; 5: 10-7

Biggs L. No bones about chiropractic? The quest for legitimacy by the Ontario chiropractic profession: 1895 to 1985. Doctoral dissertation, Department of Behavioural Sciences, University of Toronto, 1989

Biggs L. Chiropractic education: a struggle for survival. Journal of Manipulative and Physiological Therapeutics 1991 (Jan); 14(1): 22-28

Biser DE. Committee on Education meets. Journal of the National Chiropractic Association 1961 (Dec); 31(12): 54

Boline PD, Kassak K, Bronfort G, Nelson C, Anderson AV. Spinal manipulation vs. amitriptyline for the treatment of chronic tension-type headaches: a randomized clinical trial. Journal of Manipulative and Physiological Therapeutics 1995 (Mar/Apr); 18(3): 148-54

Bonham LC. Letter to W.C. Schulze. National (College) Journal of Chiropractic 1932 (June); 15(2):10

Booth ER. History of osteopathy and twentieth-century medical practice. Memorial Edition. Cincinnati OH: Caxton Press, 1924

Breen AC. Chiropractors and the treatment of back pain. Rheumatology and Rehabilitation 1977; 16: 46

Brennan MJ. Perspectives on chiropractic education in medical literature, 1910-1933. Chiropractic History 1983; 3: 24-30

Brennan PC. Ethical dimensions in chiropractic research. Journal of Chiropractic Humanities 1995; 5: 8-18

Brennan PC, Kokjohn K, Kaltinger CJ et al. Enhanced phagocytic cell respiratory burst induced by spinal manipulation: potential role of substance P. Journal of Manipulative and Physiological Therapeutics 1991; 14(7): 399-408

Brennan PC, Graham MA, Triano JJ, Hondras MA, Anderson RJ. Lymphocyte profiles in patients with chronic low back pain enrolled in a clinical trial. Journal of Manipulative and Physiological Therapeutics 1994 (May); 17(4): 219-27

A brief discourse on chiropractic and PSCC. San Lorenzo CA: Pacific States Chiropractic College, undated (circa 1980; brochure)

A brief history of the Association of Chiropractic Colleges; undated, circa 1972 (CCE Archives)

Brief resume of the activities of the International Chiropractic Congress, held in Brown Palace Hotel, Denver, Colorado, July 6-11, 1930 (Cleveland papers, Cleveland Chiropractic College of Kansas City)

Briggs OJ. Membership recruitment letter for the American Drugless Association, August 1924 (Cleveland papers, Cleveland Chiropractic College of Kansas City)

Bromley WH. Testimonial to Dr. George Haynes: a man of vision. ACA Journal of Chiropractic 1975 (Jan); 12(1): 14, 51

Bronfort G. Chiropractic versus general medical treatment of low back pain: a small scale controlled clinical trial. American Journal of Chiropractic Medicine 1989 (Dec); 2(4):145-50

Brown DM. CMCC's hazardous journey, 1945 to 1968. Journal of the Canadian Chiropractic Association 1988 (Sept); 32(3): 147-50

Brown DM. A. Earl Homewood, DC, chiropractic educator. Journal of the Canadian Chiropractic Association 1989 (Sept); 33(3): 142-6

Brown DM. CMCC's persistent pursuit of university affiliation: Part 1. Journal of the Canadian Chiropractic Association 1992 (Mar); 36(1): 33-7

Brown DM. CMCC's persistent pursuit of university affiliation: Part II: Knocking on doors and heads in Ontario, 1969 to 1988. Journal of the Canadian Chiropractic Association 1994 (Mar); 38(1): 41-54

Budden WA. Medical propaganda aided by B.J. Palmer, defeats healing arts amendment. The Chiropractic Journal (NCA) 1935a (Feb); 4(2):9, 10, 38

Budden WA. Letter. Fountain Head News 1935b [A.C. 40] (Nov); 22(12): 1

Budden WA. An outline of research projects. National Chiropractic Journal 1947 (Oct); 17(10): 11-2

Budden WA. Comments on a proposal. National Chiropractic Journal 1948 (Dec); 18(12): 24, 60

Budden WA. An analysis of recent chiropractic history and its meaning. Journal of the National Chiropractic Association 1951 (June); 21(6): 9-10

Budden WA. Two years preprofessional study. Journal of the National Chiropractic Association 1954 (Mar); 24(3): 13

Bull JP. The historical development of clinical therapeutic trials. Journal of Chronic Diseases 1959; 10: 218-48

Bulletin of the American Chiropractic Association 1927 (Sept 1); 4(5): 5

California. ACA Journal of Chiropractic 1975 (Aug); 12(8): 26

Canadian Chiropractic College, Prospectus, 1922, Toronto (CMCC Archives)

Canterbury R, Krakos G. Thirteen years after Roentgen: the origins of chiropractic radiology. Chiropractic History 1986; 6: 24-9

Carter WE. Letter to U.C.C. stockholders. Fountain Head News 1916 [A.C. 22] (Sept); 6(2): 18-20

Carver-Colorado-University of Natural Healing Arts. Chiropractic History 1994 (Dec); 14(2): 32-3

Carver W. Carver's chiropractic analysis. Oklahoma City: Carver Chiropractic College, 1909

Carver W. The open forum: letter to the Editor. Chirogram 1931 (Feb); 6(12): 10

Carver W. History of chiropractic. Oklahoma City: unpublished, mimeographed, 1936

Casey MP. Letter to William N. Coggins, D.C., 12 February 1973 (CCE Archives)

Catalogue, Lincoln Chiropractic College, for the academic year, 1943-1944. Indianapolis: the College

Catalog 1992-94. Western States Chiropractic College. Portland OR

CCA Bulletin 1931 (Dec); 1(3): 7, 13-4

CCE asked to define position on practice building, management and promotion courses. ACA Journal of Chiropractic 1976 (May); 13(5): 26

Center DB, Leach RA. The multiple baseline across subjects design: proposed use in research. Journal of Manipulative and Physiological Therapeutics 1984; 7:231-6

Certificate in Logan Universal Health-Basic Technique, awarded to S.L. Ashworth, D.C., 7 June 1935, Lincoln, Nebraska (Ashworth papers, Cleveland Chiropractic College of Kansas City)

Chance MA. Chiropractic in Denmark. Journal of the Australian Chiropractors' Association 1986 (Mar); 16(1): 8-11

Cheatham WG. Letter to T.F. Ratledge, D.C., 8 February 1939 (Ratledge papers, Cleveland Chiropractic College of Kansas City)

Cheatham WG. Letter to L.M. Rogers, D.C., 17 August 1943 (CCE Archives, #35-08-1941)

Chirogram 1925; March: 5

Chirogram 1963a (Sept/Oct); 30(8): 17

Chirogram 1963b (Nov); 30(9): 2

Chirogram 1969a (Aug); 36(8): 241

Chirogram 1969b (Aug); 36(10): 262-3

Chirogram 1974 (Nov); 41(11): 11-121

Chirogram 1975 (June); 42(6): 19

ChiroLoan - a boon to students and colleges. Dynamic Chiropractic April 22, 1996, pp. 1, 8, 33

Chiropractic diagnosis. Lincoln Bulletin, June/July, 1929, p. 1

Chiropractic education in Canada: the early decades. Chiropractic History 1985; 5: 17

Chiropractic included in the new draft law. ICA International Review of Chiropractic 1951 (July); 6(1): 11

Chiropractic colleges to be recognized by accrediting agency. Journal of the California Chiropractic Association 1952 (Apr); 8(9): 16

Chiropractic Polio Clinic Foundation. ICA International Review of Chiropractic 1954; July: 8, 31-2

Chiropractic Institute of New York, Academic Years 1962 and 1963. New York (brochure), 1962

Chiropractic loses a leader. ACA Journal of Chiropractic 1969 (June); 6(6): 23

Chiropractic education in Canada: the early decades. Chiropractic History 1985; 5: 17

Cleveland Chiropractic College in Kansas City, Missouri. Digest of Chiropractic Economics 1977 (July/Aug); 20(1): 22-3

Cleveland College. Today's Chiropractic 1975 (Mar/Apr); 4(2): 42

Cleveland CS. Letter to L.S. Hunter, D.C., 3 November 1922 (Cleveland papers, Cleveland Chiropractic College of Kansas City)

Cleveland CS. Letter to B.J. Palmer, D.C., 3 August 1926a (Cleveland papers, Cleveland Chiropractic College of Kansas City)

Cleveland CS. Letter to R.S. Marlowe, D.C., 22 October 1932 (Cleveland papers, Cleveland Chiropractic College of Kansas City)

Cleveland CS. Letter to T.F. Ratledge, D.C., 12 October 1942 (Ratledge papers, Cleveland Chiropractic College of Kansas City)

Cleveland CS. Letter to T.F. Ratledge, D.C., 10 July 1944 (Ratledge papers, Cleveland Chiropractic College of Kansas City)

Cleveland CS, Jr. Letter to B.J. Palmer clarifying content of speech by John J. Nugent to Cleveland College homecoming, circa 1949 (Cleveland papers, Cleveland Chiropractic College of Kansas City)

Cleveland CS, Jr. Letter to John J. Nugent, D.C., 2 January 1950 (Cleveland papers, Cleveland Chiropractic College of Kansas City)

Cleveland CS, Jr. Letter to Thure C. Peterson, D.C., 28 February 1952a (Cleveland papers, Cleveland Chiropractic College of Kansas City)

Cleveland CS. Letter to the National Association of Chiropractic Schools and Colleges, 21 July 1952b (Cleveland papers, Cleveland Chiropractic College of Kansas City)

Cleveland CS, Jr. Researching the subluxation on the domestic rabbit: a pilot research program conducted at the Cleveland Chiropractic College, Kansas City, Missouri. ICA Science Review of Chiropractic 1965 (Aug); 19(12): 5-28

Cleveland CS, Jr. Interview with Dorothy Marra, 7 October 1986, Los Angeles

Cleveland CS, Jr. Personal communication with the authors

Cleveland CS III. Spinal correction effects on motor and sensory functions. In Mazarelli JP (Ed.): Chiropractic interprofessional research. Torino, Italy: Edizioni Minerva Medica, 1982

Cleveland CS III. Biennial report, February 1994 - January, 1996. Scottsdale AZ: Council on Chiropractic Education, 1996

Cleveland CS III. Personal communication with the authors 26 May 1998

Cleveland CS, III, Keating JC. The postwar years, 1945-1975. Chapter 7 in Peterson D, Wiese G (Eds.): Chiropractic: an illustrated history. St. Louis: Mosby-Year Book, 1995

Cleveland postgraduate course calendar 1981. ACA Journal of Chiropractic 1981 (July); 18(7): 8

Clum G. Interview with A.K. Callender, 19 August 1998, Davenport, Iowa

CMCC curriculum undergoes transformation. Primary Contact (CMCC Alumni Newsletter) 1996 (Apr/May); 18(2): 11

Coburn D. Legitimacy at the expense of narrowing of scope of practice: chiropractic in Canada. Journal of Manipulative and Physiological Therapeutics 1991 (Jan); 14(1): 14-21

Coggins WN. Letter to Carl S. Cleveland, Jr., D.C., 29 September 1952 (Cleveland papers, Cleveland Chiropractic College of Kansas City)

Coggins WN. Letter to C. Robert Hastings, D.C., 1 August 1972 (CCE Archives)

Coggins WN, Frogley HR, McCarrel T. General statement from the Association of Chiropractic Colleges, August 1972 (CCE Archives)

Coggins WN. Letter to C. Robert Hastings, D.C., (FCLB), 26 March 1974 (CCE Archives)

College of Chiropractic Physicians and Surgeons. Announcements, 1934. Los Angeles

College directory. Today's Chiropractic 1995 (May/June); 24(3): 104-115

Collins FW. Letter to the field. 26 March 1923 (Cleveland papers, Cleveland Chiropractic College, Kansas City)

Collins FW. Letter to Roy S. Neal, 17 October 1924 (Cleveland papers, Cleveland Chiropractic College of Kansas City)

Collins FW. The naturopathic method of reducing dislocations after the great French physician LeGrange. Newark NJ: United States School of Naturopathy, 1924b

Collins JE. A report on the Louisiana case in the federal court. Journal of the National Chiropractic Association 1959 (July); 29(7): 24, 52, 54

Columbia and Atlantic States colleges merge. Digest of Chiropractic Economics 1964a; September/October: 9

Columbia and Atlantic States colleges merge: consolidation of both institutions achieved on September 21, 1964. ACA Journal of Chiropractic 1964b (Nov); 1(11): 24

Columbia Institute of Chiropractic...fifty years of progress. Digest of Chiropractic Economics 1969 (Sept/Oct); 12(2): 26-7

Conlin JF. Letter to the membership of the Massachusetts Medical Society, 26 March 1953

Conquest R. The Jefferson lecture: history, humanity and truth. National Review, 7 June 1993, pp. 28-35

Consolidation. American Drugless Healer 1913 (Aug); 3(4): 324

Contract for binding arbitration, unpublished, 10-11 November 1973 (CCE Archives)

Convention news. The Scientific Chiropractor 1939 (June); 5(1): 8-10

Cooley CS. At the crossroads! A dynamic presentation of future possibilities. Part 1. The Chiropractic Journal (NCA) 1935a (Nov); 4(11): 5-8, 20, 38

Cooley CS. At the crossroads! A dynamic presentation of future possibilities. Part 2. The Chiropractic Journal (NCA) 1935b (Dec); 4(12): 11, 12, 38

Cooper GS. The attitude of organized medicine toward chiropractic: a sociohistorical perspective. Chiropractic History 1985; 5: 18-25

Cooperstein R. Chiropraxis. Oakland CA: the author, 1990

Corporate Health Policies Group. An evaluation of federal funding policies and programs and their relationship to the chiropractic profession. Arlington VA: Foundation for Chiropractic Education and Research, December, 1991

Coulter ID. Of clouds and clocks and chiropractors: towards a theory of irrationality. American Journal of Chiropractic Medicine 1990; 3: 84-92

Coulter ID. Alternative philosophical and investigatory paradigms for chiropractic. Journal of Manipulative and Physiological Therapeutics 1993; 16: 419-25

Council on Chiropractic Education. The historical development of important aspects of chiropractic accreditation. Des Moines IA: the Council, 1984 (see Appendix B)

Council on Chiropractic Education. Annual Report, 1985. Des Moines IA: the Council, 1985.

Council on Chiropractic Education. Annual Report, 1986. Des Moines IA: the Council, 1986.

Council on Chiropractic Education. Biennial Report, 1988. Des Moines IA: the Council, 1988.

Council on Chiropractic Education. Biennial Report, 1990. Des Moines IA: the Council, 1990.

Council on Chiropractic Education. Biennial Report, 1992. West Des Moines IA: the Council, 1992.

Council on Chiropractic Education. Biennial Report, 1994. West Des Moines IA: the Council, 1994.

Council on Chiropractic Education. Biennial Report, 1996. Scottsdale AZ: the Council, 1996.

Council on Chiropractic Education. Biennial Report, 1998. Scottsdale AZ: the Council, 1998.

Coyle BA. Letter to George P. McAndrews, Esq., 27 May 1992

CRAC/Chiropractic Research Archives Collection, Volune 1, 1984

Cramp AJ. Nostrums and quackery. Chicago: American Medical Association, 1921

Crawford ME. Letter to Carl S. Cleveland, III, 29 February 1996

CRF/Chiropractic Research Foundation (Advertisement). National Chiropractic Journal 1945 (Aug); 15(8): 33

Crider WF. State boards to meet - aggressive program to be outlined. The Chiropractic Journal (NCA) 1935a (July); 4(7):7

Crider WF. Accredited colleges: definite action on standard curricula. The Chiropractic Journal (NCA) 1936 (Jan); 5(1): 10, 36, 38, 40

Crider WF. The Metropolitan College of Cleveland. Report dated 26 April 1941 (CCE Archives, #35-18-1941)

Cuneo GF. CCE's role in the evolution of chiropractic in California. California Chiropractic Journal 1990; January: 6, 8, 10

Current status of colleges related to CCE. ACA Journal of Chiropractic 1975 (June); 12(6): 26

Curtis PH. Letter to John W. Frymoyer, M.D., 23 July 1987

Dallas WH. Clinical trials: a new chiropractic research priority. ACA Journal of Chiropractic 1975 (Jul); 12(7):13-4

Davenport HW. Doctor Dock: teaching and learning medicine at the turn of the century. New Brunswick NJ: Rutgers University Press, 1987

Davis AP. Neuropathy. Dallas TX: the author, 1905

Davis AP. Neuropathy illustrated: the philosophy and practical application of drugless healing. Long Beach CA: Gaves and Hersey, 1915

Davis BP (Ed.): Advances in conservative health science. Volume 1. Proceedings of the 1982 Logan/CRC Conference on Manipulation, Diagnosis and Therapy, Logan College of Chiropractic, St. Louis, Missouri

DE is where it is!! Today's Chiropractic 1976 (Mar/Apr); 5(2): 58

DeBoer KF. An attempt to induce vertebral lesions in rabbits with vertebral lesions: preliminary report. Journal of Manipulative and Physiological Therapeutics 1981; 4:119-27

DeBoer KF. Commentary: notes from the (chiropractic college) underground. Journal of Manipulative and Physiological Therapeutics 1983; 6: 147-50

DeBoer KF. Eine kleine nacht musing. American Journal of Chiropractic Medicine 1988 (March); 1(1):41-3

Dedication of Health Research Foundation. The Oregon Chiropractor 1938 (Dec); 1(9): 1-2

Dedicatory service, Canadian Memorial Chiropractic College. Programme (pamphlet). Toronto: the College, 26 September 1947 (Archives of the Canadian Memorial Chiropractic College)

Design of the medical curriculum in relation to the health needs of the nation. A statement on the educational goals of the Texas College of Osteopathic Medicine. Fort Worth TX: the College, 1980

Digest of Chiropractic Economics 1960 (Mar/Apr); 2(5); 14-5

Digest of Chiropractic Economics 1964; March/April, pp. 24-5

Dintenfass J. Letter to J. Keating, 28 September 1995

Directory of chiropractors. American Drugless Healer 1911a (Oct); 1(2): 26

Directory of chiropractors. American Drugless Healer 1911b (Oct); 1(6): 26

Directory of chiropractors. American Drugless Healer 1911c (Nov); 1(7): 26-7

Directory of chiropractors. American Drugless Healer 1911d (Dec); 1(8): 24-5

Directory of chiropractors. American Drugless Healer 1912a (Jan); 1(9): 24-5

Directory of chiropractors. American Drugless Healer 1912b (Feb); 1(10): 28-9

Distance medicine could draw health care community closer. Outreach (National College of Chiropractic) 1996 (Feb); 12(2): 4

Division of Professional Education, State Education Department. Report to National College of Chiropractic on its Application for Registration, April 8, 1969; Albany, New York (National College Library, Special Collections)

Dock G. A visit to a chiropractic school. Journal of the American Medical Association 1922 (Jan 7); 78(1): 60-3

Doll R. Darwin Lecture: Development of controlled trials in preventive and therapeutic medicine. Journal of. Biosocial Sciences 1991; 23: 365-78

Donahue JH. D.D. Palmer and Innate Intelligence: development, division, and derision. Chiropractic History 1986; 6:30-6 (a)

Donahue JH. D.D. Palmer and the metaphysical movement in the 19th century. Chiropractic History 1987; 7(1):22-7 (b)

Doyle KC. Science vs. chiropractic. Public affairs pamphlet No. 191. New York, Public Affairs Committee, Incorporated, 1953

Dr. Dave Palmer speaks at 1968 homecoming: "The state of the chiropractic union." Digest of Chiropractic Economics 1968; September/October: 38, 40

Dr. Garrow, founder and president of Pasadena Chiropractic College, steps down. Dynamic Chiropractic 1987 (Nov 15); 5(21): 1

Dr. Goldstein of NINCDS speaks at CCE meeting. ACA Journal of Chiropractic 1975 (Sept); 12(9): 20-1

Dr. Hugh B. Logan is held on postal violation charge. The Chiropractic Journal (NCA) 1937 (Nov); 6(11): 36

Dr. James W. Parker explains motivation for new chiropractic college. World-Wide Report 1981 (Mar); 23(3): 6

Dr. Leon Coelho of Palmer appointed to PSCC presidency. World-Wide Report 1978 (Oct); 20(10): 1

Dr. Napolitano of Columbia resigns from ICA Board, requests ACA accreditation. Digest of Chiropractic Economics 1964; March/April: 40

Dr. Sid E. Williams: the defender of chiropractic. Life College, internet materials, 1995

Drain JR. Letter to B.J. Palmer. Fountain Head News 1920 [A.C. 25] (April 17); 9(31): 11

Drain JR. Letter to Homer G. Beatty, D.C., N.D., 1 May 1935a (Cleveland papers, Cleveland Chiropractic College of Kansas City)

Drain JR. Letter to Carl S. Cleveland, Sr., D.C., 1 May 1935b (Cleveland papers, Cleveland Chiropractic College of Kansas City)

Drake EM. LACC in the 1980s, unpublished, circa 1994

Dunn WH. Fountain Head News 1920 [A.C. 25] (June 26); 9(41): 6-7

Dunn M, Slaughter RL, Edington KG. Is there a chiropractic science? Journal of Manipulative and Physiological Therapeutics 1990 (Sept); 13(7):412-7

Dye AA. The evolution of chiropractic. Philadelphia: the author, 1939

Dzaman F et al. (Eds.): Who's who in chiropractic. Second Edition. Littleton CO: Who's Who in Chiropractic International Publishing Co., 1980

Ebrall PS. Mechanical low-back pain: a comparison of medical and chiropractic management within the Victorian workcare scheme. Chiropractic Journal of Australia 1992 (June); 22(2): 47-53

Ebrall PS. 1945: the half-way point (or, it was fifty years ago today). Chiropractic Journal of Australia 1995 (Mar); 25(1): 6-12

Ebrall P. Chiropractic and the second hundred years: a shiny new millenium or the return of the dark ages? Journal of Manipulative and Physiological Therapeutics 1995b (Nov/Dec); 18(9): 631-5

Ebrall P. Defensible statements: an ethical consideration for scholarly writing. Journal of Chiropractic Humanities 1995c; 5: 19-27

Edited and condensed record of proceedings of the Interstate Chiropractic Congress, held at the Continental Hotel, Kansas City, Mo., June 28, 29 and 30th, 1943. Distributed by the International Chiropractors' Association, July 22, 1943 (Cleveland papers, Cleveland Chiropractic College of Kansas City)

Editorial. Chirogram 1970 (Feb); 37(2): 6

Eighth Annual Announcement, The Chiropractic University and The American Hospital, Session 1915-16. Kansas City, Missouri

Eleventh annual catalog. Chicago: National School of Chiropractic, 1918

Elliott FW. Letter to the editor. ACA Journal of Chiropractic 1968 (June); 5(6): 8

Elliott FW. Letter to Stanley Hayes, D.C., 14 October 1963 (Collected papers of Stanley Hayes, Palmer Archives)

England v. Louisiana State Board of Medical Examiners. Federal Supplement, 246 F. Supp. 993 (1965), pp. 993-7

Evaluative criteria for chiropractic colleges. Bulletin No. 1. Association of American Chiropractic Colleges, 1968 (CCE Archives, #31-01-1968)

Everyone can benefit from the January Life D.E. meeting. Digest of Chiropractic Economics 1968 (Nov/Dec); 11(3): 39

Exclusive interview with President Simon of Lincoln Chiropractic College. Digest of Chiropractic Economics 1968 (Nov/Dec); 11(3): 58-9

Extract of Hearings before the Subcommittee of the Committee on Appropriations, House of Representatives, 78th Congress, First Session on the Navy Department Appropriation Bill for 1944; Statement of Lawrence L. Gourley, Counsel, Department of Public Relations, American Osteopathic Association, Washington, D.C., correlative to Commissioning Osteopaths In The Navy. 28 April 1943 (Cleveland papers, Cleveland Chiropractic College of Kansas City)

Faculty member receives advanced degree. ACA Journal of Chiropractic 1970 (July); 7(7): 18

Fay LE. Letter to O.L. Hidde, D.C., J.D., G.H. Haynes, D.C., M.A., J. Fisher, Ph.D. and A. Steinhilder, 19 March 1973a (CCE Archives, #37523-5)

Fay LE. Letter to Ronald S. Pugsley (USOE), 21 March 1973 (CCE Archives, #37553-4)

Fay LE. The 1986 Lee-Homewood award. Chiropractic History 1986; 6: 85-6

Fay LE. Interview with A.K. Callender, 4 August 1998

Federal accreditation... a priority for chiropractic colleges. A report to the profession concerning the Association of Chiropractic Colleges. Digest of Chiropractic Economics 1970; May/June: 8-9

Ferguson A, Wiese G. How many chiropractic schools? An analysis of institutions that offered the D.C. degree. Chiropractic History 1988 (July); 8(1): 26-36

Fine PG, Roberts WJ, Gillette RG, Child TR. Slowly developing placebo responses confound tests of intravenous phentolamine to determine mechanisms underlying idiopathic chronic low back pain. Pain 1994; 56:235-42.

First students to get diplomas in chiropractics. Newspaper clipping, undated (CMCC Archives, #35-041)

Firth JN. Letter to Wilma Churchill Wood, D.C., N.D. 19 February 1941 (Ratledge papers, Cleveland Chiropractic College of Kansas City)

Fischer WH (Texas Board of Chiropractic Examiners). Letter to William N. Coggins, D.C., and Orval L. Hidde, D.C., J.D., 27 March 1972 (CCE Archives)

Fisk GA. Editorial. Chirogram 1923 (June); 2(2): 2

Flexner A. Medical education in the United States and Canada. New York: Carnegie Foundation, 1910 (reprinted 1967, Times/Arno Press, New York)

Follick E. Interview with J.C. Keating, 9 January 1996

Foreign chiropractors attend Lincoln P.G. Lincoln Bulletin, November/December, 1929, p. 2

Foreword. Lincoln Bulletin, August, 1928, p. 1

Forster AL. Principles and practice of spinal adjustment. Chicago: National School of Chiropractic, 1915

Forster AL. Higher chiropractic standards. National (College) Journal of Chiropractic 1923 (Feb); 11(6): 10-18

Founder of Pacific States College passes on. Dynamic Chiropractic 1998 (Feb 23); 16(5):30

Frankly speaking: basic science defended by Janse. ICA International Review of Chiropractic 1949 (May); 3(11): 25-6

Freedom of health...an editorial saga. St. Paul MN: Northwest News Publishing Co., undated (circa 1943)

Frogley HR. Memo to David D. Palmer, D.C., 23 May 1972a (CCE Archives)

Frogley HR. Letter to Ernest G. Napolitano, D.C., 22 August 1972b (CCE Archives)

Frogley HR. Letter to C.S. Cleveland, Sr., D.C., C.S. Cleveland, Jr., D.C., W.N. Coggins D.C., and E.G. Napolitano, D.C., 6 September 1972c (CCE Archives)

Frogley HR. Memo to David D. Palmer, D.C., 4 December 1972d (CCE Archives)

Frogley HR. Letter to Victory L. Marty D.C., (FCLB), 9 February 1973a (CCE Archives)

Frogley HR. Letter to George H. Haynes, D.C., 9 February 1973b (CCE Archives)

Frogley HR. Letter to A.D. Bogden, 4 June 1973c (CCE Archives)

Future plans for a school in New York. ACA Journal of Chiropractic 1965 (Mar); 2(3): 8

Gardner EH. California: Dr. Nugent stresses education. National Chiropractic Journal 1946 (May); 16(5): 34-5

Garrow AJ. Letter to Ernest G. Napolitano, D.C., 8 January 1974 (CCE Archive)

Gatterman MI. W.A. Budden: the transition through proprietary education, 1924-1954. Chiropractic History 1982; 2: 20-5

Gaucher-Peslherbe PL. Chiropractic: early concepts in their historical setting. Lombard IL: National College of Chiropractic, 1994

Gaucher-Peslherbe PL. Letter to the editor. Journal of Manipulative and Physiological Therapeutics 1996 (Mar); 19(3): 219

Gauthier CE. Letter to Archie W. Macfie, 6 December 1943 (Archives of the Canadian Memorial Chiropractic College, #84-229 through 84-235)

Gautvig M, Hviid A. Chiropractic in Denmark. Copenhagen: Danish Pro-Chiropractic Association, 1975

Gelardi TA. Letter to E.G. Napolitano, D.C., 18 September 1972 (CCE Archives)

Gelardi TA. New college in South Carolina: Sherman. Today's Chiropractic 1973 (Apr/May); 2(2): 16-7

Gelardi TA. Letter to March Bach, Ph.D., 19 June 1986

Gelardi TA. A very brief history of Sherman College of Straight Chiropractic. Unpublished, 12 May 1995

General requirements for graduate degrees. Chirogram 1950 (Mar); 19(3): 17

Gerlt EC. Activities of the ACA Council on Chiropractic Physiotherapy. ACA Journal of Chiropractic 1965 (Mar); 2(3): 25, 48

Gevitz N. The D.O.'s: osteopathic medicine in America. Baltimore: Johns Hopkins University Press, 1982

Gevitz N. "A coarse sieve"; basic science boards and medical licensure in the United States. Journal of the History of Medicine and Allied Sciences 1988; 43: 36-63

Gibbons RW. The evolution of chiropractic: medical and social protest in America. Notes on the survival years. Chapter One in Haldeman S. (Ed.): Modern developments in the principles and practice of chiropractic. New York: Appleton-Century-Crofts, 1980a

Gibbons RW. The rise of the chiropractic educational establishment, 1897-1980. In Dzaman F, Scheiner S, Schwartz L. Who's Who in Chiropractic, International. Second Edition. Littleton CO: Who's Who in Chiropractic International Publishing Co., 1980b

Gibbons RW. Solon Massey Langworthy: keeper of the flame during the "lost years" of chiropractic. Chiropractic History 1981a; 1: 14-21

Gibbons RW. Physician-chiropractors: medical presence in the evolution of chiropractic. Bulletin of the History of Medicine 1981b; 55: 233-45

Gibbons RW. Forgotten parameters of general practice: the chiropractic obstetrician. Chiropractic History 1982; 2: 26-33

Gibbons RW. Chiropractors as interns, residents and staff: the hospital experience, 1910-1960. Chiropractic History 1983; 3: 50-7

Gibbons RW. Chiropractic's Abraham Flexner: the lonely journey of John J. Nugent, 1935-1963. Chiropractic History 1985; 5: 44-51

Gibbons RW. Vision to action: a history of ICA: the first 60 years. ICA Review 1986 (Mar/Apr); 42(2): 33-64 (Supplement)

Gibbons RW. Fred Collins and his New Jersey "Mecca." Chiropractic History 1989 (June); 9(1): 41

Gibbons RW. Joy Loban and Andrew P. Davis: itinerant healers and "schoolmen," 1910-1923. Chiropractic History 1991 (June); 11(1): 22-8

Gibbons RW. Minnesota, 1905: who killed the first chiropractic legislation? Chiropractic History 1993 (June); 13(1): 26-32

Gibbons RW. Miscellany: the "Steam from the Fountainhead": a 1920 report by AMA's Council on Medical Education. Chiropractic History 1993 (June); 13(1): 8-11

Gibbons RW. "With malice aforethought:" revisiting the BJ Palmer "patricide" controversy. Chiropractic History 1994 (June); 14(1): 28-34

Gielow V. Old Dad Chiro: a biography of D.D. Palmer, founder of chiropractic. Davenport IA: Bawden Brothers, 1981

Giesen JM, Center DB, Leach RA. An evaluation of chiropractic manipulation as a treatment of hyperactivity in children. Journal of Manipulative and Physiological Therapeutics 1989 (Oct); 12(5): 353-63

Gillespie G. Historical aspects of drugless therapy. Address before the National Convention of the American Naturopathic Association in Los Angeles, California, November 21, 1924. Naturopath 1925; 30: 557-62

Gillett CF. A manual of the eye, ear, nose and throat. San Francisco: Kohnke Printing, 1928a

Gillett CF. The ear. The California Chiropractor, September, 1928b, pp. 16-7

Gillett CF. Examining the drumhead. The California Chiropractor 1929 (May); 1(7): 14-5

Gillett CF. The ear. The Scientific Chiropractor 1938 (Feb); 3(9): 26

Gillette RG, Kramis RC, Roberts WJ. Spinal projections of cat primary afferent fibers innervation of lumbar facet joint and multifidus muscle. Neuroscience Letters 1993a; 157:67-71.

Gillette RG, Kramis RC, Roberts WJ. Characterization of spinal somatosensory neurons having receptive fields in lumbar tissues of cats. Pain 1993b; 54:85-98.

Gingerich W. Chiropractic in your state: California. International Chiropractic News (ICA), March, 1948: no page number

Gitelman R. The history of chiropractic research and the challenge of today. Journal of the Australian Chiropractors' Association 1984 (Dec); 14(4): 142-6

Godzway AT. "That old medical fool!" said the Old Master with great disdain! The Chiropractic Journal (NCA) 1934 (Apr); 3(4): 5, 30

Goldschmidt AM. Letter to J.C. Keating, 20 January 1992

Goldstein M (Ed.): The research status of spinal manipulative therapy: a workshop held at the National Institutes of Health, February 2-4, 1975. Bethesda MD: DHEW Publication No. (NIH) 76-998, 1975

Gonthier AM. Letter to Herbert J. Vear, 28 November 1995

Goodfellow GM. Letter to T.F. Ratledge, D.C., 16 May 1940 (Ratledge papers, Cleveland Chiropractic College of Kansas City)

Goodfellow GM. National Chiropractic Journal 1945 (Jan); 15(1): 37

Graduate catalog, 1994-1995, University of Bridgeport. Bridgeport CT: the University, 1994

Green BN. A review and critique of Chiropractic History. Chiropractic History 1995 (Dec); 15(2): 9-11

Gregory AA. Spinal treatment: auxiliary method of treatment. Second Edition. Oklahoma City: Palmer-Gregory College, 1912

Griffin LK. Merger almost: ICA unity efforts and formation of the American Chiropractic Association. Chiropractic History 1988 (Dec); 8(2): 18-22

Griffin PB. Letter to prospective students, 6 January 1923 (Cleveland papers, Cleveland Chiropractic College of Kansas City)

Gruber B. Anatomist, scholar and gentleman: Arthur V. Nilsson - a legend in his own time. Chiropractic History 1984; 4:24-38

Guidelines for authors. Journal of the American Chiropractic Association 1995 (Sept); 32(9): 86

Haas M, Peterson D, Hoyer D, Ross G. The reliability of muscle testing response to a provocative vertebral challenge. Journal of Manipulative and Physiological Therapeutics 1993a; 16: 95-100

Haas M, Peterson D, Panzer D et al. Reactivity of leg alignment to articular pressure testing: evaluation of a diagnostic test using a randomized cross-over clinical trial approach. Journal of Manipulative and Physiological Therapeutics 1993b; 16: 220-7

Haas M, Peterson D, Rothman EH et al. Responsiveness of leg alignment associated with articular pressure testing to spinal manipulation: the use of a randomized clinical trial design to evaluate a diagnostic test with a dichotomous outcome. Journal of Manipulative and Physiological Therapeutics 1993c; 16: 306-11

Haas M, Panzer D, Peterson D, Raphael R. Short-term responsiveness of manual thoracic end-play assessment to spinal manipulation: a randomized controlled trial of construct validity. Journal of Manipulative and Physiological Therapeutics 1995 (Nov/Dec); 18(9): 582-9

Haldeman S. Importance of record keeping in evaluation of chiropractic results. ACA Journal of Chiropractic 1975 (Sept); 12(9): 36-42 (Vol. IX, S-108-114)

Haldeman S. Proposal for the establishment of an institution for chiropractic research and postgraduate education. Unpublished, June 1977

Haldeman S (Ed.): Modern developments in the principles and practice of chiropractic. New York: Appleton-Century-Crofts, 1980

Haldeman S. Letter from the editor-in-chief. Journal of the Neuromusculoskeletal System 1993 (Spr); 1(1): v

Haldeman S, Chapman-Smith D, Petersen DM (Eds.): Guidelines for chiropractic quality assurance and practice parameters. Gaithersburg MD: Aspen Publishers, 1993

Hancock AA. History of chiropractic orthopedics. Journal of the National Chiropractic Association 1963 (Feb); 30(2): 13-4, 72

Hariman G. Letter to Vinton F. Logan, D.C., 25 April 1952 (Cleveland papers, Cleveland Chiropractic College of Kansas City)

Hariman GE. A history of the evolution of chiropractic education. Grand Forks ND: the author, 1970

Harper WD. In tribute to Dr. Joseph Janse. ACA Journal of Chiropractic 1965 (May); 2(5): 18, 44

Harper WD. Additional commentary on accreditation, the elusive dream. Digest of Chiropractic Economics 1972; September/October: 50-1

Harring HC. Letter to Carl S. Cleveland, D.C., 18 December 1924 (Cleveland papers, Cleveland Chiropractic College of Kansas City)

Harring HC. Letter to Carl S. Cleveland, D.C., 27 January 1925a (Cleveland papers, Cleveland Chiropractic College of Kansas City)

Harring HC. A solution. Bulletin of the American Chiropractic Association 1925b (June); 2(5): 8

Harring HC. Modern trends. Journal of the National Chiropractic Association 1950 (Jan); 20(1): 28, 56

Harris W. Interview with Alana Callender, August 15, 1998

Harris W, Wagnon RJ. The effects of chiropractic adjustments on distal skin temperature. Journal of Manipulative and Physiological Therapeutics 1987; 10:57-60

Hastings CR (Federation of Chiropractic Licensing Boards). Resolution, 20 August 1972 (CCE Archives)

Hayes S. Prior arts rights. Lincoln Bulletin, August 1928, pp. 1-4

Hayes S. The schools have spoken. The Chirogram 1931a (Mar); 7(1): 18, 21-2

Hayes S. The future of chiropractic. Bulletin of the West Virginia Chiropractors' Society 1931b (May/June); 3(6): 1-10

Hayes S. Letter to Frank W. Elliott, D.C., 5 May 1963 (Collected papers of Stanley Hayes, Palmer Archives)

Hayes S. The leopard cannot change his spots. Bulletin of Rational Chiropractic 1965 (May); 3(5): 6-9

Haynes GH. Letter to Loran M. Rogers, D.C., 11 July 1962 (CCE Archives, #45167)

Haynes GH. Letter to "All members of the Council," 28 October 1969 (CCE Archives; see Appendix B)

Haynes GH. Approval of chiropractic colleges. ACA Journal of Chiropractic 1970 (May); 7(5): 20-2

Haynes GH. The evolution of chiropractic educational accreditation. Unpublished, Council on Chiropractic Education, circa 1972 (CCE Archives, pages 37575-37587)

Haynes GH. Letter to Arthur M. Schierholz, D.C., 28 February 1972a (CCE Archives, #37445)

Haynes GH. The Council on Chiropractic Education, 1947-1973. Unpublished, submitted to the Department of Health, Education and Welfare, 1973 (CCE Archives)

Haynes GH. Comparison of allopathic and chiropractic curricula in California. ACA Journal of Chiropractic 1975 (Sept); 12(9): 16-8

Hearn EB. Letter to John J. Nugent, D.C., 15 October 1958 (CCE Archives)

Heese N. Major Bertrand DeJarnette: six decades of sacro occipital research, 1924-1984. Chiropractic History 1991 (June); 11(1):12-5

H.E.W. eligibility received. WSCC Reporter 1974; October: 1

Hidde OL. Letter to Ernest G. Napolitano, D.C., 5 June 1972a (CCE Archives)

Hidde OL. Letter to William N. Coggins, D.C., 7 November 1972 (CCE Archives)

Hidde OL. Letter to William N. Coggins, D.C., 11 September 1973 (CCE Archives)

Hidde OL. Accreditation and state action. ACA Journal of Chiropractic 1975a (Feb); 12(2): 18-20

Hidde OL. Resolution. WSCC Reporter 1975b: May: 1

Higley HG. Proposal for the establishment of research in chiropractic colleges. Presentation to the NCA Council of Education, 1953, Los Angeles

Higley HG. The intervertebral disc syndrome. Webster City IA: National Chiropractic Association, 1960

Hildebrandt RW. The science of chiropractic. ACA Journal of Chiropractic 1967 (Oct); 4(10): 58-65

Hildebrandt RW. Why a Journal of Manipulative and Physiological Therapeutics? Journal of Manipulative and Physiological Therapeutics 1978 (Mar); 1(1):1-6

Hildebrandt RW. Scientific journal indexing and its effects on the chiropractic profession. Journal of Manipulative and Physiological Therapeutics 1981a (Mar); 4(1):1-4

Hildebrandt RW. Working and winning within the system. Journal of Manipulative and Physiological Therapeutics 1981b (Sept); 4(3):117-8

Himes HM. Policy talk to P.S.C. student body, January 4, 1956

Hinz DG. Diversified chiropractic: Northwestern College and John B. Wolfe, 1941-1984. Chiropractic History 1987 (July); 7(1): 34-41

Hocking T. Unpublished list of presidents of the Texas Chiropractic College, March, 1996

Hodgins FE, Royal Commission on Medical Education. Report and supporting statements on medical education. Toronto: A.T. Wilgress, 1918

Holman GL. Report on National Board of Chiropractic Examiners. ACA Journal of Chiropractic 1970 (Aug); 7(8): 26-7

Holman GL. The National Board of Chiropractic Examiners, 1963-71. Digest of Chiropractic Economics 1971a (Mar/Apr); 13(5): 12, 31

Holman GL. National Board of Chiropractic Examiners report. ACA Journal of Chiropractic 1971b (Apr); 8(4): 20-2

Holman GL. Memorandum to Association of Chiropractic College, Council on Chiropractic Education and Chiropractic College contacts, 8 February 1974 (CCE Archives)

Holmes AT. Letter to H.B. Logan. The Chiropractic Journal (NCA) 1934 (Feb); 3(2): 28

Homewood AE. The neurodynamics of the vertebral subluxation. 3rd edition. Toronto: Chiropractic Publishers, 1961/1979

Homewood AE. The chiropractor and the law. Toronto: Chiropractic Publishers, 1965

Homewood AE. 64 years of progress. Chirogram 1975 (Aug); 42(8): 19

Homola S. Bonesetting, chiropractic and cultism. Panama City FL: Critique Books, 1963

Hopkins WH. The chiropractic college crisis can be solved by chiropractic day. Lincoln Bulletin 1942; October/November: 4-6

Howard EB. Letter to Ewald Nyquist, New York State Commissioner of Education, 13 July 1972 (National College Library, Special Collections)

Hsieh CY, Phillips RB, Adams AH, Pope MH. Functional outcomes of low back pain: comparison of four treatment groups in a randomized controlled trial. Journal of Manipulative and Physiological Therapeutics 1992; 15(1): 4-9

Humphreys CR, Triano JJ, Brandl MJ. Sensitivity study of H-reflex alterations in idiopathic low back pain patients vs. a healthy population. Journal of Manipulative and Physiological Therapeutics 1989 (Apr); 12(2):71-8

Hurley JL. Letter to H.O. Langford, D.C., 14 February 1942 (Archives of the Canadian Memorial Chiropractic College)

Hurley JL. Report on the case of Hurley vs. Logan; pamphlet. Ft. Lauderdale FL: Aquarian-Age Healing Institute, undated-a, circa 1942 (National College Library, Special Collections)

Hurley JL. Letter to "Dear Doctor" and brochure. Ft. Lauderdale FL: Aquarian-Age Healing Institute, undated-b, circa 1943 (Cleveland papers, Cleveland Chiropractic College of Kansas City)

Hurley JL, Sanders HE. Aquarian age healing for you. Two volumes. Los Angeles: Haynes Corporation, 1932

Hviid H. A Scandinavian chiropractic education: yesterday and today. European Journal of Chiropractic 1990; 38: 35-40

ICA International Review of Chiropractic 1949 (Oct); 4(4): 18

ICA (International Chiropractors' Association). Vision to action: a history of ICA, the first 60 years. ICA Review 1986 (Mar/Apr); 42(2):33-64 (Supplement)

Important announcement. Fountain Head News 1919 [A.C. 25] (Nov 1); 9(7): 8

Important warning to GI students of chiropractic. National Chiropractic Journal 1948 (Sept); 18(9): 27

In memoriam. ACA Journal of Chiropractic 1975 (Sept); 12(9): 21

It's up to you to make the next move...Life D.E. meeting. Digest of Chiropractic Economics 1968 (Sept/Oct); 11(2): 51

Jackson RB. Letter to J.C. Keating, 25 February 1993

Jackson RB. Willard Carver, LL.B., D.C., 1866-1943: doctor, lawyer, Indian chief, prisoner and more. Chiropractic History 1994 (Dec); 14(2): 12-21

Jacobs G. Editorial. Journal of Chiropractic Education 1987; 1(1):2.

Jamison JR. Looking to the future: from chiropractic philosophy to the philosophy of chiropractic. Chiropractic Journal of Australia 1991; 21: 168-75

Janse J. National-Lincoln Colleges sign affiliation agreement. Digest of Chiropractic Economics 1971 (Sept/Oct); 14(2): 56-7

Janse J. Letter to A.E. Anderson, 26 July 1972 (National College Library, Special Collections)

Janse J. Memorandum to all staff members to include administration, faculty and clinic staff, 24 August 1978 (National College Library, Special Collections)

Jarvis KB, Phillips RB, Morris EK. Cost per case comparison of back injury claims of chiropractic versus medical management for conditions with identical diagnostic codes. Journal of Occupational Medicine 1991; 33(8): 847-52

Jensen B. Doctor-patient handbook. Escondido CA: Bernard Jensen Enterprises, 1976

Jensen K. Chiropractic expansion: Palmer buys California College. Quad-City Times, September 19, 1980, p. 9

Jochims L. Allopathic medicine in Kansas, 1950-1900. Archives of the California Chiropractic Association 1982; 6(1): 67-79

Johnson AC. Chiropractic physiological therapeutics. 5th edition. Palm Springs CA: the author, 1977

Johnson MR, Ferguson AC, Swank LL. Treatment and cost of back or neck injury: a literature review. Research Forum 1985 (Spring); 1(3): 68-78

Johnson MR, Schultz MK, Ferguson AC. A comparison of chiropractic, medical and osteopathic care for work-related sprains and strains. Journal of Manipulative and Physiological Therapeutics 1989; 12(5): 335-44

Joseph B. Strauss, D.C. elected president. Cactus Flower 1979 (Nov); 2(4): 3

Journal of the International Chiropractic Congress 1932 (Feb); 1(3): 6, 16

Journal of the California Chiropractic Association 1949 (Nov); 6(5): 17

Journal of the California Chiropractic Association 1951 (Mar); 7(9): 15-6

Julander SE. Letter to Cleveland Chiropractic College, 25 February 1935 (Cleveland papers, Cleveland Chiropractic College of Kansas City)

Kaminski M, Boal R, Gillette RG, Peterson DH, Villnave TJ. A model for the evaluation of chiropractic methods. Journal of Manipulative and Physiological Therapeutics 1987 (Apr); 10(2):61-4

Kaminski M, Boal R. An effect of ascorbic acid on delayed-onset muscle soreness. Pain 1992; 50: 317-21

Kansas State Board of Healing Arts, Chiropractic Division. A brief commentary on the comparative analysis of the criteria, procedures and rules of the C.C.E. and the A.C.C.; undated, circa 1972 (CCE Archives)

Keating JC. C.O. Watkins: pioneer advocate for clinical scientific chiropractic. Chiropractic History 1987 (Dec); 7(2):10-5

Keating JC. C.O. Watkins, D.C., F.I.C.C., Doctor of Humanities. Journal of the Canadian Chiropractic Association 1988 (Dec); 32(4):199-202

Keating JC. Priorities in chiropractic historical research and preservation. American Journal of Chiropractic Medicine 1990a (Mar); 3(1):36-9

Keating JC. Letter to the editor: Lincoln walkout: was it prompted by the NCM? Chiropractic History 1990b (June); 10(1): 8

Keating JC. Introducing the neurocalometer: a view from the Fountain Head. Journal of the Canadian Chiropractic Association 1991a (Sept); 35(3):165-78

Keating JC. The embryology of chiropractic thought. European Journal of Chiropractic 1991b (Dec); 39(3): 75-89

Keating JC. Toward a philosophy of the science of chiropractic: a primer for clinicians. Stockton CA: Stockton Foundation for Chiropractic Research, 1992a

Keating JC. Letter to the editors re: Chiropractic instrumentation. Chiropractic Journal of Australia 1992b (June); 22(2): 66-7

Keating JC. At the crossroads: the National Chiropractic Association celebrates chiropractic's fortieth anniversary. Chiropractic Technique 1993a (Nov); 5(4): 152-67

Keating JC. Old Dad Chiro comes to Portland, 1908-10. Chiropractic History 1993b (Dec); 13(2): 36-44

Keating JC. The influence of World War 1 upon the chiropractic profession. Journal of Chiropractic Humanities 1994a; 4: 36-55

Keating JC. Letter to the editor: addenda to the patricide controversy. Chiropractic History 1994b (Dec); 14(2): 6

Keating JC. Shhh!!!...Radiophone station WOC is on the air, 1922-1932. European Journal of Chiropractic 1995 (Aug); 43(2): 21-37

Keating JC, Booher JA, Door FA. JMPT: a 1987-88 update. Chiropractic Technique 1989 (Nov); 1(4):146-9

Keating JC, Brown RA, Smallie P. Tullius de Florence Ratledge: the missionary of straight chiropractic in California. Chiropractic History 1991 (Dec); 11(2): 26-38

Keating JC, Brown RA, Smallie P. One of the roots of straight chiropractic: Tullius de Florence Ratledge. In Sweere JJ (Ed.): Chiropractic Family Practice, Volume 1. Gaithersburg MD: Aspen Publishers, 1992

Keating JC, Cleveland CS. Sylva L. Ashworth, D.C., the "Grand Old Lady of Chiropractic." Chiropractic History 1992 (Dec); 12(2): 14-23

Keating JC, Cleveland CS. Cleveland chiropractic: the early years, 1917-1933. Journal of Manipulative and Physiological Therapeutics 1996 (June); 19(5): 324-43

Keating JC, Dishman RW. A happy warrior passes: Ralph J. Martin, D.C., Ph.C., N.D., 1904-1994. Dynamic Chiropractic, April 22, 1994, pp. 40-1

Keating JC, Dishman RW, Oliva M, Phillips RB. Roots of the LACC: the Southern California College of Chiropractic. Journal of Chiropractic Humanities 1993; 3: 21-41

Keating JC, Giljum K, Menke JM, Lonczak RS, Meeker WC. Toward an experimental chiropractic: time-series designs. Journal of Manipulative and Physiological Therapeutics 1985 (Dec); 8(4):185-9

Keating JC, Green BN, Johnson CD. "Research" and "science" in the first half of the chiropractic century. Journal of Manipulative and Physiological Therapeutics 1995 (July/Aug); 18(6): 357-78

Keating JC, Haldeman S. Joshua N. Haldeman, D.C.: the Canadian years, 1926-1950. Journal of the Canadian Chiropractic Association 1995 (Sept); 39(3): 172-86

Keating JC, Hansen DT. Quackery vs. accountability in the marketing of chiropractic. Journal of Manipulative and Physiological Therapeutics 1992 (Sept); 15(7): 459-70

Keating JC, Jackson RB, Oliva M, Phillips RB. Origins of the LACC, 1901-1922. Journal of Manipulative and Physiological Therapeutics 1994 (Feb); 17(2): 93-106

Keating JC, Larson K, Stephens M, Mick TJ. The Journal of Manipulative and Physiological Therapeutics: a bibliographic analysis. Journal of Manipulative and Physiological Therapeutics 1989 (Feb); 12(1):15-20

Keating JC, Nelson JM, Mootz RD. A model for clinical, scientific and educational development. Research Forum 1986 (Sum); 2(4):103-14

Keating JC, Rehm WS. The origins and early history of the National Chiropractic Association. Journal of the Canadian Chiropractic Association 1993 (Mar); 37(1): 27-51

Keating JC, Rehm WS. William C. Schulze, M.D., D.C. (1870-1936): from mail-order mechano-therapists to scholarship and professionalism among drugless physicians, Part I. Chiropractic Journal of Australia 1995a (Sept); 25(3): 82-92

Keating JC, Rehm WS. William C. Schulze, M.D., D.C. (1870-1936): from mail-order mechano-therapists to scholarship and professionalism among drugless physicians, Part II. Chiropractic Journal of Australia 1995b (Dec); 25(4): 122-8

Keating JC, Young MA. Who is the chiropractic scientific community? Journal of the Australian Chiropractors' Association 1987 (Sept); 17(3):84-6

Kennedy K. Reflections and experiences in the early days of CMCC. In: Fortieth Year Celebration. Toronto: Canadian Memorial Chiropractic College, 1985, pp. 4-5

Key C. Letter to L.M. Rogers, D.C., 23 August 1949a (CCE Archives, #35-18-1941)

Key C. Letter to John J. Nugent, D.C., 23 August 1949b (CCE Archives, #35-18-1941)

Kightlinger CM. Reprint of letter to the Officers and Board of Directors of the UCA. Bulletin of the American Chiropractic Association 1925 (June); 2(5): 14

Kightlinger CM. Natural law. Bulletin of the American Chiropractic Association 1928 (Jan); 5(1): 9-10

Kightlinger CM. Letter to C.S. Cleveland, D.C., 23 March 1936 (Cleveland papers, Cleveland Chiropractic College of Kansas City)

Kightlinger CM. Chiropractic education: the day of short professional course is over. National Chiropractic Journal 1940 (Nov); 9(11): 9, 56

Kightlinger CM. Letter to John J. Nugent, D.C., 13 September 1943 (CCE Archives, #35-12-1938)

Kightlinger CM. Letter to the Board of Directors and officers of the N.C.A., and Dr. John J. Nugent, 24 January 1944 (CCE Archives, #35-12-1938)

Kimmel EH. Junior ACA day at CINY. ACA Journal of Chiropractic 1965 (July); 2(7): 21, 50

Kindig DA. Letter to Reginald R. Gold, 30 January 1976; cited in Strauss JB. Refined by fire: the evolution of straight chiropractic. Levittown PA: Foundation for the Advancement of Chiropractic Education, 1994, p. 230

Kirby JD. Psychosomatic aspects of practice. ACA Journal of Chiropractic 1964 (Nov); 1(11): 18-9, 56

Kirby JD. Editorial. Chirogram 1974 (Nov); 41(11): 6-7

Kirby JD. A special tribute. The Chiro-Practor 1979 (May/June); 2(4): 28

Kirchfeld F, Boyle W. Nature doctors: pioneers in naturopathic medicine. Portland OR: Medicina Biologica, 1994

Korr IM (Ed.): The neurobiologic mechanisms in manipulative therapy. New York: Plenum Press, 1978

Kranz KC. The public bootstrapping of physical therapy to a provider profession, 1919-86. Chiropractic History 1986; 6: 38-48

LACC's red-letter dates. LACC News and Alumni Report, Diamond Jubilee Issue 1986; 9(3):21-5

LACC, subsidiary of California Chiropractic Colleges. Chirogram 1971 (Jan); 38(1):1

Laing BL. Chiropractic society of ear, nose and throat. Chirogram 1951 (July); 20(7): 12

Lasagna L. The controlled clinical trial: theory and practice. Journal of Chronic Diseases 1955 (Apr); 1(4): 353-67

LaValley, John E. The biography of Dr. John E. La'Valley, Portland Oregon, May 25th, 1955. (Archives of Western States Chiropractic College)

Leach RA. The chiropractic theories: principles and clinical applications. Third Edition. Baltimore: Williams and Wilkins, 1994

Leboeuf C, Brown P, Herman A Leembruggen K, Walton D, Crisp TC. Chiropractic care of children with nocturnal enuresis: a prospective outcome study. Journal of Manipulative and Physiological Therapeutics 1991 (Feb); 14(2): 110-5

Lee HK. Honoring the founder in his country: conception and struggle for Canada's Memorial College. Chiropractic History 1981; 1: 42-5

Lee HK. Anecdotes and recollections: chiropractic pioneers I have known. Journal of the Canadian Chiropractic Association 1981c (June): 25(2): 75

Lee HK. Anecdotes and recollections: chiropractic pioneers I have known. Journal of the Canadian Chiropractic Association 1981d (Dec): 25(4):161

Lee HK. The establishment and early years of the Canadian Memorial Chiropractic College; unpublished and undated (Archives of the Canadian Memorial Chiropractic College)

Lee LE. Force the issue. Bulletin of the American Chiropractic Association 1927 (Mar); 4(2): 11-2

Lehman DJ. Letter to Reubin Askew, D.C., Governor of Florida, 16 December 1977 (CCE Archives, #21360)

Lehman DJ. Letter to John R. Proffitt (USOE), 19 January 1978 (CCE Archives, #21358)

Lerner C. Report on the history of chiropractic. 1954, unpublished manuscript in 8 volumes (Lyndon E. Lee Papers, Palmer College Archives)

Lessons in chiropractic. Davenport IA: Palmer School of Correspondence, 1911

Levine MR, Meyer JJ, Esch CH, Mason WR. Multiple interrupted time-series designs as a diagnostic tool: a case study of the relationship between caffeine ingestion and chronic benign premature ventricular contractions. American Journal of Chiropractic Medicine 1990 (Mar); 3(1):9-13

"Liberal" versus "straight" in California: Steele court action. National College Journal of Chiropractic 1933 (Sept); 16(3):12

Life Chiropractic College opens January 20. Today's Chiropractic 1975a (Jan/Feb); 4(1): 10

Life Chiropractic College has formal opening. Today's Chiropractic 1975b (Mar/Apr); 4(2): 24-5

Life Chiropractic College. Today's Chiropractic 1975c (May/June); 4(3): 32

Life at Life College shows expansion of the profession. World-Wide Report 1981 (Mar); 23(3): 5

Life College. ICA International Review of Chiropractic 1995a (Sept/Oct); 51(5): 137-8

Life Chiropractic College West. ICA International Review of Chiropractic 1995a (Sept/Oct); 51(5): 138-9

Lillard H. Deaf seventeen years. The Chiropractic 1897a (Jan); Number 17, p. 3 (Palmer College Archives)

Lillienfeld AM. Ceteris Parabus: the evolution of the clinical trial. Bulletin of the History of Medicine 1982; 56: 1-18

Lincoln Bulletin, November, 1927, p. 1

Lincoln College enlarges quarters. Lincoln Bulletin, June/July, 1929, p. 2

Lincoln men in the armed service. Lincoln Bulletin 1942; October/November: 2

Locklar JH. Letter to friends of Carver Chiropractic College, January 1954 (Cleveland papers, Cleveland Chiropractic College of Kansas City)

Logan HB. Medicine vs. physicians. The California Chiropractor 1928a (Aug); 1(2): 14

Logan VF. Specific adjustment applied to spinal balance. The California Chiropractor 1928b (Dec); 1(6): 10-11

Logan Basic College of Chiropractic; brochure, June, 1943 (Cleveland papers, Cleveland Chiropractic College of Kansas City)

Logan Basic College of Chiropractic, Catalog, 1952-1953. St. Louis

Logan VF. The issue must be met. ICA International Review of Chiropractic 1949 (June); 3(12): 16-8

Logan VF. Letter to C.S. Cleveland Jr., D.C., 29 December 1952 (Cleveland papers, Cleveland Chiropractic College of Kansas City)

Lombardo DM. William H. Werner and the American Bureau of Chiropractic: organizing a lay constituency. Chiropractic History 1990 (June); 10(10: 24-9

Los Angeles College of Chiropractic, 1995 annual progress report. Submitted to the Western Association of Schools and Colleges. Whittier CA: April, 1995

Los Gatos campus progress report. Chirogram 1975a (Sept); 42(9): 22-3

Los Gatos campus progress report. Chirogram 1975b (Oct); 42(10): 22-3

Los Gatos campus progress report. Chirogram 1975c (Dec); 42(12): 16-20

Louisiana's 'England' case nears court date. Digest of Chiropractic Economics 1959 (July/Aug); 2(1): 19

Lupica B. Editorial. Chirogram 1947 (Aug); 16(10): 5, 7

Lyceum, Life Chiropractic College, over $857,840 pledged. Today's Chiropractic 1974 (Aug/Sept); 3(4): 6-8

Maher TF. Letter. The Chiropractic Journal (NCA) 1934 (Aug); 3(8): 29

Mannello DM, Lawrence DJ, Mootz RD. The evolution of chiropractic research: a foundation for technology assessment. Topics in Clinical Chiropractic 1996 (Mar); 3(1): 52-64

Margetts FR. Does chiropractic need a saviour? Bulletin of the American Chiropractic Association 1924 (Sept); 1(4): 1

Marsh TH. Letter to J.C. Keating, 19 April 1991

Martin P. Interview with J.C. Keating, 29 May 1992 (Library Archives, Palmer College of Chiropractic-West)

Martin RJ. ACA gives new emphasis to research. ACA Journal of Chiropractic 1969 (Oct); 6(10): 51-4

Martin RJ. The objectives of research. ACA Journal of Chiropractic 1970 (Sept); 7(9): 19

Martin RJ. Federal recognition of chiropractic accreditation agency: a story of vision and supreme effort. Chirogram 1974 (Nov); 41(11): 6-21

Martin RJ. The practice of correction of abnormal function. "Neurovascular Dynamics" (NVD). First Edition. Sierra Madre CA: self-published, 1977

Martin RJ. The LACC story: fifty years in chiropractic. August 8, 1986; unpublished paper prepared for presentation to the LACC Alumni meeting in October, 1986

Martin SC. "The only truly scientific method of healing": chiropractic and American science, 1895-1990. Isis 1994; 85: 207-27

Marty VL. Letter to H.R. Frogley, D.C., 7 February 1973 (CCE Archives)

Mawhiney RB. Chiropractic in Wisconsin, 1900-1950. Madison WI: Wisconsin Chiropractic Association, 1984

Mazzarelli JP. Chiropractic interprofessional research. Torino, Italy: Edizioni Minerva Medica, 1982

McAndrews JF. Letter to E.S. Ambrose, 8 July 1974 (CCE Archives)

McAndrews JF, McAndrews GP. Chiropractic's renaissance. Chapter 8 in Peterson D, Wiese G (Eds.): Chiropractic: an illustrated history. St. Louis MO: Mosby-Yearbooks, 1995

McAndrews JF. Letter to J.C. Keating, 8 January 1996

McAndrews JF. Interview with A.K. Callender, 4 August 1998

McCall FB. Baruch group proves drugless therapy. National Chiropractic Journal 1945 (Apr); 15(4): 15, 58

McCarrel T. Letter to William N. Coggins, D.C., 24 March 1974 (CCE Archives)

McGinn FW (Utah Department of Registration). Letter to the Los Angeles College of Chiropractic, 25 July 1972 (CCE Archives)

McIlroy HK. National Chiropractic Journal 1945 (Jan); 15(1): 36

McLeese JM. What constitutes a good chiropractic education? National (School) Journal of Chiropractic 1919; December: 14-7

McMurrin SM (U.S. Commissioner of Education). Letter to John J. Nugent, D.C., 22 May 1961 (CCE Archive, document #26752)

McNamee KP (Ed.): The chiropractic college directory, 1994-95. 4th edition. Los Angeles: KM Enterprises, 1994

Meeker WC. Reflections on the creation of a research agenda for chiropractic. Dynamic Chiropractic, September 23, 1996, p. 35

Mellott S, Coyle BA. Interview with J.C. Keating, 29 April 1992

Memo: A.C.C. and C.C.E. unofficial meeting, 2 November 1972 (CCE Archives)

Mesmer A. On the influence of the planets upon the human body by means of a magnetic force. Doctoral dissertation, University of Vienna, 1776

Metz M. Fifty years of chiropractic recognized in Kansas. Abilene KS: the author, 1965

Meyer JJ, Zachman ZJ, Traina AD, Keating JC. Effectiveness of chiropractic management for patellofemoral pain syndrome's symptomatic control phase: a single-subject experiment. Journal of Manipulative and Physiological Therapeutics 1990 (Nov/Dec); 13(9):539-49

Mighton FC. Chiropractic care for civilians in wartime. Lincoln Bulletin 1942; October/November: 9

Miller J. Interview with A.K. Callender, 22 July 1998

Miller RG. Program cost analysis of chiropractic colleges. Des Moines IA: Council on Chiropractic Education, unpublished, 22 June 1978

Miller RG. History of chiropractic accreditation. ACA Journal of Chiropractic 1981 (Feb); 18 (2): 38-44

Miller RG. Memorandum to F.A. Zolli, 17 April 1995

Minutes of a special meeting of the Dominion Council of the Canadian Chiropractors' Association, held in the Clubroom of the Royal York Hotel, Toronto, Ontario, on Thursday, March 2nd, 1944a, and called for 8:00 p.m. (Haldeman papers)

Minutes of the second annual meeting of the Dominion Council of the Canadian Chiropractors' Association, Toronto, 23-24 October 1944b (CCA Archives)

Minutes of the semi-annual meeting of the Council on Education held in Chicago, 23-25 January 1948 (Appendix B)

Minutes of the Council on Education of the National Chiropractic Association, 1-3 February 1950 (National College Library, Special Collections); see also Appendix B

Minutes of the Council on Education of the National Chiropractic Association, 23-26 June 1952 (National College Library, Special Collections); see also Appendix B

Minutes of the semi-annual meeting of the National Council on Education of the National Chiropractic Association, 11-13 February 1954 (National College Library, Special Collections); see also Appendix B

Minutes of the mid-year meeting of the National Council on Education of the National Chiropractic Association, 9-11 February 1955, New York (National College Library, Special Collections); see also Appendix B

Minutes of the meeting of the Council on Education of the NCA, 11-17 June 1961, Las Vegas (CCE Archives); see also Appendix B

Minutes of the NCA Council on Education, midyear meeting, 19-22 February 1962, Los Angeles (CCE Archives); see Appendix B

Minutes of the meeting of the Council on Education of the A.C.A., Las Vegas, Nevada, 1-4 February 1968 (CCE Archives); see Appendix B

Minutes of meeting between representatives of the Council on Chiropractic Education and the Association of Chiropractic Colleges, May 21, 1972 (CCE Archives)

Miscellany: Earl Bebout and the Central States College circa 1922-23. Chiropractic History 1983; 3: 41

Miscellany I: A university and hospital circa 1914. Chiropractic History 1988 (Dec); 8(2): 7

Miscellany: The "Steam from the Fountainhead": a 1920 report by AMA's Council on Medical Education. Chiropractic History 1993 (June); 13(1): 8-11

Monroe JN. Preventive chiropractic. Lincoln Bulletin, May, 1929, p. 4

Montgomery DP, Nelson JM. Evolution of chiropractic theories of practice and spinal adjustment. Chiropractic History 1985; 5: 70-6

Moore JS. Chiropractic in America: the history of a medical alternative. Baltimore: Johns Hopkins University Press, 1993

Mootz RD. The impact of health policy on chiropractic. Journal of Manipulative and Physiological Therapeutics 1996 (May); 19(4): 257-64

Mootz RD, Shekelle PG, Hansen DT. The politics of policy and research. Topics in Clinical Chiropractic 1995; 2(2): 56-70

Mootz RD, Hess JA, McMillin AD. Valuation of chiropractic services: a status report and overview of the challenges of standardization. Topics in Clinical Chiropractic 1996 (Mar); 3(1): 20-31

Moss JA. Letter to J.C. Keating, 1 April 1996

Moss JA. Letter to J.C. Keating, 13 September 1996

Moyer PC. Letter to Craig M. Kightlinger, D.C., 19 July 1943 (CCE Archives, file #35-18-1941)

Muilenburg JW. Science is our friend. ACA Journal of Chiropractic 1970 (Oct); 7(10): S-71-72

Murphy EJ, Smith MC. Officers Reserve Corps for chiropractors in armed forces is our goal. National Chiropractic Journal 1940 (Apr); 10(4): 11-2

Murphy EJ. U.S. Congress gives chiropractic full recognition in new draft act. Journal of the National Chiropractic Association 1951a (Apr); 21(4): 18

Murphy EJ. Full chiropractic recognition in draft act is a major professional victory. Journal of the National Chiropractic Association 1951b (July); 21(7): 10

Musick JE. Chiropractic education: two colleges in conflict. A report to the Board and Attorneys of the Northern California College of Chiropractic, November, 1979; unpublished (LACC Rare Books Collection)

Nansel DD, Peneff AL, Jansen RD, Cooperstein R. Interexaminer concordance in detecting joint-play asymmetries in the cervical spines of otherwise asymptomatic subjects. Journal of Manipulative and Physiological Therapeutics 1989a; 12: 428-33

Nansel DD, Cremata E, Carlson J, Szlazak M. Effect of unilateral spinal adjustments on goniometrically assessed cervical lateral-flexion end-range asymmetries in otherwise asymptomatic subjects. Journal of Manipulative and Physiological Therapeutics 1989b (Dec); 12(6): 419-27

Nansel DD, Peneff AL, Cremata E, Carlson J. Time course considerations for the effects of unilateral lower cervical adjustments with respect to the amelioration of cervical lateral-flexion passive end-range asymmetry. Journal of Manipulative and Physiological Therapeutics 1990 (Jul/Aug); 13(6): 297-304

Nansel DD. Peneff A, Quitoriano J. Effectiveness of upper versus lower cervical adjustments with respect to the amelioration of passive rotational versus lateral-flexion end-range asymmetries in otherwise asymptomatic subjects. Journal of Manipulative and Physiological Therapeutics 1992 (Feb); 15(2): 99-105

Nansel DD, Waldorf T, Cooperstein R. Effect of cervical spine adjustments on lumbar spine muscle tone: evidence for facilitation of intersegmental tonic neck reflexes. Journal of Manipulative and Physiological Therapeutics 1993 (Feb); 16 (2): 91-5

Nansel DD, Szlazak. Somatic dysfunction and the phenomenon of visceral disease simulation: a probable explanation for the apparent effectiveness of somatic therapy in patients presumed to be suffering from true visceral disease. Journal of Manipulative and Physiological Therapeutics 1995 (July/Aug); 18(6): 379-97s

Napolitano EG, Peterson TC. Future plans for a school in New York. ACA Journal of Chiropractic 1965 (Mar); 2(3): 8

Napolitano EG. Letter to O.L. Hidde, D.C., J.D., 15 June 1972 (CCE Archives)

Napolitano EG. Letter to H.R. Frogley, D.C., 1 June 1973a (CCE Archives)

Napolitano EG. Letter to H.R. Frogley, D.C., 15 June 1973b (CCE Archives)

Napolitano EG. Letter to John O. Stoutenburg (Arizona State board of Chiropractic Examiners), 18 January 1974 (CCE Archives)

National meeting of drugless professions. Bulletin of the American Chiropractic Association 1926 (May/June); 3(5-6): 3

National (College) Journal of Chiropractic 1928 (Dec); 5(14): 12

National news. National (College) Journal of Chiropractic 1933 (June); 16(2): 12

National convention and clinical symposium. The Chiropractic Journal (NCA) 1934 (July); 3(7): 13

National Council on Education visits L.A.C.C. Chirogram 1951 (Mar); 20(3): 20

National and Lincoln amalgamate. ACA Journal of Chiropractic 1971 (Oct); 8(10): 10-11

National becomes third college to receive federal grant. Dynamic Chiropractic 1994; 12(26): 1

Naturopathic scandals threaten chiropractic! ICA International Review of Chiropractic 1957 (May); 11(11): 6-12

Naturopathy "out" at National School. ICA International Review of Chiropractic 1950 (Oct); 5(4): 2

NCA news notes. The Chiropractic Journal (NCA) 1935 (Sept); 49(9): 37

NCA Director of Education flies some 180,000 miles in pursuit of duties. Journal of the National Chiropractic Association 1951 (Aug); 21(8): 10, 70-1

NCIC donates another $50,000.00 to FACE. ACA Journal of Chiropractic 1965 (Nov); 2(11): 20

Nelson WA. Scientific symposium: the National-Affiliated goes to town! The Chiropractic Journal (NCA) 1938 (Nov); 7(11): 17, 55

Nelson WA. Interview with J.C. Keating and Richard A.. Brown, D.P.M., October 24, 1991

New campus is a gem!! Northwestern Bulletin and Alumni News 1983; Summer: 3

News flashes: CANADA: Canadian army says no chiros. National Chiropractic Journal 1943 (Mar); 12(3): 26-7

News flashes: California: Dr. Nugent stresses education. National Chiropractic Journal 1946 (May); 16(5): 34-5

Newspaper clipping, February-March 1923 (Cleveland papers, Cleveland Chiropractic College of Kansas City)

New York State Education Department. SED registers first chiropractic school; new release, January 7, 1972

Nilsson AV. Letter to J.D. Kirby. Chirogram 1972 (Dec); 39(12): 17

Nilsson AV. Progression. Chirogram 1975 (Oct); 42(10): 21-2

Norcross LH. The educational and specialty societies. Chirogram 1948 (Feb); 17(2): 13-5

Norcross LH. The dean of the graduate school reports to the profession. Chirogram 1949 (Apr); 18(4): 14-5

Norcross LH. Graduate school approved for veterans training. Chirogram 1951 (Oct); 10(10): 21

Northern California College of Chiropractic, Status Study Book 1. Sunnyvale CA: the College, April, 1980

Nostrums and quackery. Chicago: American Medical Association, 1912

Not seceders, but protesters. Lincoln Herald, June 17, 1921; reprinted in Fountain Head News 1921 [A.C. 26] (Aug 6); 10(47): 5-6

Nugent JJ. Chiropractic education: outline of a standard course. Webster City IA: National Chiropractic Association, 1941

Nugent JJ. New York school situation. Memorandum to the Executive Board, NCA officials and Committee on Educational Standards, December 30, 1943 (CCE Archives, #35-12-1938)

Nugent JJ. Universal and Lincoln College merge. National Chiropractic Journal 1944 (May); 14(5): 30-1

Nugent JJ. Canadian Memorial College. National Chiropractic Journal 1945 (Oct); 15(10): 15, 62

Nugent JJ. Quoting - Dr. John J. Nugent at Cleveland Chiropractic College Homecoming, 1949 (Cleveland papers, Cleveland Chiropractic College of Kansas City)

Nugent JJ. Letter to the field, 6 July 1951a (Cleveland papers, Cleveland Chiropractic College of Kansas City)

Nugent JJ. How chiropractic was recognized by Congress in the National Draft Act. Journal of the National Chiropractic Association 1951b (Aug); 21(8): 9

Nugent JJ. Educational standards for chiropractic schools. 4th edition. Webster City IA: Council on Education of the National Chiropractic Association, 1953

Nugent JJ. A tribute. Journal of the National Chiropractic Association 1954 (Sept); 24(9): 4

Nugent JJ. Memorandum to the NCA Council on Education, 12 September 1959 (Collected papers of Joseph Janse)

Nugent JJ. Copy of application for accreditation of the National Council on Education of the National Chiropractic Association,

submitted to the Department of Health, Education and Welfare, Office of Education, Washington, D.C., January 1961 (CCE Archive, documents 26751-26774)

Nyiendo J. Disabling low back Oregon workers' compensation claims. Part II: time loss. Journal of Manipulative and Physiological Therapeutics 1991a (May); 14(4): 231-9

Nyiendo J. Disabling low back Oregon workers' compensation claims. Part III: diagnostic and treatment procedures and associated costs. Journal of Manipulative and Physiological Therapeutics 1991b (June); 14(5): 287-97

Nyiendo J, Haldeman S. A prospective study of 2,000 patients attending a chiropractic college teaching clinic. Medical Care 1987; 25:516-27

Nyiendo J, Olsen E. Visit characteristics of 217 children attending a chiropractic college teaching clinic. Journal of Manipulative and Physiological Therapeutics 1988; 11:78-84

Nyiendo J, Phillips RB, Meeker WC, Konsler G, Jansen RD, Menon M. A comparison of patients and patient complaints at six chiropractic college teaching clinics. Journal of Manipulative and Physiological Therapeutics 1989 (Apr); 12(2):79-85

O'Malley JN. Toward a reconstruction of the philosophy of chiropractic. Journal of Manipulative and Physiological Therapeutics 1995 (June); 18(5): 285-92

O'Neill A. Enemies within and without: educating chiropractors, osteopaths and traditional acupuncturists. Bundoora, Victoria, Australia: LaTrobe University Press, 1994

Ontario Ministry of Health recommends funding chiropractic education: report supports university affiliation. Dynamic Chiropractic 1995 (Aug 15); 13(17): 31

Ottina J (U.S. Commissioner of Education-designate). Letter to George H. Haynes, D.C., M.A., 22 May 1971 (CCE Archives)

Ottina J. Letter to George H. Haynes, D.C., M.A., 2 May 1973a (CCE Archives)

Ottina J. Letter to George H. Haynes, D.C., M.A., 6 December 1973b (CCE Archives)

Our first graduating class. Lincoln Bulletin, May 1928, p. 3

Our chiropractic colleges: Texas. Today's Chiropractic 1972-73 (Dec/Jan); 1(6): 26

Pacific Chiropractic College. Catalog. Portland OR: the college, 1922

Pacific States: Dr. Leonard Rudnick is new dean. World-Wide Report 1978 (Oct); 20(10): 1

Palmer BJ. The Chiropractor 1911 (Jan); 7(1): 3

Palmer BJ. Fountain Head News 1917 [A.C. 23] (Nov 3); 7(8): 2

Palmer BJ. This makes me laugh. Fountain Head News 1918 [A.C. 23] (July 13); 7(44): 1-2

Palmer BJ. I agree, with a proviso. Fountain Head News 1919a [A.C. 25] (Nov 1); 9(7): 9-14

Palmer BJ. Does Willard Carver tell the truth? Fountain Head News 1919b [A.C. 25] (Nov 22); 9(10): 1-2

Palmer BJ. Now for all the facts. Fountain Head News 1920 [A.C. 25] (May 8); 9(34): 1-10

Palmer BJ. Conflicts clarify. Fountain Head News 1920b [A.C. 25] (June 26); 9(41): 4

Palmer BJ. The Palmer School of Chiropractic has no branch schools. Fountain Head News 1921 [A.C. 26] (Feb 19); 10(23): 16

Palmer BJ. Letter to Major H.H. Antles, Secretary, Department of Public Welfare, Nebraska. 9 February 1922 (Ashworth papers, Cleveland Chiropractic College of Kansas City)

Palmer BJ. The hour has struck. Davenport IA: Palmer School of Chiropractic, 1924a

Palmer BJ. Times change men. Fountain Head News 1924b (Nov 22); 14(9): 3

Palmer BJ. The ACA-UCA Union - what does it actually mean? Fountain Head News 1931a (Feb) [A.C. 35]; 18(3): 5-11

Palmer BJ. Letter to C.S. Cleveland, D.C., 7 January 1941 (Cleveland papers, Cleveland Chiropractic College of Kansas City)

Palmer BJ. Chiropractic controlled clinical trials. Davenport IA: Palmer School of Chiropractic, 1951

Palmer College. Today's Chiropractic 1975 (May/June); 4(3): 42

Palmer DD. The Magnetic Cure 1896 (Jan); Number 15, p. 2 (Palmer College Archives)

Palmer DD. The Chiropractic 1897a (Jan); Number 17, p. 2 (Palmer College Archives)

Palmer DD. The Chiropractic 1897b (March); Number 18, p. 2 (Palmer College Archives)

Palmer DD. The Chiropractic 1899; Number 26 (Palmer College Archives)

Palmer DD. The Chiropractic 1900; Number 26 (Palmer College Archives)

Palmer DD. The Chiropractic 1902; Number 29 (Palmer College Archives)

Palmer DD. Who discovered that the body is heated by nerves during health and disease. The Chiropractor: a Monthly Journal Devoted to the Interests of Chiropractic 1904b (Dec); 1(1): 12

Palmer DD (ed): The Chiropractor Adjuster 1909a (Jan); Vol. 1, No. 2

Palmer DD (ed): The Chiropractor Adjuster 1909d (Dec); Vol. 1, No. 7

Palmer DD. The chiropractor's adjuster: the science, art and philosophy of chiropractic. 1910a, Portland Printing House, Portland, Oregon

Palmer DD. The chiropractor. Los Angeles: Beacon Light Printing Company, 1914

Palmer David D. Letter to Stanley Hayes, D.C., 28 June 1963 (Collected papers of Stanley Hayes, Palmer Archives)

Palmer David D. Excerpts from the President's report delivered at the Palmer Homecoming. Digest of Chiropractic Economics 1969 (Sept/Oct); 12(2): 34-6

Palmer homecoming, etc. Today's Chiropractic 1975 (Nov/Dec); 4(6): ???

Palmer homecoming '76. Today's Chiropractic 1976 (Sept/Oct); 5(5): 48-9

Parker College of Chiropractic: background and history. Dallas TX: the college, undated fact sheet

Parker RJ. Letter to the editor. Lincoln Bulletin 1992 (Oct); 6(3): 3

Parr PO. News release to all chiropractors, chiropractic organizations and chiropractic publications, 1 March 1952a (Cleveland papers, Cleveland Chiropractic College of Kansas City)

Parr PO. Letter to R.O. McClintock, D.C., 7 March 1952b (Cleveland papers, Cleveland Chiropractic College of Kansas City)

Parr PO. Letter to all members of the North American Association of Chiropractic Schools and Colleges, 1 April 1952c (Cleveland papers, Cleveland Chiropractic College of Kansas City)

Pefley GV. Journal of the National Chiropractic Association 1961 (June); 31(6): 35-6

Pennsylvania College of Chiropractic: records retention agreement. Dynamic Chiropractic, October 23, 1995, p. 28

Peters RE. Letter re: Chiropractic instrumentation. Chiropractic Journal of Australia 1992 (June); 22(2): 67-8

Peters RE, Chance MA. Milestones in spinography: an Australian perspective. Chiropractic Journal of Australia 1993 (Mar); 23(1): 15-28

Peters RE, Chance MA. Murder they wrote: the death of D.D. Palmer and its aftermath. Chiropractic Journal of Australia 1993 (Dec); 23(4): 143-8

Peterson D, Wiese G. Chiropractic schools and colleges. In Chiropractic: an illustrated history. St. Louis: Mosby Yearbooks, 1995

Peterson TC. Great victory for Institute! Journal of the National Chiropractic Association 1949 (Apr); 19(4): 26, 58

Peterson TC. Letter to Carl S. Cleveland, Jr., D.C., 27 December 1950 (Cleveland papers, Cleveland Chiropractic College of Kansas City)

Peterson TC. Letter to Carl S. Cleveland, Jr., D.C., 1 February 1952 (Cleveland papers, Cleveland Chiropractic College of Kansas City)

Phillips RB. Politics, policies and problems: a presidential perspective on chiropractic education. Journal of the American Chiropractic Association 1995a (Dec); 32(12): 69-71

Phillips RB. Philosophy and chiropractic divisions. Journal of Chiropractic Humanities 1995b; 5: 2-7

Phillips RB. Letter to J.C. Keating, 27 January 1996

Plamondon RL. Mainstreaming chiropractic: tracing the American Chiropractic Association. Chiropractic History 1993 (Dec); 13(2): 30-5

Plaugher G, Lopes MA (Eds.): Textbook of clinical chiropractic: a specific biomechanical approach. Baltimore MD: Williams and Wilkins, 1993

Post graduate appreciation resolutions adopted by the post-graduate class, August, 1929. Lincoln Bulletin, November/December, 1929, p. 4

Preferred status admissions policy for bachelor's degrees or bachelor's candidates: effective as needed to limit enrollment to 1,300 students. Parker Parade 1996; 27: 644

Proceedings of the 1989 International Conference on Spinal Manipulation. Arlington VA: Foundation for Chiropractic Education and Research, 1989

Proffitt JR. Letter to George H. Haynes, D.C., M.A., 31 May 1973a (CCE Archives)

Proffitt JR. Letter to William N. Coggins, D.C., 27 June 1973b (CCE Archives)

Progress. The Missouri News 1922 (June); 1(1): 4-5

PSC Enrollment form (contract #8485; August 23, 1921) and transcripts for John J. Nugent (Cleveland papers, Cleveland Chiropractic College of Kansas City)

PSCC meets with CCE. PSCC News 1981 (Mar); 23(3): 1, 2

Pugsley RS. Letter to Melvin J. Rosenthal, 17 February 1978. FSCO Impulse 1978 (May/June); 1(1): 9

Quigley WH. The last days of B.J. Palmer: revolutionary confronts reality. Chiropractic History 1989 (June); 9(2): 10-19

Quigley WH. Interview with J.C. Keating, 30 December 1995

Quigley WH. Letter to J.C. Keating, 13 January 1996

Ransom JF. The origins of chiropractic physiological therapeutics: Howard, Forster and Schulze. Chiropractic History 1984; 4: 46-52

Ratledge TF. Letter to R.E. Mathis, D.C., 14 September 1915 (Ratledge papers, Cleveland Chiropractic College of Kansas City)

Ratledge TF. Letter to W.E. Hickman, Registrar, Universal Chiropractic College, 29 May 1934 (Ratledge papers, Cleveland Chiropractic College of Kansas City)

Ratledge TF. Letter to C.E. Barrows, D.C., 11 June 1935a. (Ratledge papers, Cleveland Chiropractic College of Kansas City

Ratledge TF. Letter to C.S. Cleveland, D.C., 7 July 1935b (Ratledge papers, Cleveland Chiropractic College of Kansas City)

Ratledge TF. Letter to C.S. Cleveland, Sr., D.C., 7 July 1935c (Ratledge papers, Cleveland Chiropractic College of Kansas City)

Ratledge TF. Letter to the NCA and L.M. Rogers, D.C., 12 July 1937 (Ratledge papers, Cleveland Chiropractic College of Kansas City)

Ratledge TF. Letter to Willard Carver, D.C., LL.B., 10 January 1938b (Ratledge papers) Cleveland Chiropractic College of Kansas City)

Ratledge TF. Typed and handwritten minutes of ACEI meetings recorded by its secretary; in the first author's possession.

Ratledge TF. Letter to Gordon M. Goodfellow, D.C., N.D., 17 July 1940a (Ratledge papers, Cleveland Chiropractic College of Kansas City)

Ratledge TF. Letter to C.S. Cleveland, D.C., 4 October 1940b (Ratledge papers, Cleveland Chiropractic College of Kansas City)

Ratledge TF. Letter to C.S. Cleveland, D.C., 16 February 1943a (Ratledge papers, Cleveland Chiropractic College of Kansas City)

Ratledge TF. Letter to C.S. Cleveland, D.C., 22 April 1943b (Ratledge papers, Cleveland Chiropractic College of Kansas City)

Ratledge TF. Letter to Carl S. Cleveland, Sr., D.C., 27 September 1950 (Ratledge papers, Cleveland Chiropractic College of Kansas City)

Ratledge TF. Correspondence with B.J. Palmer, D.C., 6 August 1951. (Ratledge papers, Cleveland Chiropractic College of Kansas City)

Ratledge TF. Correspondence with Russell R. Robbins, D.C. of Mason, Michigan, 15 January 1955 (Ratledge papers, Cleveland Chiropractic College of Kansas City)

Reed LS. The healing cults: a study of sectarian medical practice: its extent, causes, and control. Publication of the Committee on the Costs of Medical Care: No. 16. Chicago: University of Chicago Press, 1932

Reed WR, Beavers S, Reddy SK, Kern G. Chiropractic management of primary nocturnal enuresis. Journal of Manipulative and Physiological Therapeutics 1994 (Nov/Dec); 17(9): 596-600

Rehm WS. Who was who in chiropractic: a necrology. In Dzaman F et al. (eds.) Who's who in chiropractic, international. Second Edition. Littleton CO: Who's Who in Chiropractic International Publishing Co., 1980

Rehm WS. Letter to the Editor. Chiropractic History 1984; 4: 67

Rehm WS. Legally defensible: chiropractic in the courtroom and after, 1907. Chiropractic History 1986; 6: 50-5

Rehm WS. Letter to J.C. Keating, 21 January 1992a

Rehm WS. Pseudo-chiropractors: the correspondence school experience, 1912-1935. Chiropractic History 1992b; 12(2): 32-7

Rehm WS. Kansas coconuts: legalizing chiropractic in the first state, 1910-1915. Chiropractic History 1995 (Dec); 15(2): 43-50

Reinert OC. Merging with honor: a history of the Missouri Chiropractic College, 1920-64. Chiropractic History 1992 (Dec); 12(2): 38-42

Report of an examination of the Cleveland Chiropractic College, Kansas City, Missouri 64109 for the Association of Chiropractic College, October 13-15, 1971 (Cleveland papers, Cleveland Chiropractic College of Kansas City); see Appendix C

Report of conference of presidents of State Associations, held on B.J.'s Porch, October 6, 1922 (Cleveland papers, Cleveland Chiropractic College of Kansas City)

Research foundation organized. The Chiropractic Journal (NCA) 1934 (Jan); 3(1): 28

Resolution of representatives of state boards of Chiropractic Examiners, August 23, 1919, Davenport, Iowa (Ashworth papers, Cleveland Chiropractic College of Kansas City)

Resolution of the Disabled American Veterans of the World War, Minneapolis Chapter, reprinted in the Fountain Head News 1924a (May 17); 13(21-22):

Resolution adopted by Nebraska Chiropractic Association at its annual convention. National (College) Journal of Chiropractic 1924b (July); 11(11): 23

Rhodes WR. The official history of chiropractic in Texas. Austin TX: Texas Chiropractic Association, 1978

Ring selling medical diplomas throughout U.S. exposed. Fountain Head News 1923 [A.C. 29] (Nov 17); 13(6): 1-2

Ritter JC. The roots of Western States Chiropractic College, 1904-1932. Chiropractic History 1991 (Dec); 11(2): 18-24

Roden ER (ACA state delegate from California). Letter to the California State Board of Chiropractic Examiners, 7 August 1972 (CCE Archives)

Rodgers EA. Shades of Benedict Arnold! The Chiropractic Journal (NCA) 1935 (Jan); 4(1):38

Rogers LM. Editorial. The Chiropractic Journal (NCA) 1937 (Oct); 6(10): 6

Rogers LM. Editorial. The Chiropractic Journal (NCA) 1938a (Mar); 7(3): 6

Rogers LM. Convention highlights: a brief summary of an historical event. The Chiropractic Journal (NCA) 1938b (Sept); 7(9): 7-13, 30-2

Rogers LM. Letter to the Registrar of the Institute of the Science and Art of Chiropractic, 10 November 1944 (CCE Archives, #35-02-1956)

Rogers LM. Editorial. Journal of the National Chiropractic Association 1961a (Aug); 31(8): 5

Rogers LM. Dr. David D. Palmer assumes presidency of Palmer College of Chiropractic: investiture ceremonies at PCC indicate professional progress. Journal of the National Chiropractic Association 1961b (Oct); 31(10): 11, 62-3

Rosenthal MJ. The structural approach to chiropractic: from Willard Carver to present practice. Chiropractic History 1981; 1: 25-8

Rudnick L. Interview with J.C. Keating, July 29, 1995

Rudnick L. Letter to J.C. Keating, 5 February 1996

Rupert RL. CHIROLARS: a modern tool for chiropractic education. Journal of Chiropractic Education 1990 (Mar); 3(4):22-4

Rupert RL. Interview with J.C. Keating and C.S. Cleveland, April 1, 1996

Rutherford LW. Letter to Ted McCarrel, 27 March 1968 (Cleveland papers, Cleveland Chiropractic College of Kansas City)

Rutherford LW. To the chiropractic profession. Letter, June, 1995

Rutherford LW, Whaley JV, Young JW. A call to action. Letter, May 1996

Sampson NH. Letter to CYJ Hsieh, 29 September 1994

Sauer BA. Editorial: a statement of fact. Bulletin of the American Chiropractic Association 1925 (Mar); 2(2): 5

Sauer BA. International Congress of Chiropractic Examining Board. Bulletin of the American Chiropractic Association 1927 (Sept); 4(5): 10

Sauer BA. Basic science - its purpose, operation, effect. 10 June 1932; unpublished letter to the officers of the NCA and state chiropractic associations (Archives, Cleveland College/KC)

Sauer BA. Letter to H.B. Logan. The Chiropractic Journal (NCA) 1934 (Nov); 3(11): 31

Saunders EM. Report on National Board examinations. ACA Journal of Chiropractic 1965 (Aug); 2(8): 25, 48

Sausser WL. Spinograph and x-ray: New spinographic technique: the full length x-ray plate is a success. The Chiropractic Journal (NCA) 1933 (July); 1(7): 18-9

Savage LJ, Canterbury R, Dallas W, Pedigo M, Poole P, Sawyer C. Criteria for quality standards of patient care for chiropractic college clinics. West Des Moines IA: Council on Chiropractic Education, 1987

Schierholz AM. Progress report. ACA Journal of Chiropractic 1965a (Feb); 2(2): 4

Schierholz AM. FACE: foundation for the future. ACA Journal of Chiropractic 1965b (Oct); 2(10): 5, 40

Schierholz AM. Foundation for Chiropractic Education and Research. ACA Journal of Chiropractic 1969 (July); 6(7): 15

Schierholz AM. Letter to George H. Haynes, D.C., M.A., 19 May 1972 (CCE Archives)

Schierholz AM. The Foundation for Chiropractic Education and Research: a history. Arlington VA: The Foundation, January, 1986 (unpublished)

Schiller F. Spinal irritation and osteopathy. Bulletin of the History of Medicine 1971; 45: 250-66

Schnick JA. Personnel of committees for 1939-40 announced by president. National Chiropractic Journal 1939 (Oct); 8(10): 14

Schnick JA. Letter to Walter T. Sturdy, D.C., 7 December 1943 (Archives of the Canadian Memorial Chiropractic College, #84-229 through 84-235)

Schools of chiropractic and of naturopathy in the United States. Journal of the American Medical Association 1928; 90(21): 1733-8

School affairs. ICA International Review of Chiropractic 1949 (Oct); 4(4): 31-2

Schultz FE. Letter to J.C. Keating, 25 January 1996a

Schultz FE. Letter to J.C. Keating, 13 February 1996b

Schultz FE. Letter to J.C. Keating, 5 April 1996c

Schultz FE. Letter to J.C. Keating, 12 April 1996d

Schulze WC. Editorially speaking...professional progress of chiropractic. National (College) Journal of Chiropractic 1933 (Mar); 16(1):10

Scrapbook, undated. Cleveland papers, Cleveland Chiropractic College of Kansas City

September date for Parker opening. World-Wide Report, 1982: July: 1

Seventh Annual Announcement, The Chiropractic University and The American Hospital, Session 1914-1915. Kansas City, Missouri

Shekelle PG, Adams AH, Chassin MR, Hurwitz EL, Phillips RB, Brook RH. The appropriateness of spinal manipulation for low-back pain: project overview and literature review. 1991a, RAND Corporation, Santa Monica, California (Document #R-4025/1-CCR/FCER)

Shekelle PG, Adams AH, Chassin MR, Hurwitz EL, Park RE, Phillips RB, Brook RH. The appropriateness of spinal manipulation for low-back pain: indications and ratings by a multidisciplinary expert panel. 1991b, RAND Corporation, Santa Monica, California (Document #R-4025/2-CCR/FCER)

Sherman LW. What about research? ICA International Review of Chiropractic 1952 (Apr); 6(10): 12, 48

Sikorski D. Personal communication with J.C. Keating, 18 March 1996

Simonsen IH, Deltoff MN, Johansen KK, Petersen JN. Dansk Kiropraktor Kursus: an historical perspective and overview of the Danish Chiropractors' School. Chiropractic History 1989 (Dec); 9(2): 20-4

Slocum JE. Letter to C.S. Cleveland, D.C., 18 October 1932 (Cleveland papers, Cleveland Chiropractic College of Kansas City)

Slocum JE. Pertinent paragraphs selected from recent national convention addresses. The Chiropractic Journal (NCA) 1935 (Oct); 4(10): 6-9

Slocum JE. Letter to H. O. Langford, D.C., 10 February 1942a (Library Archives, Canadian Memorial Chiropractic College)

Slocum JE. Letter to H. O. Langford, D.C., 3 March 1942b (Library Archives, Canadian Memorial Chiropractic College)

Smallie P. The guiding light of Ratledge. Stockton CA: World-Wide Books, 1963

Smallie P. Encyclopedia chiropractica. 3rd edition, Stockton CA: World-Wide Books, 1990a

Smallie P, Smallie DD. New California Chiropractic College: a personal impression. Chirogram 1975 (Nov); 42(11): 17-22

Smith EJ. Letter to Carl S. Cleveland, Sr., D.C., 29 September 1932 (Cleveland papers, Cleveland Chiropractic College of Kansas City)

Smith JE. Letter to Carl S. Cleveland III, 5 March 1996

Smith OG. Naprapathic genetics: being a study of the origin and development of naprapathy. Chicago: the author, 1932

Smith RL. At your own risk: the case against chiropractic. New York: Pocket Books, 1969

Smithers TE. Letter to J.C. Keating, 8 March 1996

Spears Postgraduate College of Chiropractic; catalog. Undated, circa 1950 (Cleveland papers, Cleveland Chiropractic College of Kansas City)

Special mention. American Drugless Healer 1911 (Oct); 1(6): 6

Stanford Research Institute. Chiropractic in California. Los Angeles: Haynes Foundation, 1960

Starr P. The social transformation of American medicine. New York: Basic Books, 1982

State Board of Chiropractic Examiners of the State of California. In the Matter of the Application of Bert Humason, Plaintiff, For the Revocation of the License to Practice Chiropractic of Hugh Benedict Logan, Defendant. Findings of fact and order. January 24, 1929 (Ratledge papers, Cleveland Chiropractic College of Kansas City)

Status study of Palmer College of Chiropractic-West. Sunnyvale CA: the College, December 1980

Steele case reversed! Appellate court vacates injunction in California case. The Chiropractic Journal (NCA) 1935 (Mar); 4(3):5-6

Steinbach LJ. Let's face the facts concerning chiropractic education in the future! The Chiropractic Journal (NCA) 1936 (Jan); 5(1): 17, 48

Stonebrink RD. Memorandum to alumni, 14 January 1974

Stout RJ. The Ph.C. degree: an affirmation of chiropractic philosophy, 1908-1968. Chiropractic History 1988 (July); 8(1): 10-3

Stowe HF. The New York schools. The Messenger of the New York State Chiropractic Society 1921 (July); 4(10): 13

Stowell CC. Lincoln College and the "big four": a chiropractic protest, 1926-1962. Chiropractic History 1983; 3: 74-8

Strauss JB. Refined by fire: the evolution of straight chiropractic. Levittown PA: Foundation for the Advancement of Chiropractic Education, 1994

Survey of chiropractic methods of practice. Bulletin of the Research Bureau, American Chiropractic Association 1928 (June); 5(6): 1-4

Sutherland DC. Trial by fire: Canadian Royal Commissions investigate chiropractic. Chiropractic History 1985; 5: 27-37

Swenson R. Education update: revitalizing the chiropractic curriculum. Alumnus (National College of Chiropractic) 1996 (Winter); 12(1): 6-7

Tegren ERF. Letter to L.M. Rogers. The Chiropractic Journal (NCA) 1934 (July); 3(7): 37

Terrett AGJ. The genius of D.D. Palmer. Journal of the Australian Chiropractors' Association 1986 (Dec); 16(4): 150-8

Terrett AGJ, Vernon H. Manipulation and pain tolerance: a controlled study of the effect of spinal manipulation on paraspinal cutaneous pain tolerance levels. American Journal of Physical Medicine 1984; 63(5):217-25

Texans declare war on "basic science": fight for separate licensing law. ICA International Review of Chiropractic 1949 (Mar); 3(9): 9

The England case: report for 1964. ACA Journal of Chiropractic 1965 (Feb); 2(2): 25, 56

The graduate school courses and special classes. Chirogram 1951 (June); 20(6): 22-3

The graduate school: graduate school plans expanded program for 1952-1953. Chirogram 1952 (July); 21(7): 16-8

The International Congress of Chiropractic Examining Boards. Lincoln Bulletin, October 1927, p. 2

The Recoil, Volume VII, June Class, 1925. Davenport IA: Palmer School of Chiropractic, 1925

Thomas C. Life College: inside an American cult; unpublished manuscript

Thompson EA. The method of determining and adjusting tipped vertebrae. Lincoln Bulletin, November/December, 1929, pp. 1-3

Thompson T. Letter to J.C. Keating, 10 July 1991

Timmins RH. FCER - its history and work. ACA Journal of Chiropractic 1976 (Apr); 13(4): 19-20

Tolar RL, Adams AH, Coyle BA. Pacific Consortium for Chiropractic Research. California Chiropractic Journal 1986 (Feb); 11(2): 18, 28, 35

Tolerance. Lincoln Bulletin, August 1927, p. 1

TraCoil (Yearbook). New York: Chiropractic Institute of New York, 1949

Trever W. In the public interest. Los Angeles: Scriptures Unlimited, 1972

Triano JJ, Schultz AB. Correlation of objective measure of trunk motion and muscle function with low back disability ratings. Spine 1987; 12:561-5

Triano JJ, McGregor MM, Hondras M et al. Manipulation therapy vs. education programs in chronic low back pain. Spine 1995; 20:948-55

Turner C. The rise of chiropractic. Los Angeles: Powell Publishing Company, 1931

Universal Chiropractors Association of 1910. The Chiropractor 1910 (Sept/Oct); 6(9): 77-134

University of Bridgeport-College of Chiropractic. ICA Review 1995a (Sept/Oct); 51(5): 155-6

Universitè du Quebec à Trois-Riviêres. ICA Review 1995b (Sept/Oct); 51(5): 156

University of Natural Healing Arts (Inc.) Catalog, 1939-1940. Denver: the University, 1939

University of Pasadena. Today's Chiropractic 1976 (Mar/Apr); 5(2): 56

University of Pasadena, Bulletin 76-77. Pasadena CA: the University, 1976-77

University of Colorado is first American medical school to offer rotations to chiropractic residents. Dynamic Chiropractic, February 12, 1996, pp. 1, 34

Vear HJ. The validity of clinical chiropractic: a critical look. Address to the Western Canada Convention, June 7, 1974, Saskatoon, Saskatchewan

Vear HJ. Memorandum to the college community, 9 November 1977 (Western States Chiropractic College)

Vear HJ. Letter to O.L. Hidde, D.C., J.D., 28 February 1979

Vear HJ. The anatomy of a policy reversal: the A.P.H.A. and chiropractic, 1969 to 1983. Chiropractic History 1987 (Dec); 7(2): 17-22

Vear HJ (Ed.): Chiropractic standards of practice and quality of care. Gaithersburg MD: Aspen Publishers, 1992

Vear HJ. Letter to J.C. Keating, 4 December 1995

Vear HJ. Letter to J.C. Keating, 18 June 1996

Vedder HE. Chiropractic recognition should be forthcoming from War Department. National Chiropractic Journal 1940 (Mar); 10(3): 11

Vernon HT, Dhami MSI, Howley TP, Annett R. Spinal manipulation and beta-endorphin: a controlled study of the effect of a spinal manipulation on plasma beta-endorphin levels in normal males. Journal of Manipulative and Physiological Therapeutics 1986 (Jun); 9(2):115-23

Vincent RE. Letter to Leonard E. Fay (8 August 1974). Chirogram 1974 (Nov); 41(11): 15-6

Virginia situation ICA International Review of Chiropractic 1949 (Mar); 3(9): 10-11

Vogel P (Florida State Board of Chiropractic Examiners). News release concerning Chapter 21D-4.01 (CCE Archives)

Waagen GN, Haldeman S, Cook G, Lopez D, DeBoer KF. Short-term trial of chiropractic adjustments for the relief of chronic low back pain. Manual Medicine 1986; 2(3):63-7

Walker G. Chiropractic preceptor associate program: strides in education. ACA Journal of Chiropractic 1981 (July); 18(7): 78-81

Walker PD. Memorandum to J. Allenburg, W. Dallas and M. Passero re: reciprocal agreements, October 4, 1995 (CCE Archives)

War resolutions. Fountain Head News 1917 [A.C. 22] (May 5); 6(34): 8

Wardwell WI. Chiropractic: history and evolution of a new profession. St. Louis: Mosby, 1992

Warning to chiropractic students. ICA International Review of Chiropractic 1949 (June); 3(12): 2

Watkins CO. Montana Chirolite, January 20, 1932a, p. 3

Watkins CO. Chiropractic's paramount need. The Montana Chirolite, June 10, 1932b, pp. 3-4

Watkins CO. The new offensive will bring sound professional advancement. The Chiropractic Journal (NCA) 1934 (June); 3(6): 5, 6, 33

Watkins CO. Facts! On educational standards. The Chirolite, n.d. (circa January 1938), pp. 8-10

Watkins CO. Guest editorial. National Chiropractic Journal 1939 (Sept); 8(9): 6, 53

Watkins CO. The basic principles of chiropractic government. Sidney, Montana: the author, 1944; reprinted as Appendix A in Keating JC. Toward a philosophy of the science of chiropractic: a primer for clinicians. Stockton, California: Stockton Foundation for Chiropractic Research, 1992a

Watkins CO. Experimental methods of science. National Chiropractic Journal 1948 (Sept); 18(9): 21, 22, 58

Watkins CO. Clinical research in chiropractic. Journal of the National Chiropractic Association 1951 (Jan); 21(1): 22, 23, 72, 74

We accuse you, Dr. John Nugent and Dr. Joseph J. Janse, for defeat of chiropractic legislation in Illinois. ICA International Review of Chiropractic 1949 (Aug); 4(2): 6-8

Weiant CW. Letter to the editor. The Chiropractic Journal (NCA) 1938 (May); 7(5): 46-7

Weiant CW. Letter to L.M. Rogers, D.C., 9 November 1943 (CCE Archives, #35-12-1938)

Weiant CW. National committee on research. National Chiropractic Journal 1946 (Dec); 16(12): 15-6, 70

Weiant CW. Letter to Stanley Hayes, D.C., 29 August 1964 (Collected papers of Stanley Hayes)

Weiant CW. Letter to Stanley Hayes, D.C., 2 February 1965 (Collected papers of Stanley Hayes)

Wentz D, Green BN. The evolution of the American Board of Chiropractic Orthopedists: a bootstrapping of clinical skills. Chiropractic History 1995 (Dec); 15(2): 92-101

Western States. Today's Chiropractic 1975 (May/June); 4(3): 42

Western States. Today's Chiropractic 1976 (Sept/Oct); 5(5): 57

Western States Chiropractic College. ACA Journal of Chiropractic 1981 (Aug); 18(8): 82)

Western States Chiropractic College, Catalog 1992-94. Portland OR: the College, 1992

Whitehead JE. CLIBCON: the Chiropractic Library Consortium. Who are we? Journal of Chiropractic Education 1990 (Mar); 3(4):18-21

Whitten W. Militant action demanded! The Chiropractic Journal (NCA) 1935 (Aug); 4(8):30

Wiese G. New questions: why did D.D. not use "Chiropractic" in his 1896 charter? Chiropractic History 1986; 6: 63

Wiese GC, Lykins MR. A bibliography of the Palmer green books in print, 1906-1985. Chiropractic History 1986; 6: 64-74

Wiese G, Peterson D. Chiropractic schools and colleges: "To teach and practice chiropractic." Chapter 12 in Peterson D and Wiese G (Eds.): Chiropractic: an illustrated history. St. Louis: Mosby Yearbooks, 1995

Wilbur RL. Report on a community rehabilitation service and center. New York: Baruch Commission on Physical Medicine, 1946

Will erect new $300,000 building. The Chiropractor 1910 (Mar); 6(3): 92-4

Williams SE. Quo vadis. Today's Chiropractic 1972 (Jan/Feb); 1(1): 2-3, 16

Winterstein JF. As I see it: winds of change. Alumnus (National College of Chiropractic) 1996 (Winter); 32(1): 4, 8

With the editor. Bulletin of the American Chiropractic Association 1926 (Apr); 3(4): 5

Wolf WB. Interview with Kerwin P. Winkler, D.C., 6 June 1993

Wolfe JB. Northwestern College achieves significant goal in chiropractic education. ACA Journal of Chiropractic 1970 (May); 7(5): 12-3

Wright R. The role of chiropractic examining boards in enforcing high educational standards. ACA Journal of Chiropractic 1972a (Aug); 9(8): 22-3

Wright R. Alterations in the A.C.C. published articles of incorporation, August 19, 1972b (CCE Archives)

Yates RG, Lamping NL, Abram C et al. The effects of chiropractic treatment on blood pressure and anxiety: a randomized, controlled trial. Journal of Manipulative and Physiological Therapeutics 1988 (Dec); 11(6):484-8

Zarbuck MV. A profession for "Bohemian Chiropractic": Oakley Smith and the evolution of naprapathy. Chiropractic History 1986; 6: 76-82

Zarbuck MV. Historical naprapathy. IPSCA Journal of Chiropractic 1987 (Jan); 8(1): 6-8

Zarbuck MV. Chiropractic parallax. Part 1. IPSCA Journal of Chiropractic 1988a (Jan); 9(1): 4-10

Zarbuck MV. Chiropractic parallax. Part 2. IPSCA Journal of Chiropractic 1988b (Apr); 9(2): 4, 5, 14-6

Zarbuck MV. Chiropractic parallax, Part 3. Illinois Prairie State Chiropractic Association Journal of Chiropractic 1988c (July); 9(3): 4-6, 17, 19

Zarbuck MV. Chiropractic parallax. Part 2. IPSCA Journal of Chiropractic 1988d (Oct); 9(4): 4-6, 17

Zarbuck MV. Chiropractic parallax. Part 6. IPSCA Journal of Chiropractic 1989 (Oct); 10(4): 7,8, 19

Zarbuck MV, Hayes MB. Following D.D. Palmer to the West Coast: the Pasadena connection, 1902. Chiropractic History 1990 (Dec); 10(2): 17-22

Zolli F. Background and history of the University of Bridgeport, College of Chiropractic; unpublished (2/20/96)

Index